Maternal-Fetal Medicine

Maternal-Fetal Medicine

Editor: Ella Gilbert

AMERICAN
MEDICAL PUBLISHERS
www.americanmedicalpublishers.com

AMERICAN
MEDICAL PUBLISHERS
www.americanmedicalpublishers.com

Cataloging-in-Publication Data

Maternal-fetal medicine / edited by Ella Gilbert.
p. cm.
Includes bibliographical references and index.
ISBN 979-8-88740-243-7
1. Obstetrics. 2. Perinatology. 3. Fetus--Diseases. 4. Pregnancy--Complications.
5. Prenatal diagnosis. 6. Fetus--Diseases. I. Gilbert, Ella.
RG526 .M38 2023
618.2--dc23

American Medical Publishers,
41 Flatbush Avenue,
1st Floor, New York,
NY 11217, USA

ISBN 979-8-88740-243-7 (Hardback)

Contents

Preface

The world is advancing at a fast pace like never before. Therefore, the need is to keep up with the latest developments. This book was an idea that came to fruition when the specialists in the area realized the need to coordinate together and document essential themes in the subject. That's when I was requested to be the editor. Editing this book has been an honour as it brings together diverse authors researching on different streams of the field. The book collates essential materials contributed by veterans in the area which can be utilized by students and researchers alike.

Maternal–fetal medicine (MFM) is a branch of medicine that is concerned with the health of the mother and fetus before, during, and immediately after pregnancy. MFM concerns those patients who fall under defined levels of maternal care such as the mother, baby or both throughout the pregnancy. Furthermore, this field of medicine is concerned with providing care to pregnant women having chronic conditions, patients at risk for pregnancy-related problems, and pregnant women with fetuses at risk. Congenital and chromosomal abnormalities, infections, maternal sickness, growth restriction and genetic diseases are the reasons causing risk for fetuses. This book includes some of the vital pieces of work being conducted across the world, on various topics related to maternal–fetal medicine. It is a valuable compilation of topics, ranging from the basic to the most complex advancements in this area of study. This book will serve as a valuable source of reference for medical professionals and students.

Each chapter is a sole-standing publication that reflects each author´s interpretation. Thus, the book displays a multi-facetted picture of our current understanding of application, resources and aspects of the field. I would like to thank the contributors of this book and my family for their endless support.

Editor

1

Feto-Maternal Microchimerism: The Pre-Eclampsia Conundrum

*Sinuhe Hahn [1], Paul Hasler [2], Lenka Vokalova [1], Shane Vontelin van Breda [1,2], Nandor Gabor Than [3], Irene Mathilde Hoesli [4], Olav Lapaire [4] and Simona W. Rossi [1]**

[1] Department of Biomedicine, University Hospital Basel, Basel, Switzerland, [2] Division of Rheumatology, Medical University Department, Kantonsspital Aarau, Aarau, Switzerland, [3] Systems Biology of Reproduction Lendulet Research Group, Institute of Enzymology, Research Centre for Natural Sciences, Hungarian Academy of Sciences, Budapest, Hungary, [4] Department of Obstetrics, University Women's Hospital Basel, Basel, Switzerland

***Correspondence:**
Simona W. Rossi
simona.rossi@unibas.ch

Feto-maternal microchimerism (FMM) involves bidirectional cross-placental trafficking during pregnancy, leading to a micro-chimeric state that can persist for decades. In this manner a pregnant woman will harbor cells from her mother, as well as, cells from her child. Historically, eclampsia, a severe disorder of pregnancy provided the basis for FMM following the detection of trophoblast cells in the lungs of deceased women. Bi-directional cell trafficking between mother and fetus is also altered in pre-eclampsia and has been suggested to contribute to the underlying etiology. FMM has been implicated in tolerance promotion, remission of auto-inflammatory disorders during pregnancy, or the development of autoimmune conditions post-partum. The underlying mechanism whereby the host immune system is modulated is unclear but appears to involve HLA class II molecules, in that incompatibility between mother and fetus promotes remission of rheumatoid arthritis, whereas feto-maternal HLA compatibility may assist in the post-partum initiation of scleroderma. Couples having a high degree of HLA class II compatibility have an increased risk for pre-eclampsia, while the occurrence of scleroderma and rheumatoid arthritis is greater in pre-eclamptic cases than in women with normal pregnancies, suggesting a long term autoimmune predisposition. Since pregnant women with pre-eclampsia exhibit significantly lower levels of maternally-derived micro-chimerism, the question arises whether pre-eclampsia and post-partum development of autoimmune conditions occur due to the failure of the grandmothers cells to adequately regulate an inappropriate micro-chimeric constellation.

Keywords: feto-maternal microchimerism, pre-eclampsia, non-inherited-maternal-antigens, cell-free DNA, autoimmunity

FMM AND PRE-ECLAMPSIA: HISTORICAL OBSERVATIONS

Granted that pre-eclampsia, a severe life-threatening disorder of pregnancy characterized by hypertension, proteinuria and organ failure is proposed to arise from dysfunctional placentation (1). It is hardly surprising that many key observations concerning feto-maternal cell trafficking and ensuing micro-chimerism were made in this context (2, 3).

In this regard, it is generally accepted that the first evidence of FMM was made at the turn of the nineteenth century by Georg Schmorl; a German pathologist in his examination of pregnant women who had succumbed to eclampsia (2, 4). Eclampsia is the fulminant form of pre-eclampsia where very severe symptoms are accompanied by seizures (1). In his report, Schmorl documented the occurrence of multi-nucleate trophoblast cells in the lungs of 14 out 17 cases with eclampsia. It is noteworthy that this feature was absent in 4 pregnant women who had died from other causes, suggestive that it may be linked to the underlying pathology of eclampsia (2, 4). Due to the potential role of the placenta as a key aetiological trigger in pre-eclampsia, the pivotal findings of Schmorl relating FMM to altered placentation proved to be worthy of more than passing interest and formed the basis of numerous other studies examining trophoblast deportation, the release of trophoblast micro-particles or even cell-free DNA from the placenta in cases with eclampsia or pre-eclampsia (5–7). Consequently, it was worthwhile reappraising Schmorl's widely-cited seminal report in translated form (4).

These were, however, not the only early reports suggesting that pre-eclampsia may be associated with altered feto-maternal cell trafficking. In 1905 Diehl postulated that pre-eclampsia may result from increased transfusion of incompatible fetal blood cells into the maternal compartment (2). This hypothesis fitted with the then current concept of pre-eclampsia being a form of *pregnancy toxemia*, triggered by toxins, possibly of placental origin during pregnancy (8). Further evidence supporting enhanced feto-maternal bleeding in pre-eclampsia was provided by epidemiological observations suggesting that the frequency of immunization due to Rhesus D incompatibility was greater in pregnancies affected by pre-eclampsia than in those with healthy deliveries (9). Since the Rhesus D antigen is expressed exclusively on cells of the erythrocyte lineage (10), such maternal immunization could not be due to the increased presence of placental trophoblast but would of necessity involve the increased presence of fetal red blood cells in the maternal circulation. This vital aspect was subsequently confirmed by the use of the then novel Kleihauer-Betke stain, which permitted the detection of fetal erythrocytes in maternal blood samples (11). This indicated that their proportion was indeed greater in pregnancies affected by pre-eclampsia (12). These data thereby provided further insight into the placental lesion in pre-eclampsia, indicating that it involved both increased trophoblast shedding, as well as leakage of fetal blood cells across the villous barrier (2, 3).

FMM: THE QUESTION OF FETAL CELLS PERSISTENCE

Possibly one of the most exciting subsequent developments was the detection of fetal leucocytes in mitogen stimulated maternal blood samples, wherein male fetal cells could be detected by the presence of a Y chromosome (13). While this finding was confirmed in a number of ensuing studies, these did highlight the possible longevity of such fetal leucocytes as they could be detected for a considerable period post-partum (14–16). Indeed, the question arose whether such persisting fetal cells could contribute to the presence of male leucocytes in maternal blood samples from pregnancies with a female fetus (14–16).

In a landmark finding the research group of Diana Bianchi reported on the detection of circulatory fetal cells with stem cell-like characteristics for a period of almost three decades post-delivery (17). Subsequent studies have revealed that fetal cell persistence is a frequent event occurring both in mouse and man, and that this affects a variety of tissues including the brain (18–20). As we shall observe in the continuation of this discourse, the longevity of trafficking fetal cells provided the impetus for a number of other investigative routes, particularly with regard to the development of autoimmune conditions since women are more prone to develop them post-partum (21).

FMM: THE QUEST FOR NON-INVASIVE PRENATAL DIAGNOSIS LEADS TO NEW DEVELOPMENTS

The advent of amniocentesis and karyotyping revolutionized obstetrical practice by facilitating the prenatal assessment of fetal chromosomal anomalies, such as trisomy 21 occurring in Down syndrome (22). A caveat of such invasive prenatal diagnostic procedures, especially that of chorionic villous sampling performed earlier in gestation, was the risk of injury to mother and potential loss of the unborn fetus (23–25). Consequently, the need was voiced for safe efficacious alternatives, thereby fuelling the quest for methods permitting non-invasive prenatal diagnosis. It was therefore a foregone conclusion that the prior reports of FMM would provide the basis for the development of such novel prenatal tests (26). Thus, most of these early studies focussed either on the detection of fetal cells in maternal blood while a few examined for the presence of trophoblast cells in the cervix of pregnant women (27). Due to their scarcity, fetal cells in maternal blood had to be enriched with most centers using either flow cytometric or magnetic cell sorting approaches (28).

The fetal erythroblast, also termed nucleated red blood cell, emerged as the target cell of choice for fetal cells in maternal blood-based strategies. This was largely due to its abundance in the fetal circulation, its short half-life that precluded any issue pertaining to longevity, as well as the availability of suitable markers for enrichment (CD71) and identification (fetal and embryonic hemoglobin) (26, 28). By the use of multi-color FISH (fluorescent *in-situ* hybridization) early studies suggested that it may be possible to detect the most common fetal aneuploidies by this approach (28, 29), while the use of single cell PCR permitted the detection of Mendelian disorders i.e., hemoglobinopathies (30, 31). These encouraging results promoted the assessment of this challenging route in two independent NIH and EU funded studies (32, 33). Unfortunately, both of these multicenter studies revealed that the paucity of fetal erythroblasts in maternal circulation rendered their use impractical in daily clinical routine since the required level of specificity and sensitivity could not be attained (32, 33).

During these explorations our group did make two pertinent observations with regard to feto-maternal cell trafficking in preeclampsia. In the first study, by the use of male singleton pregnancies and multi-color FISH for the X and Y chromosomes we could irrevocably demonstrate a significantly increased presence of male fetal erythroblasts in the maternal circulation in cases that manifest pre-eclampsia when compared to matching healthy control pregnancies (34). Furthermore, in an examination of maternal blood samples collected from an at-risk cohort we observed an increase in male fetal erythroblasts in samples from cases that subsequently developed pre-eclampsia (35). Therefore, these results confirmed that the underlying placental lesion in pre-eclampsia facilitated leakage across the usually tight feto-maternal barrier and that this defect was an early event in the course of this disorder occurring prior to clinical manifestation of symptoms (2, 3).

FMM: NOT RESTRICTED TO CELLS BUT ALSO INCLUDES CELL-FREE DNA

During the "NIH NIFTY" study that explored the use of fetal cells for non-invasive prenatal diagnosis the discovery of fetal cell-free DNA (cfDNA) in maternal plasma or serum was reported by Dennis Lo and colleagues in Oxford using Y chromosome specific PCR (36). The basis for the Oxford study were reports on the presence of tumor-derived cfDNA in cancer patient sera (37, 38). In an extension of their original findings they observed that maternally-derived cfDNA fragments could be detected in cord blood samples indicating that FMM was not restricted to the cross placental traffic of cells but could also involve cellular cfDNA fragments (39).

The use of real-time PCR permitted a rapid and precise assessment of the concentration of cfDNA in maternal blood samples. This indicated a progressive increase during pregnancy, peaking at term and ending with rapid clearance post-partum (40). Due to our interest in pre-eclampsia we performed several detailed investigations using qRT-PCR assays. These indicated that manifestation of pre-eclampsia was associated with a significant increase in the concentration of both fetal and maternally-derived cfDNA, which correlated with disease severity and being greatest in cases complicated with HELLP (hemolysis, elevated liver, low platelet) syndrome or eclampsia (41). Furthermore, we observed that when the blood samples were drawn early during pregnancy prior to the onset of clinical symptoms only the level of fetal cfDNA but not maternal cfDNA was elevated (42, 43). Since fetal cfDNA was determined to arise from the placenta this provided further evidence that the underlying etiology of pre-eclampsia involved placental lesions that occurred early in the cascade of events leading to clinical manifestation (3). It is still unclear whether or not elevations in the amount of fetal cfDNA contribute to the development of pre-eclampsia or other pregnancy-related disorders, such as preterm labor (44). The reason for this was that by its hyper-methylated status, fetal cfDNA could trigger an inflammatory response via TLR (toll like receptor) activation, thereby playing a crucial initiatory role (44). Unfortunately no clear data exists to support this enticing hypothesis (45). The question as to the source of elevated maternal cfDNA molecules was more complex to answer and took a rather unexpected turn when it was finally revealed to be derived from excessive generation of neutrophil extracellular traps (NETS) in pre-eclampsia (46, 47).

The advantage of cfDNA over fetal cells in maternal blood for prenatal diagnostic approaches quickly became apparent, particularly when examining for fetal genetic loci absent from the maternal genome, such as the Y chromosome for male fetuses, or the Rhesus D gene in Rhesus D pregnant women (48). Furthermore, the exploitation of the post-genomic advent of massive parallel sequencing permitted the reliable detection of fetal chromosomal abnormalities, such as trisomies, thereby ushering this long sought goal into clinical practice (48, 49).

FMM: RHEUMATOID ARTHRITIS—AMELIORATION, PREVENTION OR PROMOTION?

Amongst the autoimmune rheumatic disorders, rheumatoid arthritis probably responds most favorably to pregnancy in that many cases exhibit amelioration or remission whilst women affected by systemic lupus erythematosus frequently have poor pregnancy outcome characterized by high rates of pre-eclampsia or even fetal loss (50, 51).

Since the beneficial effect of pregnancy on rheumatoid arthritis disease status was determined not to be due to the action of immune-suppressive hormones, Lee Nelson and colleagues examined whether an HLA-based interaction between mother and fetus could contribute to disease improvement (52, 53). For their study they focussed on HLA Class II antigens due to the predisposing effect of certain alleles on rheumatoid arthritis incidence. In their analysis of 57 pregnancies from 41 women with rheumatoid arthritis remission was noted in 22 and amelioration in 12 instances. In 12 pregnancies no improvement of rheumatoid arthritis symptoms were noted (52). Their data indicated that a disparity in MHC class II alleles existed between mother and fetus in those pregnancies exhibiting a remission or improvement of rheumatoid arthritis symptoms. These were most pronounced for HLA-DRB1, DQA and DQB. Limited allelic differences were noted in the 12 rheumatoid arthritis cases where no improvement of symptoms was offered by pregnancy. This association between MHC class II disparity and disease activity was also evident in instances in women having successive pregnancies where rheumatoid arthritis symptoms were reduced in one instance but not the other. At the time that these studies were conducted, no conclusions could be drawn as to the operative mechanism although the question of trafficking fetal cells and FMM were raised (52).

Pregnancy may, however, not only afford some temporary respite from rheumatoid arthritis but may prevent or reduce the onset of this debilitating disorder post-partum (54). In order to examine whether pregnancy provided a protective effect against the development of rheumatoid arthritis, Guthrie and colleagues examined 310 women with newly diagnosed rheumatoid arthritis in comparison to 1,418 control women (54). This study indicated that the occurrence of rheumatoid arthritis was indeed lower in women who had been pregnant and delivered healthy babies by a factor of almost 40% when compared to non-parous women. It was furthermore observed that no reduction in the risk of developing rheumatoid arthritis was evident in women who had been pregnant but had not continued with the pregnancy until delivery (54). There was also no evidence for a cumulative protective effect offered by multiple deliveries. In contrast it appeared that the greatest protective effect offered by pregnancy was in a period of 5 years or less after delivery, and that this effect diminished significantly by 15 years post-partum. The authors proposed that the protective effect offered by a completed pregnancy may be attributable to persisting fetal cells. This could account for the diminished influence observed in pregnancies not completed to term, as cross-placental cell trafficking would be limited in these instances. The mechanism whereby micro-chimeric fetal cells would favorably modulate the maternal immune system to prevent rheumatoid arthritis onset may be by the provision of disparate MHC class I alleles as described above. Furthermore, in parous women deemed to be at high risk for rheumatoid arthritis due to the presence of two copies of HLA alleles, such as certain HLA-DRB1 loci, micro-chimeric fetal cells may be able to offset disease development by the provisional protective HLA molecules, such as the "DERAA" HLA-DRB1 locus. Evidence that such a mechanism may be operative is provided by the report of Pietsma and colleagues who observed that the protective "DERAA" locus in the form of a non-maternally inherited allele (NIMA) lead to a diminished risk for rheumatoid arthritis (55). The NIMA mechanism is discussed in more detail below.

On the other hand, FMM could assist with the initiation of an auto-inflammatory condition by provision of the necessary genetic background (56). An example of this is the "shared epitope" of certain HLA-DRB1 alleles associated with an increased incidence of rheumatoid arthritis (57). This "shared epitope" is a highly similar five amino acid peptide sequence contained in the HLA-DRB1*04 allele. In an elegant study Yan and colleagues set out to address whether FMM could contribute to the development of rheumatoid arthritis in women who were genetically "shared epitope" negative (58). In this study they examined 52 cases with rheumatoid arthritis and 34 healthy controls; 84% of cases and 92% of controls had at least one live birth. The mean age of cases was 51 and that of controls 42 years. By the use of "shared epitope" specific PCR assays they assessed the degree of microchimerism for such alleles in their study and control groups. Although some degree of "shared epitope" specific signals could be detected in both cohorts, the extent was significantly greater in cases with rheumatoid arthritis (58). In addition, the level of FMM for these "shared epitopes" was higher in rheumatoid arthritis cases than controls. Therefore, FMM, can contribute to the subsequent development of an autoimmune condition i.e., rheumatoid arthritis by the provision of necessary HLA haplotypes it via the inheritance of fetal cells or maternal cells during pregnancy (58).

FMM: CELLS FROM GRANDMA ARE MISSING IN PRE-ECLAMPSIA

During pregnancy, the pregnant woman exhibits a complex micro-chimeric phenotype, hosting cells from her current fetus, cells from previous pregnancies as well as cells from her mother (56, 59). Following the discovery of persisting fetal cells and their possible role in autoimmune conditions like systemic sclerosis, Maloney and colleagues investigated the behavior of trafficking maternal cells. Their examination, which employed HLA specific PCR assays as well as the use of XY FISH to detect female cells in male offspring revealed that cells of maternal origin can persist for numerous decades well into adulthood (59). In most instances maternal cells were HLA class I and II disparate from those of the host offspring (59). To study whether trafficking maternal cells play a role during pregnancy, Gammil et al. examined maternal blood samples collected in each trimester of pregnancy and post-partum (60). In some instances, they also had access to samples drawn prior to conception. By the use of quantitative PCR for specific HLA loci they were able to assess the extent of microchimerism attributable to trafficking maternal cells. In their examination of 86 maternal blood samples obtained from 27 healthy pregnant women with normal deliveries, no trafficking maternal cells were detected pre-conception or in samples obtained in the first trimester of pregnancy. On the other hand, such cells could be detected in 16% of second trimester, 29% of third trimester and 14% of post-partum samples. The degree of trafficking maternal cells microchimerism was greatest in samples collected close to term (60) (**Figure 1**). A startling finding made during this study was that no evidence of microchimerism due to trafficking maternal cells could be detected in any of the samples obtained from 20 pregnant women with manifest pre-eclampsia, in contrast to matching healthy control pregnant women, where such micro-chimeric cells could be detected in 30% of cases (60). This result could have profound implications since trafficking maternal cells are potentially important immune modulators due to their expression of NIMA (see below).

FMM: THE ROLE OF NIMA

A number of early reports indicated that cross-placental cell traffic was not restricted to the fetus but could also be derived from the mother. Pioneering works performed by Owen and colleagues in 1954 observed that Rh-negative girls born from Rh-positive mothers develop very low amount of antibodies to Rh suggesting the existence of a tolerance mechanism to NIMA (61). Later and in the setting of solid organ transplantation tolerance, Claas et al. observed that 50% of the patients receiving several blood transfusions showed selective anergy to non-inherited HLA haplotypes (62). Similarly, Burlingham and colleagues describe that graft survival between

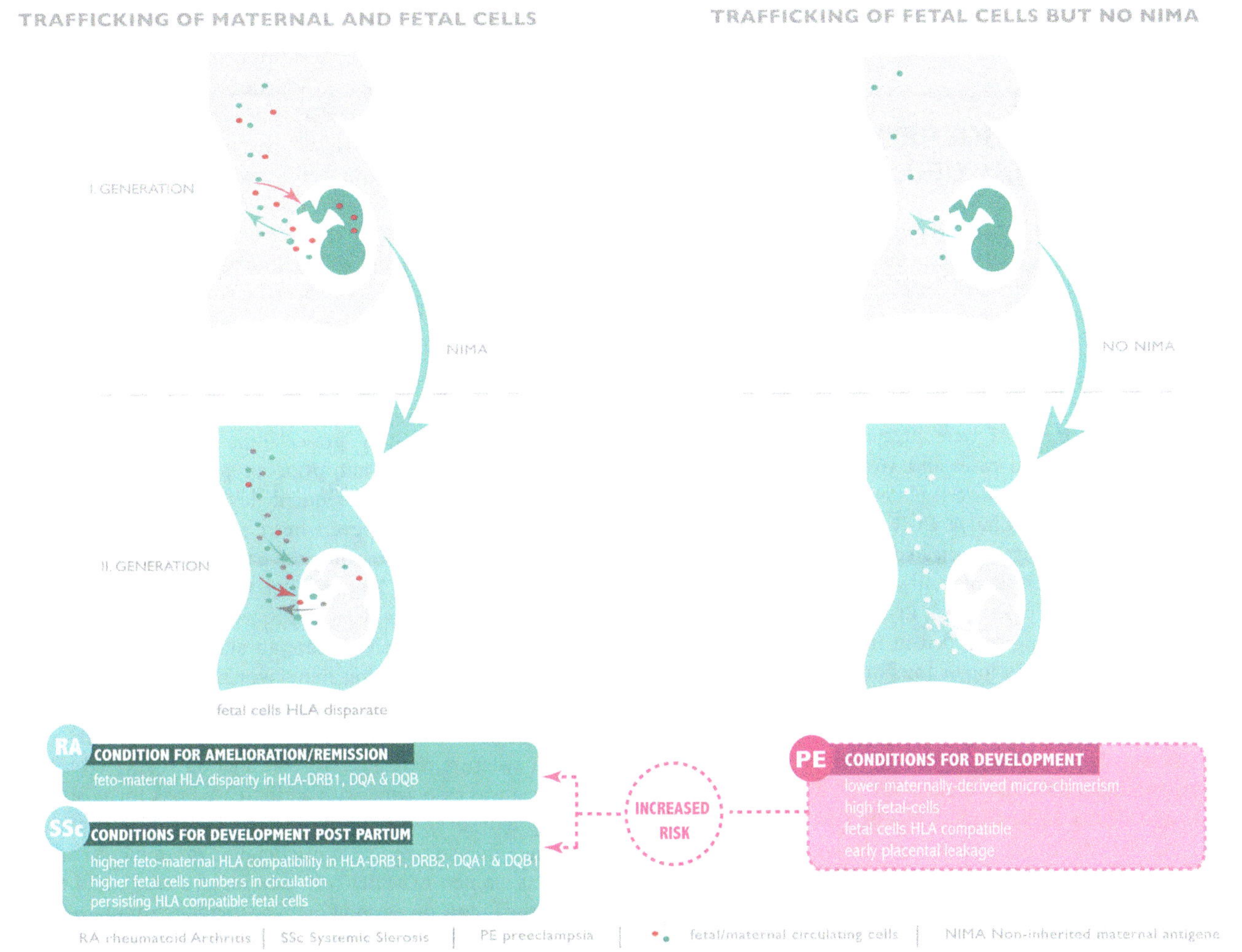

FIGURE 1 | Microchimerism throughout generations and risk of pre-eclampsia, RA and SSc development. Compatible or disparate expression of HLA of non-inherited antigen present in subsequent generation seam to promote or ameliorate autoimmunity or favor pre-eclampsia.

siblings who are mismatched with the recipient for one HLA haplotype results in higher graft survival when the donor has maternal HLA antigens not inherited by the recipient than when the donor has paternal antigens not inherited by the recipient suggesting and highlighting an important role for NIMA (63). More works performed in this direction conclude that the risk of graft vs. host disease among NIMA-matched stem cell transplants is reduced, suggesting possible clinical benefits of NIMA-specific tolerance that persists in individuals through to adulthood (64, 65). Post-natal persistence of genetically foreign chimeric maternal cells in offspring was originally described in infants with severe combined immune deficiency. In a study of 121 infants with defective T and B lymphocyte development, 40% had engrafted maternal T cells and a similar proportion developed clinically apparent graft-vs.-host disease caused by anti-fetal-allo-immunity (66, 67). Mother to offspring transfer and persistence of maternal cells is likely an unavoidable by-product of a porous placental interface. In this scenario, post-natal persistence of NIMA-specific tolerance represents an expendable developmental remnant of immune suppressive mechanisms essential for *in utero* survival (68). Very interesting is the role of NIMA during fetal life: Kinder and colleagues showed that the developmental exposure to foreign maternal cells primes the expansion and accumulation of NIMA-specific immune suppressive regulatory T cells that help establishing better tolerance (68, 69). The persistence of those regulatory T cells could then reinforce fetal tolerance during the next generation pregnancies sired by males with overlapping MHC haplotype specificity, conferring a reproductive advantage.

Taken together, genetic fitness is not restricted to chromosome transmission but is expanded through vertical transfer and survival of tolerogenic cells that establish microchimerism in offspring favoring in return the preservation of NIMA. On the other hand, cross-generational reproductive advantages that preserve post-natal retention of microchimeric maternal cells may also perpetuate auto-inflammatory or autoimmune diseases in offspring (56).

FMM: SYSTEMIC SCLEROSIS—TRIGGERED BY PERSISTING FETAL CELLS?

Unlike rheumatoid arthritis where the risk is diminished post-partum, systemic sclerosis, an autoimmune disorder characterized by graft-vs.-host disease like symptoms has a strong predilection in women post-partum (21). It was therefore hypothesized that persisting fetal cells may play a role in initiation of systemic sclerosis (21). In order to address this possibility, a group of 40 women who had previously given birth to a son were recruited. Of these, 17 were affected by systemic sclerosis, 7 were sisters of affected cases and 16 were healthy matching controls. The degree of fetal cell persistence in the circulation was assessed by a quantitative PCR assay specific for the Y chromosome. This analysis indicated that the median level of male positive cells was significantly higher in the circulation of systemic sclerosis cases than in matching controls, with intermediate levels being recorded in the 7 siblings (21). Since rheumatoid arthritis remission or amelioration during pregnancy involves a disparity in HLA class II, the role of such an interaction between mother and fetus was examined also in the systemic sclerosis cases. This indicated that a high degree of compatibility between mother and child existed for HLA $DRB1_1$, $DRB1_2$, DQA1, and DQB1 in systemic sclerosis cases (21). Since this feature was not evident in the healthy controls group, it is possible that microchimerism due to persisting HLA compatible fetal cells may contribute to the development of systemic sclerosis post-partum (**Figure 1**).

FMM: WHAT IS THE INFLUENCE OF PRE-ECLAMPSIA ON INCIDENCE OF SYSTEMIC SCLEROSIS OR RHEUMATOID ARTHRITIS?

As our report on elevated trafficking of fetal cells in pre-eclampsia (34) was published at around the same time as that of persisting fetal cells in systemic sclerosis (21), we queried whether the incidence of systemic sclerosis was higher in women who had pre-eclamptic pregnancies (26). Unfortunately, we did not have the correct epidemiological data set at our disposal at the time and so this hypothesis lay resting for almost two decades to finally be addressed in two recent reports (70, 71). In the first van Wyk and colleagues examined whether a relationship existed between the incidence of pre-eclampsia and subsequent development of systemic sclerosis (70). In their study cohort ($n = 103$), the incidence of systemic sclerosis post-first delivery was in mean after 27 years. The authors also determined that systemic sclerosis occurred with greater frequency in women who had pregnancies affected by pre-eclampsia or fetal growth restriction. A limitation of this study was that no information was available concerning potential HLA compatibility, a facet which would have been most interesting to investigate; on one hand in view of previous findings reporting on FMM (21), on the other hand due to reports indicating that pre-eclampsia may occur with greater frequency in instances where a high degree of MHC compatibility for the HLA-DR, -DP, and -DQ alleles occurs between spouses (72). In the second study, which made use of the Danish national register from which the pregnancy outcome and co-incidence of systemic sclerosis for 778,758 women was obtained (71). This indicated that the occurrence of pre-eclampsia is associated with a 69% risk of developing systemic sclerosis. Once again, unfortunately no details concerning HLA types could be obtained.

In the instance of post-partum development of rheumatoid arthritis, the issue is somewhat more complex with a major difference existing with regard as whether the pregnancy was healthy or disturbed by pre-eclampsia. As discussed above, it is widely accepted that prior pregnancy has a beneficial effect on reducing the subsequent development of rheumatoid arthritis. Indeed, it has even been suggested that parity may serve as a vaccine to prevent post-partum rheumatoid arthritis, especially in the first 5 years after the last delivery (54). This is in stark contrast to what is observed if the pregnancy was affected by pre-eclampsia, where an alternate scenario emerges in that such a constellation may favor post-partum rheumatoid arthritis. Evidence of such a feature was initially obtained by epidemiological data mining of the Danish National Patient Register where a retrospective examination suggested that pre-eclampsia was associated with an increased risk for post-partum development of rheumatoid arthritis (73). This feature was confirmed in a subsequent more detailed examination of 55,752 pregnant women of which 169 developed rheumatoid arthritis during the follow up period (74). The incidence of pre-eclampsia was greater in the rheumatoid arthritis study group (6.5%) than in the control cohort (3.6%) suggesting that pre-eclampsia lead to an increased risk for rheumatoid athritis (R.H = 1.96). On the basis of these findings the authors argued that rheumatoid arthritis may be associated with a long pre-clinical phase prior to symptom manifestation, a feature which may affect pregnancy outcome and thereby promote pre-eclampsia, or that a shared predisposition for pre-eclampsia and rheumatoid arthritis may exist (74) (**Figure 1**). In an independent study Ma and colleagues examined whether adverse pregnancy outcome as measured by extreme ($\leq$1,000 g) or very low birth weight ($\leq$1,500), a common feature of severe pre-eclampsia, was associated with subsequent clinical manifestation of rheumatoid arthritis (75). In their study they examined 202 cases with rheumatoid arthritis and 1,102 controls. This analysis indicated that both extreme and very low birth weight had a 3- to 5-fold greater risk of rheumatoid arthritis, particularly for the rheumatoid factor positive form (75).

FMM: THE PRE-ECLAMPSIA CONUNDRUM AND THE ROLE OF NIMA

The incidence of pre-eclampsia, particularly the severe form involving a defect in placenta development and spiral artery modification is associated with a high degree of HLA class II compatibility between spouses specifically for the HLA-DR, -DP, and -DQ alleles (72). Since trans-placental fetal cell traffic is enhanced in cases with pre-eclampsia (34), this would lead to a high level of microchimerism involving HLA class II compatible fetal cells of the type previously observed in cases with systemic sclerosis, autoimmune condition characterized by graft-vs.-host disease-like lesions (21). In this context it is worth noting that previous studies have suggested that pre-eclampsia exhibits traits of an autoimmune condition with placental features akin to graft-vs.-host disease (76). The question, hence, arises if a histo-compatible FMM state contributes to the etiology of pre-eclampsia. It is also plausible that the presence of this high grade pro-autoimmune microchimeric setting in pre-eclampsia, involving a greater than normal dosage of fetal cells, contributes to the subsequent increased risk for systemic sclerosis and rheumatoid arthritis occurring years later in an extended post-partum period (71, 74).

As pointed out above, microchimerism in a pregnant woman not only involves cells from the current fetus, but also that of any previous pregnancies as well as trafficking maternal cells the proband inherited from her mother (60). Due to their expression of NIMA, these trafficking maternal cells are important in inducing tolerance. A striking feature of pre-eclampsia is the apparent lack of trafficking maternal cells (60). It is therefore possible that the immunological effect of the microchimeric imbalance occurring in pre-eclampsia due to an influx of fetal cells may be further skewed by the apparent lack of trafficking maternal cells in the proband. Consequently, there is no mechanism in place to check or dampen the deleterious action of FMM derived haplo-identical or similar HLA alleles. Since pregnancy is an inflammatory process characterized by basal activation of circulatory neutrophils (77), this could in combination with a micro-chimeric aberrancy provide the necessary stimulus for the dysregulation observed in pre-eclampsia. In a similar manner, the combination of a lack or reduced level of trafficking maternal cells and high grade fetal microchimerism of disease associated HLA alleles could contribute to post-partum onset of rheumatoid arthritis or systemic sclerosis.

SUMMARY AND CONCLUSIONS

While feto-maternal exchange in pregnancy was previously viewed as rare and innocuous event, a vast body of work in the interim has shown that it is a common feature of mammalian pregnancy being readily discernible from mouse to man. The effects of this exchange are far reaching and can persist into adulthood and possibly even old age. In this review we have highlighted the potential anomaly regarding FMM occurring in pre-eclampsia and how this could contribute to the etiology of this enigmatic disorder, but also to the development of autoimmune diseases years post-partum. Should an imbalance between trafficking maternal cells and newly acquired fetal microchimerism prove to be a pivotal trigger driving these developments, then it is highly likely that an altering of the microchimeric milieu could be used to modulate or steer the maternal immune system away from this destructive direction. Evidence that such a mechanism may be viable is provided by reports indicating that the incidence of pre-eclampsia is reduced in women who have received blood transfusions, an event known to lead to a microchimeric state (78). It could therefore transpire that we are on the cusp of new era in the field of microchimerism, whereby this phenomenon provides the basis for new cell-based therapies geared at immune modulation and if so, what better target than pre-eclampsia.

AUTHOR CONTRIBUTIONS

SH and SR wrote the manuscript. LV prepared the figure. SH, PH, SvB, LV, NT, IH, OL, and SR discussed and revised the manuscript.

FUNDING

SH and SR are founded by the Department of Obstetrics, University Hospital Basel.

REFERENCES

1. Brosens I, Pijnenborg R, Vercruysse L, Romero R. The "Great Obstetrical Syndromes" are associated with disorders of deep placentation. *Am J Obstet Gynecol.* (2011) 204:193–201. doi: 10.1016/j.ajog.2010.08.009
2. Hahn S, Holzgreve W. Fetal cells and cell-free fetal DNA in maternal blood: new insights into pre-eclampsia. *Hum Reprod Update.* (2002) 8:501–8. doi: 10.1093/humupd/8.6.501
3. Hahn S, Huppertz B, Holzgreve W. Fetal cells and cell free fetal nucleic acids in maternal blood: new tools to study abnormal placentation? *Placenta.* (2005) 26:515–26. doi: 10.1016/j.placenta.2004.10.017
4. Lapaire O, Holzgreve W, Oosterwijk JC, Brinkhaus R, Bianchi DW. Georg Schmorl on trophoblasts in the maternal circulation. *Placenta.* (2007) 28:1–5. doi: 10.1016/j.placenta.2006.02.004
5. Attwood HD, Park WW. Embolism to the lungs by trophoblast. *J Obstet Gynaecol Br Commonw.* (1961) 68:611–7. doi: 10.1111/j.1471-0528.1961.tb02778.x
6. Johansen M, Redman CW, Wilkins T, Sargent IL. Trophoblast deportation in human pregnancy–its relevance for pre-eclampsia. *Placenta.* (1999) 20:531–9. doi: 10.1053/plac.1999.0422
7. Lo YM, Leung TN, Tein MS, Sargent IL, Zhang J, Lau TK, et al. Quantitative abnormalities of fetal DNA in maternal serum in preeclampsia. *Clin Chem.* (1999) 45:184–8.
8. Chesley LC, Annitto JE, Cosgrove RA. The familial factor in toxemia of pregnancy. *Obstet Gynecol.* (1968) 32:303–11.
9. Pilkington R, Knox EG, Russell JK, Walker W. Foetal-maternal transfusion and rhesus sensitization. *J Obstet Gynaecol Br Commonw.* (1966) 73:909–16. doi: 10.1111/j.1471-0528.1966.tb06113.x
10. Avent ND, Ridgwell K, Tanner MJ, Anstee DJ. cDNA cloning of a 30 kDa erythrocyte membrane protein associated with Rh (Rhesus)-blood-group-antigen expression. *Biochem J.* (1990) 271:821–5. doi: 10.1042/bj2710821
11. Kleihauer E, Braun H, Betke K. Demonstration of fetal hemoglobin in erythrocytes of a blood smear. *Klin Wochenschr.* (1957) 35:637–8. doi: 10.1007/BF01481043

12. Jones P, McNay A, Walker W. Association between foeto-maternal bleeding and hypertension in pregnancy. *Br Med J.* (1969) 3:738–42. doi: 10.1136/bmj.3.5673.738
13. Walknowska J, Conte FA, Grumbach MM. Practical and theoretical implications of fetal-maternal lymphocyte transfer. *Lancet.* (1969) 1:1119–22. doi: 10.1016/S0140-6736(69)91642-0
14. Schroder J, De la Chapelle A. Fetal lymphocytes in the maternal blood. *Blood.* (1972) 39:153–62.
15. Schroder J, Tiilikainen A, De la Chapelle A. Fetal leukocytes in the maternal circulation after delivery. I. Cytological aspects. *Transplantation.* (1974) 17:346–54. doi: 10.1097/00007890-197404000-00003
16. Tiilikainen A, Schroder J, De la Chapelle A. Fetal leukocytes in the maternal circulation after delivery. II. Masking of HL-A antigens. *Transplantation.* (1974) 17:355–60. doi: 10.1097/00007890-197404000-00004
17. Bianchi DW, Zickwolf GK, Weil GJ, Sylvester S, DeMaria MA. Male fetal progenitor cells persist in maternal blood for as long as 27 years postpartum. *Proc Natl Acad Sci USA.* (1996) 93:705–8. doi: 10.1073/pnas.93.2.705
18. Chan WF, Gurnot C, Montine TJ, Sonnen JA, Guthrie KA, Nelson JL. Male microchimerism in the human female brain. *PLoS ONE.* (2012) 7:e45592. doi: 10.1371/journal.pone.0045592
19. Rijnink EC, Penning ME, Wolterbeek R, Wilhelmus S, Zandbergen M, van Duinen SG, et al. Tissue microchimerism is increased during pregnancy: a human autopsy study. *Mol Hum Reprod.* (2015) 21:857–64. doi: 10.1093/molehr/gav047
20. Stelzer IA, Thiele K, Solano ME. Maternal microchimerism: lessons learned from murine models. *J Reprod Immunol.* (2015) 108:12–25. doi: 10.1016/j.jri.2014.12.007
21. Nelson JL, Furst DE, Maloney S, Gooley T, Evans PC, Smith A, et al. Microchimerism and HLA-compatible relationships of pregnancy in scleroderma. *Lancet.* (1998) 351:559–62. doi: 10.1016/S0140-6736(97)08357-8
22. Simpson JL, Martin AO. Prenatal diagnosis of cytogenetic disorders. *Clin Obstet Gynecol.* (1976) 19:841–53. doi: 10.1097/00003081-197612000-00013
23. Jackson LG, Wapner RA, Barr MA. Safety of chorionic villus biopsy. *Lancet.* (1986) 1:674–5. doi: 10.1016/S0140-6736(86)91741-1
24. Sundberg K, Bang J, Smidt-Jensen S, Brocks V, Lundsteen C, Parner J, et al. Randomised study of risk of fetal loss related to early amniocentesis versus chorionic villus sampling. *Lancet.* (1997) 350:697–703. doi: 10.1016/S0140-6736(97)02449-5
25. Jauniaux E, Rodeck C. Use, risks and complications of amniocentesis and chorionic villous sampling for prenatal diagnosis in early pregnancy. *Early Pregnancy.* (1995) 1:245–52.
26. Hahn S, Sant R, Holzgreve W. Fetal cells in maternal blood: current and future perspectives. *Mol Hum Reprod.* (1998) 4:515–21. doi: 10.1093/molehr/4.6.515
27. Holzgreve W, Hahn S. Fetal cells in cervical mucus and maternal blood. *Baillieres Best Pract Res Clin Obstet Gynaecol.* (2000) 14:709–22. doi: 10.1053/beog.1999.0106
28. de la Cruz F, Shifrin H, Elias S, Simpson JL, Jackson L, Klinger K, et al. Prenatal diagnosis by use of fetal cells isolated from maternal blood. *Am J Obstet Gynecol.* (1995) 173:1354–5. doi: 10.1016/0002-9378(95)91393-9
29. Bianchi DW, Mahr A, Zickwolf GK, Houseal TW, Flint AF, Klinger KW. Detection of fetal cells with 47, XY, +21 karyotype in maternal peripheral blood. *Hum Genet.* (1992) 90:368–70. doi: 10.1007/BF00220460
30. Cheung MC, Goldberg JD, Kan YW. Prenatal diagnosis of sickle cell anaemia and thalassaemia by analysis of fetal cells in maternal blood. *Nat Genet.* (1996) 14:264–8. doi: 10.1038/ng1196-264
31. Di Naro E, Ghezzi F, Vitucci A, Tannoia N, Campanale D, D'Addario V, et al. Prenatal diagnosis of beta-thalassaemia using fetal erythroblasts enriched from maternal blood by a novel gradient. *Mol Hum Reprod.* (2000) 6:571–4. doi: 10.1093/molehr/6.6.571
32. Bianchi DW, Simpson JL, Jackson LG, Evans MI, Elias S, Holzgreve W, et al. Fetal cells in maternal blood: NIFTY clinical trial interim analysis. DM-STAT. NICHD fetal cell study (NIFTY) group. *Prenat Diagn.* (1999) 19:994–5.
33. Chitty LS, van der Schoot CE, Hahn S, Avent ND. SAFE–the Special Non-invasive Advances in Fetal and Neonatal Evaluation Network: aims and achievements. *Prenat Diagn.* (2008) 28:83–8. doi: 10.1002/pd.1929
34. Holzgreve W, Ghezzi F, Di Naro E, Ganshirt D, Maymon E, Hahn S. Disturbed feto-maternal cell traffic in preeclampsia. *Obstet Gynecol.* (1998) 91:669–72.
35. Holzgreve W, Li JJ, Steinborn A, Kulz T, Sohn C, Hodel M, et al. Elevation in erythroblast count in maternal blood before the onset of preeclampsia. *Am J Obstet Gynecol.* (2001) 184:165–8. doi: 10.1067/mob.2001.108861
36. Lo YM, Corbetta N, Chamberlain PF, Rai V, Sargent IL, Redman CW, et al. Presence of fetal DNA in maternal plasma and serum. *Lancet.* (1997) 350:485–7. doi: 10.1016/S0140-6736(97)02174-0
37. Chen XQ, Stroun M, Magnenat JL, Nicod LP, Kurt AM, Lyautey J, et al. Microsatellite alterations in plasma DNA of small cell lung cancer patients. *Nat Med.* (1996) 2:1033–5. doi: 10.1038/nm0996-1033
38. Anker P, Lefort F, Vasioukhin V, Lyautey J, Lederrey C, Chen XQ, et al. K-ras mutations are found in DNA extracted from the plasma of patients with colorectal cancer. *Gastroenterology.* (1997) 112:1114–20. doi: 10.1016/S0016-5085(97)70121-5
39. Lo YM, Lau TK, Chan LY, Leung TN, Chang AM. Quantitative analysis of the bidirectional fetomaternal transfer of nucleated cells and plasma DNA. *Clin Chem.* (2000) 46:1301–9.
40. Lo YM, Tein MS, Lau TK, Haines CJ, Leung TN, Poon PM, et al. Quantitative analysis of fetal DNA in maternal plasma and serum: implications for noninvasive prenatal diagnosis. *Am J Hum Genet.* (1998) 62:768–75. doi: 10.1086/301800
41. Zhong XY, Laivuori H, Livingston JC, Ylikorkala O, Sibai BM, Holzgreve W, et al. Elevation of both maternal and fetal extracellular circulating deoxyribonucleic acid concentrations in the plasma of pregnant women with preeclampsia. *Am J Obstet Gynecol.* (2001) 184:414–9. doi: 10.1067/mob.2001.109594
42. Zhong XY, Holzgreve W, Hahn S. The levels of circulatory cell free fetal DNA in maternal plasma are elevated prior to the onset of preeclampsia. *Hypertens Pregnancy.* (2002) 21:77–83. doi: 10.1081/PRG-120002911
43. Zhong XY, Holzgreve W, Hahn S. Circulatory fetal and maternal DNA in pregnancies at risk and those affected by preeclampsia. *Ann N Y Acad Sci.* (2001) 945:138–40. doi: 10.1111/j.1749-6632.2001.tb03874.x
44. Hahn S, Giaglis S, Buser A, Hoesli I, Lapaire O, Hasler P. Cell-free nucleic acids in (maternal) blood: any relevance to (reproductive) immunologists? *J Reprod Immunol.* (2014) 104–105:26–31. doi: 10.1016/j.jri.2014.03.007
45. Conka J, Konecna B, Laukova L, Vlkova B, Celec P. Fetal DNA does not induce preeclampsia-like symptoms when delivered in late pregnancy in the mouse. *Placenta.* (2017) 52:100–5. doi: 10.1016/j.placenta.2017.02.008
46. Gupta AK, Hasler P, Holzgreve W, Gebhardt S, Hahn S. Induction of neutrophil extracellular DNA lattices by placental microparticles and IL-8 and their presence in preeclampsia. *Hum Immunol.* (2005) 66:1146–54. doi: 10.1016/j.humimm.2005.11.003
47. Sur Chowdhury C, Hahn S, Hasler P, Hoesli I, Lapaire O, Giaglis S. Elevated levels of total cell-free DNA in maternal serum samples arise from the generation of neutrophil extracellular traps. *Fetal Diagn Ther.* (2016) 40:263–7. doi: 10.1159/000444853
48. Chiu RW, Lo YM. Clinical applications of maternal plasma fetal DNA analysis: translating the fruits of 15 years of research. *Clin Chem Lab Med.* (2013) 51:197–204. doi: 10.1515/cclm-2012-0601
49. Hui L, Bianchi DW. Noninvasive prenatal DNA testing: the vanguard of genomic medicine. *Annu Rev Med.* (2017) 68:459–72. doi: 10.1146/annurev-med-072115-033220
50. Ostensen M, Brucato A, Carp H, Chambers C, Dolhain RJ, Doria A, et al. Pregnancy and reproduction in autoimmune rheumatic diseases. *Rheumatology (Oxford).* (2011) 50:657–64. doi: 10.1093/rheumatology/keq350
51. Soh MC, Nelson-Piercy C. High-risk pregnancy and the rheumatologist. *Rheumatology (Oxford).* (2015) 54:572–87. doi: 10.1093/rheumatology/keu394
52. Nelson JL, Hughes KA, Smith AG, Nisperos BB, Branchaud AM, Hansen JA. Maternal-fetal disparity in HLA class II alloantigens and the pregnancy-induced amelioration of rheumatoid arthritis. *N Engl J Med.* (1993) 329:466–71. doi: 10.1056/NEJM199308123290704
53. Nelson JL, Hughes KA, Smith AG, Nisperos BB, Branchaud AM, Hansen JA. Remission of rheumatoid arthritis during pregnancy and maternal-fetal class II alloantigen disparity. *Am J Reprod Immunol.* (1992) 28:226–7. doi: 10.1111/j.1600-0897.1992.tb00798.x
54. Guthrie KA, Dugowson CE, Voigt LF, Koepsell TD, Nelson JL. Does pregnancy provide vaccine-like protection against rheumatoid arthritis? *Arthritis Rheum.* (2010) 62:1842–8. doi: 10.1002/art.27459

55. Feitsma AL, Worthington J, van der Helm-van Mil AH, Plant D, Thomson W, Ursum J, et al. Protective effect of noninherited maternal HLA-DR antigens on rheumatoid arthritis development. *Proc Natl Acad Sci USA.* (2007) 104:19966–70. doi: 10.1073/pnas.0710260104
56. Nelson JL. The otherness of self: microchimerism in health and disease. *Trends Immunol.* (2012) 33:421–7. doi: 10.1016/j.it.2012.03.002
57. Holoshitz J. The rheumatoid arthritis HLA-DRB1 shared epitope. *Curr Opin Rheumatol.* (2010) 22:293–8. doi: 10.1097/BOR.0b013e328336ba63
58. Yan Z, Aydelotte T, Gadi VK, Guthrie KA, Nelson JL. Acquisition of the rheumatoid arthritis HLA shared epitope through microchimerism. *Arthritis Rheum.* (2011) 63:640–4. doi: 10.1002/art.30160
59. Maloney S, Smith A, Furst DE, Myerson D, Rupert K, Evans PC, et al. Microchimerism of maternal origin persists into adult life. *J Clin Invest.* (1999) 104:41–7. doi: 10.1172/JCI6611
60. Gammill HS, Adams Waldorf KM, Aydelotte TM, Lucas J, Leisenring WM, Lambert NC, et al. Pregnancy, microchimerism, and the maternal grandmother. *PLoS ONE.* (2011) 6:e24101. doi: 10.1371/journal.pone.0024101
61. Owen RD, Wood HR, Foord AG, Sturgeon P, Baldwin LG. Evidence for actively acquired tolerance to Rh antigens. *Proc Natl Acad Sci USA.* (1954) 40:420–4. doi: 10.1073/pnas.40.6.420
62. Claas FH, Gijbels Y, van der Velden-de Munck J, van Rood JJ. Induction of B cell unresponsiveness to noninherited maternal HLA antigens during fetal life. *Science.* (1988) 241:1815–7. doi: 10.1126/science.3051377
63. Burlingham WJ, Grailer AP, Heisey DM, Claas FH, Norman D, Mohanakumar T, et al. The effect of tolerance to noninherited maternal HLA antigens on the survival of renal transplants from sibling donors. *N Engl J Med.* (1998) 339:1657–64. doi: 10.1056/NEJM199812033392302
64. Eikmans M, van Halteren AG, van Besien K, van Rood JJ, Drabbels JJ, Claas FH. Naturally acquired microchimerism: implications for transplantation outcome and novel methodologies for detection. *Chimerism.* (2014) 5:24–39. doi: 10.4161/chim.28908
65. Ichinohe T, Uchiyama T, Shimazaki C, Matsuo K, Tamaki S, Hino M, et al. Feasibility of HLA-haploidentical hematopoietic stem cell transplantation between noninherited maternal antigen (NIMA)-mismatched family members linked with long-term fetomaternal microchimerism. *Blood.* (2004) 104:3821–8. doi: 10.1182/blood-2004-03-1212
66. Muller SM, Ege M, Pottharst A, Schulz AS, Schwarz K, Friedrich W. Transplacentally acquired maternal T lymphocytes in severe combined immunodeficiency: a study of 121 patients. *Blood.* (2001) 98:1847–51. doi: 10.1182/blood.V98.6.1847
67. Kinder JM, Jiang TT, Ertelt JM, Xin L, Strong BS, Shaaban AF, et al. Tolerance to noninherited maternal antigens, reproductive microchimerism and regulatory T cell memory: 60 years after 'Evidence for actively acquired tolerance to Rh antigens'. *Chimerism.* (2015) 6:8–20. doi: 10.1080/19381956.2015.1107253
68. Kinder JM, Stelzer IA, Arck PC, Way SS. Immunological implications of pregnancy-induced microchimerism. *Nat Rev Immunol.* (2017) 17:483–94. doi: 10.1038/nri.2017.38
69. Kinder JM, Jiang TT, Ertelt JM, Xin L, Strong BS, Shaaban AF, et al. Cross-generational reproductive fitness enforced by microchimeric maternal cells. *Cell.* (2015) 162:505–15. doi: 10.1016/j.cell.2015.07.006
70. van Wyk L, van der Marel J, Schuerwegh AJ, Schouffoer AA, Voskuyl AE, Huizinga TW, et al. Increased incidence of pregnancy complications in women who later develop scleroderma: a case control study. *Arthritis Res Ther.* (2011) 13:R183. doi: 10.1186/ar3510
71. Kamper-Jorgensen M, Gammill HS, Nelson JL. Preeclampsia and scleroderma: a prospective nationwide analysis. *Acta Obstet Gynecol Scand.* (2018) 97:587–90. doi: 10.1111/aogs.13296
72. Ooki I, Takakuwa K, Akashi M, Nonaka T, Yokoo T, Tanaka K. Studies on the compatibility of HLA-Class II alleles in patient couples with severe pre-eclampsia using PCR-RFLP methods. *Am J Reprod Immunol.* (2008) 60:75–84. doi: 10.1111/j.1600-0897.2008.00592.x
73. Jorgensen KT, Pedersen BV, Jacobsen S, Biggar RJ, Frisch M. National cohort study of reproductive risk factors for rheumatoid arthritis in Denmark: a role for hyperemesis, gestational hypertension and pre-eclampsia? *Ann Rheum Dis.* (2010) 69:358–63. doi: 10.1136/ard.2008.099945
74. Jorgensen KT, Harpsoe MC, Jacobsen S, Jess T, Frisch M. Increased risk of rheumatoid arthritis in women with pregnancy complications and poor self-rated health: a study within the Danish National Birth Cohort. *Rheumatology (Oxford).* (2014) 53:1513–9. doi: 10.1093/rheumatology/keu150
75. Ma KK, Nelson JL, Guthrie KA, Dugowson CE, Gammill HS. Adverse pregnancy outcomes and risk of subsequent rheumatoid arthritis. *Arthritis Rheumatol.* (2014) 66:508–12. doi: 10.1002/art.38247
76. Gleicher N. Why much of the pathophysiology of preeclampsia-eclampsia must be of an autoimmune nature. *Am J Obstet Gynecol.* (2007) 196:5 e1–7. doi: 10.1016/j.ajog.2006.09.016
77. Sacks GP, Studena K, Sargent K, Redman CW. Normal pregnancy and preeclampsia both produce inflammatory changes in peripheral blood leukocytes akin to those of sepsis. *Am J Obstet Gynecol.* (1998) 179:80–6. doi: 10.1016/S0002-9378(98)70254-6
78. Feeney JG, Tovey LA, Scott JS. Influence of previous blood-transfusion on incidence of pre-eclampsia. *Lancet.* (1977) 1:874–5. doi: 10.1016/S0140-6736(77)91199-0

2

Immune Profile of the Normal Maternal-Fetal Interface in Rhesus Macaques and its Alteration Following Zika Virus Infection

Matilda J. Moström[1,2], Elizabeth A. Scheef[1], Lesli M. Sprehe[1], Dawn Szeltner[1], Dollnovan Tran[1], Jon D. Hennebold[3], Victoria H. J. Roberts[3], Nicholas J. Maness[2,4], Marissa Fahlberg[1] and Amitinder Kaur[1,2]*

[1] Division of Immunology, Tulane National Primate Research Center, Covington, LA, United States, [2] Department of Microbiology and Immunology, Tulane School of Medicine, New Orleans, LA, United States, [3] Division of Reproductive and Developmental Sciences, Oregon National Primate Research Center, Beaverton, OR, United States, [4] Division of Microbiology, Tulane National Primate Research Center, Covington, LA, United States

***Correspondence:**
Amitinder Kaur
akaur@tulane.edu

The maternal decidua is an immunologically complex environment that balances maintenance of immune tolerance to fetal paternal antigens with protection of the fetus against vertical transmission of maternal pathogens. To better understand host immune determinants of congenital infection at the maternal-fetal tissue interface, we performed a comparative analysis of innate and adaptive immune cell subsets in the peripheral blood and decidua of healthy rhesus macaque pregnancies across all trimesters of gestation and determined changes after Zika virus (ZIKV) infection. Using one 28-color and one 18-color polychromatic flow cytometry panel we simultaneously analyzed the frequency, phenotype, activation status and trafficking properties of $\alpha\beta$ T, $\gamma\delta$ T, iNKT, regulatory T (Treg), NK cells, B lymphocytes, monocytes, macrophages, and dendritic cells (DC). Decidual leukocytes showed a striking enrichment of activated effector memory and tissue-resident memory CD4+ and CD8+ T lymphocytes, CD4+ Tregs, CD56+ NK cells, CD14+CD16+ monocytes, CD206+ tissue-resident macrophages, and a paucity of B lymphocytes when compared to peripheral blood. t-distributed stochastic neighbor embedding (tSNE) revealed unique populations of decidual NK, T, DC and monocyte/macrophage subsets. Principal component analysis showed distinct spatial localization of decidual and circulating leukocytes contributed by NK and CD8+ T lymphocytes, and separation of decidua based on gestational age contributed by memory CD4+ and CD8+ T lymphocytes. Decidua from 10 ZIKV-infected dams obtained 16-56 days post infection at third (n=9) or second (n=1) trimester showed a significant reduction in frequency of activated, CXCR3+, and/or Granzyme B+ memory CD4+ and CD8+ T lymphocytes and $\gamma\delta$ T compared to normal decidua. These data suggest that ZIKV induces local immunosuppression with reduced immune recruitment and impaired cytotoxicity. Our study adds to the immune characterization of the maternal-fetal interface in a translational nonhuman primate model of congenital infection and provides novel insight in to putative mechanisms of vertical transmission.

Keywords: fetal-maternal immunity, decidua, Zika, gammadelta T cells, dNK, decidual T cells, Treg, congenital viral infection

INTRODUCTION

Successful maintenance of pregnancy requires a balance between sustaining an immune tolerant state to prevent rejection of foreign paternal-origin fetal antigens and at the same time protect the fetus against vertical transmission of microbial pathogens (1). The maternal-fetal interface is a rich and complex immune environment essential to fetal growth and survival that consists of maternal decidual tissue and fetal-origin cells such as placental trophoblasts, endothelial cells and Hofbauer cells (2, 3). The decidua contains a myriad of immune cells including antigen-presenting cells (DC and macrophages), stromal cells, NK cells, neutrophils, mast cells, regulatory T (Treg) cells, and adaptive T lymphocytes that are geared towards a dual role of establishing a tolerogenic environment conducive to placental embedding while maintaining local immunity against infections (1, 4, 5). Decidual leukocytes are phenotypically and functionally distinct from peripheral blood and change with gestational age. Most of the data in humans are from first trimester pregnancy with fewer studies in the second or third trimester (6–8). Studies in the first trimester of pregnancy in humans have shown that NK cells account for 50-90% of the decidual leukocyte population and predominantly have a CD56bright CD16– phenotype (7, 9). Despite the presence of cytolytic granules, decidual NK are poorly cytotoxic and differ from circulating NK cells in their functionality, expression of inhibitory and cytotoxicity receptors, and at the level of gene expression (7, 10–13). A similar dominant population of CD56+ NK cells has been described in rhesus macaque decidua (14–16). Along with decidual NK cells, Tregs and macrophages play a key role in maintaining an anti-inflammatory environment in the decidua (17, 18). Among adaptive immune subsets, CD3+ T lymphocytes constitute 5-20% of the decidual leukocyte population in early pregnancy and increase with gestational age; in contrast, B lymphocytes are rare (6, 19). Decidual T lymphocytes are enriched for differentiated CD8+ effector memory T cells that have reduced cytotoxic granule content and a transcriptional profile of exhaustion and activation genes distinct from circulating effector memory CD8+ T lymphocytes (20, 21). Decidual CD8+ T cells are also key players in recognition of foreign antigen and have been shown to contain fetal-specific CD8+ T cells (22–25). It is not known however whether decidual CD8+ T lymphocytes mount an antigen-specific response against pathogens; one study demonstrating decidual CD8+ T cells binding to EBV-specific tetramers was not conclusive (26, 27). Although the maternal-fetal interface has been extensively investigated for mechanisms underlying preterm birth and preeclampsia, relatively little is known about factors that prevent or allow maternal-fetal transmission of pathogens. We are using the rhesus macaque nonhuman primate (NHP) model to study factors predisposing to placental transmission of congenital infections such as cytomegalovirus (CMV) and Zika virus (ZIKV) (28–30).

Important similarities in placental biology make NHPs a suitable animal model to study vertical transmission of pathogens. Rhesus macaque placentation resembles humans in consisting of a hemochorial placenta with trophoblast invasion of the uterine wall (31, 32). However, macaque placentation is less deep with trophoblast invasion restricted to spiral arteries in the decidua and only occurring *via* the endovascular route (33). Macaque extravillous trophoblasts express the HLA-G ortholog, Mamu-AG, which has features of a nonclassical MHC class I molecule and was shown to be a ligand for the inhibitory killer immunoglobulin-like receptor Mamu-KIR3DL05 (34, 35). A recent transcriptomic analysis of human and macaque placenta revealed that the majority of human placental marker genes were shared between the two species, further validating the relevance of the NHP model (36). Of particular interest to the current study are the immune determinants at the maternal-fetal interface that protect against vertical transmission. A single-cell transcriptomics study of normal human pregnancy demonstrated the complexity of the immune populations in the maternal-fetal interface (37). The maternal-fetal interface of NHPs is less well delineated. Currently data are lacking on the decidual T lymphocyte phenotype, presence of nontraditional T cells, NK cell subsets, B cells, and myeloid cells in rhesus macaques across different gestational ages and their comparison to peripheral blood. The aim of this study was to conduct a comprehensive analysis of the immune composition of decidual and circulating leukocytes in normal rhesus macaque pregnancies throughout gestation and investigate changes in congenital infection. To this end we developed one 28-color and one 18-color flow cytometry panel to simultaneously analyze multiple innate and adaptive immune subsets in the decidua and blood of healthy rhesus macaques in the first, second and third trimester of pregnancy. We compared the frequency, phenotype, function and trafficking properties of decidual leukocytes with that of circulating leukocytes. In addition, we correlated changes in the decidual leukocyte composition with increasing gestational age. We then investigated changes following ZIKV infection in pregnancy by comparing normal decidua with decidual leukocytes and peripheral blood mononuclear cells from a previously reported study on ZIKV infection in pregnant rhesus macaques (29).

MATERIALS AND METHODS

Animals and Study Design

Rhesus macaque dams of Indian ancestry from the Tulane National Primate Research Center (TNPRC) and the Oregon National Primate Research Center (ONPRC) were used for this study. All macaques were from the specific pathogen free (SPF) colonies of the respective primate centers. SPF macaques are CMV-seropositive but free of SIV, STLV, Type D retrovirus, and herpes B virus. At both institutions all animal procedures were performed according to approved Institutional Animal Care and Use Committee protocols. Peripheral blood (n=24) and decidua (n=11) from normal pregnant dams aged 3.6-17.0 years (mean=7.7 years, median=6.7 years) were collected for cross-sectional analysis of first, second, and third trimester gestation (**Table 1**). Information regarding timed-mating, housing, and mode of sampling are detailed in **Supplemental Table 1.** Decidua was obtained in 1st trimester from day 44-50 gestation (n=3), 2nd trimester at day 100 gestation (n=3), and 3rd trimester from day 130-167 gestation (n=5) (**Supplemental Table 1**).

Blood and decidua were also collected close to or at the time of Caesarian section (C-section) from a cohort of ZIKV-infected dams (n=10) enrolled in a separate previously published study (29). The group consisted of pregnant Indian-ancestry rhesus macaques inoculated subcutaneously with a single dose of $1x10^4$ PFU ZIKV Rio-U1 at the first (n=1), second (n=3), or third trimester (n=6) gestation followed by C-section and decidua collection at 2nd or 3rd trimester gestation (**Table 1** and **Supplemental Table 2**). Peripheral blood was obtained 5-41 days post ZIKV infection while placenta was collected at the time of study C-section or spontaneous abortion which ranged from 16-56 days post ZIKV infection (**Supplemental Table 2**). One decidua was collected in the second trimester at 64 days gestation age while the remaining 9 decidua samples were collected in the third trimester at 142 to 157 days gestation age (**Table 1** and **Supplemental Table 2**).

Isolation of Leukocytes From Blood and Decidual Tissue

Peripheral blood mononuclear cells (PBMC) were isolated from blood collected in anticoagulant EDTA or heparin tubes by density gradient centrifugation with Lymphocyte Separation Medium (LSM; MP Biomedicals) or Lymphoprep (Stemcell Technologies). Isolated PBMC were cryopreserved using serum-free Bambanker cryopreservation media (Bulldog Bio) and stored in liquid nitrogen until use.

Following C-section, decidua from ONPRC study animals was dissected from the maternal side of the placenta and shipped overnight to TNPRC in R10 media (RPMI supplemented with Hepes, L-glutamine, and 10%FBS) on ice for decidual leukocyte isolation. Placental samples collected at TNPRC were immediately processed for decidual leukocyte isolation. Blood clots were removed from the maternal side of the placenta and decidual tissue carefully dissected away from the placenta. Visible blood vessels were removed and decidual tissue pieces were then washed extensively with sodium chloride 0.9% (Hanna Pharmaceutical Supply Co.) to remove any debris and remaining blood. Clean decidua was dissected into 2 mm^2 pieces and subjected to three rounds of digestion by shaking at 60 RPM at 37°C for 30 minutes in digestion media containing 0.1mg/mL DNAse I (Millipore Sigma 11284932001) and collagenase IV 1 mg/mL (Millipore Sigma C5138-100MG). Released cells in solution were collected in between each digestion and washed. After the last digestion, residual cells were passed repeatedly through a sterile 18-gauge animal feeding needle (Fisherbrand™) for gentle mechanical sheering before straining through sterile 70μm filters. Cells from each digestion were pooled. The resulting single cell suspension was layered over a density gradient LSM (MP Biomedicals) and spun at 1500 rpm for 45 minutes with no brakes. Lymphocytes were carefully collected from the top layer, washed, and cryopreserved in DMSO supplemented with 90% FBS or in serum-free Bambanker cryopreservation medium (Bulldog Bio).

Phenotyping by Multicolor Flow Cytometry

Two flow cytometry panels were used to phenotype the leukocytes, one adaptive 28-color panel, and one innate 18-color panel (**Supplemental Table 3**). In the same batch experiment, decidual leukocytes and PBMC from normal and ZIKV-infected animals were gently thawed using standard protocols supplemented with 17.5μg/mL DNAse I (Millipore Sigma 11284932001). 1-3 million live lymphocytes were used for staining. Briefly, cells were stained with live/dead discriminating dye for 20min at room temperature (RT). Cell suspensions were washed with 2% FBS/PBS buffer and the 28-color panel was stained sequentially with anti-Vα24-PE and BV421-CD1d tetramer first (20 minutes incubation at RT), followed by addition of the chemokine receptor antibodies anti-CCR5-BUV737 and anti-CXCR3-PE-Cy7 (20 minutes incubation at 37°C), and finally by addition of the chemokine receptor antibodies anti-CCR4-BV510 and anti-CCR6-BV650 (20 minutes incubation at 37°C) with no washes in between. Last, the remaining surface cocktail was added and the tubes incubated for 20 minutes at RT with antibodies outlined in **Supplemental Table 3**. Cells were then washed with 2% FBS/PBS prior to incubating with BD Cytofix/Cytoperm™ solution (BD Biosciences) for 20 minutes at RT followed by washing with BD Perm/Wash™ buffer (BD Biosciences). Intracellular antibodies

TABLE 1 | Description of study cohort.

Trimester	1st Trimester		2nd Trimester		3rd Trimester	
Sample type	Decidua	PBMC	Decidua	PBMC	Decidua	PBMC
Uninfected (n)	3	6	3	11	5	7
Zika (n)	0	0	1	1	9	8

were then added for a 20-minute incubation at RT. The 18-color panel was stained using the same applicable steps. Cells were fixed with Stabilizing Fixative (BD Biosciences; Cat# 338036) and acquired the next day on the BD FACSymphony A5 and BD LSRFortessa X-20 using BD FACSDiva version 9.1 and 9.0 respectively. A mean of 244,000 (50,000 to 718,000) Time/CD45+/Live events were collected. FMO controls included in the experiments were BB700-PD-1, BV650-CCR6, PE-Cy7-CXCR3, AL647-CX3CR1, PE-Vα24, and APC-NKG2D. Single color controls were acquired in all experiments and compensation and analysis was performed in FlowJo software v10.7 (BD Biosciences).

Data Analysis

Flow cytometry data was analyzed using FlowJo v10.7 (BD Biosciences). Statistical analysis was performed using GraphPad Prism version 9.0.1 (GraphPad Software Inc.) and R (CRAN). tSNEs were calculated in FlowJo using the default settings for opt-SNE. An equal number of cells per tissue were used when analyzing PBMC *versus* decidua in uninfected animals. An equal number of cells per condition were used when analyzing ZIKV-infection *versus* uninfected decidua. Boxplots and tSNE renderings were created using the tidyverse and ggpubr packages in R. Data throughout the result section are reported as mean ± standard deviation (SD) unless noted.

RESULTS

Circulating and Decidual Leukocyte Composition in Normal Pregnancy

To examine immune cell populations at the maternal-fetal interface in normal rhesus macaques, we conducted a cross-sectional analysis of first (n=3), second (n=3), and third (n=5) trimester decidua obtained at the time of C-section in healthy pregnancy and compared it with blood obtained from gestation-matched healthy, uninfected dams experiencing normal pregnancies (**Table 1**). PBMC and decidual leukocytes were evaluated with two flow cytometry panels, one 28-color panel focused on adaptive immunity, and one 18-color innate cell focused panel (**Supplemental Table 3**). T lymphocytes, NK cells, B lymphocytes, and cells of the myeloid lineage were enumerated using the gating strategy in **Figures 1A–C**. Definitions used in this study for each analyzed cell type in the two flow panels were based on markers in NHPs that are equal to their human counterparts (**Table 2**). For example, NK cells which are CD3− $CD16^{bright}$ $CD56^{dim}$ or $CD16^{-/dim}$ $CD56^{bright}$ in humans are defined as CD3− $HLA\text{-}DR^{lo/-}$ CD8+ in rhesus macaques (38). T lymphocytes were the predominant leukocytes in both PBMC (mean ± SD; 48.0 ± 14.7%) and decidua (54.2 ± 12.6%) but not significantly different between the two compartments (**Figures 2A, B**). NK cells were significantly increased in the decidua with ~3-fold greater frequency compared to PBMC, and were highest in the 2nd trimester (**Figures 2A, B**). No relationship between NK cells and gestational age was found in the decidua (**Supplemental Figure 1**). B lymphocytes were close to absent in decidual tissue in contrast to PBMC where they made up 25.3 ± 10.8% of the live CD45+ leukocytes (**Figures 2A, B**). In the myeloid antigen presenting compartment, which was defined as CD3− CD20− $CD8^{lo/-}$HLA-DR+ (**Table 2**), a population of CD14+ tissue macrophages expressing both CD163+ and CD206+ were found in the decidua (**Figures 2C, D**). This population was virtually absent in PBMC (0.1 ± 1.2%) but represented 28.1 ± 14.7% of HLA-DR+ leukocytes in the decidua (**Figure 2D**). CD14+ CD163+ CD206− myeloid cells were found in PBMC and decidua at 54.1 ± 25.8% and 18.3 ± 12.8% respectively of myeloid HLA-DR+ expressing cells (**Figure 2D**). These cells are a mix of classical and intermediate monocytes in the PBMC and recently infiltrated monocytes and macrophages in tissues (39, 40). CD14+ CD163− CD206− cells were significantly increased in the decidua compared to PBMC (**Figure 2D**). Plasmacytoid DC (pDC) frequency ranged between 0.3 to 14.7% of HLA-DR-expressing cells in decidua but were not significantly different from PBMC (**Figure 2D**). CD14− CD123− HLA-DR+ leukocytes, which can be either conventional DCs or CD14− CD16+ non-classical monocytes in circulation, were similar between PBMC and decidua (34.4 ± 21.3% and 29.8 ± 15.8% respectively of HLA-DR-expressing cells).

To further probe differences and assess global changes of PBMC *vs.* decidua that may have been missed during manual gating, we performed an unbiased clustering analysis by t-distributed stochastic neighbor embedding (tSNE) using CD45+ live+ single cells in the 28-color panel focused on T, NK, and B cells. There were clear differences in leukocyte populations between sample types (**Figure 3**). Gradients colored by MFI depicted distinct CD3+ CD4+ (clusters 3 and 6) and CD3+ CD8+ T cells (clusters 8, 9, and 10) between the circulation and the decidual T cells (**Figure 3**). The near absence of B cells in decidua observed by manual gating was confirmed by the cluster of HLA-DR+ CD20+ (cluster 2) events only found in PBMC (**Figure 3**). CD95/Fas receptor, a marker of T cell memory in NHPs, was found in cluster 9, representing CD8+ T cells, which was predominantly found in the decidua. Granzyme B was found in both tissues but in different clusters which represented unique types of NK cells (**Figure 3**). An additional 17 more markers used to perform the tSNE algorithm are found in **Supplemental Figure 2**.

Classical and Unconventional T Lymphocytes Distribution in PBMC and Decidua

αβ T and γδ T cells were distinguished by expression of the pan-γδ T cell marker on total CD3+ T lymphocytes (**Figure 1A**). In classical αβ T lymphocytes, the CD4+ T cells were reduced in decidua compared to PBMC from 37.4 ± 12.0% to 20.7 ± 4.1% (**Figure 4A**). Consistent with human data, CD8+ T cells were the dominant T lymphocyte population in macaque decidua and present at significantly higher frequencies (63.1 ± 7.4%) compared to PBMC (47.5 ± 11.6%) (6, 19). No significant differences were found in double-positive (DP) or double-negative (DN) T cells (**Figure 4A**). In the non-classical T lymphocyte subset, γδ T cells were increased in decidua compared to PBMC but did not reach statistical significance

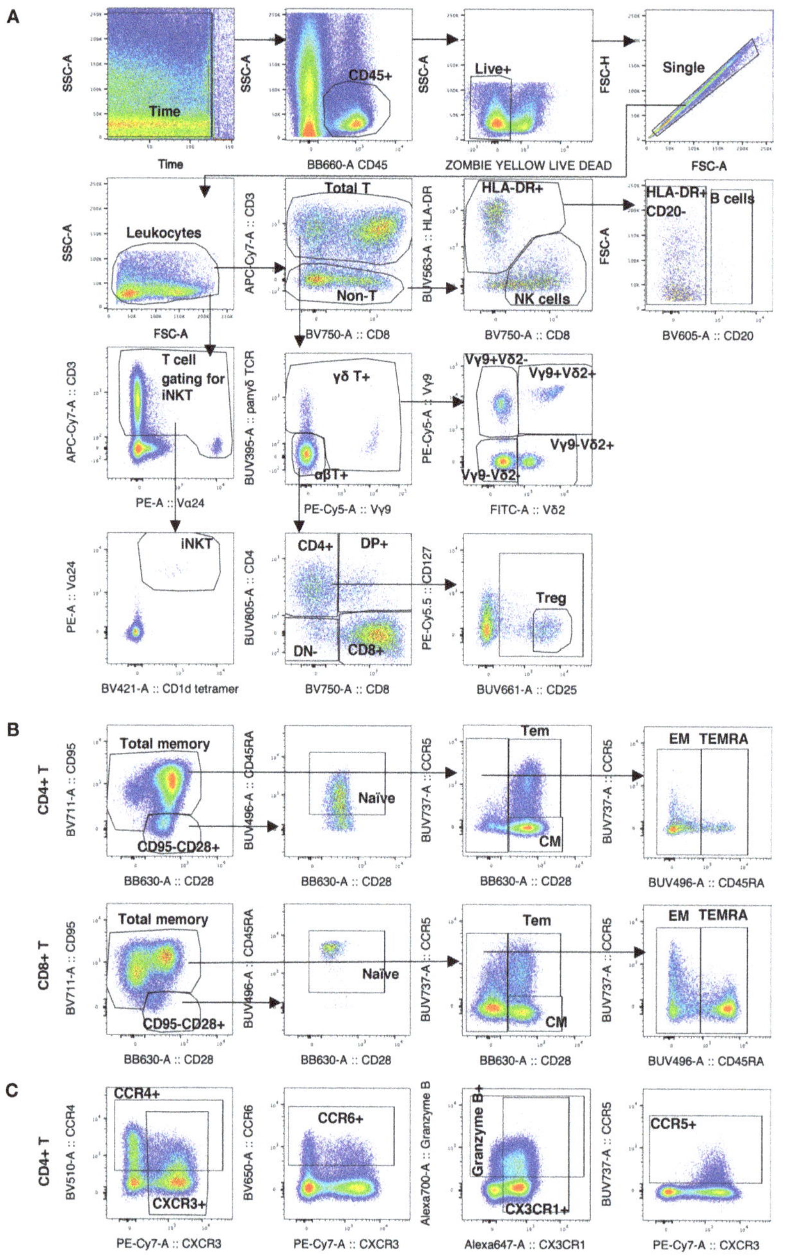

FIGURE 1 | Gating strategy of decidual leukocytes and PBMC in normal rhesus macaques. **(A)** Gating strategy in 28-color panel to identify αβ T cells, NK cells, B cells, myeloid cells (HLA-DR+ CD20-), iNKTs, γδ T cells, Tregs. **(B)** Gating strategy in CD4+ T and CD8+ T to delineate the naïve memory T cells subsets of CM, Tem, EM, and TEMRA. **(C)** Gating strategy of chemokine receptor expression.

unless only third trimester animals were compared (two-tailed unpaired t-test, p-value = 0.0008) (**Figure 4A**).

Among unconventional T lymphocytes, we evaluated invariant natural killer T (iNKT) cells. iNKT are an innate subset of T lymphocytes that respond to glycolipid antigens presented on CD1d molecules. These cells have been reported in human decidua but there are no data in NHPs (41, 42). Here, we sought to identify their presence in rhesus macaque decidua using the stringent identifying criteria of Vα24 TCR-expressing T lymphocytes binding to α-galactoslyceramide (αGC)-loaded CD1d tetramers (41–44). A detectable but sparse population of iNKTs with frequencies ranging between 0.036 to 0.918% of CD3+ T lymphocytes were detected in 6 of 9 decidua samples and at frequencies ranging between 0.005 to 4.4% in 17 out of 24 PBMC samples. We did not detect any difference in iNKT frequency between PBMC and decidua (**Figure 4A**).

In agreement with data from humans (6, 19), the decidua had a significantly increased frequency of CD4+ T regulatory cells

TABLE 2 | Flow cytometric definition of cell types.

Cell type*	Definition	Panel
αβ T cells	CD3$^+$ panγδ$^-$ CD4+: CD4$^+$ CD8$^-$ CD8+: CD4$^-$ CD8$^+$ Double Positive (DP+): CD4+ CD8+ Double Negative (DN–): CD4– CD8–	Adaptive 28-color
γδ T cells	CD3+ panγδ+ Vγ9+ Vδ2+ Vγ9+ Vδ2– Vγ9– Vδ2+ Vγ9– Vδ2–	Adaptive 28-color
iNKT	CD3+ Vα24+ CD1d tetramer+	Adaptive 28-color
T regulatory cells	CD3+ CD4+ CD127– CD25^{hi}	Adaptive 28-color
Memory T cells In CD4+ αβ T In CD8+ αβ T In γδ T	Naïve: CD95– CD28+ CD45RA+ Total Memory: CD95+ CD28+/– Central Memory (CM): CD95+ CD28+ CCR5– Transitional Effector Memory (Tem): CD95+ CD28+ CCR5+ Effector Memory (EM): CD95+ CD28– CD45RA– Terminal Effector Memory (TEMRA): CD95+ CD28– CD45RA+ Tissue Resident Memory (Trm): CD95+ CD28+/– CD103+ CD69+	Adaptive 28-color
T helper subsets	CD3+ CD4+ CXCR3+ CCR5+/– Th1-like CCR4+ Th2-like CCR6+ Th17-like	Adaptive 28-color
NK cells	CD3– HLA-DR$^{lo/-}$ CD8+ CD16+ CD56– CD16– CD56+ CD16+ CD56+ CD16– CD56–	Innate 18-color and adaptive 28-color
B cells	CD3– HLA-DR^{hi} CD20+	Adaptive 28-color
Macrophages in Decidua	CD3– CD20– HLA-DR+ CD8– CD14+ CD163+ CD206+ CD163+ CD206– CD163– CD206–	Innate 18-color
Monocytes in PBMC	CD3– CD20– HLA-DR+ CD8– Classical monocytes: CD14+ CD16– Intermediate monocytes: CD14+ CD16+ Non-classical monocytes and DCs: CD14– CD16+	Innate 18-color
Dendritic cells (DC)	CD3– CD20– HLA-DR+ CD14– Conventional DC, myeloid DC, and non-classical monocytes: CD123– Plasmacytoid DC: CD123+	Innate 18-color

Cells are pre-gated as Live+ Single CD45+ Leukocytes.

(Tregs) when compared to PBMC (**Figure 4A**). In this study, CD4+ Tregs were defined based on low CD127 expression on CD25hi CD4+ T lymphocytes, a population that has previously been shown in both humans and macaques to be FoxP3-positive and display Treg functionality of suppressive activity (45). Tregs accounted for 7.9 ± 5.5% of decidual CD4+ T lymphocytes while they were present in only 0.5 ± 0.4% of circulating CD4+ T lymphocytes. If assessed as a fraction of T cells, Tregs were 1.7 ± 1.4% in decidua and 0.2 ± 0.2% in PBMC. Decidual Tregs increased with gestation as a positive correlation (R^2 = 0.5392, p-value = 0.0243) between Treg frequency and days of gestation was detected (**Supplemental Figure 1**).

Memory CD4+ and CD8+ T Lymphocytes in PBMC and Decidua

Using a combination of CD95, CD28, CCR5, CD45RA, CD69, and CD103 we delineated naïve (CD95– CD28+ CD45RA+) and five populations of CD95+ memory CD4+ T or CD8+ T lymphocytes (**Table 2** and **Figure 1B**). Memory subsets included CD95+ CD28+ CCR5–CD45RA– central memory (CM), CD95+ CD28– CCR5+/- CD45RA– effector memory (EM), CD95+ CD28+ CCR5+ CD45RA–transitional effector memory (Tem), CD95+ CD28– CCR5+/- CD45RA+ terminally differentiated effector memory (TEMRA), and CD95+ CD69+ CD103+ tissue-resident memory (Trm).

The decidua exhibited a distinct phenotype of memory cells and a near absence of naïve cells (**Figure 4B**). The majority of CD4+ T memory lymphocytes in decidua and PBMC were CM but PBMC had an increased frequency of CM CD4+ T compared to decidua, whereas decidua had higher frequencies of EM and Tem CD4+ T lymphocytes (**Figure 4C**). CD4+ Trm were present at a small frequency of 0.7 ± 0.5% of CD4+ memory while no cells of this phenotype were found in PBMC (**Figure 4C**). Effector memory (EM) constituted the predominant subset of CD8+ T memory lymphocytes in decidua at a frequency of 67.0 ± 13.4% that was significantly higher than PBMC. Conversely, in

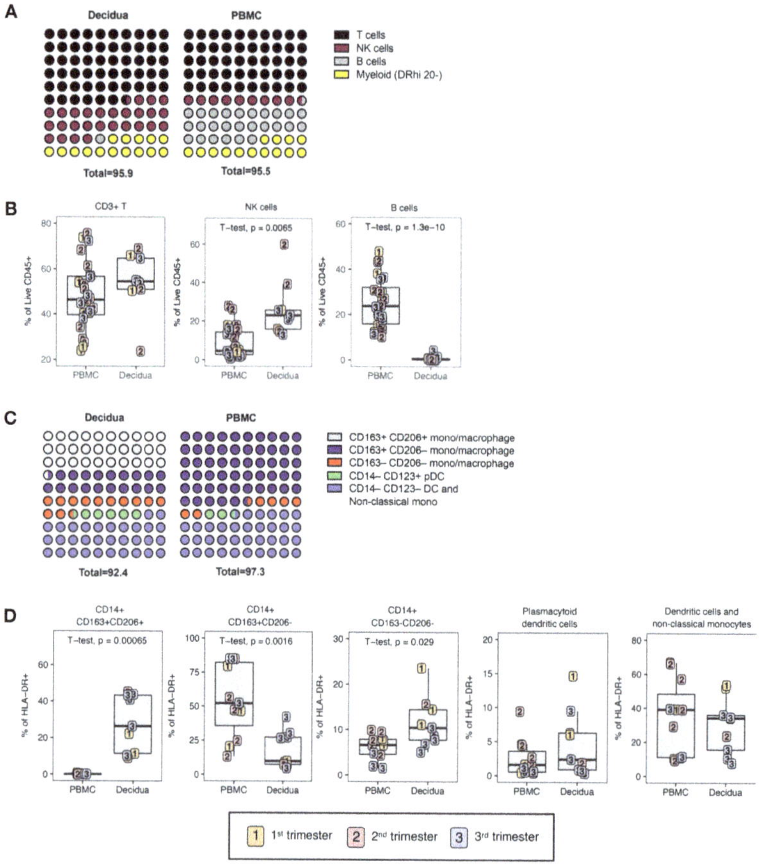

FIGURE 2 | Leukocyte composition of PBMC and decidua in normal rhesus macaques. **(A)** Comparison of relative proportions of the CD45+ leukocytes in decidua and PBMC. **(B)** Frequency of total T lymphocytes, NK cells, and B lymphocytes in PBMC and decidua during the first (yellow), second (red) and third trimester (blue) of pregnancy in normal rhesus macaques. **(C)** Comparison of relative proportions of the myeloid cells (CD3-CD20-HLA-DR+) in decidua and PBMC. **(D)** Frequency of myeloid cells (CD3-CD20-HLA-DR+) in PBMC and decidua of monocyte/macrophages subsets, and dendritic cells (DC). P-values <0.05 (unpaired t-test) shown on the plots.

PBMC, the majority of CD8+ memory T cells showed a terminally differentiated TEMRA phenotype of 65.6 ± 16.7%. The decidua had a reduced frequency of CD8+ T CM at 13.1 ± 4.9% compared to 18.7 ± 9.4% in the PBMC, which is similar to what was seen in the CD4+ T lymphocyte memory compartment (**Figure 4D**). Decidua also had a clear population of CD8+ Trm cells (6.8 ± 5.4%), which was completely absent in the PBMC (**Figure 4D**).

To evaluate the functional potential of circulatory T cells to those at the maternal-fetal interface, markers related to exhaustion, cytotoxicity, and activation were investigated using the gating strategy shown in **Supplemental Figure 3**. The exhaustion marker PD-1 was significantly elevated in decidual CD4+ and CD8+ T lymphocytes compared to PBMC with roughly 4-fold higher frequencies of PD-1+ CD4 + or CD8+ T lymphocytes in the decidua (**Figures 5A, B**). This is similar to what has been observed for effector memory T lymphocytes in humans between PBMC and decidual T lymphocytes (25). Despite high expression levels of PD-1, memory CD4+ and CD8+ T lymphocytes in the decidua were highly activated with significantly increased frequencies of CD69+ and HLA-DR+ cells as compared to PBMC (**Figures 5A, B**). CD25, a marker of activation, was significantly increased on CD4+ T lymphocytes in the decidua compared to PBMC (**Figure 5A**).

To investigate cytotoxic potential, we examined granzyme B expression in memory CD4+ and CD8+ memory T lymphocytes. Although decidual CD8+ memory T cells as a whole had lower frequencies of granzyme B-positive cells compared to PBMC (38.6 ± 9.9 *versus* 48.4 ± 17.4), these differences did not reach statistical significance (**Figure 5B**). However, evaluation of memory subsets yielded clear differences between PBMC and decidua. Among circulating CD8+ memory T lymphocytes, TEMRA contained the highest frequency of granzyme B-positive cells (62.0 ± 15.9) followed by EM at 55.5 ± 17.2%, and Tem and CM at <50% (**Figure 5C**). Comparison between the two compartments showed significantly higher frequency of granzyme B-positive Tem and CM CD8+ T lymphocytes in the decidua compared to PBMC (**Figure 5C**). No difference was found in CD8+ EM or

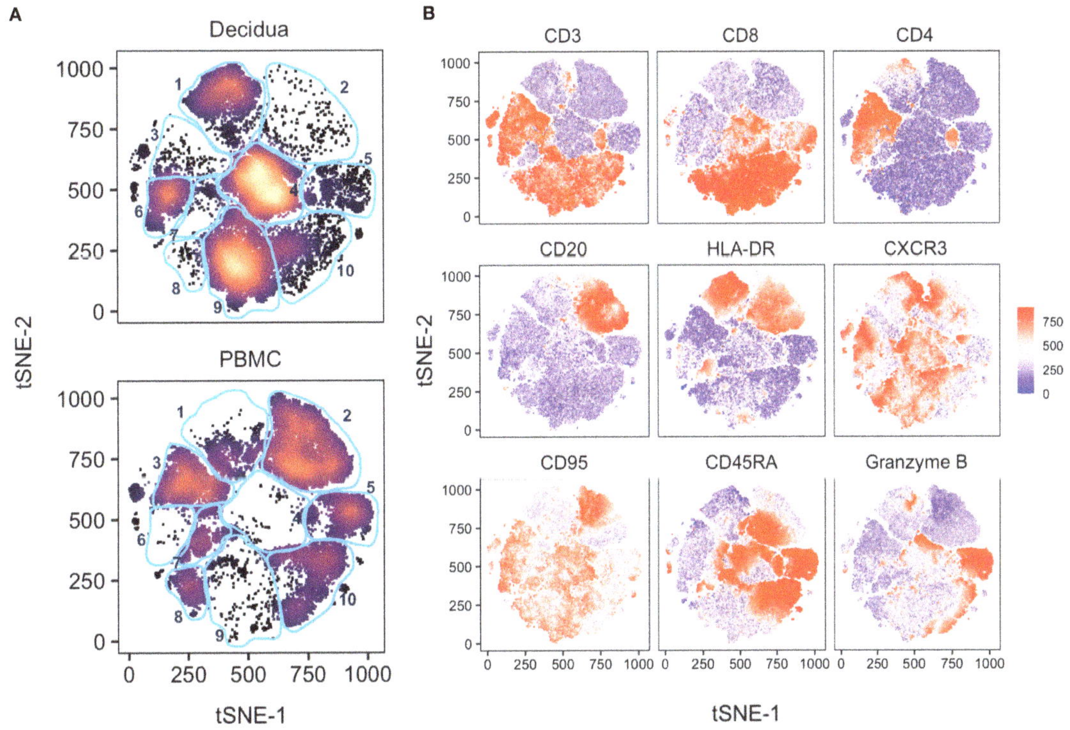

FIGURE 3 | tSNE analysis of PBMC and decidua in normal rhesus macaques. **(A)** tSNE plot representing an equal number of CD45+/live/single cell/leukocytes from decidua (n = 9) and PBMC (n = 24) of normal pregnant rhesus macaque samples. The 28-color adaptive panel was used to generate this plot. Blue gates were manually drawn based on clustering patterns. **(B)** Individual MFI gradients of nine markers on the tSNE map. Red coloring represents high MFI and blue coloring represents low MFI. Remaining gradients are found in **Supplemental Figure 2**.

TEMRA. To further assess granzyme B expression in decidual and PBMC CD8+ T lymphocytes, we measured the median fluorescence intensity (MFI) of granzyme B in the different CD8+ T lymphocyte memory subsets as an approximation of granzyme B content. Across the memory subsets of TEMRA, EM and CM, granzyme B MFI in decidual leukocytes was significantly lower compared to their circulating counterparts (**Figure 5D**). Therefore, despite similar frequencies of granzyme B-positive cells, the predominant decidual subsets of EM and TEMRA CD8+ T memory have reduced granzyme B content and are potentially less cytotoxic compared to the corresponding memory subsets in circulation. It is noteworthy that the granzyme B content as measured by MFI was significantly lower in decidual CM compared to PBMC CM despite the frequency of granzyme B-positive CM CD8+ T lymphocytes being significantly higher in decidua (**Figures 5C, D**).

In memory T cells, the trafficking phenotype was also investigated by Th-subset associated receptors CXCR3, CCR6, CCR5, and CCR4 (**Figures 1C, 5E, F**). Consistent with previous reports in humans (25), decidual memory CD4+ T lymphocytes have an increased frequency of CXCR3 expression in contrast to the peripheral leukocytes from 87.3 ± 7.5% in decidua to 52.7 ± 10.8% in PBMC indicating Th1 skewing (**Figure 5E**). The same is true for CD8+ T lymphocytes where 90.0 ± 7.6% expressed CXCR3 and only 66.2 ± 13.6% did so in PBMC (**Figure 5F**). CCR5 was also increased in decidual CD4+ and CD8+ T lymphocytes compared to PBMC. Little to no CCR4 and CCR6 expression was found in the decidua, which was significantly different from PBMC where these chemokines were well-expressed (**Figures 5E, F**).

γδ T Lymphocytes in PBMC and Decidua

Next, the non-classical T lymphocytes were investigated. There are limited data on γδ T at the maternal-fetal interface. In one study in humans, γδ T cells were shown to be increased in the decidua in contrast to peripheral blood while having a reduced Vδ2 frequency (46). We investigated the frequency, CD4/CD8 phenotype, memory phenotype, and activation status of total γδ T lymphocytes detected by the pan- γδ TCR antibody. We also evaluated γδ T subsets based on TCR chain usage of total γδ T by using NHP cross-reactive antibodies against the Vγ9 TCR and Vδ2 TCR chain.

The majority of both decidual and peripheral blood γδ T lymphocytes were CD8+ or DN for CD4 and CD8 (**Figure 6A**). They were nearly entirely of a memory phenotype in both PBMC and decidua; however, CD8+ EM predominated in the decidua (42.6 ± 10.0) and TEMRA were most abundant in the PBMC (49.9 ± 14.8%) (**Figure 6B**). As expected, tissue resident Trm were detected in the decidua (5.5 ± 4.1%) but not in PBMC (**Figure 6B**). Similar to what was observed in αβ T lymphocytes,

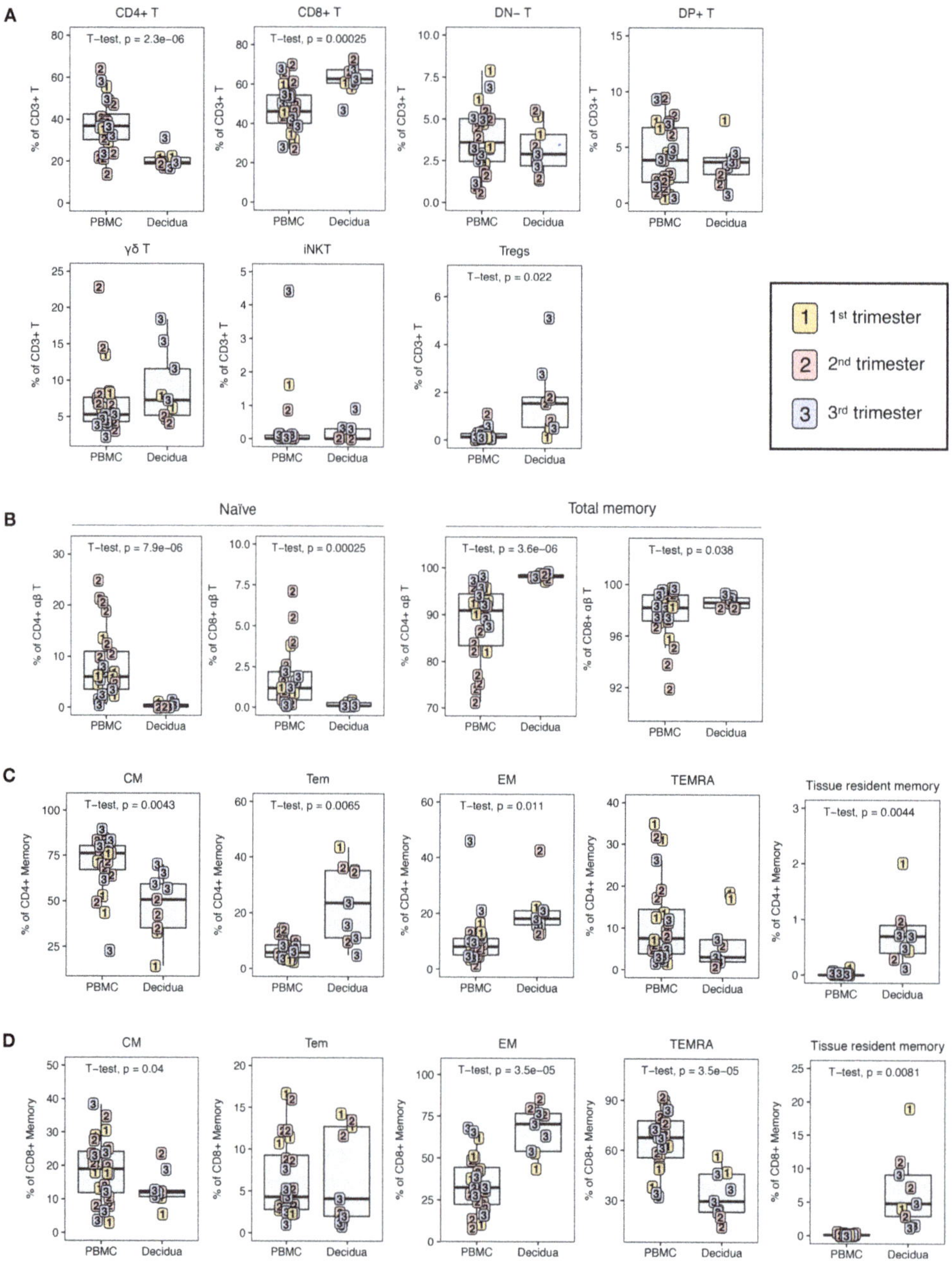

FIGURE 4 | T lymphocyte composition in PBMC and decidua from first to third trimester in normal pregnant rhesus macaques. **(A)** Frequency of conventional and innate T cells in first (yellow), second (red) and third trimester (blue) of pregnancy in PBMC and decidua of normal rhesus macaques. **(B)** CD4+ T and CD8+ T naive and total memory. **(C)** CD4+ T memory subsets. **(D)** CD8+ T memory subsets. P-values <0.05 (unpaired t-test) shown on the plots.

total γδ T lymphocytes appeared to be more activated in the decidua. Expression of CD25, CD69 and HLA-DR were significantly increased compared to PBMC, and this was accompanied with a concurrent increase of PD-1 expression in the decidua (**Figure 6C**). Like the αβ T lymphocytes, there was a significant reduction in the frequency of CCR6-expressing cells in the decidual γδ T cells (**Figure 6C**).

Using the individual gamma and delta TCR chains, four subsets of γδ T cells could be distinguished. The double positive, Vγ9+ Vδ2+ was present at significantly lower frequencies in the decidua compared to PBMC (**Figure 6D**). The single positive Vγ9+ Vδ2− and Vγ9− Vδ2+ γδ T were minor populations in both PBMC and decidua ranging in frequency from 1.0 to 21.8% of γδ T cells (**Figure 6D**). The innate-like

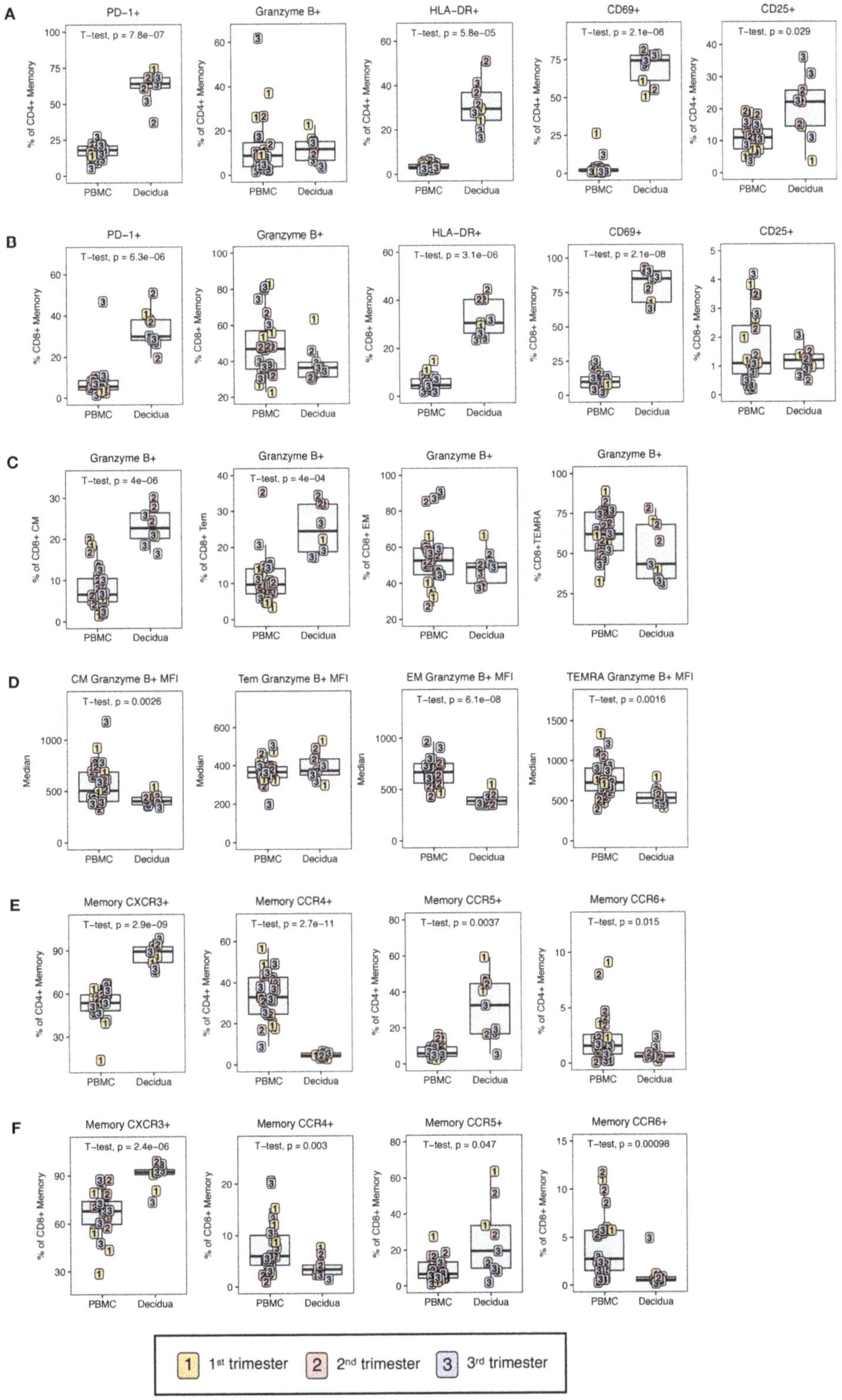

FIGURE 5 | Phenotypic characterization of T lymphocyte memory. **(A)** Phenotype of CD4+ T cell and **(B)** CD8+ T cell memory by PD-1, Granzyme B, HLA-DR, CD69, and CD25 in first (yellow), second (red) and third trimester (blue) of pregnancy in PBMC and decidua of normal rhesus macaques. **(C)** Cytotoxic potential in CD8+ T memory subsets by Granzyme B frequency in CM, Tem, EM, and TEMRA. **(D)** MFI of Granzyme B in CD8+ T memory subsets. **(E)** Chemokine receptor expression on memory CD4+ and **(F)** CD8+ T cells. P-values < 0.05 (unpaired t-test) shown on the plots.

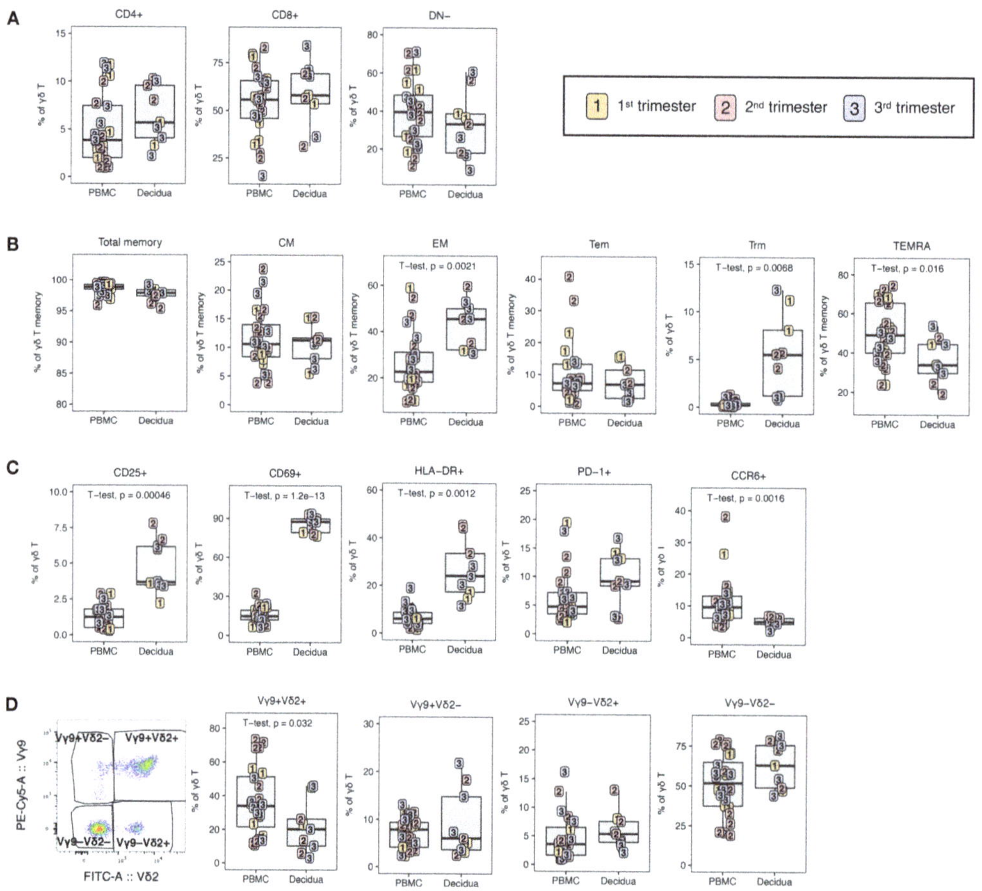

FIGURE 6 | γδ T lymphocytes in PBMC and decidua of normal rhesus macaque pregnancies. **(A)** CD4 and CD8 expression on γδ T lymphocytes in PBMC and decidua in first (yellow), second (red) and third trimester (blue) of pregnancy of normal rhesus macaques. **(B)** Memory phenotype of γδ T lymphocytes. **(C)** Phenotype of activation, exhaustion, cytotoxic potential and chemokine receptor expression in γδ T lymphocytes. **(D)** Representative flow plot of Vγ9 and Vδ2 chains and the Vγ9 and Vδ2 subsets in PBMC and decidua. P-values < 0.05 (unpaired t-test) shown on the plots.

double negative Vγ9− Vδ2− subset was increased in the decidua, although not significantly (**Figure 6D**).

Global Analysis of Innate Immune Cells in Decidua and PBMC

To analyze global differences of innate leukocytes of the peripheral blood compared to decidua, we performed a tSNE analysis on the 18-color innate cell panel. Only live CD45+ CD3− CD20−cells were included in the computation. Stark differences could be observed between the PBMC and the decidual cells (**Figure 7A**). The top half of the tSNE shows clusters 1,2,3,4,5 which consist of NK cells based on their CD8+ and HLA-DRlo/− expression (**Figures 7A, B**). In decidua, cluster 4 was a dominant cluster of CD16− CD56+ NK cells which was absent in the PBMC tSNE. On the other hand, peripheral blood NK cells like those present in cluster 3 exhibited a CD16+ CD56− or CD16− CD56− phenotype (**Figures 7A, B**). The lower half of the tSNE expresses HLA-DR+ which by the removal of CD20+ cells in the gating preceding tSNE analysis is consistent with myeloid antigen-presenting cells (APCs). Cluster 8 is the major myeloid APC subset in the decidua which is absent in PBMC and is likely mostly comprised of monocytes or macrophages based on CD14 and CD163 expression (**Figures 7A, B**). In the PBMC, clusters 7 and 9 are predominant subsets which are rare in the decidua. Based on gradient expression of CD14, CD16, and CD163, cluster 7 is likely classical monocytes based on CD14+ CD16− CD163+ events, while cluster 9 is consistent with intermediate, non-classical monocytes, or conventional DCs (**Figures 7A, B**). Cluster 10 appears to be a pDC population based on CD123 expression. Four additional markers used to perform the tSNE clustering algorithm are shown in **Supplemental Figure 4**.

NK Cells in PBMC and Decidua

The decidual tissue has been reported to be enriched with innate cells such as NK cells in previous non-human primate studies (15). Here, we sought to complement these data by identifying the activation status of innate cells and their unique phenotypes. A distinct phenotype of CD16− CD56+ single-positive NK cells was found to predominate in the decidua (55.3 ± 16.1%), in stark contrast to PBMC where the major NK cell subset identified were

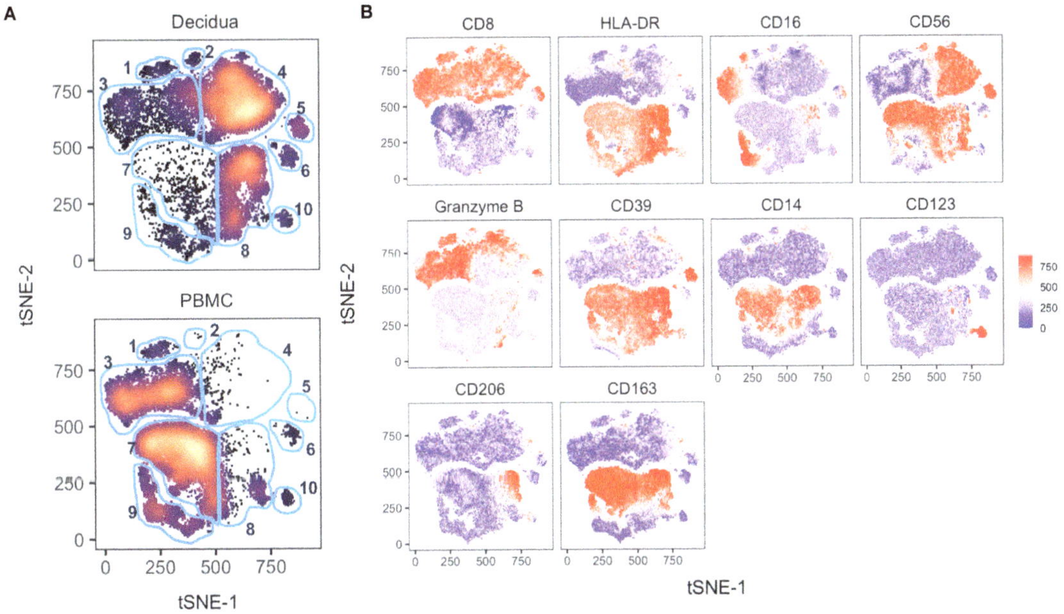

FIGURE 7 | tSNE of 14 innate cell markers of PBMC and decidual leukocytes in normal pregnant rhesus macaques. **(A)** tSNE plot representing an equal number of CD45+/live/single cells/CD3-CD20- cells from decidua (n = 8) and PBMC (n = 11) of rhesus macaques experiencing a normal pregnancy. The 18-color innate panel was used to generate this plot. Blue gates were manually drawn based on clustering patterns. **(B)** Individual MFI gradients of ten markers on the tSNE map. Red coloring represents high MFI and blue coloring represents low MFI. Remaining gradients are found in **Supplemental Figure 4**.

CD16+ CD56– cells (48.2 ± 20.2%) (**Figures 8A, B**). Interestingly, a distinct CD16+ CD56+ population of NK cells was found in the decidual tissue (8.4 ± 5.2%) which was virtually absent in PBMC (**Figure 8B**). These have been described in human decidua as CD56bright and CD16+/dim NK cells (9). In addition, double-negative CD16– CD56– NK cells were significantly increased in the PBMC compared to decidua (**Figure 8B**). NKG2A and NKG2D dual positivity also defined a subset of NK cells found almost exclusively in the decidua (62.9 ± 12.1%) (**Figures 8C, D**). NKG2D+ NKG2A– cells were greatly reduced in decidual NK cells as compared to peripheral NK cells (**Figures 8C, D**).

To analyze the cytotoxic capacity of these cells, we measured the frequency of granzyme B+ cells as well as the MFI, a proxy of intracellular granzyme B content. The frequency and MFI of granzyme B in the cytotoxic CD16+ CD56– and the double-positive CD16+ CD56+ NK subsets were significantly lower in the decidua compared to PBMC (**Figure 8E**). Interestingly, the frequency of granzyme B-positive CD16– CD56+ NK cells was significantly higher in the decidua compared to PBMC; however, the granzyme B MFI of this decidual subset was significantly lower as was true of the other decidual NK subsets (**Figure 8E**). These data show that the dominant decidual CD16– CD56+ NK subset contain high proportions of cytotoxic NK, albeit with less cytotoxicity. It is noteworthy that the frequency of the granzyme B-positive cells in all the NK subsets was highest in third trimester decidua (**Figure 8E**).

Similar to T lymphocytes, decidual NK cells expressed more CXCR3 in both CD56– and CD56+ subsets compared to PBMC (**Figure 8F**). We also evaluated expression of CX3CR1, a chemokine receptor which is upregulated in cells that home to sites experiencing endothelial inflammation and is elevated on a subset of memory CD8+ T lymphocytes and myeloid cells (47). We found decreased expression of CX3CR1 on CD56– NK cells of the decidua (47.8 ± 4.6) compared to PBMC (71.1 ± 11.1) but not in CD56+ NK cells where similar expression levels were found (**Figure 8F**). All of the NK cells in the decidua expressed high levels of the activation marker CD69 ranging from 42.7% to 94.9%, which is similar to levels observed in αβ and γδ T cells (**Figures 5A, B, 6C, 8F**). In contrast, CD69 expression on peripheral blood NK cells never exceeded 39.3% (**Figure 8F**). We also evaluated expression of the sialo-adhesin molecule CD169, a marker of activation, which has been previously reported to be present on >60% of CD16+ decidual NK cells in macaques (48). The frequency of CD169+ NK cells was significantly higher in decidua compared to PBMC, but was only found on 0.4-4.4% of total NK cells in our study (**Figure 8F**).

In a recent single cell RNA sequencing analysis of human first trimester maternal-fetal interface, three NK cells subsets were defined by combinations of NKG2A, NKG2C, CD39, Granzyme B, and CD103 expression (37). These were termed dNK1, dNK2, and dNK3 where dNK1 expressed many HLA-C binding molecules and was the only subset to express LILRB1 that can bind dimeric HLA-G. dNK1 was found to be the subset with most cytotoxic potential by granzyme A, granzyme B, perforin, and granulysin followed by dNK2 and dNK3. We defined dNK1 as NKG2A+, CD39+, granzyme B+ NK; dNK2 as NKG2A+, CD39–, Granzyme B+ NK; and dNK3 as CD103+ granzyme B– NK (**Figure 8G**). Between the 28-color and 18-color flow panels, we

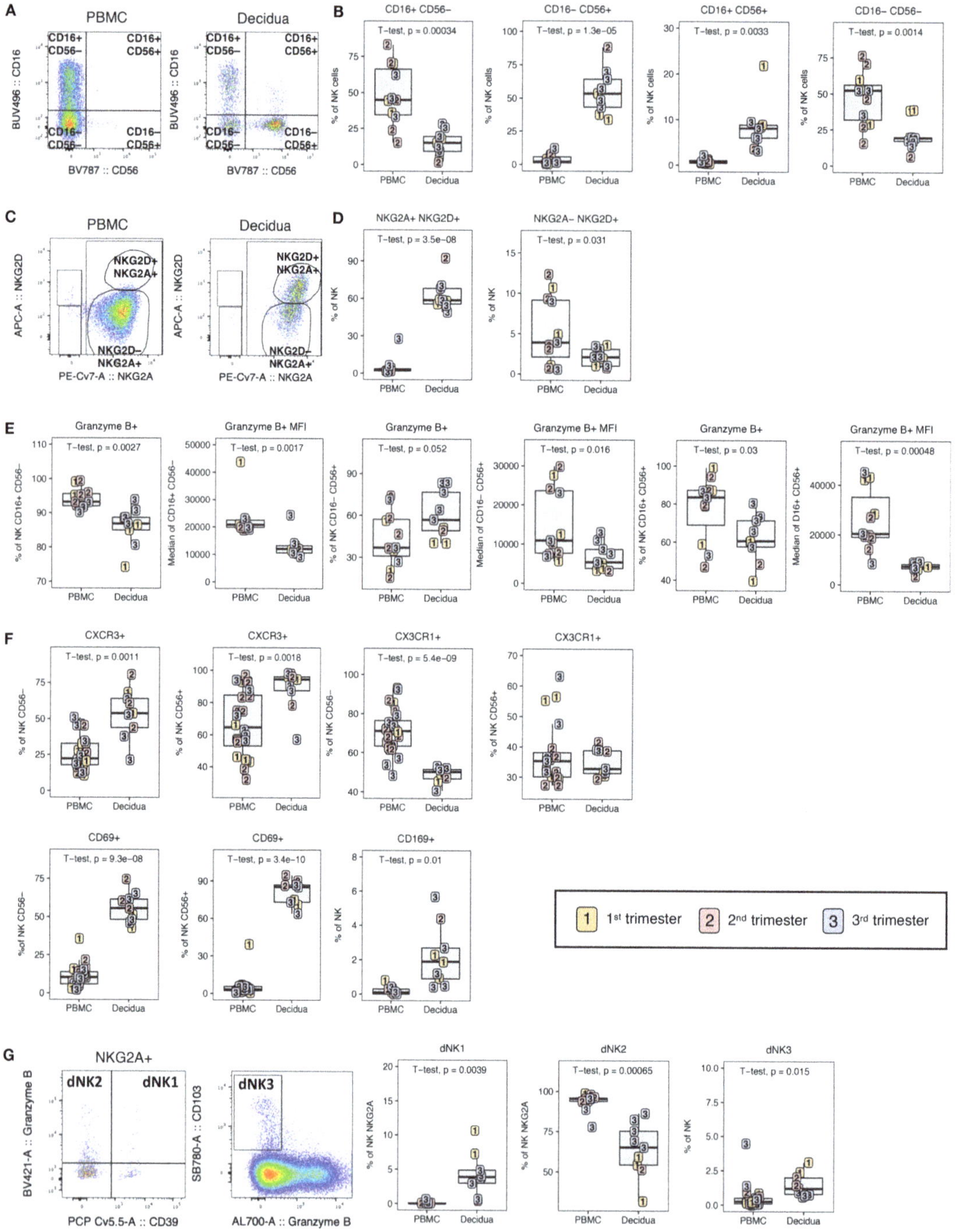

FIGURE 8 | NK cell composition in PBMC and decidua of normal rhesus macaque pregnancies. **(A)** Representative flow plots of NK cells CD16/CD56 subsets. **(B)** NK cell subset frequencies in PBMC and decidua first (yellow), second (red) and third trimester (blue) of normal pregnant rhesus macaques. **(C)** NKG2A/NKG2D flow plots with representative gating of PBMC and decidua. **(D)** Frequency of NKG2A+NKG2D+ and NKG2A-NKG2D+ NK cells in PBMC and decidua. **(E)** Granzyme B expression frequency and MFI on NK cell subsets. **(F)** CD56- *vs* CD56+ NK cell expression of CXCR3, CX3CR1, CD69 and the CD169 on total NK cells. **(G)** Representative flow plot of dNK1, dNK2, and dNK3 subsets with box plots showing their frequency in PBMC and decidua. P-values < 0.05 (unpaired t-test) shown on the plots.

could readily identify all three dNK subsets in decidua samples from the rhesus macaques (**Figure 8G**). dNK2 was the most common phenotype in both PBMC and decidua while dNK1 and dNK3 were only consistently found in decidua (**Figure 8G**).

Myeloid Cells in PBMC and Decidua

Using the gating strategy shown in **Figure 9A** on HLA-DR+ CD3– CD20– CD45+ leukocytes in the 18-color innate panel, we identified a similar proportion of classical monocytes or macrophages (CD14+ CD16–) in PBMC and decidua (**Figure 9B**). CD14+ CD16+ intermediate monocytes were significantly increased in the decidua while non-classical monocytes and dendritic cells (CD14– CD16+/– CD123–) were found at a higher frequency in the PBMC compared to decidua (**Figure 9B**). pDCs, which express CD123, were more abundant in the decidua compared to the PBMC, though not significantly. CD14+ CD163+ CD206+ macrophages were detected at high frequency in the decidua (44.7 ± 16.2%) and were not detected in PBMC (**Figure 9B**). In contrast, single positive CD14+ CD163+ CD206– myeloid cells were predominantly found in the PBMC (84.4 ± 11.3%). Double negative CD14+ CD163– CD206– myeloid cells were highest at the first and second trimester of gestation but were not significantly different between PBMC and decidua (**Figure 9B**). We also assessed the expression of CD169 and CD69 on myeloid cells to determine their activation status. We found that the decidual classical and intermediate monocytes had an increased expression of CD169 (34.2% ± 21.5% and 70.5% ± 20.7 respectively) compared to PBMC (1.0% ± 1.7 and 11.8% ± 9.4 respectively) (**Figure 9C**). DC and monocyte/macrophage subsets (HLA-DR+ CD14– CD123–) in decidua also contained significantly higher frequencies of CD69+ and CX3CR1+ cells when compared to PBMC (**Figure 9C**). These data support increased activation status and migration capability of decidual macrophages and DC populations.

Changes in Decidual Leukocytes With Gestation Age

To assess temporal gestational effects on decidual immune cell composition, the frequency of major decidual cell populations were correlated with gestational age in days (**Supplemental Figure 1**). Neither T nor B lymphocytes showed a change with gestation (**Supplemental Figure 1**). In contrast, Tregs had a correlative increase with gestation while γδ T cells and iNKTs trended towards an increase (**Supplemental Figure 1**). In the innate compartment, neither total NK cell frequency nor any NK cell subset proportion were significantly different with gestation (**Supplemental Figure 1**). We identified a significant increase in CD14+ CD163+ CD206– decidual macrophages cells with gestation, with a corresponding decrease of CD14+ CD163– CD206– macrophages (**Supplemental Figure 1**). Both pDCs and DC/non-classical monocytes decreased with gestation, though the decrease in pDCs was not significant (**Supplemental Figure 1**).

Among naïve and memory T lymphocyte subsets, several memory CD4+ T lymphocyte subsets showed significant changes with gestational age (**Supplemental Figure 5**). These included gestational dependency of central memory CD4+ T lymphocytes with a highly significant positive correlation (R^2 0.8267; p-value >0.001) with increasing gestation age (**Supplemental Figure 5**). This coincided with significant declines in CD4+ Tem, CD4+ TEMRA and activated/proliferating Ki67+ memory CD4+ T lymphocytes in the decidua (**Supplemental Figure 5**). Expression of CCR5 on CD4+ and CD8+ T memory cells also showed significant negative correlation with gestational age (**Supplemental Figure 5**). For Th1-like cells assessed by CXCR3 expression, Th2-like cells assessed by CCR4 expression, and Th17-like cells assessed by CCR6, no correlative relationships were observed with gestational age (**Supplemental Figure 5**). A significant positive correlation between CD4+ memory T lymphocytes PD-1 and HLA-DR expression was observed in the PBMC but not the decidua (**Supplemental Figure 5**) indicating a discordance of activated/exhausted memory CD4+ T between the two compartments.

PCA Analysis of PBMC and Decidual Leukocytes

To help interpret what most distinguishes the PBMC and decidual leukocytes in normal rhesus macaques, a Principal Component Analysis (PCA) was performed using all of the populations manually gated from samples stained with both the 28-color adaptive panel and 18-color innate focused panel (**Figure 10**). Despite a range in gestation, the PBMC samples from pregnant macaques clustered tightly in the right-hand quadrant. The decidual leukocytes clustered away from the PBMC by principal component 1 (PC1) and were more spread, indicating their lack of similarity to PBMC and highlighting the heterogeneity of the tissue. Populations which contributed most prominently to PC1 were innate NK cells and many types of T lymphocytes expressing the activation marker CD69. This coincides with differences manifest in the tSNE analysis in **Figures 3, 7**. By principal component 2 (PC2), the decidual leukocytes are less well-clustered together while a longitudinal pattern of gestational age is apparent. The major contributors to PC2 are memory CD4+ T lymphocyte proliferation markers and frequencies of different innate cells (**Figure 10**).

ZIKV Impact on Maternal Immunity

To investigate the impact of ZIKV on the leukocytes of the peripheral blood and decidua, we studied dams infected with ZIKV during pregnancy in comparison to normal, uninfected rhesus macaques. Placenta was collected from 10 ZIKV-infected dams either at second trimester spontaneous abortion (n=1) or at near term C-section (n=9); details are described in **Supplementary Table 2**. We found that the frequency of total T lymphocytes out of live CD45+ leukocytes was increased in the ZIKV-infected dams compared to the uninfected dams (**Figure 11A**). Within the traditional αβ T cells there were no indications of changes in CD4/CD8 proportions or their memory subtypes to explain the increase in T cells (data not shown).

To determine whether ZIKV infection affected immune function, we assessed the expression of HLA-DR (activation), CXCR3 (activation and trafficking), Ki67 (activation and proliferation), and granzyme B (cytotoxicity) on decidual T lymphocytes in ZIKV-infected dams and compared with decidua of normal pregnancies. A significant decline in HLA-DR+ activated memory CD4+ and CD8+ T lymphocytes was observed in ZIKV-infected decidua as compared to normal decidua (**Figures 11B, C**). Coinciding with the lack of HLA-DR, Ki67+ memory CD4+ T lymphocytes were also significantly decreased in the infected animals compared to normal decidua (**Figure 11B**). Other notable changes on memory T lymphocytes in decidua of ZIKV-infected dams including a significant decrease in frequency of CXCR3 positive cells in both CD4+

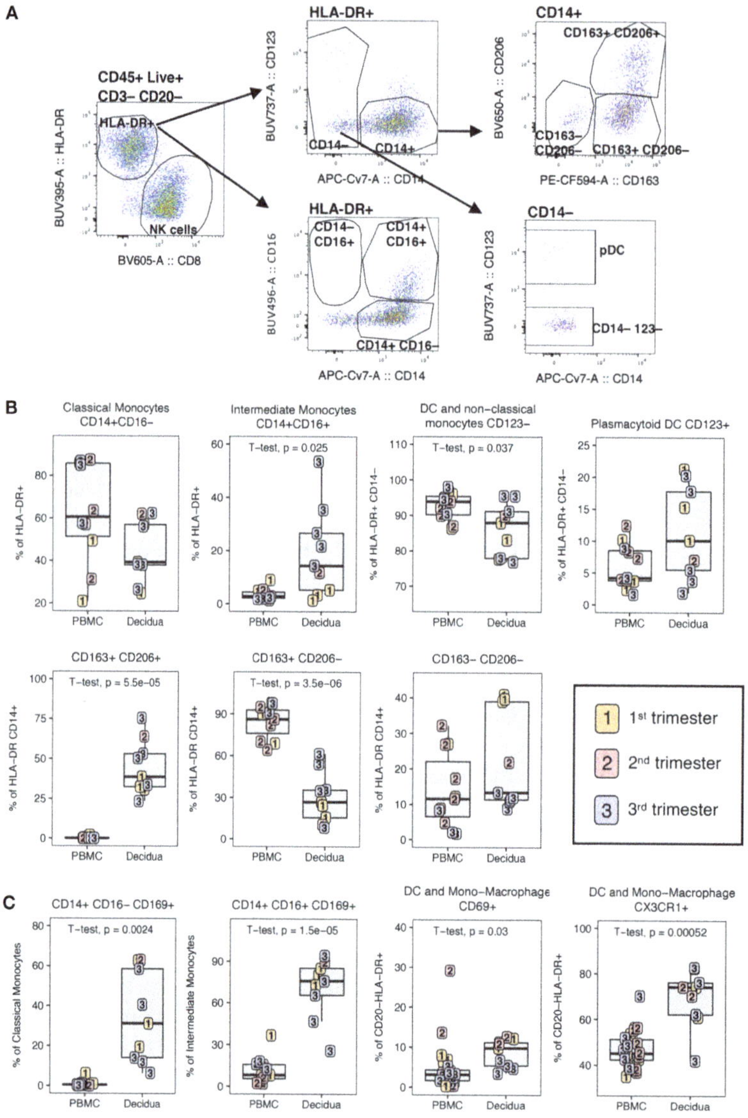

FIGURE 9 | Phenotype of dendritic cells and monocyte/macrophage in PBMC and decidua of normal pregnant rhesus macaques. **(A)** Representative flow plot and gating of HLA-DR+ myeloid cells. **(B)** Frequency of monocyte/macrophage and DC subsets in PBMC and decidua first (yellow), second (red) and third trimester (blue) of normal pregnant rhesus macaques. **(C)** Phenotype of monocyte/macrophages and DCs with box plots showing their frequency. P-values < 0.05 (unpaired t-test) shown on the plots.

and CD8+ T lymphocytes, and reduced frequency of granzyme B-positive CD4+ T memory cells compared to uninfected decidua (**Figures 11B, C**). A similar pattern of perturbation was observed in decidual γδ T cells of ZIKV-infected dams, namely a significant decrease in HLA-DR, Ki67, PD-1, and granzyme B, indicative of inhibition of activation, proliferation and cytotoxicity of γδ T (**Figure 11D**). Vγ9 and Vδ2 subsets likewise showed a general reduction of proliferative and activation potential by Ki67+ suggesting that the effect was global and not confined to a particular subset of γδ T (**Figure 11E**). In contrast to Ki67, decreased granzyme B expression was confined to the Vγ9+ Vδ2+ subset of γδ T (**Figure 11E**). This subset was recently shown to have the greatest cytotoxic potential and cytokine secretory capacity in healthy adults (49). In addition, decreased PD-1 expression and HLA-DR was confined to the Vγ9+ Vδ2− and Vγ9− Vδ2+ subsets respectively.

To study changes in the innate compartment, we found a loss of total NK cells in ZIKV-infected compared to uninfected dams (**Figure 12A**). These decreases were subset specific, in that the decidual CD16+ CD56+ NK subset showed a significant decrease whereas the CD16− CD56− NK cell subset showed a proportional increase in frequency in ZIKV-infected compared to uninfected macaques (**Figure 12A**). We observed an increase in dNK2 in ZIKV-infected dams while dNK1 and dNK3 were comparable to normal decidua (**Figure 12**). Similar to the changes observed in T cells of ZIKV-infected macaques, CD69

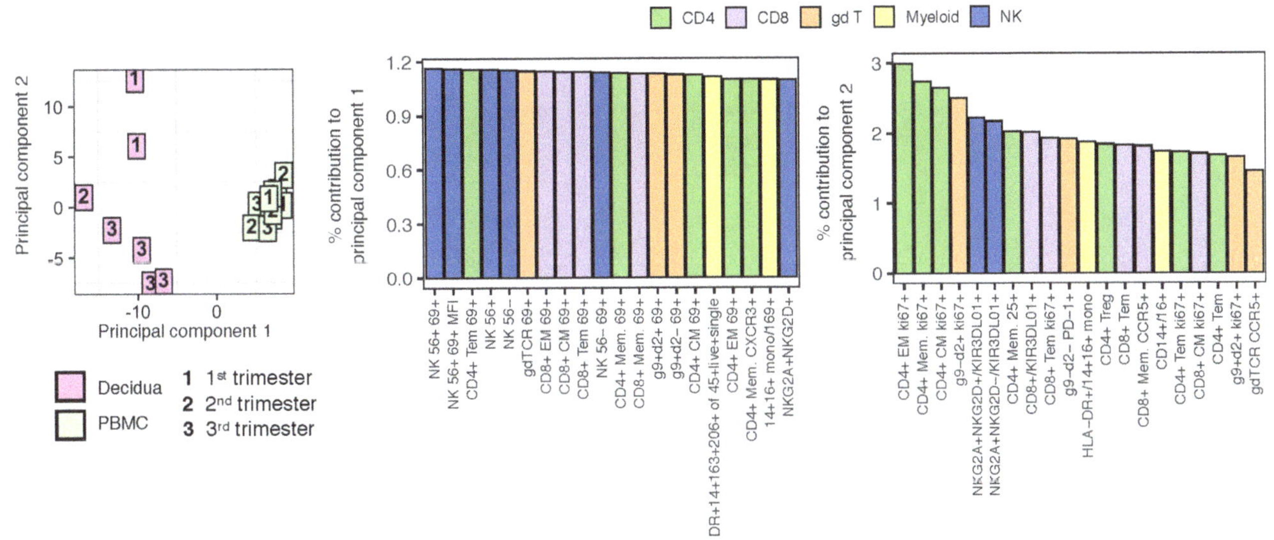

FIGURE 10 | PCA plot using adaptive and innate cell data of PBMC and decidual leukocytes in normal rhesus macaques. A PCA plot was generated using a combination of adaptive and innate immune cells and their features. 217 variables describing frequencies of unique cell types and MFI when applicable (e.g. Granzyme B MFI) were used to contrast PBMC (n = 9) (green) to decidua (n = 7) (pink) samples across 1st, 2nd, and 3rd trimester (left). The top 20 contributing variables to principal component 1 (middle) and principal component 2 (right) are shown and color coded according to major cell populations, CD4+ T (green), CD8+ T (purple), γδ T (orange), myeloid CD20-HLA-DR+ (yellow), and NK cells (blue).

expression on both CD56– and CD56+ NK cells were reduced compared to normal decidua (**Figure 12A**). We did not observe increased CD169 expression on NK cells contrary to a recent study that reported an increase in CD169-positive CD16+ NK cells in the decidua of ZIKV-infected dams (48). Few changes in myeloid cell proportions were observed following ZIKV-infection, although CD14+ CD163– CD206– cells were higher in the decidua of uninfected macaques compared to ZIKV-infected macaques (22.0 ± 13.1% and 8.5 ± 6.4%, respectively, p = 0.025).

Similar to changes observed in the decidua, the majority of changes observed in PBMC of ZIKV-infected dams were confined to the T lymphocyte compartment and manifest as a decrease in markers of activation of HLA-DR, Ki67, and PD-1 expression on CD4+ and CD8+ T lymphocyte subsets compared to normal pregnant macaques (**Supplemental Table 4**). In addition to the reduced activation of αβ T lymphocytes, γδ T lymphocytes appeared to be more differentiated by increased TEMRA memory phenotype and the Vγ9+ Vδ2+ had a reduced activation status. Both the CD56– NK cells, and myeloid cells (HLA-DR+ CD20–) showed decreased Ki67 compared to uninfected macaques (**Supplemental Table 3**).

Global Analysis of the Impact of ZIKV on the Maternal-Fetal Interface

To further understand the impact of ZIKV on pregnancy and specifically in the decidua, we performed tSNE and PCA analysis of the decidual leukocytes in comparison to uninfected animals (**Figures 13A–C**). A tSNE analysis of decidual cells computed with data from a 28-color panel focused on the adaptive immune system resolved several notable differences (**Figures 13A, B**). In particular, clusters 2 and 8 appear to be affected by ZIKV infection (**Figure 13A**). Cluster 2 is consistent with CD8 memory T cells by CD3+ CD8+ CD95+ CD28– cells, and cluster 8 are likely myeloid cells defined by CD3– HLA-DR+ CD20– expression (**Figure 13B** and **Supplemental Figure 6**). An additional 16 markers used to compute the tSNE are found in **Supplemental Figure 6**.

tSNE analysis of innate markers using an 18-color panel focusing on the innate immune system further highlighted differences in decidual immune composition after Zika virus infection (**Figures 13C, D**). Prior to computing the tSNE map, dead cells and CD45+ CD3+ or CD45+ CD20+ cells were excluded. The most notable differences appear in clusters 4, 6, and 7. Cluster 4 are tissue macrophages defined by their HLA-DR+ CD14+ CD163+ CD206+ CD39+ CD169+ phenotype (**Figures 13C, D** and **Supplemental Figure 7**). Cluster 7 are CD16– CD56+ NK cells defined by the presence of CD8+ HLA-DR–/lo CD16– and CD56+, and cluster 6 are also NK CD16– CD56+ NK cells with the additional expression of CD39 (**Figures 13C, D** and **Supplemental Figure 7**).

PCA analysis shown in **Figure 13E** determined immune cell subsets that most contributed to the separation between infected and uninfected decidua. The uninfected decidua is found to cluster away from infected tissues by PC1. The top contributors to PC1 were memory T lymphocytes expressing activation and proliferation markers (**Figure 13F**). PC2 did not well separate uninfected from infected samples (**Figure 13E**). Little to no clustering effect was observed between animals with congenital transmission and no congenital transmission of ZIKV (**Figure 13E**). Like the uninfected decidua, there was also wide heterogeneity among ZIKV-infected decidua.

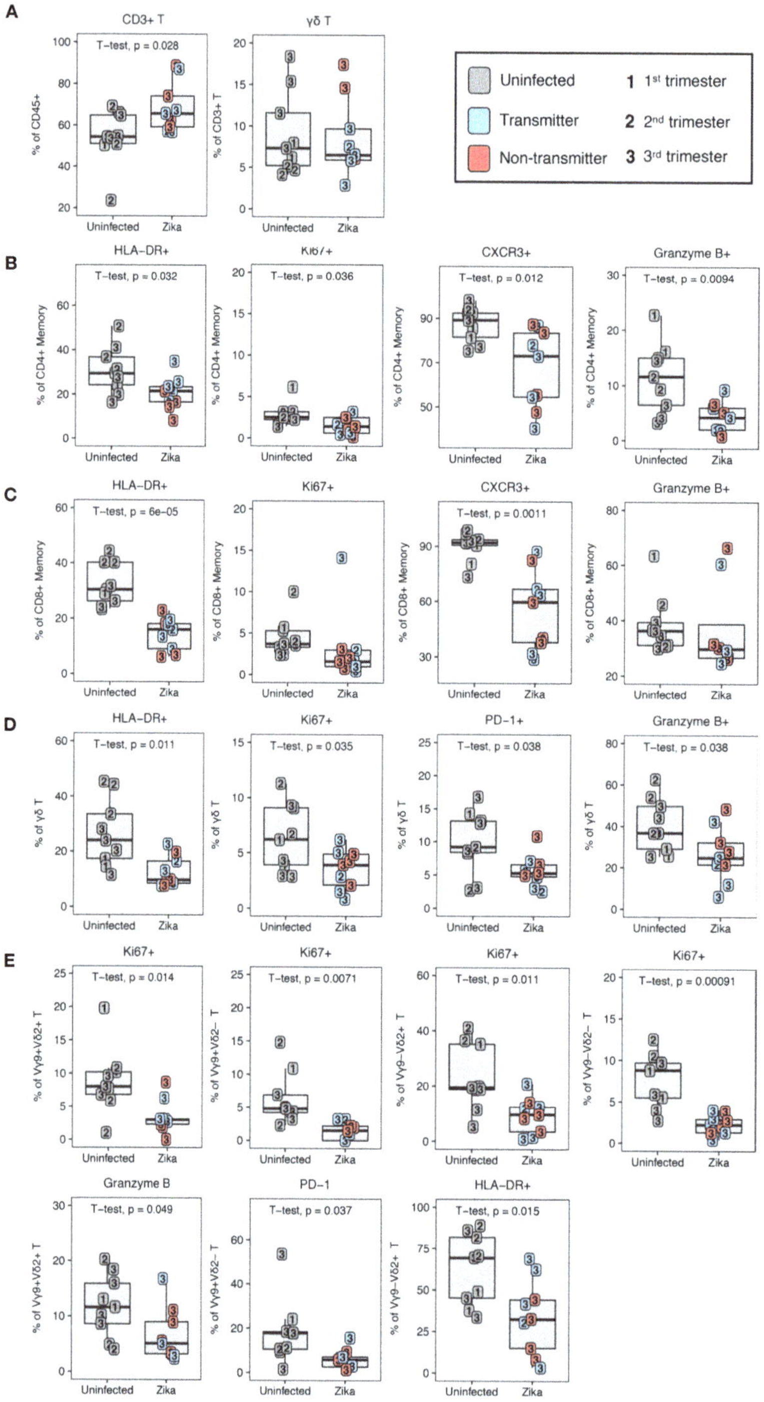

FIGURE 11 | T lymphocyte changes in ZIKV-infected macaques. **(A)** T and γδ T lymphocytes in uninfected (n = 9) (grey) and ZIKV-infected (n = 9) decidual leukocytes. In the ZIKV-infected group, animals with detected amniotic fluid transmission displayed in blue and non-transmitters in red **(B)** Decreased activation of CD4+ T memory in the ZIKV-infected group. **(C)** Decreased activation of CD8+ T memory in the ZIKV-infected group. **(D)** Decreased activation of γδ T lymphocytes in the ZIKV-infected group. **(E)** Decreased decidual γδ T lymphocyte subset activation in ZIKV-infected macaques. P-values < 0.05 (unpaired t-test) shown on the plots.

ZIKV Non-Transmitters Compared to Transmitters

Five of the 10 ZIKV-infected dams had ZIKV RNA detected by PCR in the amniotic fluid. Although we cannot definitively exclude absence of placental transmission in the PCR-negative dams, we compared immune parameters in the amniotic fluid ZIKV PCR positive (transmitters) and negative (non-transmitters) dams. The frequency of single positive CD16–

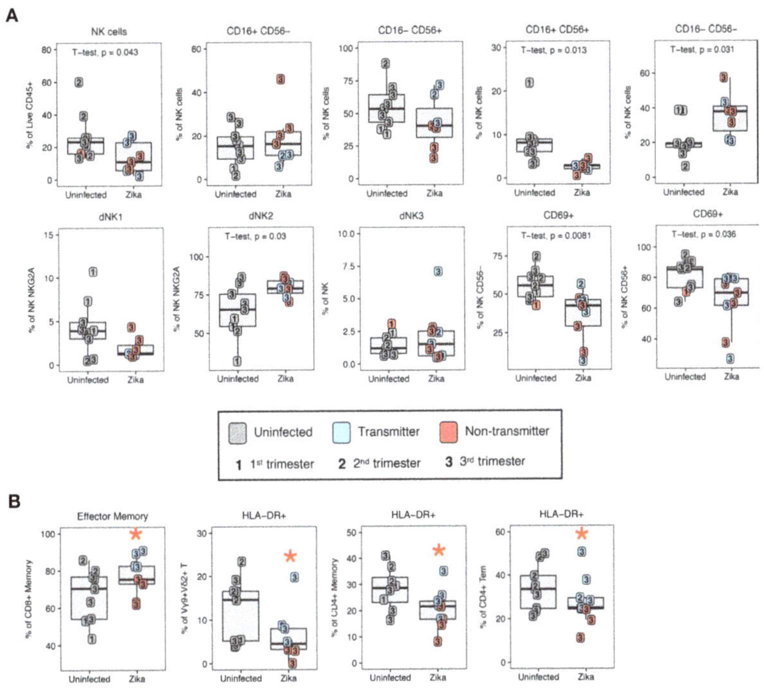

FIGURE 12 | Changes in decidual NK cells in ZIKV-infected dams and immune correlates of transmission. **(A)** Altered NK cell subsets by CD16/CD56, granzyme B, KIR3DL01, and CD169 in the decidual leukocytes of uninfected (n=9) (grey) and ZIKV-infected (n=9) dams. In the ZIKV-infected group, animals with detected amniotic fluid transmission displayed in blue and non-transmitters in red. P-values < 0.05 (unpaired t-test) shown on the plots. **(B)** Immune parameters significantly different between transmitter and non-transmitter dams. P-value <0.05 between transmitters and non-transmitters shown as red asterisk. Normal decidual leukocytes are displayed for comparison.

CD56+ NK cells in the non-transmitter dams (24.4 ± 14.1%) was reduced compared to the transmitter dams (59.7 ± 12.2% (**Figure 12A**). Animals that transmitted also had higher frequencies of CD8+ T effector memory cells compared to non-transmitters (83.5 ± 6.3% compared to 68.2 ± 5.9%, respectively) (**Figure 12B**). Interestingly, macaques that did not transmit ZIKV had the greatest reduction of T cell activation compared to both uninfected and ZIKV-transmitters (**Figure 12B**). For example, HLA-DR expression in Vγ9+ Vδ2+ was reduced from 9.2 ± 5.6% to 2.4 ± 1.4% in non-transmitters, and HLA-DR expression on total CD4+ memory T cells was reduced from 24.6 ± 6.0% to 15.2 ± 4.8% in non-transmitters (**Figure 12B**). CD4+ Tem cells also had a reduced expression of HLA-DR in non-transmitters compared to transmitters (**Figure 12B**).

DISCUSSION

This is the first comprehensive single-cell phenotypic analysis of multiple immune cell subsets in the decidua and peripheral blood of healthy rhesus macaques across the three trimesters of pregnancy. By simultaneously probing conventional T lymphocytes, iNKT, Tregs, γδ T, B lymphocytes, NK cells, monocytes, macrophages and dendritic cells (DC), we could evaluate components of both the innate and adaptive immune system and study their interaction in the setting of normal pregnancy and after ZIKV infection of pregnant macaque. Several findings reported in blood and decidua of human pregnancy were recapitulated in normal rhesus macaque pregnancy reinforcing the value of this NHP model for the study of congenital viral infections. Notable among the similarities between human and NHP decidua were the predominance of the CD16–CD56+ phenotype of NK cells, enrichment of CD4+ Tregs, enrichment of memory CD4+ and CD8+ T lymphocytes, increased activation but decreased cytotoxicity of decidual NK cells and CD8+ T lymphocytes, a predominance of CD206+ macrophages, and a paucity of B lymphocytes (6, 20, 50–52). tSNE analysis of CD45+ live leukocytes on the 28-color adaptive lymphocyte-focused flow cytometry panel and on CD3–CD20–CD45+ live leukocytes on the 18-color innate cell-focused flow panel revealed several clusters representing populations of CD4+ and CD8+ T lymphocytes, NK cells, monocytes or macrophages and DCs that were unique to either peripheral blood or decidua. The immune cell diversity between decidua and PBMC was similar to what was recently reported in humans using a similar approach (53).

Memory T lymphocytes comprise roughly 5-20% of the CD45+ leukocyte population in human decidua from the first trimester and increase with gestational age. As part of the adaptive immune system they are key players in mounting an immune response against foreign antigens in pregnancy (10, 22). Decidual CD8+ T lymphocytes are unique in that they recognize

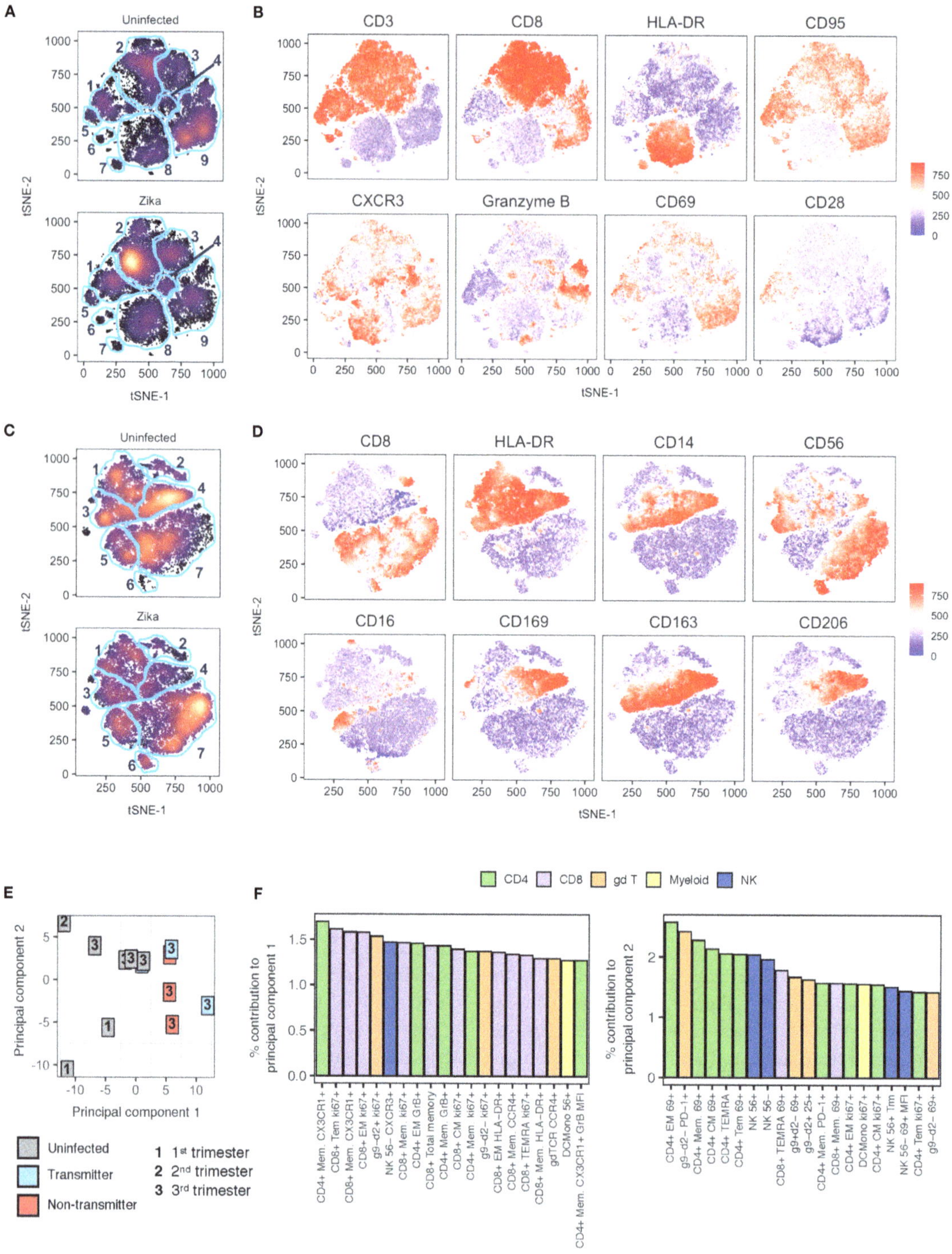

FIGURE 13 | tSNE and PCA analysis of decidual leukocytes of uninfected and ZIKV-infected rhesus macaques. **(A)** tSNE plot representing an equal number of CD45+/live/single cells/leukocytes cells from decidua of rhesus macaques experiencing a normal pregnancy (n = 9) or after ZIKV infection (n = 8). The 28-color adaptive panel was used to generate this plot. Blue gates were manually drawn based on clustering patterns. **(B)** Individual MFI gradients of eight markers on the tSNE map. Red coloring represents high MFI and blue coloring represents low MFI. **(C)** tSNE plot representing an equal number of CD45+/live/single cells/CD3-/CD20- cells from decidua of rhesus macaques experiencing a normal pregnancy (n = 8) or after ZIKV infection (n = 7). The 18-color innate panel was used to generate this plot. Blue gates were manually drawn based on clustering patterns. **(D)** Individual MFI gradients of eight markers on the tSNE map. Red coloring represents high MFI and blue coloring represents low MFI. **(E)** PCA plot of decidual leukocytes of uninfected and ZIKV-infected dams. **(F)** The top 20 contributing variables to principal component 1 (left) and principal component 2 (right) are shown and color coded according to major cell populations, CD4+ T (green), CD8+ T (purple), $\gamma\delta$ T (orange), myeloid CD20-HLA-DR+ (yellow), and NK cells (blue).

fetal antigens but remain tolerant to avoid fetal rejection. However, their role in pathogen-specific immunity and the properties of the immune response necessary to clear infections without harming the fetus are not known (23). In our study, we performed an extensive evaluation of the memory phenotype, activation status, cytotoxic granule content, and chemokine receptor expression on memory subsets of both circulating and decidual CD4+ and CD8+ T lymphocytes in pregnancy. T lymphocytes were the dominant leukocyte population in the decidua across all three trimesters with the exception of one second trimester dam in whom NK cells comprised roughly 60% of the decidual leukocyte population (**Figure 2B**). Reciprocally, we did not find NK cells as the dominant decidual population in first trimester. Neither was there a clear trend of decidual NK cells declining with gestation age. These findings are in contrast with humans where NK cells are the dominant leukocyte population in first trimester decidua. Whether this observation represents a species-specific difference in decidual leukocyte composition will require further study in a larger cohort of animals.

Relative to studies on decidual NK cells, data on decidual T lymphocytes are limited particularly for rhesus macaque decidua. A recent study in rhesus macaques at the third trimester of pregnancy used mass cytometry to examine multiple immune subsets including memory T lymphocytes in choriodecidual cells in decidua parietalis as well as in placental villi (54). The decidual leukocytes evaluated in our study were primarily isolated from tissue removed from the maternal surface of the placenta (decidua basalis) and stripped away from chorionic tissue. Using a combination of CD95, CD28, CCR5, CD45RA, CD69 and CD103, we delineated CM, EM, TEM, TEMRA, and tissue-resident Trm memory. Rhesus macaques had significantly higher proportions of EM CD8+ and CD4+ T in the decidua compared to peripheral blood consistent with human data (20, 25, 55). Less clear is the concordance between rhesus macaque and human decidua for other memory subsets. CM CD8+ and CD4+ T lymphocytes were present at significantly lower frequencies in rhesus macaque decidua. One study showed higher frequencies of CM CD4+ and CD8+ T lymphocytes in term human decidua compared to peripheral blood (55). CD4+ TEMRA lymphocytes did not differ between peripheral blood and decidua; however, CD8+ TEMRA were significantly lower in the decidual compartment, contrary to human studies showing a higher proportion of CD8+ TEMRA in the decidua (22). It is noteworthy that in rhesus macaques, the proportion of decidual CM CD4+ T was lowest in the first trimester and highest in the third trimester, a finding that has not previously been reported. The increase in decidual CM CD4+ T with increasing gestation age was associated with a decline in Ki67+ activated memory CD4+ T (both CM and EM subsets) and a decline in CCR5+ CD4 memory and CD8 memory. These changes with gestational age were confined to the decidua and not observed in circulating lymphocytes. Reduced decidual CCR5+ memory CD4+ T with gestation age may have implications for the relative risk of mother-to-child transmission of HIV in different trimesters of pregnancy (56).

Consistent with findings in humans, decidual EM, CM and TEMRA CD8+ T had lower granzyme B content compared to their circulating memory counterparts (20). Of note, the proportion of granzyme B+ TEM and CM CD8+ T lymphocytes was significantly higher in the decidua but their granzyme B content measured by MFI was lower. Thus, decidual CD8+ T contain substantial proportions of Granzyme B-positive cells but likely are less cytotoxic compared to circulating memory CD8+ T lymphocytes. With respect to effector function, the majority of decidual memory CD4+ and CD8+ T were highly activated and skewed to a Th1 phenotype as evidenced by high proportions expressing CD69, HLA-DR, and CXCR3. This was in striking contrast to circulating memory T lymphocytes that were less activated and showed a mixture of Th1 (CXCR3+), Th2 (CCR4+), and Th17 (CCR6+, CCR4+) cells and is similar to findings in humans (55). In concert with high levels of activation, decidual CD4+ and CD8+ T lymphocytes contained significantly higher levels of PD-1+ cells compared to circulating memory T lymphocytes but not in a correlative manner like the PBMC. This is not surprising in light of studies showing expression of immune inhibitory check-point receptors on human decidual T lymphocytes as one likely mechanism by which decidual T lymphocytes maintain concurrent effector function and a tolerogenic phenotype during pregnancy (21, 57).

In addition to conventional T lymphocytes, CD4+ Tregs, iNKT and γδ T lymphocytes accounted for roughly 20% of the total decidual T (CD3+) lymphocyte population. Tregs play an essential immunosuppressive role in inhibiting alloreactive T cells and maintaining tolerance during normal pregnancy. As in humans, CD4+ CD25bright CD127lo Tregs in rhesus macaques were present at significantly higher frequencies in the decidua compared to peripheral blood and showed a significant increase with gestation age. Human studies of normal pregnancy have shown that decidual Treg frequencies remain unchanged (d. basalis) or increase (d. parietalis) at term gestation (51, 58–60). A recent study provided evidence for clonally expanded effector Tregs, likely containing fetal antigen-specific Tregs, increasing in the 3rd trimester of normal pregnancy but decreasing in preeclampsia (61). While we did not characterize the type of decidual Tregs in this study, the findings of CD4+ Tregs enrichment in macaque decidua and its relationship to gestation age appear similar to human decidua.

Among other immunomodulatory T lymphocytes, low frequencies of decidual iNKT were detected at levels comparable to peripheral blood. It should be noted that the method of iNKT detection is an important consideration for comparison with studies reporting on NKT lymphocytes. Several publications including one on macaque decidua have defined NKT as CD3+CD56+ T lymphocytes (62). This is erroneous and does not represent genuine iNKT lymphocytes (63). We used T lymphocyte expression of the Vα24 TCR along with binding to α-galactoslyceramide(GC)-loaded CD1d tetramers for specific and stringent identification of iNKT lymphocytes as described in humans and nonhuman primates (43, 64). In our study, CD3+CD56+ T lymphocytes were enriched in the decidua with mean frequency of 21.7% of T lymphocytes as compared to <5%

of T lymphocytes in peripheral blood. Yet, less than 1% of decidual CD56+ T were genuine iNKT as defined by Vα24+ T lymphocytes binding to αGC-loaded CD1d tetramer. Moreover, all Vα24+ CD1d-tetramer-positive iNKT lymphocytes did not express CD56. In two studies in humans that used stringent criteria for identification, iNKT were detected in first trimester decidua at low frequencies of <0.5% of CD3+ decidual leukocytes and were present at significantly higher frequencies in the decidua compared to peripheral blood (41, 42).

γδ T lymphocytes are another unconventional T lymphocyte subset that recognize non-peptide antigens in an MHC-independent manner and respond to bacterial and viral infections (65). Early trimester decidua is enriched for γδ T but their role in pregnancy is not well understood (46). In utero CMV infection is associated with expansion of fetal Vγ9− γδ T lymphocytes (66). In one study ZIKV infection in humans was associated with expansion of Vδ2+ γδ T in the peripheral blood (67). To our knowledge there are no published data on decidual γδ T in rhesus macaques. Using a NHP cross-reactive pan-γδ TCR antibody along with antibodies specific for the Vγ9 and Vδ2 TCR chain, four populations of γδ T were defined of which the Vγ9−Vδ2− subset formed the bulk of the γδ T lymphocytes in the decidua and peripheral blood. γδ T lymphocytes showed higher frequencies in the decidua particularly at third trimester gestation. Of total γδ T cells, the Vδ2 subset is significantly higher in blood of healthy human donors compared to early gestation decidua (46). The same conclusion can be inferred in rhesus macaques as the dominant Vγ9+Vδ2+ population was significantly higher in the peripheral blood compared to the decidua. Similar to the conventional T lymphocytes, decidual γδ T were highly activated and enriched for effector memory cells in the decidua. These data suggest that despite being a relatively small population, decidual γδ T also have the capability to be potent effectors. Their role in protective immunity at the maternal-fetal interface remains to be determined. Of interest, ZIKV-infected pregnant dams in our study had increased levels of circulating Vδ2+ γδ T compared to normal pregnancies. In the ZIKV-infected dams, the decidual γδ T had a reduced proliferation potential similar to the memory CD4+ T but also reduced PD-1 expression. This may suggest that decidual γδ T are less exhausted and could have effector function in the face of a viral infection.

Among innate leukocytes we evaluated NK cells, monocytes/macrophages and dendritic cells in the decidua and peripheral blood of normal pregnancy. Based on co-expression of the scavenger receptor CD163 and the mannose receptor CD206, three populations of decidual macrophages were detected of which the dual positive CD163+ CD206+ subset was only seen in the decidua. A CD163+ CD206− decidual macrophage population was present but at a significantly lower frequency compared to peripheral blood where this monocyte subset was dominant. The two populations of CD163+ decidual macrophages appear to be phenotypically analogous to the CD11c(lo) and CD11c(hi) subsets with distinct gene expression profiles described in humans (50). Although neither subset is precisely M1- or M2-polarized, the gene profile of the CD11c(lo) CD206+ subset resembles M2-polarized macrophages. It is noteworthy that the CD163+CD206− decidual macrophage population increased with gestational age as did the frequency of CD14+CD16+ inflammatory monocytes. These changes likely reflect the plasticity of the decidual macrophages moving to a more inflammatory phenotype as pregnancy progresses to term.

NK cells are the most abundant decidual leukocyte population in the first trimester of pregnancy and essential for implantation of the placenta through their interactions with extravillous trophoblasts. Decidual NK cells are phenotypically and functionally distinct from NK cells in the circulation and at other tissue sites and constitute a diverse population of tissue-resident innate lymphoid cells (68). Recent studies on first trimester human decidua using single cell RNAseq and mass cytometry have revealed several novel populations including dNK1, dNK2, and dNK3 based on their gene expression profile, phenotypic markers and function (11, 37). In this study we complemented evaluation of macaque NK subsets based on CD16 and CD56 co-expression patterns with NKG2A, CD39, CD103 and Granzyme B to define putative dNK1, dNK2 and dNK3 populations in macaques. These definitions were adapted from and based on the single cell gene expression, flow cytometry and mass cytometry profile of human first trimester decidua (11, 37). By flow cytometry, we defined dNK1 as NKG2A+ CD39+ granzymeB+ NK; dNK2 as NKG2A+ CD39+ granzymeB+ NK; and dNK3 as CD103+ granzymeB− NK. CD39 is a surface bound ectonucleosidase enzyme which is upregulated during inflammatory conditions. It is constitutively expressed in the placenta and is found on many immune cell subsets such as Tregs, NK cells, monocyte/macrophages, and dendritic cells. CD39 along with CD73 can convert ATP to adenosine leading the extracellular environment from a proinflammatory to immunosuppressive environment (69). tSNE analysis of the 28-color and 18-color flow cytometry panel revealed several unique non-overlapping clusters for NK cells in decidual and circulating leukocytes. With manual gating, several expected and novel observations were made. Consistent with previous studies in humans and macaques, the majority of decidual NK cells were CD56+CD16− (7, 9, 15, 16). This was in contrast to circulating NK cells in macaques that are predominantly CD16+CD56− (38). Macaque decidua also contained a clearly discernible population of CD16+ CD56+ double-positive NK cells that were not detected in peripheral blood. A similar double-positive NK population has been reported in vaginal and rectal mucosal tissues of rhesus macaques (70). To our knowledge this is the first report of CD16+CD56+ NK cells in macaque decidua. Similar to humans, granzyme B content in the decidual NK subsets was lower than their circulating phenotypic counterparts. When analyzed for dNK1-3 subsets on the basis of CD39, granzyme B and CD103 expression, the dominant dNK2 population was significantly lower in the decidua compared to peripheral blood. The dNK1 and dNK3 subsets constituted a small population of NK cells which was present at higher frequencies in the decidua. The dNK1 and dNK3 decidual populations were lower in the third trimester compared to the first trimester, whereas the dNK2 decidual population increased from the first to the third trimester. These data are consistent with the known functions of human dNK1 cells expressing high levels of KIRs and interacting with HLA-C molecules on extra-villous trophoblasts to promote placentation in the first trimester (11). Macaque decidual NK cells also contained a high frequency of NKG2A+NKG2D+ NK cells that were absent or detected at low frequencies in the circulation. NKG2D is a C-type lectin-like activating receptor expressed on NK cells and T lymphocyte subsets. In a study of first trimester human decidua, NKG2D was expressed on all CD56+ decidual NK and surface expression of the NKG2D ligands, UL16 binding protein and the stress-inducible MHC-Class I related chain molecules (MIC), was detected on extra-villous trophoblasts, villous trophoblasts, and decidual macrophages (71). A significant increase in NKG2D expression was observed in second trimester decidual NK as compared to first trimester (72). NKG2D was also shown to be involved in the cytotoxic effector function that decidual NK acquire *in vitro* on exposure to human CMV-infected autologous fibroblasts (73). Because the anti-NKG2A antibody in rhesus macaques does not differentiate between the inhibitory receptor NKG2A and the activating receptor NKG2C, we cannot be certain whether the NKG2D+ decidual NK cells co-express NKG2A or NKG2C (74). However, in light of the human data, it is likely that the NKG2A+NKG2D+ NK population in macaque decidua is a cytotoxic population. Similar to the T lymphocyte subsets in macaque decidua, the majority of decidual NK cells were significantly more activated than circulating NK cells as evidenced by surface expression of CD69, CXCR3 and CD169 molecules. The chemokine receptor CX3CR1 was also expressed on decidual NK cells but at lower frequencies compared to circulating NK cells.

Our analysis of decidual and circulating leukocytes from a ZIKV infection study in pregnancy in comparison to normal decidua yielded unexpected and interesting findings. In human studies, patients with ZIKV infection are reported to have increased DN T cells and increased activated CD8+ T cells when compared to healthy controls. Furthermore, nonclassical T cell subsets such as double negative (CD4-CD8-) Vδ2 TCR+ T cells are increased in ZIKV infected individuals which correlate with acute resolution of symptoms. This suggests that Vδ2 TCR+ T cells play a role in resolution in ZIKV symptoms (67). Based on these data, ZIKV could potentially disturb the balance at the maternal-fetal interface, as early gestation decidua has an increased frequency of γδ T cells compared to matched maternal blood (46). *In vitro* studies have shown that ZIKV can infect and replicate in human placental macrophages or Hofbauer cells, viral replication coincides with type I interferon induction, and anti-viral gene expression and pro-inflammatory cytokines (75). The mechanism of transmission is thought to by direct infection of Hofbauer cells and disrupting placental barrier. The role of decidual immunity is unknown as few studies have investigated tissue level cellular immunity to ZIKV despite its broad tissue trophism (76). To our surprise, the most striking finding in decidual cells from ZIKV-infected dams was a decrease in NK cells and increase in total T lymphocytes with significant reduction in activated (HLA-DR+ and/or Ki67+) memory CD4+ and CD8+ T and γδ T lymphocytes, reduced frequency of decidual Granzyme B+ CD4+ T and γδ T lymphocytes and reduction in CXCR3+ memory CD4+ and CD8+ T lymphocytes. We also saw a reduction in circulating DN T lymphocytes and a significant reduction in activated, proliferating, and PD-1-positive memory CD4+ T, memory CD8+ T, γδ T, and NK cells in ZIKV-infected dams as compared to healthy pregnant macaques. Overall, these data suggest an immunosuppressive effect with suppression of inflammation and decreased immune recruitment of decidual memory T cells at the maternal-fetal interface. Our findings raise the possibility that the prolonged ZIKV viremia reported in pregnant humans and macaques (29, 77, 78) is related to the immunosuppressive effect of ZIKV infection. Immunosuppression has been reported with Asian-lineage ZIKV related to suppression of type I interferon responses and induction of a M2 anti-inflammatory type transcription phenotype of monocytes ex vivo. But no changes in T cell phenotype were observed in this study (79).

The immunosuppressive effects we have observed in this study are in contrast to the autoimmunity (loss of immune suppression) type of symptoms by Guillain-Barré syndrome that may arise in conjunction with ZIKV infection (76). It is possible that ZIKV induces autoimmunity of the circulating leukocytes while at the tissue-level of the already tolerant maternal-fetal interface, the immune cell environment is silenced by loss of T cell activation and reduced infiltration of CXCR3-expressing CD4+ and CD8+ T lymphocytes which are inflammation-homing T cells. The CXCL10-CXCR3 axis is important in attracting effector T cells to decidual tissue (23). In mice epigenetic silencing of T cell chemoattractant genes in decidual stromal cells led to impaired accumulation of decidual effector T lymphocytes (80). CXCR3 blockade eliminated decidual CD8+ T cell infiltration and protected against in utero fetal infection and immunopathogenesis in a murine model of Listeria infection (81). The question of whether or not the immunosuppressive effects in the maternal decidua reflected an impaired virus-specific cellular immune response or protected against immunopathology are unresolved and will require future prospective studies.

The overall picture of the NHP maternal-fetal interface emerging from our study is that of a complex, dynamic immune environment with capability of robust effector activity balanced with features of a tolerogenic phenotype. Normal macaque decidua is populated with a dominance of memory T lymphocytes, CD8+ more than CD4+, throughout the gestation period with a subset showing markers of tissue-resident memory. The majority of memory CD4+ and CD8+ T, and γδ T lymphocytes are highly activated with a CXCR3+ Th1 phenotype but a significant proportion also express PD-1. Higher frequencies of cytotoxic memory T lymphocytes with less granzyme B content at the single cell level compared to their circulating counterparts are detected in the decidua. Decidual

NK cells are phenotypically distinct with a dominance of cytotoxic CD56+ NK cells that co-express NKG2D and NKG2a/c. Similar to memory T lymphocytes, the majority of decidual NK cells are activated and express CXCR3 but have lower granzyme B content compared to their circulating counterparts. In the myeloid lineage, we found a population of tissue-resident CD163+ CD206+ macrophages which were unique to the decidual environment. We also found a strong presence of tolerogenic CD4+ Tregs which correlated with gestational age in the decidua. In all, these features identify the maternal-fetal interface as a distinct and unique environment that pathogens need to navigate for vertical transmission to the fetus. Our findings of reduced activation, reduced CXCR3 expression and reduced cytotoxicity of decidual memory T lymphocytes in ZIKV infection indicate local immunosuppression and impaired immune recruitment as possible mechanisms of vertical transmission.

In conclusion, we have reported on the first deep and comprehensive analysis of immune cells at the maternal-fetal interface and its comparison to circulating leukocytes in a normal rhesus macaque pregnancy model. By extending our analysis to an investigation of changes in the maternal decidua in a cohort of ZIKV-infected dams, we provide novel insights in to immune perturbations following a congenital viral infection. The stark contrasts of the circulating to decidual leukocytes highlights the immunological barrier formed by the maternal-fetal interface and the need to study this in the context of pathogenic infections that can be transmitted from mother to fetus. Such studies are needed to find vaccine targets against congenital infections.

ETHICS STATEMENT

The animal study was reviewed and approved by TNPRC and ONPRC IACUC.

AUTHOR CONTRIBUTIONS

MM and AK conceived the study. MM, MF, and AK wrote the manuscript. MM, AK, MF, JH, VR, and NM reviewed the manuscript. MM, LS, ES, DT, DS, JH, and VR helped procure and process samples. MM, LS, and ES performed the experiment. MM, MF, and AK analyzed the data. MM and MF prepared and processed the data for presentation. AK, JH, VR, and NM were responsible for the support of experiments. All authors contributed to the article and approved the submitted version.

FUNDING

Funding was provided by NIH by 1P01AI129859, TNPRC Base Grant OD011104, and ONPRC Base Grant OD011092. Additional funding for the ZIKV-infected study group was provided by the Bill and Melinda Gates Foundation (OPP1152818). Animal samples were available through the ONPRC Pathology tissue distribution program, which is supported by ONPRC NIH Base Grant OD011092.

ACKNOWLEDGMENTS

The authors would like to acknowledge the TNPRC Flow Core, Megan Varnado, Natalie Guy, and Kaitlin Didier for the flow cytometry support. Both the TNPRC and ONPRC veterinary medicine teams provided animal care and procured samples. Teresa Beechwood for shipping samples from OHSU to Tulane. In addition, Blake Schouest is acknowledged for assisting with literature references. The authors would like to thank the NIH Tetramer Core facility for provision of the CD1dTM conjugated to BV421.

REFERENCES

1. Mor G, Aldo P, Alvero AB. The Unique Immunological and Microbial Aspects of Pregnancy. *Nat Rev Immunol* (2017) 17(8):469–82. doi: 10.1038/nri.2017.64
2. Ander SE, Diamond MS, Coyne CB. Immune Responses at the Maternal-Fetal Interface. *Sci Immunol* (2019) 4(31):1–10. doi: 10.1126/sciimmunol.aat6114
3. Schumacher A, Sharkey DJ, Robertson SA, Zenclussen AC. Immune Cells at the Fetomaternal Interface: How the Microenvironment Modulates Immune Cells To Foster Fetal Development. *J Immunol* (2018) 201(2):325–34. doi: 10.4049/jimmunol.1800058
4. Robson A, Harris LK, Innes BA, Lash GE, Aljunaidy MM, Aplin JD, et al. Uterine Natural Killer Cells Initiate Spiral Artery Remodeling in Human Pregnancy. *FASEB J* (2012) 26(12):4876–85. doi: 10.1096/fj.12-210310
5. Tessier DR, Yockell-Lelievre J, Gruslin A. Uterine Spiral Artery Remodeling: The Role of Uterine Natural Killer Cells and Extravillous Trophoblasts in Normal and High-Risk Human Pregnancies. *Am J Reprod Immunol* (2015) 74 (1):1–11. doi: 10.1111/aji.12345
6. Bartmann C, Segerer SE, Rieger L, Kapp M, Sutterlin M, Kammerer U. Quantification of the Predominant Immune Cell Populations in Decidua Throughout Human Pregnancy. *Am J Reprod Immunol* (2014) 71(2):109–19. doi: 10.1111/aji.12185
7. Koopman LA, Kopcow HD, Rybalov B, Boyson JE, Orange JS, Schatz F, et al. Human Decidual Natural Killer Cells Are a Unique NK Cell Subset With Immunomodulatory Potential. *J Exp Med* (2003) 198(8):1201–12. doi: 10.1084/jem.20030305
8. Williams PJ, Searle RF, Robson SC, Innes BA, Bulmer JN. Decidual Leucocyte Populations in Early to Late Gestation Normal Human Pregnancy. *J Reprod Immunol* (2009) 82(1):24–31. doi: 10.1016/j.jri.2009.08.001
9. Nishikawa K, Saito S, Morii T, Hamada K, Ako H, Narita N, et al. Accumulation of CD16-CD56+ Natural Killer Cells With High Affinity

Interleukin 2 Receptors in Human Early Pregnancy Decidua. *Int Immunol* (1991) 3(8):743–50. doi: 10.1093/intimm/3.8.743

10. Crespo AC, van der Zwan A, Ramalho-Santos J, Strominger JL, Tilburgs T. Cytotoxic Potential of Decidual NK Cells and CD8+ T Cells Awakened by Infections. *J Reprod Immunol* (2017) 119:85–90. doi: 10.1016/j.jri.2016.08.001
11. Huhn O, Ivarsson MA, Gardner L, Hollinshead M, Stinchcombe JC, Chen P, et al. Distinctive Phenotypes and Functions of Innate Lymphoid Cells in Human Decidua During Early Pregnancy. *Nat Commun* (2020) 11(1):381. doi: 10.1038/s41467-019-14123-z
12. Jabrane-Ferrat N. Features of Human Decidual NK Cells in Healthy Pregnancy and During Viral Infection. *Front Immunol* (2019) 10:1397. doi: 10.3389/fimmu.2019.01397
13. Siewiera J, Gouilly J, Hocine HR, Cartron G, Levy C, Al-Daccak R, et al. Natural Cytotoxicity Receptor Splice Variants Orchestrate the Distinct Functions of Human Natural Killer Cell Subtypes. *Nat Commun* (2015) 6:10183. doi: 10.1038/ncomms10183
14. Dambaeva SV, Breburda EE, Durning M, Garthwaite MA, Golos TG. Characterization of Decidual Leukocyte Populations in Cynomolgus and Vervet Monkeys. *J Reprod Immunol* (2009) 80(1-2):57–69. doi: 10.1016/j.jri.2008.12.006
15. Dambaeva SV, Durning M, Rozner AE, Golos TG. Immunophenotype and Cytokine Profiles of Rhesus Monkey CD56bright and CD56dim Decidual Natural Killer Cells. *Biol Reprod* (2012) 86(1):1–10. doi: 10.1095/biolreprod.111.094383
16. Slukvin II, Watkins DI, Golos TG. Phenotypic and Functional Characterization of Rhesus Monkey Decidual Lymphocytes: Rhesus Decidual Large Granular Lymphocytes Express CD56 and Have Cytolytic Activity. *J Reprod Immunol* (2001) 50(1):57–79. doi: 10.1016/S0165-0378(00)00090-5
17. Laskarin G, Kammerer U, Rukavina D, Thomson AW, Fernandez N, Blois SM. Antigen-Presenting Cells and Materno-Fetal Tolerance: An Emerging Role for Dendritic Cells. *Am J Reprod Immunol* (2007) 58(3):255–67. doi: 10.1111/j.1600-0897.2007.00511.x
18. Vacca P, Cantoni C, Vitale M, Prato C, Canegallo F, Fenoglio D, et al. Crosstalk Between Decidual NK and CD14+ Myelomonocytic Cells Results in Induction of Tregs and Immunosuppression. *Proc Natl Acad Sci U S A* (2010) 107(26):11918–23. doi: 10.1073/pnas.1001749107
19. Tilburgs T, Claas FH, Scherjon SA. Elsevier Trophoblast Research Award Lecture: Unique Properties of Decidual T Cells and Their Role in Immune Regulation During Human Pregnancy. *Placenta* (2010) 31 Suppl:S82–6. doi: 10.1016/j.placenta.2010.01.007
20. Tilburgs T, Schonkeren D, Eikmans M, Nagtzaam NM, Datema G, Swings GM, et al. Human Decidual Tissue Contains Differentiated CD8+ Effector-Memory T Cells With Unique Properties. *J Immunol* (2010) 185(7):4470–7. doi: 10.4049/jimmunol.0903597
21. van der Zwan A, Bi K, Norwitz ER, Crespo AC, Claas FHJ, Strominger JL, et al. Mixed Signature of Activation and Dysfunction Allows Human Decidual CD8 (+) T Cells to Provide Both Tolerance and Immunity. *Proc Natl Acad Sci U S A* (2018) 115(2):385–90. doi: 10.1073/pnas.1713957115
22. Kieffer TEC, Laskewitz A, Scherjon SA, Faas MM, Prins JR. Memory T Cells in Pregnancy. *Front Immunol* (2019) 10:625. doi: 10.3389/fimmu.2019.00625
23. Lissauer D, Kilby MD, Moss P. Maternal Effector T Cells Within Decidua: The Adaptive Immune Response to Pregnancy? *Placenta* (2017) 60:140–4. doi: 10.1016/j.placenta.2017.09.003
24. Lissauer D, Piper K, Goodyear O, Kilby MD, Moss PA. Fetal-Specific CD8+ Cytotoxic T Cell Responses Develop During Normal Human Pregnancy and Exhibit Broad Functional Capacity. *J Immunol* (2012) 189(2):1072–80. doi: 10.4049/jimmunol.1200544
25. Powell RM, Lissauer D, Tamblyn J, Beggs A, Cox P, Moss P, et al. Decidual T Cells Exhibit a Highly Differentiated Phenotype and Demonstrate Potential Fetal Specificity and a Strong Transcriptional Response to IFN. *J Immunol* (2017) 199(10):3406–17. doi: 10.4049/jimmunol.1700114
26. Parker EL, Silverstein RB, Verma S, Mysorekar IU. Viral-Immune Cell Interactions at the Maternal-Fetal Interface in Human Pregnancy. *Front Immunol* (2020) 11:522047. doi: 10.3389/fimmu.2020.522047
27. van Egmond A, van der Keur C, Swings GM, Scherjon SA, Claas FH. The Possible Role of Virus-Specific CD8(+) Memory T Cells in Decidual Tissue. *J Reprod Immunol* (2016) 113:1–8. doi: 10.1016/j.jri.2015.09.073
28. Bialas KM, Tanaka T, Tran D, Varner V, Cisneros de la Rosa E, Chiuppesi F, et al. Maternal CD4+ T Cells Protect Against Severe Congenital Cytomegalovirus Disease in a Novel Nonhuman Primate Model of Placental Cytomegalovirus Transmission. *Proc Natl Acad Sci U S A* (2015) 112 (44):13645–50. doi: 10.1073/pnas.1511526112
29. Magnani DM, Rogers TF, Maness NJ, Grubaugh ND, Beutler N, Bailey VK, et al. Fetal Demise and Failed Antibody Therapy During Zika Virus Infection of Pregnant Macaques. *Nat Commun* (2018) 9(1):1624. doi: 10.1038/s41467-018-04056-4
30. Schouest B, Beddingfield BJ, Gilbert MH, Bohm RP, Schiro F, Aye PP, et al. Zika Virus Infection During Pregnancy Protects Against Secondary Infection in the Absence of CD8(+) Cells. *Virology* (2021) 559:100–10. doi: 10.1016/j.virol.2021.03.019
31. Carter AM, Enders AC, Pijnenborg R. The Role of Invasive Trophoblast in Implantation and Placentation of Primates. *Philos Trans R Soc Lond B Biol Sci* (2015) 370(1663):20140070. doi: 10.1098/rstb.2014.0070
32. Furukawa S, Kuroda Y, Sugiyama A. A Comparison of the Histological Structure of the Placenta in Experimental Animals. *J Toxicol Pathol* (2014) 27(1):11–8. doi: 10.1293/tox.2013-0060
33. Carter AM. Comparative Studies of Placentation and Immunology in Non-Human Primates Suggest a Scenario for the Evolution of Deep Trophoblast Invasion and an Explanation for Human Pregnancy Disorders. *Reproduction* (2011) 141(4):391–6. doi: 10.1530/REP-10-0530
34. Banerjee P, Ries M, Janaka SK, Grandea AG3rd, Wiseman R, O'Connor DH, et al. Diversification of Bw4 Specificity and Recognition of a Nonclassical MHC Class I Molecule Implicated in Maternal-Fetal Tolerance by Killer Cell Ig-Like Receptors of the Rhesus Macaque. *J Immunol* (2018) 201(9):2776–86. doi: 10.4049/jimmunol.1800494
35. Boyson JE, Iwanaga KK, Urvater JA, Hughes AL, Golos TG, Watkins DI. Evolution of a New Nonclassical MHC Class I Locus in Two Old World Primate Species. *Immunogenetics* (1999) 49(2):86–98. doi: 10.1007/s002510050467
36. Rosenkrantz JL, Gaffney JE, Roberts VHJ, Carbone L, Chavez SL. Transcriptomic Analysis of Primate Placentas and Novel Rhesus Trophoblast Cell Lines Informs Investigations of Human Placentation. *BMC Biol* (2021) 19(1):127. doi: 10.1186/s12915-021-01056-7
37. Vento-Tormo R, Efremova M, Botting RA, Turco MY, Vento-Tormo M, Meyer KB, et al. Single-Cell Reconstruction of the Early Maternal-Fetal Interface in Humans. *Nature* (2018) 563(7731):347–53. doi: 10.1038/s41586-018-0698-6
38. Webster RL, Johnson RP. Delineation of Multiple Subpopulations of Natural Killer Cells in Rhesus Macaques. *Immunology* (2005) 115(2):206–14. doi: 10.1111/j.1365-2567.2005.02147.x
39. Cai Y, Sugimoto C, Arainga M, Alvarez X, Didier ES, Kuroda MJ. *In Vivo* Characterization of Alveolar and Interstitial Lung Macrophages in Rhesus Macaques: Implications for Understanding Lung Disease in Humans. *J Immunol* (2014) 192(6):2821–9. doi: 10.4049/jimmunol.1302269
40. Takahashi N, Sugimoto C, Allers C, Alvarez X, Kim WK, Didier ES, et al. Shifting Dynamics of Intestinal Macrophages During Simian Immunodeficiency Virus Infection in Adult Rhesus Macaques. *J Immunol* (2019) 202(9):2682–9. doi: 10.4049/jimmunol.1801457
41. Boyson JE, Rybalov B, Koopman LA, Exley M, Balk SP, Racke FK, et al. CD1D and Invariant NKT Cells at the Human Maternal-Fetal Interface. *Proc Natl Acad Sci U S A* (2002) 99(21):13741–6. doi: 10.1073/pnas.162491699
42. Tsuda H, Sakai M, Michimata T, Tanebe K, Hayakawa S, Saito S. Characterization of NKT Cells in Human Peripheral Blood and Decidual Lymphocytes. *Am J Reprod Immunol* (2001) 45(5):295–302. doi: 10.1111/j.8755-8920.2001.450505.x
43. Rout N, Else JG, Yue S, Connole M, Exley MA, Kaur A. Paucity of CD4+ Natural Killer T (NKT) Lymphocytes in Sooty Mangabeys Is Associated With Lack of NKT Cell Depletion After SIV Infection. *PLoS One* (2010) 5(3):e9787. doi: 10.1371/journal.pone.0009787

44. Rout N, Greene J, Yue S, O'Connor D, Johnson RP, Else JG, et al. Loss of Effector and Anti-Inflammatory Natural Killer T Lymphocyte Function in Pathogenic Simian Immunodeficiency Virus Infection. *PLoS Pathog* (2012) 8 (9):e1002928. doi: 10.1371/journal.ppat.1002928
45. Hartigan-O'Connor DJ, Poon C, Sinclair E, McCune JM. Human CD4+ Regulatory T Cells Express Lower Levels of the IL-7 Receptor Alpha Chain (CD127), Allowing Consistent Identification and Sorting of Live Cells. *J Immunol Methods* (2007) 319(1-2):41–52. doi: 10.1016/j.jim.2006.10.008
46. Terzieva A, Dimitrova V, Djerov L, Dimitrova P, Zapryanova S, Hristova I, et al. Early Pregnancy Human Decidua Is Enriched With Activated, Fully Differentiated and Pro-Inflammatory Gamma/Delta T Cells With Diverse TCR Repertoires. *Int J Mol Sci* (2019) 20(3):1–18. doi: 10.3390/ijms 20030687
47. Bottcher JP, Beyer M, Meissner F, Abdullah Z, Sander J, Hochst B, et al. Functional Classification of Memory CD8(+) T Cells by CX3CR1 Expression. *Nat Commun* (2015) 6:8306. doi: 10.1038/ncomms9306
48. Hirsch AJ, Roberts VHJ, Grigsby PL, Haese N, Schabel MC, Wang X, et al. Zika Virus Infection in Pregnant Rhesus Macaques Causes Placental Dysfunction and Immunopathology. *Nat Commun* (2018) 9(1):263. doi: 10.1038/s41467-017-02499-9
49. Papadopoulou M, Dimova T, Shey M, Briel L, Veldtsman H, Khomba N, et al. Fetal Public Vgamma9Vdelta2 T Cells Expand and Gain Potent Cytotoxic Functions Early After Birth. *Proc Natl Acad Sci U S A* (2020) 117(31):18638–48. doi: 10.1073/pnas.1922595117
50. Houser BL, Tilburgs T, Hill J, Nicotra ML, Strominger JL. Two Unique Human Decidual Macrophage Populations. *J Immunol* (2011) 186(4):2633–42. doi: 10.4049/jimmunol.1003153
51. Tilburgs T, Roelen DL, van der Mast BJ, van Schip JJ, Kleijburg C, de Groot-Swings GM, et al. Differential Distribution of CD4(+)CD25(bright) and CD8 (+)CD28(-) T-Cells in Decidua and Maternal Blood During Human Pregnancy. *Placenta* (2006) 27(Suppl A):S47–53. doi: 10.1016/j.placenta.2005.11.008
52. Vacca P, Pietra G, Falco M, Romeo E, Bottino C, Bellora F, et al. Analysis of Natural Killer Cells Isolated From Human Decidua: Evidence That 2b4 (CD244) Functions as an Inhibitory Receptor and Blocks NK-Cell Function. *Blood* (2006) 108(13):4078–85. doi: 10.1182/blood-2006-04-017343
53. Vazquez J, Chavarria M, Li Y, Lopez GE, Stanic AK. Computational Flow Cytometry Analysis Reveals a Unique Immune Signature of the Human Maternal-Fetal Interface. *Am J Reprod Immunol* (2018) 79(1):1–9. doi: 10.1111/aji.12774
54. Toothaker JM, Presicce P, Cappelletti M, Stras SF, McCourt CC, Chougnet CA, et al. Immune Cells in the Placental Villi Contribute to Intra-Amniotic Inflammation. *Front Immunol* (2020) 11:866. doi: 10.3389/fimmu. 2020.00866
55. Feyaerts D, Benner M, van Cranenbroek B, van der Heijden OWH, Joosten I, van der Molen RG. Human Uterine Lymphocytes Acquire a More Experienced and Tolerogenic Phenotype During Pregnancy. *Sci Rep* (2017) 7(1):2884. doi: 10.1038/s41598-017-03191-0
56. Johnson EL, Chakraborty R. HIV-1 at the Placenta: Immune Correlates of Protection and Infection. *Curr Opin Infect Dis* (2016) 29(3):248–55. doi: 10.1097/QCO.0000000000000267
57. Meggyes M, Miko E, Szigeti B, Farkas N, Szereday L. The Importance of the PD-1/PD-L1 Pathway at the Maternal-Fetal Interface. *BMC Pregnancy Childbirth* (2019) 19(1):74. doi: 10.1186/s12884-019-2218-6
58. Erlebacher A. Immunology of the Maternal-Fetal Interface. *Annu Rev Immunol* (2013) 31:387–411. doi: 10.1146/annurev-immunol-032712-100003
59. Salvany-Celades M, van der Zwan A, Benner M, Setrajcic-Dragos V, Bougleux Gomes HA, Iyer V, et al. Three Types of Functional Regulatory T Cells Control T Cell Responses at the Human Maternal-Fetal Interface. *Cell Rep* (2019) 27(9):2537–47 e5. doi: 10.1016/j.celrep.2019.04.109
60. Tilburgs T, Roelen DL, van der Mast BJ, de Groot-Swings GM, Kleijburg C, Scherjon SA, et al. Evidence for a Selective Migration of Fetus-Specific CD4 +CD25bright Regulatory T Cells From the Peripheral Blood to the Decidua in Human Pregnancy. *J Immunol* (2008) 180(8):5737–45. doi: 10.4049/jimmunol.180.8.5737
61. Tsuda S, Zhang X, Hamana H, Shima T, Ushijima A, Tsuda K, et al. Clonally Expanded Decidual Effector Regulatory T Cells Increase in Late Gestation of Normal Pregnancy, But Not in Preeclampsia, in Humans. *Front Immunol* (2018) 9:1934. doi: 10.3389/fimmu.2018.01934
62. Presicce P, Senthamaraikannan P, Alvarez M, Rueda CM, Cappelletti M, Miller LA, et al. Neutrophil Recruitment and Activation in Decidua With Intra-Amniotic IL-1beta in the Preterm Rhesus Macaque. *Biol Reprod* (2015) 92(2):56. doi: 10.1095/biolreprod.114.124420
63. Boyson JE, Aktan I, Barkhuff DA, Chant A. NKT Cells at the Maternal-Fetal Interface. *Immunol Invest* (2008) 37(5):565–82. doi: 10.1080/08820130802191409
64. Lee PT, Benlagha K, Teyton L, Bendelac A. Distinct Functional Lineages of Human V(alpha)24 Natural Killer T Cells. *J Exp Med* (2002) 195(5):637–41. doi: 10.1084/jem.20011908
65. Lawand M, Dechanet-Merville J, Dieu-Nosjean MC. Key Features of Gamma-Delta T-Cell Subsets in Human Diseases and Their Immunotherapeutic Implications. *Front Immunol* (2017) 8:761. doi: 10.3389/fimmu.2017.00761
66. Vermijlen D, Brouwer M, Donner C, Liesnard C, Tackoen M, Van Rysselberge M, et al. Human Cytomegalovirus Elicits Fetal Gammadelta T Cell Responses In Utero. *J Exp Med* (2010) 207(4):807–21. doi: 10.1084/jem.20090348
67. Cimini E, Castilletti C, Sacchi A, Casetti R, Bordoni V, Romanelli A, et al. Human Zika Infection Induces a Reduction of IFN-Gamma Producing CD4 T-Cells and a Parallel Expansion of Effector Vdelta2 T-Cells. *Sci Rep* (2017) 7 (1):6313. doi: 10.1038/s41598-017-06536-x
68. Bjorkstrom NK, Ljunggren HG, Michaelsson J. Emerging Insights Into Natural Killer Cells in Human Peripheral Tissues. *Nat Rev Immunol* (2016) 16(5):310–20. doi: 10.1038/nri.2016.34
69. Antonioli L, Pacher P, Vizi ES, Hasko G. CD39 and CD73 in Immunity and Inflammation. *Trends Mol Med* (2013) 19(6):355–67. doi: 10.1016/j.molmed.2013.03.005
70. Reeves RK, Gillis J, Wong FE, Yu Y, Connole M, Johnson RP. CD16- Natural Killer Cells: Enrichment in Mucosal and Secondary Lymphoid Tissues and Altered Function During Chronic SIV Infection. *Blood* (2010) 115(22):4439–46. doi: 10.1182/blood-2010-01-265595
71. Apps R, Gardner L, Traherne J, Male V, Moffett A. Natural-Killer Cell Ligands at the Maternal-Fetal Interface: UL-16 Binding Proteins, MHC Class-I Chain Related Molecules, HLA-F and CD48. *Hum Reprod* (2008) 23(11):2535–48. doi: 10.1093/humrep/den223
72. Zhang J, Dunk CE, Kwan M, Jones RL, Harris LK, Keating S, et al. Human dNK Cell Function Is Differentially Regulated by Extrinsic Cellular Engagement and Intrinsic Activating Receptors in First and Second Trimester Pregnancy. *Cell Mol Immunol* (2017) 14(2):203–13. doi: 10.1038/cmi.2015.66
73. Siewiera J, El Costa H, Tabiasco J, Berrebi A, Cartron G, Le Bouteiller P, et al. Human Cytomegalovirus Infection Elicits New Decidual Natural Killer Cell Effector Functions. *PLoS Pathog* (2013) 9(4):e1003257. doi: 10.1371/journal.ppat.1003257
74. Biassoni R, Fogli M, Cantoni C, Costa P, Conte R, Koopman G, et al. Molecular and Functional Characterization of NKG2D, Nkp80, and NKG2C Triggering NK Cell Receptors in Rhesus and Cynomolgus Macaques: Monitoring of NK Cell Function During Simian HIV Infection. *J Immunol* (2005) 174(9):5695–705. doi: 10.4049/jimmunol.174.9.5695
75. Quicke KM, Bowen JR, Johnson EL, McDonald CE, Ma H, O'Neal JT, et al. Zika Virus Infects Human Placental Macrophages. *Cell Host Microbe* (2016) 20(1):83–90. doi: 10.1016/j.chom.2016.05.015
76. Miner JJ, Diamond MS. Zika Virus Pathogenesis and Tissue Tropism. *Cell Host Microbe* (2017) 21(2):134–42. doi: 10.1016/j.chom.2017.01.004
77. Driggers RW, Ho CY, Korhonen EM, Kuivanen S, Jaaskelainen AJ, Smura T, et al. Zika Virus Infection With Prolonged Maternal Viremia and Fetal Brain Abnormalities. *N Engl J Med* (2016) 374(22):2142–51. doi: 10.1056/NEJMoa1601824
78. Dudley DM, Aliota MT, Mohr EL, Weiler AM, Lehrer-Brey G, Weisgrau KL, et al. A Rhesus Macaque Model of Asian-Lineage Zika Virus Infection. *Nat Commun* (2016) 7:12204. doi: 10.1038/ncomms 12204
79. Foo SS, Chen W, Chan Y, Bowman JW, Chang LC, Choi Y, et al. Asian Zika Virus Strains Target CD14(+) Blood Monocytes and Induce M2-Skewed

Immunosuppression During Pregnancy. *Nat Microbiol* (2017) 2(11):1558–70. doi: 10.1038/s41564-017-0016-3

80. Nancy P, Tagliani E, Tay CS, Asp P, Levy DE, Erlebacher A. Chemokine Gene Silencing in Decidual Stromal Cells Limits T Cell Access to the Maternal-Fetal Interface. *Science* (2012) 336(6086):1317–21. doi: 10.1126/science.1220030
81. Chaturvedi V, Ertelt JM, Jiang TT, Kinder JM, Xin L, Owens KJ, et al. CXCR3 Blockade Protects Against Listeria Monocytogenes Infection-Induced Fetal Wastage. *J Clin Invest* (2015) 125(4):1713–25. doi: 10.1172/JCI78578

3

Memory T Cells in Pregnancy

Tom E. C. Kieffer[1], Anne Laskewitz[2], Sicco A. Scherjon[1], Marijke M. Faas[2] and Jelmer R. Prins[1*]*

[1] Department of Obstetrics and Gynecology, University Medical Center Groningen, University of Groningen, Groningen, Netherlands, [2] Division of Medical Biology, Department of Pathology and Medical Biology, University Medical Center Groningen, University of Groningen, Groningen, Netherlands

***Correspondence:**
Tom E. C. Kieffer
t.e.c.kieffer@umcg.nl
Jelmer R. Prins
j.r.prins@umcg.nl

Adaptations of the maternal immune response are necessary for pregnancy success. Insufficient immune adaption is associated with pregnancy pathologies such as infertility, recurrent miscarriage, fetal growth restriction, spontaneous preterm birth, and preeclampsia. The maternal immune system is continuously exposed to paternal-fetal antigens; through semen exposure from before pregnancy, through fetal cell exposure in pregnancy, and through microchimerism after pregnancy. This results in the generation of paternal-fetal antigen specific memory T cells. Memory T cells have the ability to remember previously encountered antigens to elicit a quicker, more substantial and focused immune response upon antigen reencounter. Such fetal antigen specific memory T cells could be unfavorable in pregnancy as they could potentially drive fetal rejection. However, knowledge on memory T cells in pregnancy has shown that these cells might play a favorable role in fetal-maternal tolerance rather than rejection of the fetus. In recent years, various aspects of immunologic memory in pregnancy have been elucidated and the relevance and working mechanisms of paternal-fetal antigen specific memory T cells in pregnancy have been evaluated. The data indicate that a delicate balance of memory T cells seems necessary for reproductive success and that immunologic memory in reproduction might not be harmful for pregnancy. This review provides an overview of the different memory T cell subtypes and their function in the physiology and in complications of pregnancy. Current findings in the field and possible therapeutic targets are discussed. The findings of our review raise new research questions for further studies regarding the role of memory T cells in immune-associated pregnancy complications. These studies are needed for the identification of possible targets related to memory mechanisms for studies on preventive therapies.

Keywords: pregnancy, reproduction, memory T cell, immunologic memory, literature review

INTRODUCTION

Immune tolerance toward paternal-fetal antigen is crucial for reproductive success since dysfunctional tolerance is implicated in the pathophysiology of pregnancy complications as infertility, recurrent miscarriage, fetal growth restriction, spontaneous preterm birth, and preeclampsia (1–4). In reproduction, the maternal immune system is exposed to paternal-fetal antigens (**Figure 1**). Firstly, the male antigen is introduced to the maternal immune system through semen exposure even before pregnancy (5). Secondly, paternal-fetal antigens are exposed at the fetal-maternal interface in pregnancy since the maternal immune cells in blood are in direct contact with fetal trophoblast cells in the placenta (6, 7). Additionally, in pregnancy, there is trafficking of

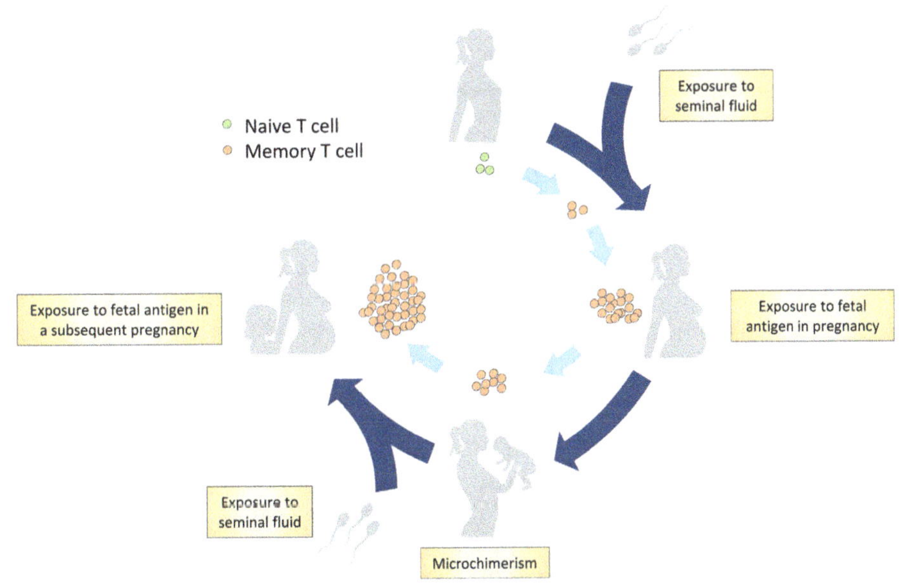

FIGURE 1 | Hypothesis on generation of the memory T cell population in reproduction through paternal-fetal antigen exposure. Firstly, naive T cells are exposed to the male antigen through antigens in seminal fluid. A subsequent encounter with the antigens occurs during pregnancy through exposure to fetal antigens on trophoblast cells and through microchimerism. Postpartum, the maternal immune system remains exposed to fetal antigens through microchimerism. In addition, postpartum, memory T cells are possibly exposed to paternal antigens through exposure to seminal fluid. In a subsequent pregnancy, the maternal memory T cells likely reaccumulate and respond to the cognate paternal-fetal antigens.

fetal cells expressing paternal-fetal antigens to maternal tissues at low levels which can recirculate in the maternal blood for years after pregnancy (8, 9). This phenomenon is called microchimerism (8, 9). It has been shown that the exposure of the maternal immune system to paternal-fetal antigens induces a memory T cell population with paternal-fetal antigen specificity (10–12).

The memory lymphocyte population is comprised of memory T lymphocytes (T cells) and memory B lymphocytes (B cells) (13, 14). Memory T cells are the most studied and appear to be the most important memory cell population in reproduction. Memory cells enable the immune system to protect the body from pathogens efficiently by generating a more adequate immune response to a known antigen, making it unnecessary to elicit a new response to an antigen that was encountered before (15). This process forms the basis for vaccination which is widely used to prevent infectious diseases and more recently to fight cancer and auto-immune diseases (16–18). In general, a more aggressive immune response toward pathogens is protective for health since the pathogen is cleared faster, however, the same aggressive response toward paternal- or fetal antigens would be disastrous for fetal and maternal health. Indeed, most studies of memory T cell populations in reproduction indicated that memory T cell subsets may exhibit a different function, proliferation pattern and migratory abilities toward paternal antigens in healthy pregnancies as compared with their function, proliferation and migratory abilities toward other antigens (12, 19, 20). In fact, specific memory cell populations have been shown to be involved in generating immune tolerance, rather than immune rejection, toward paternal-fetal antigens (12, 21–23).

In recent years, the implication and relevance of memory T cells in pregnancy and complications of pregnancy have been revealed. Major conceptual breakthroughs were seen in the T cell field, showing the role of memory T cells in reproductive fitness in mouse studies (11, 12, 21). Since increasing numbers of human studies on memory T cells have been published, this review gives an overview of the current literature on the different memory T cell subtypes and their adaptation in pregnancy and the implication of memory T cells in different complications of pregnancy. We will mainly focus on human studies and refer to mouse studies if needed. Current research gaps, controversies, and possible therapeutic targets will also be discussed.

MEMORY T CELLS

The memory T cell population is formed during a primary antigen response (24). In the primary response, antigens are presented to T cells through major histocompatibility complex (MHC) molecules (25). Depending on the type of MHC molecule, either type I or type II, CD8 positive or CD4 positive T cells respectively are activated through the T cell receptor (TCR) on the cell membrane (25). Additional co-stimulatory molecules can connect to co-stimulatory receptors on the T cell such as CD28 and CD70, for extra induction of the T cell response (25, 26). Depending on the cytokine environment, $CD4^+$ cells differentiate into either different T helper (Th) subsets (Th1, Th2, and Th17) which help in inducing/activating immune responses through secretion of cytokines, or into T regulatory (Treg) cells which exert regulatory effects on other immune cells after activation (27). After the primary response, most $CD4^+$ cells die, but some $CD4^+$ cells differentiate into $CD4^+$ memory T cells (24, 28). $CD8^+$ cells also differentiate into different subpopulations; i.e., effector $CD8^+$ cells which are ready to release cytotoxic cytokines or induce apoptosis via cell surface interaction, and a small population of regulatory $CD8^+$ cells which exhibit an immune regulatory function (29). Once the pathogen is cleared, most $CD8^+$ cells die, however some proliferate into memory $CD8^+$ cells (29).

Several memory T cell subsets are known, and can be distinguished by various markers (**Tables 1, 2**). The main markers are CD45RO expression, and lack of CD45RA expression (52, 53). The $CD45RO^+CD45RA^-$ phenotype has been linked to long living memory T cells (52, 53). It should be noted that CD45RO expression and lack of CD45RA expression are not conclusive markers for memory T cells, since their expression does not predict long time survival and rapid effector function upon secondary exposure *per se* (54). In addition, it has been shown that $CD45RO^+$ T cells can be reprogrammed and go back to a $CD45RO^-$ naive phenotype (55, 56). So far there are no other reliable markers of phenotype memory T cells in clinical experiments, therefore, phenotypic characterization of the memory cell population by CD45RO expression is widely used. Memory $CD4^+$ and $CD8^+$ cells can be divided into subsets based on their migration pattern, cytokine secretion abilities, and protein expression profile. The main memory cell subsets are the central memory (CM) cells and the effector memory (EM) cells, although the number of subsets is expanding rapidly (**Tables 1, 2**). The CM cell subset differentiates into effector cells upon secondary antigen exposure and is characterized by CCR7 expression which makes them home to secondary lymphoid organs (53, 57). The EM cell subset is characterized by their presence in peripheral tissue and direct pro-inflammatory effector function upon secondary antigen encounter with the cognate antigen (53). Below, an overview of the current knowledge of the various memory T cell subsets in pregnancy is reviewed (**Supplementary Material**).

$CD4^+$ MEMORY CELLS IN PREGNANCY

Within the $CD4^+$ memory cell population, a subdivision has been made based on migration pattern and effector function; i.e., $CD4^+$ effector memory ($CD4^+$ EM) cells, $CD4^+$ central memory ($CD4^+$ CM) cells, $CD4^+$ tissue resident memory ($CD4^+$ TRM) cells, $CD4^+$ T follicular helper memory ($CD4^+$ FHM) cells, $CD4^+$ regulatory memory cells, and $CD4^+$ memory stem cells (58–65).

It has been known for many years that pregnancy and some pregnancy complications affect the general $CD4^+$ memory T cell population. In 1996, it was shown that general $CD4^+$ memory cell ($CD4^+CD45RO^+$) proportions in peripheral blood were lower from the second trimester onwards until 2–7 days postpartum compared to proportions in non-pregnant controls (66). These findings have been followed up by studies in preeclampsia (67–69), gestational diabetes (70), and preterm labor (71) in which higher proportions of total memory T cells in peripheral blood have been found compared to healthy pregnant controls. Early studies also showed $CD4^+CD45RO^+$ memory cells in the decidua and showed that CD45RO expression on $CD4^+$ cells is upregulated in the decidua compared to $CD4^+$ cells in peripheral blood (72, 73). Later, Gomez-Lopez et al. suggested a role for $CD4^+$ memory cells in human term parturition by showing an increase of $CD4^+$ memory cells ($CD4^+CD45RO^+$) using immunohistochemistry on choriodecidual tissue from women in spontaneous labor at term compared to women with term scheduled cesarean sections (74). The early data already indicated that memory T cells are affected by pregnancy and its complications. In more recent years, studies have focused on specific subsets of $CD4^+$ memory cells. These data are reviewed per memory T cell subset below.

$CD4^+$ Effector Memory Cells in Pregnancy

Th1, Th2, and possibly Th17 effector cells can differentiate into $CD4^+$ EM cells (75–77). $CD4^+$ EM cell characterization is based on the lack of expression of lymph node homing receptors CC-chemokine receptor-7 (CCR7) and CD62L (L-selectin), which enables them to migrate to peripheral tissue (59). EM cells are the memory cells with the fastest immune response on a secondary encounter. Within several hours after re-stimulation with a memorized antigen, $CD4^+$ EM cells produce a variety of cytokines as interferon-gamma (IFN-gamma), tumor necrosis factor (TNF), interleukin-4 (IL4), and IL5 (53, 77, 78). A specific subtype of $CD4^+$ EM cell can re-express CD45RA after antigen stimulation (TEMRA) (79). These cells are poorly studied and there are no published investigations on $CD4^+$ TEMRA cells in reproduction to our knowledge.

In the second and third trimesters of pregnancy, two studies showed higher $CD4^+$ EM cell ($CD45RA^-CCR7^-$ and $CD45RO^+CCR7^-$) proportions in peripheral blood, compared to proportions of these cells in non-pregnant women (23, 30), while another study found decreased numbers of $CD4^+$ EM cells in peripheral blood during pregnancy (34). Differences between the studies could be due to the fact that that hormonal fluctuations during the menstrual cycle were not taken into account in the latter study. Not only is the proportion of $CD4^+$ EM cells increased during pregnancy, these cells also showed increased expression of CD69 (30), as well as decreased expression of programmed death-1 (PD-1) (23). This suggests that there is increased activation of $CD4^+$ EM cells, and that these cells are less susceptible to apoptosis. The increase of $CD4^+$ EM cells is not only seen during pregnancy, but also years after when $CD4^+$ EM cell proportions remained increased, i.e., at gestation levels as compared with women that have never been pregnant (30). These cells also showed increased CD69 expression after pregnancy, which could suggest persistent activation through exposure to antigen. This could be related to microchimerism, although it remains to be investigated whether the increased EM cell proportion is due to an increase in cells specific for paternal-fetal antigens.

Whereas, in blood the proportion of $CD4^+$ EM cells of the total $CD4^+$ cell population was about 20–30% (19, 30, 31), locally, in the decidua, the proportion of $CD4^+$ EM cells ($CD45RA^-CCR7^-$) was higher with 50–60% of the total $CD4^+$ cell population being EM cells (19, 31). This may indicate

TABLE 1 | $CD4^+$ memory T cells in pregnancy.

Memory T cell		Markers (human)	Cytokines	Findings in pregnancy	Findings in complications of pregnancy
$CD4^+$	EM	$CD45RO^+$, $CD45RA^-$, $CD44^+$, $CCR7^-$, $CD62L^-$, $CD28^+$	IFN-$gamma^+$, TNF^+, $IL4^+$, $IL5^+$	- Higher proportion in peripheral blood in pregnancy (23, 30) - Higher proportions in decidua compared to peripheral blood (19, 31) - Increased IFN-gamma, IL4, PD-1, Tim-3, CTLA-4, and LAG-3 expression in decidua compared to peripheral blood (19) - Lower PD-1 expression in peripheral blood in pregnancy (23) - Higher proportion and higher activated proportion in peripheral blood postpartum compared to nulliparous women (30)	- Comparable proportions in peripheral blood in preeclampsia and healthy controls (32) - Higher proportions in peripheral blood in women with recurrent miscarriages compared to healthy controls (not specified CD4/CD8) (33)
	TEMRA	$CD45RO^-$, $CD45RA^+$, $CCR7^-$, $CD62L^-$, $CD28^-$	$Perforin^+$, granzyme B^+	Not studied in pregnancy	Not studied in complications of pregnancy
	CM	$CD45RO^+$, $CD45RA^-$, $CD44^+$, $CCR7^+$, $CD62L^+$, $CD28^+$	$IL2^+$, IFN-$gamma^-$, and TNF^-	- Higher proportion in peripheral blood compared to menstrual blood (31) - Comparable proportions and HLA-DR and CD38 expression in peripheral blood in non-pregnant and pregnant women (23, 30, 34) - Higher proportions in decidua compared to peripheral blood (31) - Higher proportion and higher activated proportion in peripheral blood postpartum compared to nulliparous women (30)	- Higher proportion in peripheral blood in preeclampsia compared to healthy controls (32) - Comparable CD27, CD28, and CD127 expression in peripheral blood in preeclampsia and healthy controls (32) - Higher proportions in peripheral blood in women with recurrent miscarriages compared to healthy controls (not specified CD4/CD8) (33, 35)
	TRM	$CD45RO^+$, $CD45RA^-$, $CCR7^-$, $CD62L^-$, $CD69^{+/-}$, $CD103^{+/-}$	IFN-$gamma^+$, $IL17^+$	Not studied in pregnancy	Not studied in complications of pregnancy
	Treg memory	$CD45RO^+$, $CD45RA^-$, $CD44^+$, $CD25^+$, $CD127^-$, $Foxp3^+$, $CTLA4^+$	$IL10^+$, $TGFB^+$	- Higher proportions in the decidua compared to peripheral blood (36) - Strong increase in peripheral blood in the first trimester (37) - Comparable proportions in peripheral blood in 3rd trimester and non-pregnant women (34) - Higher immune regulating capabilities upon stimulation with umbilical cord blood (36) - HLA-DR^+ proportion in pregnancy showed decreased suppressive activity compared to HLA-DR^+ proportion in non-pregnant women (37) - Differentiated from RTE Treg cells in first trimester peripheral blood (38) - Remain high during pregnancy, decreased with onset of labor, and at preconception levels postpartum (38) - In mice, paternal-specific Treg memory is generated in gestation, remaining at lower levels postpartum, and lowering resorption rates in a subsequent pregnancy (12, 39, 40)	- Higher proportion in peripheral blood in preeclampsia compared to healthy controls (32) - Higher proportion of RTE Treg cells in peripheral blood in preeclampsia differentiate into $CD31^+$ Treg memory cells (38). - $CD31^+$ Treg memory cells in peripheral blood in preeclampsia have decreased immune suppressive capacity compared to $CD31^+$ memory Treg cells in healthy women (38). - HLA-DR^- memory Treg cells were increased in gestational diabetes with dietary adjustment (41) - HLA-DR^- memory Treg cells were strongly increased in gestational diabetes with insulin therapy (41)
	FHM	$CXCR5^+$, $CD45RA^-$, $CD45RO^+$, $CD62L^+$, $CCR7^+$, $FR4^+$	$IL21^+$, $IL10^+$	- Increased in the uterus and placenta toward late gestation in mice (42)	- Higher PD-1^+CCR7^+ and PD-1^+ICOS^+ proportions in decidual tissue but not in peripheral blood from spontaneous miscarriages compared to elective terminations in healthy controls (43)
	Memory stem cell	$CD45RO^-$, $CD45RA^+$, $CCR7^+$, $CD62L^+$, $CD28^+$, $CD27^+$, $CD95^+$, $IL2RB^+$	IFN-$gamma^-$, $IL2^{+/-}$	Not studied in pregnancy	Not studied in complications of pregnancy

EM, effector memory; TEMRA, effector memory CD45RA revertant; CM, central memory; TRM, tissue resident memory; Treg, T regulatory; FHM, follicular helper memory; CCR7, CC-chemokine receptor 7; CD62-L, L-selectin; Foxp3, forkhead box P3; CXCR5, chemokine receptor type 5; FR4, folate receptor-4; IFN-gamma, interferon-gamma; TNF, tumor necrosis factor; IL, interleukin; TGFB, transforming growth factor B; PD-1, programmed death-1; Tim-3, T cell immunoglobulin and mucin domain 3; CTLA-4, cytotoxic T lymphocyte antigen; LAG-3, lymphocyte activation gene 3; HLA-DR, Human Leukocyte Antigen-DR; ICOS, inducible T cell co-stimulator; RTE, recent thymic emigrant.

TABLE 2 | $CD8^+$ memory T cells in pregnancy.

Memory T cell			Markers (human)	Cytokines	Findings in pregnancy	Findings in complications of pregnancy
$CD8^+$	EM	General	$CD45RO^+$, $CD45RA^-$, $CD44^+$, CCR7-, CD62L-	Combination of cytokines produced by EM1, EM2, EM3, and EM4	- Higher proportions in peripheral blood postpartum compared to nulliparous women (30) - Higher proportion in decidua compared to peripheral blood (19, 22, 31) - Comparable proportions and $PD\text{-}1^+$ and $PDL\text{-}1^+$ proportions in peripheral blood in pregnant and non-pregnant women (30, 34) - Higher CD38 and HLA-DR expression in peripheral blood in 3rd trimester compared to non-pregnant women (34, 44) - Higher proportions of $IFN\text{-}gamma^+$ and $IL4^+$ in the decidua compared to peripheral blood (19, 22) - Higher expression of PD-1, Tim-3, CTLA-4, and LAG-3 in the decidua compared to peripheral blood (19, 45, 46) - Elevated gene expression in genes involved in chemotaxis, co-inhibitory receptors, T cell activation, galectin 1, and the IFN-gamma pathway, in decidua compared to peripheral blood (19, 46) - Comparable gene expression in decidua in 1st and 3rd trimester (46)	- Comparable proportions in peripheral blood in preeclampsia and healthy controls (32) - Higher proportions in peripheral blood in women with recurrent miscarriages compared to healthy controls (not specified CD4/CD8) (33)
		EM1	$CD45RO^+$, $CD45RA^-$, $CD44^+$, $CCR7^-$, $CD62L^-$, $CD27^+$, $CD28^+$, $CD127^+$	Granzyme K^+, Granzyme B^-, Perforin $^{+/-}$, $IFN\text{-}gamma^+$, $IL4^+$, $IL5^+$	- Higher proportions in the decidua compared to peripheral blood (19, 22)	- Comparable proportions in peripheral blood in preeclampsia and healthy controls (32) - Lower proportions in pregnant CMV+ women compared to pregnant CMV- women (44)
		EM2	$CD45RO^+$, $CD45RA^-$, $CD44^+$, $CCR7^-$, CD62L-, $CD27^+$, $CD28^-$, $CD94^+$	$Perforin^{+/-}$, Granzyme $B^{+/-}$, $IFN\text{-}gamma^+$	- Higher proportions in the decidua compared to peripheral blood (19, 22) Lower proportion of $perforin^+$ and granzyme B^+ in the decidua compared to peripheral blood (22, 47)	- Comparable proportions in peripheral blood in preeclampsia and healthy controls (32)
		EM3	$CD45RO^+$, $CD45RA^-$, $CD44^+$, $CCR7^-$, $CD62L^-$, $CD27^-$, $CD28^-$, $CD94^+$	$Perforin^+$, Granzyme B^+, $IFN\text{-}gamma^+$	- Higher proportions in the decidua compared to peripheral blood (19, 22) Lower proportion $perforin^+$ and granzyme B^+ in the decidua compared to peripheral blood (22, 47)	- Comparable proportions in peripheral blood in preeclampsia and healthy controls (32) - Higher proportions in pregnant CMV+ women compared to pregnant CMV- women (44)
		EM4	$CD45RO^+$, $CD45RA^-$,$CD44^+$, $CCR7^-$, $CD62L^-$, $CD27^-$, $CD28^+$, $CD127^+$	Granzyme K^+, Granzyme B^-, Perforin $^{+/-}$, $IFN\text{-}gamma^+$	- Higher proportions in the decidua compared to peripheral blood (19, 22)	- Comparable proportions in peripheral blood in preeclampsia and healthy controls (32) - Higher proportions in pregnant CMV+ women compared to pregnant CMV- women (44)
		TEMRA	$CD45RO^-$, $CD45RA^+$, $CCR7^-$, $CD62L^-$, $CD28^-$		- Higher proportions in the decidua compared to peripheral blood (22) Higher CD38 expression in peripheral blood in pregnancy compared to non-pregnant women (44)	- Higher proportions in pregnant CMV+ women compared to pregnant CMV- women (44)

(Continued)

TABLE 2 | Continued

Memory T cell	Markers (human)	Cytokines	Findings in pregnancy	Findings in complications of pregnancy
CM	$CD45RO^+$, $CD45RA^-$, $CD44^+$, $CCR7^+$, $CD62L^+$, $CD28^+$, $CD27^+$, $CD127^+$	$Perforin^-$, Granzyme B^-, IFN-$gamma^-$, $IL2^+$	- Low proportions in decidua, peripheral blood and menstrual blood (22, 31) - Higher proportions in peripheral blood compared to menstrual blood (31) - Comparable proportions and $CD38^+$, $CD28^+$, and $CD27^+$ proportions in peripheral blood in pregnant and non-pregnant women (23, 30, 34) - Higher HLA-DR^+ expression in peripheral blood in 3rd trimester compared to non-pregnant women (34)	- Comparable $CD28^+$ proportions in peripheral blood in preeclampsia and healthy controls (32) - Higher proportions in peripheral blood in women with recurrent miscarriages compared to healthy controls (not specified CD4/CD8) (33)
TRM	$CD45RO^+$, $CD45RA^-$, $CD103^{+/-}$, $CD69^+$, $CCR7^-$, $CD62L^-$, $CD49A^+$	Granzyme B^+, IFN-$gamma^+$, $perforins^+$	- Present in the reproductive tract (48, 49) - In the reproductive tract do not require IL15 for maintenance and work independently from $CD4^+$ cells (48–50)	- Comparable proportions in endometrial tissue from women with recurrent miscarriages compared to healthy controls (51)
Treg memory	Unknown	Unknown	- Not studied in pregnancy	- Not studied in pregnancy
FHM	$CD45RO^+$, $CXCR5^+$	$IL21^+$, $IL4^+$, IFN-$gamma^+$	- Not studied in pregnancy	- Not studied in pregnancy
Memory stem cell	$CD45RO^-$, $CD45RA^+$, $CCR7^+$, $CD62L^+$, $CD28^+$, $CD27^+$, $CD95^+$,	IFN-$gamma^+$, $IL2^+$	- Not studied in pregnancy	- Not studied in pregnancy

EM, effector memory; TEMRA, effector memory CD45RA revertant; CM, central memory; TRM, tissue resident memory; Treg, T regulatory; FHM, Follicular Helper Memory; CCR7, CC-chemokine receptor 7; CD62-L, L-selectin; CXCR5, chemokine receptor type 5; IFN-gamma, interferon-gamma; IL, interleukin; PD-1, programmed death-1; PDL-1, programmed death ligand-1; Tim-3, T cell immunoglobulin and mucin domain 3; CTLA-4, cytotoxic T lymphocyte antigen; LAG-3, lymphocyte activation gene 3; CMV, cytomegalovirus; HLA-DR, human leukocyte antigen-DR.

accumulation of CD4$^+$ EM cells in the decidua, although it can also be simply due to the fact that naive T cells do not accumulate in peripheral tissue (80). Important for the function of memory T cells is the expression of co-stimulatory molecules like CD28 (81). Such molecules are important for the recall response of memory T cells (82). Interestingly, within the CD4$^+$ EM cell population in the decidua, the proportion of the EM subset not expressing co-stimulatory molecules is highly increased compared to peripheral blood (19), suggesting that the CD4$^+$ EM cells in the decidua may not be able to mount a secondary response comparable to CD4$^+$ EM cells in peripheral blood. Despite this, increased IFN-gamma and IL4 expressions were found in decidual CD4$^+$ EM cells compared to CD4$^+$ EM cells in peripheral blood *in vitro* following mitogen stimulation (19). This may be related to the high local progesterone concentrations at the fetal maternal interface (19). The decidual EM cells were not only able to respond to mitogen stimulation, they were also able to respond to fetal antigens (19). The fact that the decidual EM cells are able to respond to fetal antigens and other stimuli suggests that there are extrinsic or intrinsic mechanisms at the fetal-maternal interface to suppress these cells. One of these mechanisms could be the presence of Treg cells (83, 84). Another mechanism may be the expression of immune inhibitory checkpoint receptors on decidual CD4$^+$ EM cells (19). Activation of these receptors inhibit immune responses to avoid autoimmunity and chronic inflammation (85). Increased expression of the immune inhibitory checkpoint receptors PD-1, T cell immunoglobulin and mucin domain 3 (Tim-3), cytotoxic T lymphocyte antigen 4 (CTLA-4), and lymphocyte activation gene 3 (LAG-3), on CD4$^+$ EM cells in the decidua was found as compared to peripheral blood (19). These findings are in line with Wang et al. who showed that the majority of CD4$^+$ EM cells (CD44$^+$CD62L$^-$) in first trimester decidual tissue from healthy terminated human pregnancies, expressed Tim-3 and PD-1 (86). A role for such immune inhibitory check point receptors in pregnancy has been shown in mouse studies (86). Blocking the Tim-3 and PD-1 pathway (not on CD4$^+$ EM cells specifically) in healthy pregnant mice showed that lower expression of Tim-3 and PD-1 increased fetal resorption rates (86). These studies propose a regulatory function for CD4$^+$ EM cells locally that could be favorable for fetal-maternal immune tolerance and prevent pregnancy loss.

The current data on CD4$^+$ EM cells in women with uncomplicated pregnancy outcomes show that during pregnancy CD4$^+$ EM cells may accumulate in the decidua and remain present at higher levels and higher activated proportions in peripheral blood postpartum (30). In addition, the CD4$^+$ EM cell population in the decidua has a different phenotype with increased IFN-gamma expression, however the CD4$^+$ EM cell population also has increased expression of immune inhibitory proteins compared to peripheral blood (19). To understand the relevance and function of CD4$^+$ EM cells in fetal-maternal tolerance and their role in the postpartum period, further research should focus on their general and more specifically on their antigen specific function, since none of the studies has shown antigen specific tolerance induction by CD4$^+$ EM cells yet.

Unfortunately, until now, CD4$^+$ EM cells have been hardly studied in complications of pregnancy. CD4$^+$ EM cells were studied in preeclampsia by Loewendorf et al. who performed flow cytometric analyses on peripheral blood and a swab from the intrauterine cavity during cesarean sections (32). They did not find differences in levels of CD4$^+$ EM cells between healthy and preeclamptic women in peripheral blood or in lymphocytes isolated from the intra uterine swab (32). However, since the specific tissue of origin of the cells from the swab cannot be defined, caution should be taken when interpreting these results. In non-pregnant women suffering recurrent spontaneous miscarriages, higher proportions of EM cells were observed in peripheral blood compared to non-pregnant fertile controls (33). This study did not further specify the CD4$^+$ or CD8$^+$ status or phenotype. With the proposed relevance of CD4$^+$ EM cells in fetal-maternal tolerance it would be of great value to gain knowledge on CD4$^+$ EM cells in complications of pregnancy.

CD4$^+$ Central Memory Cells in Pregnancy

CD4$^+$ CM cells circulate in the blood and are home to lymph nodes through expression of lymph node homing receptors CCR7 and CD62L (57–59). CD4$^+$ CM cells secrete IL2 and only very low levels of effector cell cytokines (28, 53). Upon secondary antigen exposure, or spontaneously, in the presence or absence of polarizing cytokines, CD4$^+$ CM cells differentiate into Th1, Th2, and CD4$^+$ EM cells, and produce effector cytokines as IFN-gamma and IL4 (53, 87–89). Furthermore, CM cells can quickly cause expansion of the antigen specific T cell population (89).

During pregnancy, as for CD4$^+$ EM cells, CD4$^+$ CM cells are studied mainly in the circulating blood and less at the fetal-maternal interface. One study looked at CD4$^+$ CM cells (CD45RA$^-$CCR7$^+$) in decidual tissue at the end of pregnancy and showed that proportions of CD4$^+$ CM cells were higher compared to peripheral blood from non-pregnant women (31). Another study evaluated first trimester decidual tissue from terminated healthy pregnancies, and showed that about 40% of CD4$^+$ CM cells (CD44$^+$CD62L$^+$) were Tim-3$^+$ and PD-1$^+$ (86). This appears to be a subset of CD4$^+$ EM cells that have a strong suppressive capacity on proliferation and preferentially produce Th2 type cytokines (86). Since blocking of PD-1 and Tim-3 in pregnancies in mice induced fetal loss (86), the Tim-3$^+$PD-1$^+$ CD4$^+$ EM cells may be important for maintaining normal pregnancy.

A number of studies in pregnancy observed that the proportions of CD4$^+$ CM cells (CD45RA$^-$CCR7$^+$) in peripheral blood are comparable between women in the second or third trimester of pregnancy and in healthy non-pregnant women (23, 30, 34). However, it seems that after pregnancy the CD4$^+$ CM cell proportions in peripheral blood are increased, since CD4$^+$ CM cells were higher in women after pregnancy compared to pregnant women and compared to women that have never been pregnant (30). Whether the CD4$^+$ CM cells are activated in the circulation of pregnant women remains to be established, since expression of the activation marker CD69 was higher during pregnancy as compared with non-pregnant women (30), whereas expression of the activation markers HLA-DR and CD38 was not affected in the CD4$^+$ CM cell population (CCR7$^+$CD45RO$^+$) in peripheral blood from 3rd trimester pregnant women compared to non-pregnant women (34). This higher $CD69^+$ proportion of $CD4^+$ CM cells in pregnancy remained high in women after pregnancy compared to women who have never been pregnant (30).

To date, $CD4^+$ CM cells are investigated in two complications of pregnancy, i.e., preeclampsia and miscarriages. In preeclampsia, slightly, but significantly higher proportions of $CD4^+$ CM cells ($CD45RO^+CCR7^+$) were found in peripheral blood from preeclamptic women compared to healthy pregnant women (32). Proportions of $CD4^+$ CM cells isolated from a swab from the intrauterine cavity during a cesarean section did not show differences between preeclamptic and healthy pregnant women (32). This study also analyzed expression of co-stimulatory molecules, CD28, CD27, and the survival receptor CD127 (IL7 receptor alpha chain), on $CD4^+$ CM cells (32). Only a difference in CD28 expression was found: in an intrauterine swab from preeclamptic women, $CD4^+$ CM cells expressed lower levels of CD28 compared to healthy pregnant women (32). In peripheral blood this difference was not observed (32). In women suffering from recurrent spontaneous miscarriages, higher levels of CM cells ($CD45RO^+CD62L^+$) have been found in peripheral blood compared to fertile women (33). It was not specified whether these CM cells were from the $CD4^+$ or the $CD8^+$ lineage. Part of this increase is likely due to $CD4^+$ CM cells, since another study reported higher levels of $CD4^+$ CM cells ($CD4^+CD45RA^-CCR7^+$) in peripheral blood from women suffering from recurrent miscarriages compared to women with proven fertility and women with no previous pregnancies (35).

As indicated above, Tim-3 and PD-1 expression on memory cells may be important for a healthy pregnancy. This suggestion is in line with the finding of decreased proportions of $Tim\text{-}3^+PD\text{-}1^+$ $CD4^+$ cells in decidua from patients who had undergone miscarriage (86). Unfortunately, these $CD4^+$ cells were not stained for memory cell markers. Further studies on $CD4^+$ CM cells in pregnancy complications in blood and at the fetal-maternal interface are needed in order to be able to show that these cells may play a role in the physiology of pregnancy and the pathophysiology of complications.

$CD4^+$ Regulatory Memory Cells in Pregnancy

Treg cells have potent immunosuppressive properties. They produce IL10 and transforming growth factor beta (TGFB), and have the capability of suppressing $CD4^+$, $CD8^+$, and B cell proliferation and cytokine secretion as well as inhibiting effects on dendritic cells and macrophages (90–93). It was long assumed that Treg cells did not survive the contraction phase of the immune response and undergo apoptotic cell death (64). Nevertheless, a long time surviving memory Treg cell subset has now been shown to persist after antigen exposure (12, 64, 94, 95). There is increasing evidence that memory Treg cells regulate the EM immune response on a secondary encounter with a memorized antigen (64). Treg memory function is implicated in many different pathological and physiological contexts such as auto-immune diseases (96), respiratory disorders (97), hepatitis (98), and pregnancy (12). Treg memory cells are complex to study, since no conclusive markers for a long-living Treg cell population are known (64). Identification of the Treg memory cell pool is therefore performed by combining Treg cell markers as [forkhead box p3 ($Foxp3^+$), $CD25^+$, and $CD127^-$ (99)] with memory cell markers [as $CD45RO^+$ and $CD45RA^-$ (52, 53)] (64).

In rodent models, Treg cells with fetal antigen specificity and a memory phenotype have been shown to accumulate in gestation and impact reproductive success in subsequent pregnancies (12, 39, 40). Rowe et al. developed a mouse model that demonstrated an increase of fetal antigen specific Treg memory cells at mid-gestation in first pregnancies that remained present at lower levels postpartum (12). The Treg memory cell population expanded substantially with accelerated kinetics in a following pregnancy as compared with the first pregnancy (12). This expansion resulted in decreased resorption rates compared to Treg memory cell ablated mice (12). The fetal antigen specific memory Treg cells, as shown by Rowe et al. seem important at mid gestation and it is hypothesized that they might be especially valuable in subsequent pregnancies to set boundaries for a secondary EM cell response toward paternal-fetal antigens (12). Chen et al. showed that in early gestation in mice (during implantation) self-antigen specific memory Treg cells and not fetal antigen specific memory Treg cells are recruited to the reproductive tract and create the tolerant environment for the implantation of the blastocyst (39).

Similar to mouse studies, in early pregnancy fetal maternal immune tolerance is probably not exclusively managed by memory Treg cells, since higher naive Treg cell subsets were associated with successful *in vitro* fertilization (IVF)/intracytoplasmic sperm injection (ICSI) treatment (37). Schlossberger et al. distinguished naive Treg ($CD45RA^+CD25^+Foxp3^+$) and memory Treg ($CD45RA^-CD25^+Foxp3^+$) subsets in blood samples from women undergoing IVF/ICSI treatment and observed higher proportions of naive Treg cells in women who became pregnant compared to the women who did not (37). This finding could indicate that in (preparation for) early pregnancy, higher levels of naive Treg cells are important for successful pregnancy. It could be speculated that these higher levels of naive Treg cells might be able to proliferate into antigen experienced memory Treg cells which are possibly beneficial in late pregnancy. This hypothesis needs to be tested in further studies, but would be in line with findings in mouse studies, in which the paternal antigen specific Treg memory cells were important at mid gestation (12).

The same group followed up on this study and showed that in healthy pregnant women, in early pregnancy (1st trimester) the decrease in naive Treg cells is most likely due to a decreased output of thymic Treg cells, since a decrease in recent thymic emigrant Treg cells was found in early pregnancy (38). They also showed that the increase in memory Treg cells in early pregnancy seems to be due to a differentiation of the recent thymic emigrant Treg cells, since an increased proportion of $CD45RA^-CD31^-$ memory Treg cells was found (38), which returned to normal non-pregnancy levels over the course of pregnancy (38). In line with their previous publication (37), this group showed again that the suppressive capacity of the naive Treg cells is increased during pregnancy and the suppressive capacity of the memory Treg cell population is decreased during pregnancy (38). At the end of pregnancy, the proportion of $CD4^+$ Treg memory cells ($CD45RA^-Foxp3^+$) in peripheral blood were present at comparable levels as in non-pregnant women (34, 38), which may suggest that memory Treg cells either undergo apoptotic cell death or reside in tissues toward the end of pregnancy. Thus, $CD4^+$ memory Treg cells are found to be favorable for pregnancy in mice, differentiate from recent thymic emigrant Treg cells in early human pregnancy, and circulate in peripheral blood. Studies on their presence and function at the fetal-maternal interface during pregnancy and studies postpartum and during a second pregnancy are lacking.

$Foxp3^+$ Treg cells are implicated in the pathophysiology of many complications of pregnancy as, preeclampsia (4, 100), recurrent miscarriage (101), and infertility (4, 102), however the potential role of the memory cell subset of the Treg cell population in different complications is not well studied. In preeclampsia, there was a decrease of naive Treg cells and an increase in memory Treg cells as compared with healthy pregnancy (32, 103). Although the naive Treg population in preeclampsia showed decreased suppressive activity compared with healthy pregnancy, this was not the case for the memory cell population (103). Further studies are needed to evaluate the role of the memory Treg population in preeclampsia.

In women with gestational diabetes, phenotypic characterization of memory Treg cell subsets showed that the proportion of naive Treg cells ($CD45RA^+HLA$-$DR^-CD127^+Foxp3^+$) was lower in women with gestational diabetes compared to healthy pregnant women, independently of whether diabetes was treated with a diet or insulin (41). The proportion of memory Treg cells, on the other hand, increased in gestational diabetes (41). Within the memory Treg cell population HLA-DR^+ and HLA-DR^- memory Treg cells are distinguished (104), in which HLA-DR^+ memory Treg cells have a more differentiated phenotype, are more suppressive and secrete lower amounts of pro-inflammatory cytokines as compared with HLA-DR^- memory Treg cells (104). Whereas, HLA-DR^- memory Treg cells were increased in gestational diabetes with dietary adjustment, HLA-DR^+ memory Treg cells were strongly increased in gestational diabetes treated with insulin therapy compared to healthy pregnant women (41). Whether this is an effect of the insulin treatment or a reflection of the pathophysiology of the disease is not known.

In summary, studies on memory Treg cells in complications of pregnancy show that memory Treg cells might be beneficial for reproductive success in subsequent pregnancies in mice (12), however human studies are inconclusive so far. The fact that some studies find higher memory Treg cell levels in pregnancy complications such as preeclampsia and gestational diabetes (32, 41, 103), whereas others find that lower levels prior to embryo transfer in IVF/ICSI treatment are associated with pregnancy success (37), could indicate specific roles depending on the phase of pregnancy. Identification of more conclusive markers for memory Treg cell function and longevity is a priority to fully elucidate the role of memory Treg cells in reproduction. In addition, since previous studies were mostly performed in peripheral blood, studies on memory Treg cells should also focus on the fetal-maternal interface, as it is known that memory T cells not only reside in peripheral tissues but also in the decidua (48, 74).

$CD4^+$ Follicular Helper Memory Cells in Pregnancy

$CD4^+$ follicular helper cells, which are located mainly in lymphoid organs and in particular in the germinal centers of lymphoid organs, also have a memory cell subset, called $CD4^+$ FHM cells (63, 105). They are known to assist B cells in their differentiation process and produce IL10 and IL21 (106). $CD4^+$ FHM cells are recognized by CXCR5, CD62L, CCR7, and Folate receptor 4 (FR4) (106). Contrary to the effector T follicular helper subset, $CD4^+$ FHM cells exhibit low B-cell lymphoma 6 (Bcl-6) expression (63, 106, 107). Bcl-6 is a transcriptional suppressor of GATA3, TBET, and RORGT, and is of major importance for T follicular helper functioning and maintenance (63). Within the $CD4^+$ FHM cell population, different $CD4^+$ FHM cell subsets can be distinguished based on PD-1, CCR7, and inducible T cell co-stimulator (ICOS) expression (63, 106, 107).

One mouse and one human study reported on $CD4^+$ FHM cells in pregnancy (42, 43). In mid gestation, in mice after allogeneic mating, T follicular helper cells ($CD4^+CXCR5^+PD$-$1^+/ICOS^+$) were shown to accumulate in the uterus and placenta (42). These $CD4^+$ T follicular helper cells could be $CD4^+$ FHM cells, since they showed an activated memory ($CD44^+$) phenotype. This putative $CD4^+$ FHM population increased abundantly toward late gestation, but this study also showed that programmed death ligand-1 (PDL-1) blockage induced abortion and increased the putative $CD4^+$ FHM cell accumulation even further (42). The study does suggest that $CD4^+$ FHM cells may be implicated in fetal-maternal tolerance and that excessive abundance might be associated with pregnancy loss (42).

In accordance with the suggestion that increased numbers of $CD4^+$ FHM cells may be implicated in pregnancy loss, a human study in recurrent miscarriage found higher decidual $CD4^+$ FHM cells ($CXCR5^+PD$-1^+CCR7^- and $CXCR5^+PD$-1^+ICOS^+) in spontaneous miscarriage decidual tissue compared to tissue from elective terminations in healthy women (43). In peripheral blood, the proportions of $CD4^+$ FHM cells ($CXCR5^+PD$-1^+CCR7^- and $CXCR5^+PD$-1^+ICOS^+) did not differ between the groups, implying a local response (43). In summary, the current data that exist on $CD4^+$ FHM cells in complications of pregnancy may suggest that pregnancy loss is associated with abundance of $CD4^+$ FHM cells. Thorough research is necessary to increase fundamental knowledge on the function of TFH memory cells in normal and complicated pregnancies.

$CD4^+$ Tissue Resident Memory Cells in Pregnancy

In the classification of memory T cells, $CD4^+$ TRM cells are distinguished from circulating cells (108, 109). Since no conclusive defining markers for the TRM cells from the $CD4^+$ compartment are known, they are difficult to investigate (62, 108,

109). Occasionally, the markers for CD8$^+$ TRM cells are used to study TRM cells in the CD4$^+$ compartment, although it is unclear whether this is correct (**Table 2**) (108, 109). To the best of our knowledge, no literature on CD4$^+$ TRM cells in reproduction is published yet.

CD4$^+$ Memory Stem Cells in Pregnancy

CD4$^+$ memory stem cells are a rare kind of memory T cell that cannot be classified according to the general differentiation of naive and memory cells using the CD45 isoforms (65). Long living cells with a naive phenotype (CD45RA$^+$CCR7$^+$CD27$^+$), but with antigen specificity and effector function, were shown in human blood years after Epstein Barr Virus infection (110). The so-called T memory stem cells exhibit almost all conventional memory cell like properties as high CXCR3, CD95, and IL2 receptor beta expression (65, 111), however they lack CD45RO expression and show similar recirculation patterns as naive T cells (65). Studies have shown that CD4$^+$ memory stem cells play a role in auto-immune diseases, Human Immunodeficiency Virus (HIV) and immune protection from a range of infections (65). To our knowledge, CD4$^+$ memory stem cells have not been studied in reproduction yet.

CD8$^+$ MEMORY CELLS IN PREGNANCY

Similar to CD4$^+$ memory cells, CD8$^+$ memory cell subsets are distinguished according to their migration pattern, cytokine secretion abilities, and protein expression (**Table 2**) (112–114). CD8$^+$ memory cells are divided in several subpopulations: CD8$^+$ effector memory cells (CD8$^+$ EM), CD8$^+$ central memory cells (CD8$^+$ CM), CD8$^+$ tissue resident memory cells (CD8$^+$ TRM), CD8$^+$ follicular helper memory cells (CD8$^+$ FHM), and CD8$^+$ memory stem cells (58–65, 115, 116). CD8$^+$ memory cells with regulatory properties are described, however there is no consensus on existence of a CD8$^+$ Treg memory subset (45). Most CD8$^+$ memory cells are generated from antigen experienced effector cells over the course of an immune response (113, 117, 118), however some CD8$^+$ memory cells may arise directly from naive T cells (119, 120). CD8$^+$ memory cells form the first line of defense in mucosal tissues and are able to produce effector cytokines and granzymes, IFN-gamma and perforin upon stimulation without the need for co-stimulatory signals (53, 121).

It has been known for many years that CD8$^+$ memory cells are present in the decidua during pregnancy (73). Higher CD45RO$^+$ proportions of CD8$^+$ cells were found in first trimester decidua compared to peripheral blood at the same time of pregnancy (72, 73). Furthermore, the proportion of CD8$^+$ memory (CD8$^+$CD45RO$^+$) cells in peripheral blood did not differ between pregnant and non-pregnant women (30, 73). In a further study, the CD8$^+$ memory T cell population was found to be influenced by seminal fluid (122). Using immunohistochemistry, CD8$^+$ memory cells (CD3$^+$CD8$^+$CD45RO$^+$) were shown to be increased in the stroma and epithelium of human cervix biopsies taken 12 h after unprotected coitus compared to biopsies after a period of abstinence and biopsies after coitus with condom use (122). Although this shows that memory CD8$^+$ cells are generated as a response toward seminal fluid, it is unknown whether these cells are specific to the paternal antigen. Furthermore, their role in preparation for pregnancy and fetal-maternal tolerance is not known. More recent studies have focused on evaluating the different CD8$^+$ memory cell subsets in reproduction. This is reviewed per subset below.

CD8$^+$ Effector Memory Cells in Pregnancy

CD8$^+$ EM cells express CD45RO, but lack CCR7 expression and are therefore bound to circulate in peripheral blood and non-lymphoid tissue (28, 112). CD8$^+$ EM cells rapidly produce effector cytokines as IL4, IL5, and IFN-gamma upon secondary encounter with the cognate antigen and therewith generate immediate protection (24). The CD8$^+$ EM cells express co-stimulatory molecules CD27 and CD28, which are gradually lost with differentiation of CD8$^+$ EM cells (47). Using these molecules, the CD8$^+$ EM cell population can be subdivided in 4 EM cell subtypes; i.e., EM1 (CD27$^+$CD28$^+$), EM2 (CD27$^+$CD28$^-$), EM3 (CD27$^-$CD28$^-$), and EM4 (CD27$^-$CD28$^+$) (**Table 2**) (47), with EM-1 being the most prominent in peripheral blood (about 70%) (47, 123). Next to a different immune phenotype, these subsets may exert different functions (47).

CD45RA expression on CD8$^+$ T cells is widely known to be lost on antigen exposure, however on one highly differentiated subpopulation of CD8$^+$ EM cells, CD45RA is again expressed despite previous antigen exposure (47, 121). These CD8$^+$ memory cells are terminally differentiated and called CD45RA revertant effector memory cells (CD8$^+$ TEMRA or sometimes abbreviated EMRA) (47, 121). CD8$^+$ TEMRA cells exhibit great cytolytic activity, but lack expansion abilities and CCR7 expression, disabling them to migrate to secondary lymphoid tissue (47, 121).

Increasing evidence shows that CD8$^+$ EM cells are involved in the establishment of functional immune tolerance toward the fetus (20, 46, 124). In peripheral blood, the total CD8$^+$ EM cell population was similar in healthy non-pregnant women compared to healthy pregnant women in the 2nd and 3rd trimesters (30, 34). Several studies showed an altered activation marker profile on CD8$^+$ EM cells in pregnancy. Higher expression of CD38$^+$ on CD8$^+$ EM (CD45RO$^+$CCR7$^-$) and CD8$^+$ TEMRA (CCR7$^-$CD45RA$^+$) cells was found in peripheral blood from pregnant women in the 3rd trimester compared to non-pregnant women (34, 44). Moreover, higher HLA-DR expression, but comparable CD69 expression, were found on CD8$^+$ EM cells (CD45RO$^+$CCR7$^-$) in peripheral blood in pregnant women compared to non-pregnant women (30, 34). Interestingly, although during pregnancy the proportions of CD8$^+$ EM cells in blood were not different from the proportion in non-pregnant women, higher proportions of CD8$^+$ EM cells (CD45RO$^+$CCR7$^-$) were found in peripheral blood from women postpartum compared to women who have never been pregnant (30). The higher expression of some of the activation markers on CD8$^+$ EM cells in pregnancy suggest that CD8$^+$ EM cells are activated in peripheral blood in pregnancy. A similar expression of inhibitory molecules PD-1 and PDL-1 on CD8$^+$ EM cells was found, suggesting that their effector function remains the same (23).

Approximately half of the $CD8^+$ cells in the decidua were found to be $CD8^+$ EM cells ($CD45RA^-CCR7^-$), which is about two-fold higher than the proportion of these cells in peripheral blood (19, 22, 31). This may be due to preferential accumulation of these cells in the decidua, but as for naive $CD4^+$ cells, it may also be due to the fact that naive $CD8^+$ cells do not accumulate in peripheral tissues (80). Not only does the proportion of $CD8^+$ EM cells differ between peripheral blood and the decidua, also substantial differences in phenotype, gene expression and function between these cells in peripheral blood and decidua have been observed (19, 22, 31, 46). $CD8^+$ EM cells ($CD45RA^-CCR7^-$) in the decidua have shown increased IFN-gamma and IL4 secretion abilities and reduced perforin and granzyme B expression compared to $CD8^+$ EM cells in peripheral blood (19, 22). Whether these specific functionalities of the decidual $CD8^+$ EM cells contribute to fetal-maternal immune tolerance remains to be established.

More evidence for altered functionality of $CD8^+$ EM cells in the decidua compared to peripheral blood was found by a study showing elevated expression of inhibitory check point receptors PD-1, Tim-3, CTLA-4, and LAG-3 on decidual $CD8^+$ EM cells compared to $CD8^+$ EM cells in peripheral blood (19, 45, 46). The higher Tim-3 and PD-1 expression on decidual $CD8^+$ T cells might be the result of interaction with trophoblasts, since co-culturing $CD8^+$ T cells with trophoblasts induced upregulation of Tim-3 and PD-1 (45), suggesting that trophoblasts may induce a function change, i.e., tolerance in $CD8^+$ EM cells in the decidua. In accordance with the increased expression of activation markers, inhibitory check point receptors, and cytokine production in decidual $CD8^+$ EM cells is the elevated gene-expression of several genes that was found in decidual $CD8^+$ EM cells compared to $CD8^+$ EM cells in peripheral blood (19, 46). Genes involved in chemotaxis, inhibitory receptors, T cell activation, Treg cell differentiation and genes associated with the IFN-gamma pathway were found higher in decidual $CD8^+$ EM cells compared to peripheral blood $CD8^+$ EM cells (19, 46). The different characteristics of decidual $CD8^+$ EM cells vs. peripheral blood $CD8^+$ EM cells might be beneficial for immune tolerance at the fetal maternal interface.

The question arises whether the changes in $CD8^+$ EM cells are due to the appearance of fetal specific $CD8^+$ EM cells. H HY tetramers are used to detect maternal T cells with specificity for Y-chromosome encoded HY-protein expressed by a male fetus (125). The proportion of HY-specific $CD8^+$ cells (not further specified which memory subtype) in peripheral blood in early pregnancy was 0.035% of the $CD8^+$ population, which almost tripled toward the end of pregnancy (10). The majority of the HY-specific $CD8^+$ memory cell population in peripheral blood and decidua showed an effector memory phenotype, being either $CD8^+$ EM ($CCR7^-CD45RA^-$) or $CD8^+$ TEMRA ($CD45RA^+CCR7^-$) (10, 125). Upon stimulation with male cells, the HY-specific T cells were cytotoxic and secreted IFN-gamma (10). The HY specific $CD8^+$ cells in the decidua expressed higher PD-1 and CD69 as compared with peripheral blood (19).

In preeclampsia, $CD8^+$ EM cell proportions and their CD27 and CD28 expression were comparable to $CD8^+$ EM cell proportions in healthy women in peripheral blood and in a swab from the intrauterine cavity (32). Contrary to preeclampsia, in non-pregnant women following recurrent spontaneous miscarriages, higher proportions of EM cells (not specified whether from the $CD4^+$ or $CD8^+$ cell compartment) were observed in peripheral blood compared to fertile non-pregnant controls (33). Lissauer et al. found that $CD8^+$ EM cell subsets are present at different proportions in pregnancy in women with latent CMV infection (44). They found that in CMV seropositive women the proportion of $CD8^+$ TEMRA cells ($CD45RA^+CCR7^-$) was higher and that the $CD8^+$ EM cell population was more differentiated with higher EM3 ($CD28^-CD27^-$) and EM4 $CD28^+CD27^-$) phenotypes and lower EM1 ($CD28^+CD27^+$) compared to CMV seronegative pregnant women (44). With the proposed important role for $CD8^+$ EM cells in successful pregnancies, it is worthwhile to investigate $CD8^+$ EM cells and their function in peripheral blood and in the decidua in complications of pregnancy to further evaluate their role in reproduction.

$CD8^+$ Central Memory Cells in Pregnancy

$CD8^+$ CM cells have little effector function and need to be converted to other cell types before effector functions can be induced (53, 112). In contrast to $CD8^+$ EM cells, they are highly proliferative upon stimulation and express the lymph node homing receptor CCR7, which allows these cells to migrate to secondary lymphoid tissue (57). $CD8^+$ CM cells have the ability to generate a diverse progeny, with different types of daughter cells like $CD8^+$ EM cells and effector cells (126). The main cytokine produced by $CD8^+$ CM cells is IL2, but they also produce low levels of IFN-gamma and TNF (112).

In reproduction, $CD8^+$ CM cells are less well studied than $CD8^+$ EM cells, this could be explained by their low prevalence, as the proportions of $CD8^+$ cells with a CM phenotype in the decidua and peripheral blood are low (about 5% of $CD8^+$ cells) (22, 30, 31). Three studies showed that $CD8^+$ CM cell proportions in peripheral blood are not altered by pregnancy (23, 30, 34). CD38, CD28, and CD27 expression on the $CD8^+$ CM cell population was also found to be similar in peripheral blood in pregnant and non-pregnant women (23), although HLA-DR expression on $CD8^+$ CM cells was found higher in peripheral blood from women in the third trimester compared to non-pregnant women (34). Investigation of male-fetus specific $CD8^+$ CM cells in peripheral blood using HY-dextramer staining, revealed that very low proportions of HY specific $CD8^+$ cells have a $CD8^+$ CM phenotype (10, 19). This could suggest that fetal antigens do not reach the secondary lymphoid tissue, less HY-specific $CD8^+$ CM cells develop, and less HY-specific $CD8^+$ CM cells recirculate into peripheral blood (10). Whether less HY-specific $CD8^+$ cells develop is not known.

Whether $CD8^+$ CM cells are present at different proportions in decidual tissue compared to peripheral blood remains to be established, since one study did not find differences, while another study found significantly lower $CD8^+$ CM cell ($CD45RA^-CCR7^+$) proportions in decidual tissue compared to peripheral blood (22, 31). A possible explanation for the discrepancy could be methodological, as only one of the studies used a viability stain. Granzyme B and perforin are very low expressed by $CD8^+$ CM cells and no differences have been found for granzyme B and perforin expression when comparing decidual and peripheral blood $CD8^+$ CM cells (22).

In preeclampsia, $CD8^+$ CM cell proportions and their CD28 and CD27 expression were comparable to the proportions in healthy women, both in peripheral blood and in a swab from the intrauterine cavity (32). In peripheral blood from non-pregnant women suffering from recurrent spontaneous miscarriage, higher proportions of $CD8^+$ CM cells ($CD45RO^+CD62L^+$) were found compared to non-pregnant fertile women (33). However, as $CD4^+$ or $CD8^+$ cell phenotype was not identified, it is not sure if this finding reflects a difference in $CD8^+$ CM cells.

$CD8^+$ Tissue Resident Memory T Cells in Pregnancy

Tissue resident memory (TRM) cells are a distinct subpopulation of $CD8^+$ memory cells which reside in peripheral tissues, including endometrium and decidua (49, 51). After the primary immune response, $CD8^+$ TRM cells reside in peripheral tissues awaiting a secondary encounter without recirculating in peripheral blood or lymph nodes (127–129). Upon reactivation, $CD8^+$ TRM cells produce IFN-gamma, granzyme B, and perforins (127). TRM cells are typically identified by the expression of different surface markers as CD103, CD69, and CD49A (127, 130–133). $CD8^+$ TRM cells are found in the entire reproductive tract and in contrast to $CD8^+$ TRM cells in the kidney, skin and salivary gland, do not require IL15 for maintenance of the cell population (48, 49, 134).

Next to this, $CD8^+$ TRM cells in the reproductive tract seem to be able to recruit circulating memory T cells, independently from their cognate antigen, into mucosal tissue of the reproductive tract and convert them to TRM cells (50). These data are suggestive of a well-functioning first line of defense of memory T cells in the reproductive tract. Presumably, TRM cells, $CD4^+$ or $CD8^+$, are the first memory T cells the male antigens on spermatozoa will encounter. Despite their presence in the reproductive tract, little information is available on their function and presence during pregnancy. One study looked at $CD8^+$ TRM in endometrial tissue and showed the presence of high proportions of memory $CD8^+$ cells in endometrial tissue, which was similar in women with recurrent miscarriages and control women (51). Part of these $CD8^+$ memory T cells expressed CD103, indicating that the cells may be $CD8^+$ TRM cells (51). The proportion of $CD8^+$ memory cells expressing CD103 was similar in women with recurrent miscarriages and control women (51). However, the percentage of $CD8^+$ memory cells expressing CD69, a TRM marker, was decreased in women with recurrent miscarriages as compared with control women (51). This might suggest a decrease in $CD8^+$ TRM cells in women with recurrent miscarriage.

$CD8^+$ Regulatory Memory, $CD8^+$ Follicular Helper Memory, and $CD8^+$ Memory Stem Cells in Pregnancy

The regulatory memory, follicular helper memory, and the memory stem cell subsets are relatively well studied in the $CD4^+$ cell compartment but only to a limited extent in the $CD8^+$ cell compartment. $CD8^+$ cells with immune regulatory abilities are described in literature (135–137), however, the existence of a memory cell subset within the $CD8^+$ Treg cell population is still uncertain (45). $CD8^+$ cells with expression of follicular helper cell marker CXCR5, and memory cell marker CD45RO, are identified in germinal centers of human tonsils, and were found to support B cells (116, 138). The presence of such $CD8^+$ follicular helper memory cells are only very recently confirmed and are not studied in pregnancy yet (116). $CD8^+$ memory stem cells, as for their $CD4^+$ counterpart, are antigen specific memory cells with a naive phenotype and are mostly studied in oncology settings (115, 139–141). Research on $CD8^+$ regulatory memory, $CD8^+$ FHM, and $CD8^+$ memory stem cells in pregnancy will be of interest, but more knowledge on their functioning in general is needed before studying their role in reproduction.

MEMORY T CELLS IN PREGNANCY AS POSSIBLE THERAPEUTIC TARGETS

Literature shows that memory T cells are likely implicated in fetal-maternal tolerance before, during and after pregnancy. Firstly, it has been shown that exposure to seminal fluid before pregnancy induces a memory T cell population in the ectocervix (122). Even though there is no evidence yet that these memory cells are paternal-antigen specific, this could be a mechanism that contributes to tolerance toward paternal-fetal antigens. This mechanism is supported by existing epidemiologic data showing an association between a longer period of exposure to seminal fluid of the future father and a lower risk of preeclampsia (142–144). Generating paternal specific memory T cells as a therapeutic target, through paternal cell immunization before conception seems obvious and has indeed been carried out by several studies (145, 146). Studies are however small, but a meta-analysis of 7 small studies showed an improvement in clinical pregnancy rate following IVF treatment when seminal plasma is used as an adjunct treatment (average pregnancy rate increased from 25% in the control group to 29% in the seminal plasma treated group), with no significant increases in live birth or ongoing pregnancy rate (146). Since in these studies, timed intercourse or deposition of untreated semen in the vagina before IVF was used, it is not known whether the positive effect of semen is due to the seminal plasma itself or to paternal-fetal antigen exposure. This should be subject of future research. In order to potentially achieve better results, additional options for priming may be tested. An additional option could be a prime and pull method, by first eliciting an immune response to recruit T cells into the reproductive tract, followed by topical vaccination, a method that has been shown to be effective in genital herpes prevention (147).

Secondly, this review indicates that tolerance mechanisms involving memory T cells are in place during pregnancy. Various alterations in memory T cell function and levels have been shown, which together likely ensure tolerance; for instance, $CD4^+$ Treg memory cells may play an important role, while also low responsive $PD\text{-}1^+Tim\text{-}3^+$ $CD8^+$ memory cells are present at the fetal-maternal interface, which may also be important. These different tolerating mechanisms and their interactions should be further investigated, while it is also important to focus on their alterations in complications of pregnancy. The lack of knowledge on these mechanisms in healthy pregnancy and how they are affected in complications of pregnancy, makes therapeutic options using immune modulation of memory T cells to treat pregnancy complications not feasible yet.

Thirdly, after pregnancy, maternal immune cells are exposed to fetal-paternal antigens through microchimerism and possibly through semen exposure (8, 9). Since $CD4^+$ memory T cells are known to require low-levels of antigen exposure for long term maintenance (60, 148, 149), it is proposed that microchimerism and semen exposure are ways to ensure persistence of the fetal-paternal specific $CD4^+$ memory cell population (150–152). Thorough investigations on possible beneficial effects of memory T cells on reproductive success and of microchimerism on memory T cell populations should point out whether this could bring forward another possible therapeutic target. Lowering pregnancy complication rates through priming and enhancing the maternal memory T cell repertoire in parous women could be considered for future therapies. These could involve similar approaches as therapeutic options before pregnancy.

CONCLUSIONS

To conclude, a delicate balance of memory T cells seems necessary for successful pregnancy and memory T cells might not be harmful for pregnancy, but in fact, they may induce tolerance. Memory T cells show different phenotypes, dynamics, and functioning in uncomplicated pregnancies compared to memory T cells outside the reproductive context. Together, these mechanisms may induce tolerance toward fetal antigens during pregnancy. More research on memory T cells in pregnancy is needed to better understand the function of these cells in pregnancy and to develop therapeutic strategies for pregnancy complications based on memory T cells.

AUTHOR CONTRIBUTIONS

TK organized financial support, built the search strategy, performed the literature study, and wrote the first draft of the manuscript. AL organized financial support, built the search strategy, performed the literature study, and reviewed and edited the manuscript. SS, MF, and JP reviewed and edited the manuscript, organized financial support, and supervised the project.

FUNDING

This study was funded by the University Medical Center Groningen, the University of Groningen, Junior Scientific Masterclass MD/PhD grants (awarded to TK and AL) and a Mandema Stipendium So: (awarded to JP).

REFERENCES

1. Cudihy D, Lee R. The pathophysiology of pre-eclampsia: current clinical concepts. *J Obstet Gynaecol.* (2009) 29:576–82. doi: 10.1080/01443610903061751
2. Larsen EC, Christiansen OB, Kolte AM, Macklon N. New insights into mechanisms behind miscarriage. *BMC Med.* (2013) 11:154. doi: 10.1186/1741-7015-11-154
3. Zenclussen AC. Adaptive immune responses during pregnancy. *Am J Reprod Immunol.* (2013) 69:291–303. doi: 10.1111/aji.12097; 10.1111/aji.12097
4. Guerin LR, Prins JR, Robertson SA. Regulatory T-cells and immune tolerance in pregnancy: a new target for infertility treatment? *Hum Reprod Update.* (2009) 15:517–35. doi: 10.1093/humupd/dmp004
5. Robertson SA, Guerin LR, Bromfield JJ, Branson KM, Ahlström AC, Care AS. Seminal fluid drives expansion of the CD4+CD25+ T regulatory cell pool and induces tolerance to paternal alloantigens in mice. *Biol Reprod.* (2009) 80:1036–45. doi: 10.1095/biolreprod.108.074658
6. Lo YM, Lo ES, Watson N, Noakes L, Sargent IL, Thilaganathan B, et al. Two-way cell traffic between mother and fetus: biologic and clinical implications. *Blood.* (1996) 88:4390–5.
7. Arck PC, Hecher K. Fetomaternal immune cross-talk and its consequences for maternal and offspring's health. *Nat Med.* (2013) 99:548–56. doi: 10.1038/nm.3160
8. Bianchi DW, Zickwolf GK, Weil GJ, Sylvester S, DeMaria MA. Male fetal progenitor cells persist in maternal blood for as long as 27 years postpartum. *Proc Natl Acad Sci USA.* (1996) 93:705–8. doi: 10.1073/pnas.93.2.705
9. Nelson JL. Your cells are my cells. *Sci Am.* (2008) 298:64–71. doi: 10.1038/scientificamerican1208-64
10. Lissauer D, Piper K, Goodyear O, Kilby MD, Moss PAH. Fetal-specific CD8+ cytotoxic T cell responses develop during normal human pregnancy and exhibit broad functional capacity. *J Immunol.* (2012) 189:1072–80. doi: 10.4049/jimmunol.1200544
11. Kahn DA, Baltimore D. Pregnancy induces a fetal antigen-specific maternal T regulatory cell response that contributes to tolerance. *Proc Natl Acad Sci USA.* (2010) 107:9299–304. doi: 10.1073/pnas.1003909107
12. Rowe JH, Ertelt JM, Xin L, Way SS. Pregnancy imprints regulatory memory that sustains anergy to fetal antigen. *Nature.* (2012) 490:102–6. doi: 10.1038/nature11462
13. Wakim LM, Bevan MJ. From the thymus to longevity in the periphery. *Curr Opin Immunol.* (2010) 22:274–8. doi: 10.1016/j.coi.2010.03.003
14. Kurosaki T, Kometani K, Ise W. Memory B cells. *Nat Rev Immunol.* (2015) 15:149–59. doi: 10.1038/nri3802
15. Ahmed R, Gray D. Immunological memory and protective immunity: understanding their relation. *Science.* (1996) 272:54–60.
16. Sallusto F, Lanzavecchia A, Araki K, Ahmed R. From vaccines to memory and back. *Immunity.* (2010) 33:451–63. doi: 10.1016/j.immuni.2010.10.008
17. Larché M, Wraith DC. Peptide-based therapeutic vaccines for allergic and autoimmune diseases. *Nat Med.* (2005) 11:S69–76. doi: 10.1038/nm1226
18. Lollini PL, Cavallo F, Nanni P, Forni G. Vaccines for tumour prevention. *Nat Rev Cancer.* (2006) 6:204–16. doi: 10.1038/nrc1815
19. Powell RM, Lissauer D, Tamblyn J, Beggs A, Cox P, Moss P, et al. Decidual T cells exhibit a highly differentiated phenotype and demonstrate potential

fetal specificity and a strong transcriptional response to IFN. *J Immunol.* (2017) 199:3406–17. doi: 10.4049/jimmunol.1700114
20. Tilburgs T, Strominger JL. CD8+ Effector T cells at the fetal-maternal interface, balancing fetal tolerance and antiviral immunity. *Am J Reprod Immunol.* (2013) 69:395–407. doi: 10.1111/aji.12094
21. Barton BM, Xu R, Wherry EJ, Porrett PM. Pregnancy promotes tolerance to future offspring by programming selective dysfunction in long-lived maternal T cells. *J Leukoc Biol.* (2017) 101:975–87. doi: 10.1189/jlb.1A0316-135R
22. Tilburgs T, Schonkeren D, Eikmans M, Nagtzaam NM, Datema G, Swings GM, et al. Human decidual tissue contains differentiated CD8+ effector-memory T cells with unique properties. *J Immunol.* (2010) 185:4470–7. doi: 10.4049/jimmunol.0903597
23. Shah NM, Herasimtschuk AA, Boasso A, Benlahrech A, Fuchs D, Imami N, et al. Changes in T cell and dendritic cell phenotype from mid to late pregnancy are indicative of a shift from immune tolerance to immune activation. *Front Immunol.* (2017) 8:1138. doi: 10.3389/fimmu.2017.01138
24. Lanzavecchia A, Sallusto F, Lanzavecchia Federica AS, Lanzavecchia A, Sallusto F. Understanding the generation and function of memory T cell subsets. *Curr Opin Immunol.* (2005) 17:326–32. doi: 10.1016/j.coi.2005.04.010
25. Rudolph MG, Stanfield RL, Wilson IA. How TCRS bind MHCS, peptides, and coreceptors. *Annu Rev Immunol.* (2006) 24:419–66. doi: 10.1146/annurev.immunol.23.021704.115658
26. Sharpe AH. Mechanisms of costimulation. *Immunol Rev.* (2009) 229:5–11. doi: 10.1111/j.1600-065X.2009.00784.x
27. Zhu J, Paul WE. CD4 T cells: fates, functions, and faults. *Blood.* (2008) 112:1557–69. doi: 10.1182/blood-2008-05-078154
28. Mueller SN, Gebhardt T, Carbone FR, Heath WR. Memory T cell subsets, migration patterns, and tissue residence. *Annu Rev Immunol.* (2013) 31:137–61. doi: 10.1146/annurev-immunol-032712-095954
29. Obar JJ, Lefrançois L. Memory CD8+ T cell differentiation. *Ann N Y Acad Sci.* (2010) 1183:251–66. doi: 10.1111/j.1749-6632.2009.05126.x
30. Kieffer TEC, Faas MM, Scherjon SA, Prins JR. Pregnancy persistently affects memory T cell populations. *J Reprod Immunol.* (2017) 119:1–8. doi: 10.1016/j.jri.2016.11.004
31. Feyaerts D, Benner M, van Cranenbroek B, van der Heijden OWH, Joosten I, van der Molen RG. Human uterine lymphocytes acquire a more experienced and tolerogenic phenotype during pregnancy. *Sci Rep.* (2017) 7:2884. doi: 10.1038/s41598-017-03191-0
32. Nguyen TA, Kahn DA, Loewendorf AI. Maternal—fetal rejection reactions are unconstrained in preeclamptic women. *PLoS ONE.* (2017) 12:e0188250. doi: 10.1371/journal.pone.0188250
33. Ramhorst R, Garcia V, Agriello E, Corigliano A, Etchepareborda E, Irigoyen M, et al. Intracellular expression of CD69 in endometrial and peripheral T cells represents a useful marker in women with recurrent miscarriage: Modulation after allogeneic leukocyte immunotherapy. *Am J Reprod Immunol.* (2003) 49:149–58. doi: 10.1034/j.1600-0897.2003.00021.x
34. Loewendorf AI, Nguyen TA, Yesayan MN, Kahn DA. Normal human pregnancy results in maternal immune activation in the periphery and at the uteroplacental interface. *PLoS ONE.* (2014) 9:e96723. doi: 10.1371/journal.pone.0096723
35. Carbone J, Sarmiento E, Gallego A, Lanio N, Navarro J, García S, et al. Peripheral blood T- and B-cell immunophenotypic abnormalities in selected women with unexplained recurrent miscarriage. *J Reprod Immunol.* (2016) 113:50–3. doi: 10.1016/j.jri.2015.11.003
36. Tilburgs T, Roelen D, van der Mast B, de Groot-Swings G, Kleijburg C, Scherjon SA, et al. Evidence for a selective migration of fetus-specific CD4+CD25bright regulatory T cells from the peripheral blood to the decidua in human pregnancy. *J Immunol.* (2008) 180:5737–45. doi: 10.4049/jimmunol.180.8.5737
37. Schlossberger V, Schober L, Rehnitz J, Schaier M, Zeier M, Meuer S, et al. The success of assisted reproduction technologies in relation to composition of the total regulatory T cell (Treg) pool and different Treg subsets. *Hum Reprod.* (2013) 28:3062–73. doi: 10.1093/humrep/det316
38. Wagner MI, Mai C, Schmitt E, Mahnke K, Meuer S, Eckstein V, et al. The role of recent thymic emigrant-regulatory T-cell (RTE-Treg) differentiation during pregnancy. *Immunol Cell Biol.* (2015) 93:858–67. doi: 10.1038/icb.2015.51
39. Chen T, Darrasse-Jeze G, Bergot A-S, Courau T, Churlaud G, Valdivia K, et al. Self-specific memory regulatory T cells protect embryos at implantation in mice. *J Immunol.* (2013) 191:2273–81. doi: 10.1016/j.micinf.2011.07.011.Innate
40. Kalekar LA, Schmiel SE, Nandiwada SL, Lam WY, Barsness LO, Zhang N, et al. CD4+ T cell anergy prevents autoimmunity and generates regulatory T cell precursors. *Nat Immunol.* (2016) 17:304–14. doi: 10.1038/ni.3331
41. Schober L, Radnai D, Spratte J, Kisielewicz A, Schmitt E, Mahnke K, et al. The role of regulatory T cell (Treg) subsets in gestational diabetes mellitus. *Clin Exp Immunol.* (2014) 177:76–85. doi: 10.1111/cei.12300
42. Zeng W, Liu Z, Zhang S, Ren J, Ma X, Qin C, et al. Characterization of T follicular helper cells in allogeneic normal pregnancy and PDL1 blockage-induced abortion. *Sci Rep.* (2016) 6:36560. doi: 10.1038/srep36560
43. Luan X, Kang X, Li W, Dong Q. An investigation of the relationship between recurrent spontaneous abortion and memory T follicular helper cells. *Am J Reprod Immunol.* (2017) 78:e12714. doi: 10.1111/aji.12714
44. Lissauer D, Choudhary M, Pachnio A, Goodyear O, Moss PAH, Kilby MD. Cytomegalovirus sero positivity dramatically alters the maternal CD8 T cell repertoire and leads to the accumulation of highly differentiated memory cells during human pregnancy. *Hum Reprod.* (2011) 26:3355–65. doi: 10.1093/humrep/der327
45. Wang S, Li Y, Piao H, Hong X, Zhang D, Xu Y, et al. PD-1 and Tim-3 pathways are associated with regulatory CD8+ T-cell function in decidua and maintenance of normal pregnancy. *Cell Death Dis.* (2015) 6:e1738. doi: 10.1038/cddis.2015.112
46. van der Zwan A, Bi K, Norwitz ER, Crespo ÂC, Claas FHJ, Strominger JL, et al. Mixed signature of activation and dysfunction allows human decidual CD8+ T cells to provide both tolerance and immunity. *Proc Natl Acad Sci USA.* (2018) 115:385–90. doi: 10.1073/pnas.1713957115
47. Romero P, Zippelius A, Kurth I, Pittet MJ, Touvrey C, Iancu EM, et al. Four functionally distinct populations of human effector-memory CD8+ T lymphocytes. *J Immunol.* (2007) 178:4112–9. doi: 10.4049/JIMMUNOL.178.7.4112
48. Schenkel JM, Masopust D. Tissue-resident memory T cells. *Immunity.* (2014) 41:886–97. doi: 10.1016/j.immuni.2014.12.007
49. Casey KA, Fraser KA, Schenkel JM, Moran A, Abt MC, Beura LK, et al. Antigen-independent differentiation and maintenance of effector-like resident memory T cells in tissues. *J Immunol.* (2012) 188:4866–75. doi: 10.4049/jimmunol.1200402
50. Beura LK, Mitchell JS, Thompson EA, Schenkel JM, Mohammed J, Wijeyesinghe S, et al. Intravital mucosal imaging of CD8+ resident memory T cells shows tissue-autonomous recall responses that amplify secondary memory article. *Nat Immunol.* (2018) 19:173–82. doi: 10.1038/s41590-017-0029-3
51. Southcombe JH, Mounce G, McGee K, Elghajiji A, Brosens J, Quenby S, et al. An altered endometrial CD8 tissue resident memory T cell population in recurrent miscarriage. *Sci Rep.* (2017) 7:41335. doi: 10.1038/srep41335
52. Michie CA, McLean A, Alcock C, Beverley PCL. Lifespan of human lymphocyte subsets defined by CD45 isoforms. *Nature.* (1992) 360:264–5. doi: 10.1038/360264a0
53. Sallusto F, Geginat J, Lanzavecchia A. Central memory and effector memory T cell subsets: function, generation, and maintenance. *Annu Rev Immunol.* (2004) 22:745–63. doi: 10.1146/annurev.immunol.22.012703.104702
54. Booth NJ, McQuaid AJ, Sobande T, Kissane S, Agius E, Jackson SE, et al. Different proliferative potential and migratory characteristics of human CD4+ regulatory T cells that express either CD45RA or CD45RO. *J Immunol.* (2010) 184:4317–26. doi: 10.4049/jimmunol.0903781
55. Henson SM, Riddell NE, Akbar AN. Properties of end-stage human T cells defined by CD45RA re-expression. *Curr Opin Immunol.* (2012) 24:476–81. doi: 10.1016/j.coi.2012.04.001
56. Dunne PJ, Belaramani L, Fletcher JM, Fernandez de Mattos S, Lawrenz M, Soares MVD, et al. Quiescence and functional reprogramming of Epstein-Barr virus (EBV)-specific CD8+ T cells during persistent infection. *Blood.* (2005) 106:558–65. doi: 10.1182/blood-2004-11-4469
57. Förster R, Schubel A, Breitfeld D, Kremmer E, Renner-Müller I, Wolf E, et al. CCR7 coordinates the primary immune response by establishing functional

microenvironments in secondary lymphoid organs. *Cell.* (1999) 99:23–33. doi: 10.1016/S0092-8674(00)80059-8
58. Cyster JG. Chemokines, sphingosine-1-phosphate, and cell migration in secondary lymphoid organs. *Annu Rev Immunol.* (2005) 23:127–59. doi: 10.1146/annurev.immunol.23.021704.115628
59. Reinhardt RL, Khoruts A, Merica R, Zell T, Jenkins MK. Visualizing the generation of memory CD4 T cells in the whole body. *Nature.* (2001) 410:101–5. doi: 10.1038/35065111
60. Seder RA, Ahmed R. Similarities and differences in CD4+ and CD8+ effector and memory T cell generation. *Nat Immunol.* (2003) 4:835–42. doi: 10.1038/ni969
61. Gebhardt T, Whitney PG, Zaid A, Mackay LK, Brooks AG, Heath WR, et al. Different patterns of peripheral migration by memory CD4+ and CD8+ T cells. *Nature.* (2011) 477:216–9. doi: 10.1038/nature10339
62. Clark RA, Watanabe R, Teague JE, Schlapbach C, Tawa MC, Adams N, et al. Skin effector memory T cells do not recirculate and provide immune protection in alemtuzumab-treated CTCL patients. *Sci Transl Med.* (2012) 4:117ra7. doi: 10.1126/scitranslmed.3003008
63. Hale JS, Ahmed R. Memory T follicular helper CD4 T cells. *Front Immunol.* (2015) 6:16. doi: 10.3389/fimmu.2015.00016
64. Rosenblum MD, Way SS, Abbas AK. Regulatory T cell memory. *Nat. Rev. Immunol.* (2015) 1:1–12. doi: 10.1038/nri.2015.1
65. Gattinoni L, Lugli E, Ji Y, Pos Z, Paulos CM, Quigley MF, et al. A human memory T cell subset with stem cell-like properties. *Nat Med.* (2011) 17:1290–7. doi: 10.1038/nm.2446
66. Matthiesen L, Berg G, Ernerudh J, Håkansson L. Lymphocyte subsets and mitogen stimulation of blood lymphocytes in normal pregnancy. *Am J Reprod Immunol.* (1996) 35:70–9. doi: 10.1111/j.1600-0897.1996.tb00010.x
67. Chaiworapongsa T, Gervasi MT, Refuerzo J, Espinoza J, Yoshimatsu J, Berman S, et al. Maternal lymphocyte subpopulations (CD45RA+ and CD45RO+) in preeclampsia. *Am J Obstet Gynecol.* (2002) 187:889–93. doi: 10.1067/mob.2002.127309
68. Darmochwal-Kolarz D, Saito S, Rolinski J, Tabarkiewicz J, Kolarz B, Leszczynska-Gorzelak B, et al. Activated T lymphocytes in pre-eclampsia. *Am J Reprod Immunol.* (2007) 58:39–45. doi: 10.1111/j.1600-0897.2007.00489.x
69. Matthiesen L, Berg G, Ernerudh J, Skogh T. Lymphocyte subsets and autoantibodies in pregnancies complicated by placental disorders. *Am J Reprod Immunol.* (1995) 33:31–9. doi: 10.1111/j.1600-0897.1995.tb01135.x
70. Mahmoud FF, Haines DD, Abul HT, Omu AE, Abu-Donia MB. Butyrylcholinesterase activity in gestational diabetes: correlation with lymphocyte subpopulations in peripheral blood. *Am J Reprod Immunol.* (2006) 56:185–92. doi: 10.1111/j.1600-0897.2006.00416.x
71. Oleszczuk J, Darmochwal-Kolarz D, Leszczynska-Gorzelak B, Rolinski J. Alterations in the immune system of patients with imminent preterm labour. *Gynecol Obstet Invest.* (2000) 49:110–3. doi: 10.1159/000010226
72. Slukvin II, Merkulova AA, Vodyanik MA, Chernyshov VP. Differential expression of CD45RA and CD45RO molecules on human decidual and peripheral blood lymphocytes at early stage of pregnancy. *Am J Reprod Immunol.* (1996) 35:16–22.
73. Saito S, Nishikawa K, Morii T, Narita N, Enomoto M, Ito A, et al. A study of CD45RO, CD45RA and CD29 antigen expression on human decidual T cells in an early stage of pregnancy. *Immunol Lett.* (1994) 40:193–7. doi: 10.1016/0165-2478(93)00019-A
74. Gomez-Lopez N, Vega-Sanchez R, Castillo-Castrejon M, Romero R, Cubeiro-Arreola K, Vadillo-Ortega F. Evidence for a role for the adaptive immune response in human term parturition. *Am J Reprod Immunol.* (2013) 69:212–30. doi: 10.1111/aji.12074
75. Pepper M, Linehan JL, Pagán AJ, Zell T, Dileepan T, Cleary PP, et al. Different routes of bacterial infection induce long-lived TH1 memory cells and short-lived TH17 cells. *Nat Immunol.* (2010) 11:83–9. doi: 10.1038/ni.1826
76. Harrington LE, Janowski KM, Oliver JR, Zajac AJ, Weaver CT. Memory CD4 T cells emerge from effector T-cell progenitors. *Nature.* (2008) 452:356–60. doi: 10.1038/nature06672
77. Pepper M, Jenkins MK. Origins of CD4(+) effector and central memory T cells. *Nat Immunol.* (2011) 12:467–71. doi: 10.1038/ni.2038
78. MacLeod MKL, Kappler JW, Marrack P. Memory CD4 T cells: generation, reactivation and re-assignment. *Immunology.* (2010) 130:10–5. doi: 10.1111/j.1365-2567.2010.03260.x
79. Tian Y, Babor M, Lane J, Schulten V, Patil VS, Seumois G, et al. Unique phenotypes and clonal expansions of human CD4 effector memory T cells re-expressing CD45RA. *Nat Commun.* (2017) 8:1473. doi: 10.1038/s41467-017-01728-5
80. Mueller DL. Mechanisms maintaining peripheral tolerance. *Nat Immunol.* (2010) 11:21–7. doi: 10.1038/ni.1817
81. Esensten JH, Helou YA, Chopra G, Weiss A, Bluestone JA. CD28 Costimulation: from mechanism to therapy. *Immunity.* (2016) 44:973–88. doi: 10.1016/j.immuni.2016.04.020
82. Langenhorst D, Haack S, Göb S, Uri A, Lühder F, Vanhove B, et al. CD28 Costimulation of T helper 1 cells enhances cytokine release *in vivo. Front Immunol.* (2018) 9:1060. doi: 10.3389/fimmu.2018.01060
83. Sasaki Y. Decidual and peripheral blood CD4+CD25+ regulatory T cells in early pregnancy subjects and spontaneous abortion cases. *Mol Hum Reprod.* (2004) 10:347–53. doi: 10.1093/molehr/gah044
84. Tilburgs T, Roelen DL, van der Mast BJ, van Schip JJ, Kleijburg C, de Groot-Swings GM, et al. Differential distribution of CD4+CD25bright and CD8+CD28- T-cells in decidua and maternal blood during human pregnancy. *Placenta.* (2006) 27:47–53. doi: 10.1016/j.placenta.2005.11.008
85. Dyck L, Mills KHG. Immune checkpoints and their inhibition in cancer and infectious diseases. *Eur J Immunol.* (2017) 47:765–79. doi: 10.1002/eji.201646875
86. Wang S, Zhu X, Xu Y, Zhang D, Li Y, Tao Y, et al. Programmed cell death-1 (PD-1) and T-cell immunoglobulin mucin-3 (Tim-3) regulate CD4+ T cells to induce Type 2 helper T cell (Th2) bias at the maternal-fetal interface. *Hum Reprod.* (2016) 31:700–11. doi: 10.1093/humrep/dew019
87. Rivino L, Messi M, Jarrossay D, Lanzavecchia A, Sallusto F, Geginat J. Chemokine receptor expression identifies pre–T helper (Th)1, Pre–Th2, and nonpolarized cells among human CD4$^+$ central memory T cells. *J Exp Med.* (2004) 200:725–35. doi: 10.1084/jem.20040774
88. Zaph C, Uzonna J, Beverley SM, Scott P. Central memory T cells mediate long-term immunity to Leishmania major in the absence of persistent parasites. *Nat Med.* (2004) 10:1104–10. doi: 10.1038/nm1108
89. Gray JI, Westerhof LM, MacLeod MKL. The roles of resident, central and effector memory CD4 T-cells in protective immunity following infection or vaccination. *Immunology.* (2018) 154:574–81. doi: 10.1111/imm.12929
90. Piccirillo CA, Shevach EM. Cutting edge: control of CD8+ T cell activation by CD4+CD25+ immunoregulatory cells. *J Immunol.* (2001) 167:1137–40. doi: 10.4049/jimmunol.167.3.1137
91. Lim HW, Hillsamer P, Banham AH, Kim CH. Cutting edge: direct suppression of B cells by CD4+ CD25+ regulatory T cells. *J Immunol.* (2005) 175:4180–3. doi: 10.4049/jimmunol.175.7.4180
92. Misra N, Bayry J, Lacroix-Desmazes S, Kazatchkine MD, Kaveri, SV. Cutting edge: human CD4+CD25+ T cells restrain the maturation and antigen-presenting function of dendritic cells. *J Immunol.* (2004) 172:4676–80. doi: 10.4049/jimmunol.172.8.4676
93. Taams LS, van Amelsfort JMR, Tiemessen MM, Jacobs KMG, de Jong EC, Akbar AN, et al. Modulation of monocyte/macrophage function by human CD4+CD25+ regulatory T cells. *Hum Immunol.* (2005) 66:222–30. doi: 10.1016/j.humimm.2004.12.006
94. Brincks EL, Roberts AD, Cookenham T, Sell S, Kohlmeier JE, Blackman MA, et al. Antigen-specific memory regulatory CD4+Foxp3+ T cells control memory responses to influenza virus infection. *J Immunol.* (2013) 190:3438–46. doi: 10.4049/jimmunol.1203140
95. Rosenblum MD, Gratz IK, Paw JS, Lee K, Marshak-Rothstein A, Abbas AK. Response to self antigen imprints regulatory memory in tissues. *Nature.* (2011) 480:538–42. doi: 10.1038/nature10664
96. Cvetanovich GL, Hafler DA. Human regulatory T cells in autoimmune diseases. *Curr Opin Immunol.* (2010) 22:753–60. doi: 10.1016/j.coi.2010.08.012
97. Kim B-S, Kim I-K, Park Y-J, Kim Y-S, Kim Y-S, Chang W-S, et al. Conversion of Th2 memory cells into Foxp3+ regulatory T cells suppressing Th2-mediated allergic asthma. *Proc Natl Acad Sci.* (2010) 107:8742–7. doi: 10.1073/PNAS.0911756107

98. Hu C-C, Jeng W-J, Chen Y-C, Fang J-H, Huang C-H, Teng W, et al. Memory regulatory T cells increase only in inflammatory phase of chronic hepatitis B infection and related to galectin-9/Tim-3 interaction. *Sci Rep.* (2017) 7:15280. doi: 10.1038/s41598-017-15527-x
99. Hori S, Nomura T, Sakaguchi S. Control of regulatory T cell development by the transcription factor Foxp3. *Science.* (2003) 299:1057–61. doi: 10.1126/science.1079490
100. Prins JR, Boelens HM, Heimweg J, Van der Heide S, Dubois AE, Van Oosterhout AJ, et al. Preeclampsia is associated with lower percentages of regulatory T cells in maternal blood. *Hypertens Pregnancy.* (2009) 28:300–11. doi: 10.1080/10641950802601237
101. Winger EE, Reed JL. Low circulating CD4+ CD25+ Foxp3+ T regulatory cell levels predict miscarriage risk in newly pregnant women with a history of failure. *Am J Reprod Immunol.* (2011) 66:320–8. doi: 10.1111/j.1600-0897.2011.00992.x
102. Jasper MJ, Tremellen KP, Robertson SA. Primary unexplained infertility is associated with reduced expression of the T-regulatory cell transcription factor Foxp3 in endometrial tissue. *Mol Hum Reprod.* (2006) 12:301–8. doi: 10.1093/molehr/gal032
103. Wagner MI, Jöst M, Spratte J, Schaier M, Mahnke K, Meuer S, et al. Differentiation of ICOS+ and ICOS- recent thymic emigrant regulatory T cells (RTE T regs) during normal pregnancy, pre-eclampsia and HELLP syndrome. *Clin Exp Immunol.* (2016) 183:129–42. doi: 10.1111/cei.12693
104. Dong S, Maiella S, Xhaard A, Pang Y, Wenandy L, Larghero J, et al. Multiparameter single-cell profiling of human CD4+FOXP3+ regulatory T-cell populations in homeostatic conditions and during graft-versus-host disease. *Blood.* (2013) 122:1802–12. doi: 10.1182/BLOOD-2013-02-482539
105. Weber JP, Fuhrmann F, Hutloff A. T-follicular helper cells survive as long-term memory cells. *Eur J Immunol.* (2012) 42:1981–8. doi: 10.1002/eji.201242540
106. Ma CS, Deenick EK, Batten M, Tangye SG. The origins, function, and regulation of T follicular helper cells. *J Exp Med.* (2012) 209:1241–53. doi: 10.1084/jem.20120994
107. He J, Tsai LM, Leong YA, Hu X, Ma CS, Chevalier N, et al. Circulating precursor CCR7(lo)PD-1(hi) CXCR5+ CD4+ T Cells indicate Tfh cell activity and promote antibody responses upon antigen reexposure. *Immunity.* (2013) 39:770–81. doi: 10.1016/j.immuni.2013.09.007
108. Clark RA. Resident memory T cells in human health and disease. *Sci Transl Med.* (2015) 7:269rv1. doi: 10.1126/scitranslmed.3010641
109. Turner DL, Farber DL. Mucosal resident memory CD4 T cells in protection and immunopathology. *Front Immunol.* (2014) 5:331. doi: 10.3389/fimmu.2014.00331
110. Long HM, Chagoury OL, Leese AM, Ryan GB, James E, Morton LT, et al. MHC II tetramers visualize human CD4 + T cell responses to Epstein–Barr virus infection and demonstrate atypical kinetics of the nuclear antigen EBNA1 response. *J Exp Med.* (2013) 210:933–49. doi: 10.1084/jem.20121437
111. Gattinoni L, Speiser DE, Lichterfeld M, Bonini C. T memory stem cells in health and disease. *Nat Med.* (2017) 23:18–27. doi: 10.1038/nm.4241
112. Sallusto F, Lenig D, Förster R, Lipp M, Lanzavecchia A. Two subsets of memory T lymphocytes with distinct homing potentials and effector functions. *J Immunol.* (2014) 192:840–4. doi: 10.1126/science.1058867
113. Harty JT, Badovinac VP. Shaping and reshaping CD8+ T-cell memory. *Nat Rev Immunol.* (2008) 8:107–19. doi: 10.1038/nri2251
114. Chang JT, Wherry EJ, Goldrath AW. Molecular regulation of effector and memory T cell differentiation. *Nat Immunol.* (2014) 15:1104–15. doi: 10.1038/ni.3031
115. Gattinoni L, Zhong X-S, Palmer DC, Ji Y, Hinrichs CS, Yu Z, et al. Wnt signaling arrests effector T cell differentiation and generates CD8+ memory stem cells. *Nat Med.* (2009) 15:808–13. doi: 10.1038/nm.1982
116. Shen J, Luo X, Wu Q, Huang J, Xiao G, Wang L, et al. A subset of CXCR5+CD8+ T cells in the germinal centers from human tonsils and lymph nodes help B cells produce immunoglobulins. *Front Immunol.* (2018) 9:2287. doi: 10.3389/fimmu.2018.02287
117. Youngblood B, Hale JS, Kissick HT, Ahn E, Xu X, Wieland A, et al. Effector CD8 T cells dedifferentiate into long-lived memory cells. *Nature.* (2017) 552:404–9. doi: 10.1038/nature25144
118. Akondy RS, Fitch M, Edupuganti S, Yang S, Kissick HT, Li KW, et al. Origin and differentiation of human memory CD8 T cells after vaccination. *Nature.* (2017) 552:362–7. doi: 10.1038/nature24633
119. Ahmed R, Bevan MJ, Reiner SL, Fearon DT. The precursors of memory: models and controversies. *Nat Rev Immunol.* (2009) 9:662–8. doi: 10.1038/nri2619
120. White JT, Cross EW, Kedl RM. Antigen-inexperienced memory CD8+ T cells: where they come from and why we need them. *Nat Rev Immunol.* (2017) 17:391–400. doi: 10.1038/nri.2017.34
121. Appay V, van Lier RAW, Sallusto F, Roederer M. Phenotype and function of human T lymphocyte subsets: consensus and issues. *Cytom. Part A.* (2008) 73A:975–83. doi: 10.1002/cyto.a.20643
122. Sharkey DJ, Tremellen KP, Jasper MJ, Gemzell-Danielsson K, Robertson SA. Seminal fluid induces leukocyte recruitment and cytokine and chemokine mRNA expression in the human cervix after coitus. *J Immunol.* (2012) 188:2445–54. doi: 10.4049/jimmunol.1102736
123. Kaech SM, Tan JT, Wherry EJ, Konieczny BT, Surh CD, Ahmed R. Selective expression of the interleukin 7 receptor identifies effector CD8 T cells that give rise to long-lived memory cells. *Nat Immunol.* (2003) 4:1191–8. doi: 10.1038/ni1009
124. van Egmond A, van der Keur C, Swings GMJS, Scherjon SA, Claas FHJ. The possible role of virus-specific CD8+ memory T cells in decidual tissue. *J Reprod Immunol.* (2016) 113:1–8. doi: 10.1016/j.jri.2015.09.073
125. Piper KP, McLarnon A, Arrazi J, Horlock C, Ainsworth J, Kilby MD, et al. Functional HY-specific CD8+ T cells are found in a high proportion of women following pregnancy with a male fetus. *Biol Reprod.* (2007) 76:96–101. doi: 10.1095/biolreprod.106.055426
126. Graef P, Buchholz VR, Stemberger C, Flossdorf M, Henkel L, Schiemann M, et al. Serial transfer of single-cell-derived immunocompetence reveals stemness of CD8+central memory T cells. *Immunity.* (2014) 41:116–26. doi: 10.1016/j.immuni.2014.05.018
127. Topham DJ, Reilly EC. Tissue-resident memory CD8+ T cells: from phenotype to function. *Front Immunol.* (2018) 9:515. doi: 10.3389/fimmu.2018.00515
128. Watanabe R. Resident memory t cells in mouse and human. *Jap J Clin Immunol.* (2016) 39:505–12. doi: 10.2177/jsci.39.505
129. Mueller SN, Mackay LK. Tissue-resident memory T cells: local specialists in immune defence. *Nat Rev Immunol.* (2016) 16:79–89. doi: 10.1038/nri.2015.3
130. Carico E, Atlante M, Giarnieri E, Raffa S, Bucci B, Giovagnoli MR, et al. E-cadherin and alpha-catenin expression in normal, hyperplastic and neoplastic endometrium. *Anticancer Res.* (2010) 30:4993–7.
131. Blechschmidt K, Mylonas I, Mayr D, Schiessl B, Schulze S, Becker K-F, et al. Expression of E-cadherin and its repressor Snail in placental tissue of normal, preeclamptic and HELLP pregnancies. *Virchows Arch.* (2007) 450:195–202. doi: 10.1007/s00428-006-0343-x
132. Hadley GA, Bartlett ST, Via CS, Rostapshova EA, Moainie S. The epithelial cell-specific integrin, CD103 (alpha E integrin), defines a novel subset of alloreactive CD8+ CTL. *J Immunol.* (1997) 159:3748–56.
133. Mackay LK, Braun A, Macleod BL, Collins N, Tebartz C, Bedoui S, et al. Cutting edge: CD69 interference with sphingosine-1-phosphate receptor function regulates peripheral T cell retention. *J Immunol.* (2015) 194:2059–63. doi: 10.4049/JIMMUNOL.1402256
134. Mackay LK, Rahimpour A, Ma JZ, Collins N, Stock AT, Hafon M-L, et al. The developmental pathway for CD103+CD8+ tissue-resident memory T cells of skin. *Nat Immunol.* (2013) 14:1294–301. doi: 10.1038/ni.2744
135. Machicote A, Belén S, Baz P, Billordo LA, Fainboim L. Human CD8+HLA-DR+ regulatory T cells, similarly to classical CD4+Foxp3+ cells, suppress immune responses via PD-1/PD-L1 Axis. *Front Immunol.* (2018) 9:2788. doi: 10.3389/fimmu.2018.02788
136. Rifa'i M, Kawamoto Y, Nakashima I, Suzuki H. Essential roles of CD8+ CD122+ regulatory T cells in the maintenance of T cell homeostasis. *J Exp Med.* (2004) 200:1123–34. doi: 10.1084/jem.20040395
137. Arruvito L, Payaslián F, Baz P, Podhorzer A, Billordo A, Pandolfi J, et al. Identification and clinical relevance of naturally occurring human CD8+HLA-DR+ regulatory T cells. *J Immunol.* (2014) 193:4469–76. doi: 10.4049/jimmunol.1401490

138. Quigley MF, Gonzalez VD, Granath A, Andersson J, Sandberg JK. CXCR5+ CCR7− CD8 T cells are early effector memory cells that infiltrate tonsil B cell follicles. *Eur J Immunol.* (2007) 37:3352–62. doi: 10.1002/eji.200636746
139. Sabatino M, Hu J, Sommariva M, Gautam S, Fellowes V, Hocker JD, et al. Generation of clinical-grade CD19-specific CAR-modified CD8+ memory stem cells for the treatment of human B-cell malignancies. *Blood.* (2016) 128:519–28. doi: 10.1182/blood-2015-11-683847
140. Guan L, Li X, Wei J, Liang Z, Yang J, Weng X, et al. Antigen-specific CD8+ memory stem T cells generated from human peripheral blood effectively eradicate allogeneic targets in mice. *Stem Cell Res Ther.* (2018) 9:337. doi: 10.1186/s13287-018-1080-1
141. Gattinoni L, Klebanoff CA, Restifo NP. Paths to stemness: building the ultimate antitumour T cell. *Nat Rev Cancer.* (2012) 12:671–84. doi: 10.1038/nrc3322
142. Robillard PY, Hulsey TC, Périanin J, Janky E, Miri EH, Papiernik E. Association of pregnancy-induced hypertension with duration of sexual cohabitation before conception. *Lancet.* (1994) 344:973–5.
143. Saftlas AF, Rubenstein L, Prater K, Harland KK, Field E, Triche EW. Cumulative exposure to paternal seminal fluid prior to conception and subsequent risk of preeclampsia. *J Reprod Immunol.* (2014) 101–102:104–10. doi: 10.1016/j.jri.2013.07.006
144. Koelman CA, Coumans AB, Nijman HW, Doxiadis II, Dekker GA, Claas FH. Correlation between oral sex and a low incidence of preeclampsia: a role for soluble HLA in seminal fluid? *J Reprod Immunol.* (2000) 46:155–66. doi: 10.1016/S0165-0378(99)00062-5
145. Wong LF, Porter TF, Scott JR. Immunotherapy for recurrent miscarriage. *Cochrane Database Syst Rev.* (2014) 1:CD000112. doi: 10.1002/14651858.CD000112.pub3
146. Crawford G, Ray A, Gudi A, Shah A, Homburg R. The role of seminal plasma for improved outcomes during *in vitro* fertilization treatment: review of the literature and meta-analysis. *Hum Reprod Update.* (2015) 21:275–84. doi: 10.1093/humupd/dmu052
147. Shin H, Iwasaki A. A vaccine strategy that protects against genital herpes by establishing local memory T cells. *Nature.* (2012) 491:463–7. doi: 10.1038/nature11522
148. Homann D, Teyton L, Oldstone MBA. Differential regulation of antiviral T-cell immunity results in stable CD8+ but declining CD4+ T-cell memory. *Nat Med.* (2001) 7:913–9. doi: 10.1038/90950
149. Nelson RW, McLachlan JB, Kurtz JR, Jenkins MK. CD4+ T Cell persistence and function after infection are maintained by low-level peptide: MHC class II presentation. *J Immunol.* (2013) 190:2828–34. doi: 10.4049/jimmunol.1202183
150. Kinder JM, Jiang TT, Clark DR, Chaturvedi V, Xin L, Ertelt JM, et al. Pregnancy-induced maternal regulatory T cells, bona fide memory or maintenance by antigenic reminder from fetal cell microchimerism? *Chimerism.* (2014) 5:16–9. doi: 10.4161/chim.28241
151. Kinder JM, Jiang TT, Ertelt JM, Xin L, Strong BS, Shaaban AF, et al. Cross-generational reproductive fitness enforced by microchimeric maternal cells. *Cell.* (2015) 162:505–15. doi: 10.1016/j.cell.2015.07.006
152. Kinder JM, Stelzer IA, Arck PC, Way SS. Immunological implications of pregnancy-induced microchimerism. *Nat Rev Immunol.* (2017) 17:483–94. doi: 10.1038/nri.2017.38

4

Early Embryonic Loss Following Intravaginal Zika Virus Challenge in Rhesus Macaques

Christina M. Newman[1], Alice F. Tarantal[2,3], Michele L. Martinez[2,3], Heather A. Simmons[4], Terry K. Morgan[5], Xiankun Zeng[6], Jenna R. Rosinski[1], Mason I. Bliss[7], Ellie K. Bohm[8], Dawn M. Dudley[1], Matthew T. Aliota[8], Thomas C. Friedrich[7], Christopher J. Miller[3,9] and David H. O'Connor[1,4]*

[1] Pathology and Laboratory Medicine, University of Wisconsin-Madison, Madison, WI, United States, [2] Pediatrics, Cell Biology and Human Anatomy, School of Medicine, University of California, Davis, CA, United States, [3] California National Primate Research Center, University of California, Davis, CA, United States, [4] Wisconsin National Primate Research Center, University of Wisconsin-Madison, Madison, WI, United States, [5] Pathology, Oregon Health and Sciences University, Portland, OR, United States, [6] Pathology Division, United States Army Medical Research Institute of Infectious Diseases, Frederick, MD, United States, [7] Pathobiological Sciences, University of Wisconsin-Madison, Madison, WI, United States, [8] Veterinary and Biomedical Sciences, University of Minnesota, Saint Paul, MN, United States, [9] Pathology, Microbiology, and Immunology, School of Veterinary Medicine, Center for Immunology and Infectious Diseases, University of California, Davis, CA, United States

***Correspondence:**
David H. O'Connor
dhoconno@wisc.edu

Zika virus (ZIKV) is an arthropod-borne virus (arbovirus) and is primarily transmitted by *Aedes* species mosquitoes; however, ZIKV can also be sexually transmitted. During the initial epidemic and in places where ZIKV is now considered endemic, it is difficult to disentangle the risks and contributions of sexual versus vector-borne transmission to adverse pregnancy outcomes. To examine the potential impact of sexual transmission of ZIKV on pregnancy outcome, we challenged three rhesus macaques (*Macaca mulatta*) three times intravaginally with 1 x 10^7 PFU of a low passage, African lineage ZIKV isolate (ZIKV-DAK) in the first trimester (~30 days gestational age). Samples were collected from all animals initially on days 3 through 10 post challenge, followed by twice, and then once weekly sample collection; ultrasound examinations were performed every 3-4 days then weekly as pregnancies progressed. All three dams had ZIKV RNA detectable in plasma on day 3 post-ZIKV challenge. At approximately 45 days gestation (17-18 days post-challenge), two of the three dams were found with nonviable embryos by ultrasound. Viral RNA was detected in recovered tissues and at the maternal-fetal interface (MFI) in both cases. The remaining viable pregnancy proceeded to near term (~155 days gestational age) and ZIKV RNA was detected at the MFI but not in fetal tissues. These results suggest that sexual transmission of ZIKV may represent an underappreciated risk of pregnancy loss during early gestation.

Keywords: Zika virus, macaques, pregnancy, intravaginal infection, embryonic loss

INTRODUCTION

Zika virus (ZIKV) emerged from relative obscurity five years ago to sweep through tropical and subtropical regions of the Western hemisphere. More than a million cases between 2015 and 2018 were reported in Pan American Health Organization (PAHO) regions alone (1). While ZIKV primarily causes mild febrile illness or asymptomatic infections in a majority of individuals, infection during pregnancy can result in a range of adverse outcomes including fetal loss and a constellation of birth defects now known as congenital Zika syndrome (CZS) (2–4). Human infection with ZIKV can occur following mosquito-borne, vertical, and sexual transmission (5–7). While mosquito-borne transmission from infected *Aedes* species mosquitoes is thought to be the most common route of infection in endemic areas, the contribution of sexual transmission in epidemics remains poorly understood, in part because during an outbreak, both transmission routes occur simultaneously and can be challenging to disentangle (8).

Sexual transmission of ZIKV was first documented in 2008 when a scientist working in Senegal became infected and, upon his return to the United States, infected his wife (9). Throughout the ZIKV outbreak in 2015 and 2016, additional sexually-transmitted infections were documented (10–14). The majority of sexually-transmitted cases in non-endemic areas are likely the result of infection of the primary cases during travel, followed by inadvertent transmission to the secondary cases upon returning home (7). As previously mentioned, sexually-transmitted ZIKV infections in endemic areas or areas experiencing active outbreaks are difficult to differentiate from mosquito-transmitted infections because there may be an individual risk of exposure by either route. Epidemiological data suggest that sexual transmission occurs primarily male-to-female through vaginal contact, even weeks after clinical symptom resolution, which suggests that sexual transmission of ZIKV does pose at least a theoretical risk to pregnant women (15). Furthermore, the ZIKV viral RNA (vRNA) load in human semen has been reported to range from the hundreds to tens of millions of copies per milliliter, with values as high as 3.98×10^8 copies/ml reported (16–18). The testes in particular, were found to be a ZIKV reservoir in animal models (19, 20). In addition, studies have recently shown that intimate partners of household index cases are more likely to also be positive or show serologic evidence of ZIKV infection relative to other members of the same household (21).

Overall, we have limited information regarding the risk of ZIKV sexual transmission to pregnant women and their developing fetuses (14). Studies have shown that other sexually transmitted ascending vaginal infections are associated with an increased risk of pre-term labor and other poor outcomes (22). Whether an ascending intravaginal ZIKV infection poses a higher risk to pregnancy than mosquito-borne infection is currently unknown. Pregnant women or women trying to become pregnant may be less likely to utilize condoms, a recommended strategy for the prevention of sexual transmission of ZIKV (23, 24). Furthermore, a woman might not be aware of a pregnancy during early gestation and unfortunately, existing data suggest that the highest risk for developmental anomalies associated with ZIKV infection is during the first trimester, a critical developmental time period (25–27). Additionally, ZIKV infection during pregnancy has also been associated with an increased risk for spontaneous abortion in both humans and nonhuman primates (28, 29).

Animal models have played a critical role in improving our understanding of the natural history and pathogenesis of ZIKV. To-date, both murine and nonhuman primate (NHP) models have been utilized to examine aspects of sexual transmission of ZIKV (19, 20, 30, 31). Studies in these models have shown persistent shedding of vRNA from the reproductive tract, infection of the female reproductive tract *via* a vaginal exposure route, and fetal effects as a result of vaginal exposure or sexual transmission in mice (20, 30–39). Although studies in pregnant olive baboons have shown that intravaginal challenge with infected baboon semen during mid-gestation can result in productive maternal infection and vRNA detection in some maternal tissues and placentas, to date, studies in NHP have not shown clear evidence of vertical transmission associated with maternal ZIKV infection by the intravaginal route (33).

Because infection during the first trimester is associated with the highest risk for adverse pregnancy outcomes and, since women may be unaware of a pregnancy and may potentially be less likely to utilize barrier methods to prevent sexually-transmitted ZIKV infections during the early first trimester (23, 24), we designed a proof-of-concept study in which we challenged three gravid rhesus macaques (*Macaca mulatta*) intravaginally with ZIKV. Our goal was to investigate the potential impact of intravaginal ZIKV challenge during the first trimester on fetal and pregnancy outcomes and to develop a model for sexual transmission during early pregnancy.

METHODS

Ethics Statement

All animal procedures conformed to the requirements of the Animal Welfare Act and protocols were approved prior to implementation by the Institutional Animal Care and Use Committee (IACUC) at the University of California, Davis. Activities related to animal care, housing, and diet were performed according to California National Primate Research Center (CNPRC) standard operating procedures (SOPs). SOPs for colony related procedures are reviewed and approved by the UC Davis IACUC.

Study Design

Female rhesus macaques (*Macaca mulatta*, N=3) were time-mated and identified as pregnant by ultrasound according to established methods (40). Prior to study assignment normal embryonic growth and development were confirmed by ultrasound. Females were challenged in the first trimester at approximately 30 days gestational age (trimesters divided by 55-day increments; term 165 ± 10 days) with 1×10^7 PFU ZIKV-DAK three times intravaginally at approximately two-hour intervals

(**Table 1** and **Figure 1**). Pregnancies were monitored by ultrasound every 3-4 days post-challenge and then weekly from day 50 onward throughout the study period. Standardized parameters were assessed including fetal growth (greatest length then biparietal and occipitofrontal diameters, head and abdominal circumferences, humerus and femur lengths) and structural development, amniotic fluid volumes and placental parameters, and compared to normal growth and developmental trajectories for the species (40). Dams were weighed at each sedation and blood samples were collected daily from day 3 through day 10 post-challenge, followed by bi-weekly until maternal plasma vRNA loads were undetectable, and then weekly until hysterotomy. Plasma and peripheral blood mononuclear cells (PBMCs) were isolated at all time points, and serum was collected on days 0, 14, and 24 post-challenge (dams 049-102 and 049-103), and on days 0, 14, 27, and 122 post-challenge for dam 049-101. Urine was collected by ultrasound-guided cystocentesis (~1 ml) on days 7, 10, 14, 21, and 24 post-challenge (dams 049-102 and 049-103) and on days 7, 10, 14, 27, and 122 post-challenge for dam 049-101. Hysterotomies were performed for dam 049-102 and 049-103 at the end of the first trimester (post-detection of nonviable embryos by ultrasound) and near term (~155 days gestational age) for dam 049-101.

Virus Challenge Preparation and Infection

ZIKV strain Zika virus/A.africanus-tc/Senegal/1984/DAK AR 41524 (ZIKV-DAK; GenBank: KX601166) was originally isolated from *Aedes luteocephalus* mosquitoes in Senegal in 1984. One round of amplification on *Aedes pseudocutellaris* cells, followed by amplification on C6/36 cells and two rounds of amplification on Vero cells, were used to prepare a master stock obtained from BEI Resources (Manassas, VA). Challenge stocks were prepared from this master stock by inoculation onto a confluent monolayer of C6/36 mosquito cells as described previously (41). Prior to administration, the ZIKV-DAK stock was diluted to $1x10^7$ PFU in 1 ml sterile saline and delivered *via* a 1 ml tuberculin syringe (37). Animals were inoculated three times intravaginally under ketamine sedation at approximately two-hour intervals using a previously described method (37).

Blood Processing and Plasma vRNA Loads

Plasma and PBMCs were isolated from blood placed in EDTA vacutainers and processed at 1500 RPM for 15 minutes according to standard protocols. Serum was isolated from whole blood collected into glass vacutainers without additives. Viral RNA was extracted from 300 µl plasma as previously described with a Maxwell 16 MDx instrument (Promega, Madison, WI) and evaluated using qRT-PCR (42). RNA concentration was determined by interpolation onto an internal standard curve of seven ten-fold serial dilutions of a synthetic ZIKV RNA segment based on Zika virus/Human/French Polynesia/10087PF/2013 (ZIKV-FP). The limit of quantification of the ZIKV qRT-PCR assay is estimated to be 100 copies vRNA/ml plasma or serum.

Hysterotomy and Tissue Collection

Dams 049-102 and 049-103 were scheduled for hysterotomies in the late first trimester (nonviable embryos detected 3 days prior to hysterotomy). The hysterotomy for dam 049-101 was performed at approximately 155 days gestational age according

TABLE 1 | Dam information on day 0 of study.

Dam ID	Weight (kg)	Age (y)	Gestational Age (days)	Scheduled hysterotomy (days)	Virus	Dose (PFU)	Challenge #
049-101	5.55	6.93	29	155	ZIKV-DAK	$1x10^7$	3
049-102	7.40	11.83	32	155	ZIKV-DAK	$1x10^7$	3
049-103	8.43	12.83	31	155	ZIKV-DAK	$1x10^7$	3

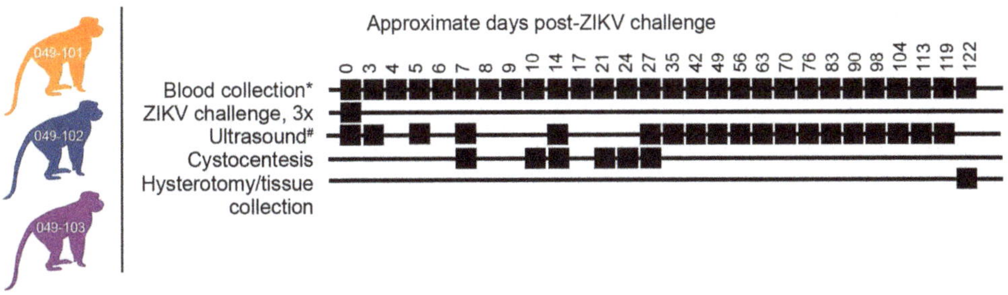

FIGURE 1 | Study design. Three female rhesus macaques were time-mated, confirmed pregnant by ultrasound, and challenged intravaginally at 30 days (+/-2) gestational age with $1x10^7$ PFU ZIKV-DAK three times at two-hour intervals. Blood collection* denotes plasma and PBMC isolation at every sampling time point while serum collection was planned only on days 0, 14, 27, and 122 post-ZIKV challenge. Ultrasound# denotes ultrasound imaging was performed every 3-4 days during early gestation, then weekly thereafter. Hysterotomies were originally planned for each animal at approximately 122 days post-ZIKV challenge.

to the original study design (**Figure 1**) and following established protocols (43). The gestational sac was removed for fetal tissue assessments, with a modified collection protocol for nonviable specimens (see below). For the fetus from dam 049-101 amniotic fluid, fetal blood, and fetal cerebrospinal fluid were collected, then fetal body weights and measures (biparietal and occipitofrontal diameters, abdominal and arm circumferences, hand and foot lengths, humerus and femur lengths, crown-rump length) were assessed. The left cerebral hemisphere and left eye were collected under aseptic conditions and shipped with cold packs to Wisconsin by overnight delivery for additional assessments (see below). Specimens collected for qRT-PCR for vRNA analysis included dura mater; right cerebral hemisphere (frontal, parietal, temporal, occipital lobes); cerebellum (right and left) and midbrain; right optic nerve; right eye (cornea, retina, sclera); spinal cord (cervical, thoracic, lumbar); right and left parotid glands, submandibular, and salivary glands; omentum; thymus; spleen; liver (right, left, quadrate, caudate lobes); pancreas; right and left adrenal glands and kidneys; right and left axillary and inguinal lymph nodes; diaphragm; tracheobronchial and mesenteric lymph nodes; right and left thyroids; trachea; esophagus; pericardium; aorta; right and left atria and ventricles; lung lobes (right and left; all lobes); reproductive tract including right and left gonads; urinary bladder; gastrointestinal tract (stomach, duodenum, jejunum, ileum, colon; meconium), skin, skeletal muscle, and bone marrow (**Table 2**). The placenta was weighed and assessed including disk measurements (primary and secondary for bidiscoid placentas; primary disk only for monodiscoid), umbilical cord and membrane insertion sites, blood vessel distribution, cut surfaces, and examined for the presence of infarcts. Decidua, membranes, umbilical cord, and multiple sections of the placental disks were collected. All specimens were quick frozen in triplicate over liquid nitrogen for qRT-PCR analysis or collected into RNAlater (cat# R0901, Sigma-Aldrich, St. Louis, MO). Multiple blocks of tissues were collected in histology cassettes fixed in 10% buffered formalin, embedded, sectioned (5-6 μm) and stained with hematoxylin and eosin (H&E) or used for *in situ* hybridization (ISH).

For dams 049-102 and 049-103 a modified collection was performed, consistent with the early developmental stage of the conceptus (**Table 2**). Decidua, membranes, umbilical cord, and multiple sections of the placental disks were collected as noted above.

Fresh samples collected from the 049-101 fetus (left cerebral hemisphere and left eye) were shipped with cold packs for additional assessments as noted above; the eye was analyzed by the Comparative Ocular Pathology Laboratory of Wisconsin

TABLE 2 | Fetal and maternal-fetal interface tissues collected at hysterotomy.

Dam ID	Organ System/Tissue	Tissue samples tested (N)	Tissue samples qRT-PCR positive (N)	Positive tissue vRNA copies/mg (± SD)
049-101	integumentary	3	0	0.0
	musculoskeletal	2	0	0.0
	nervous	14	0	0.0
	endocrine	7	0	0.0
	lymphatic	8	0	0.0
	cardiovascular	4	0	0.0
	respiratory	10	0	0.0
	digestive	12	0	0.0
	urinary	3	0	0.0
	reproductive	3	0	0.0
	other	8	0	0.0
	primary placental disk	3	2	$0.66x10^{2a}$ ($\pm$ $0.51x10^{2}$)
	primary placental disk	3	3	$1.59x10^{3a}$ ($\pm$ $1.20x10^{3}$)
	placenta with decidua	18	3	$8.13x10^{2a}$ ($\pm$ $3.97x10^{2}$)
	placenta without decidua	18	6	$6.45x10^{2a}$ ($\pm$ $6.10x10^{2}$)
	decidua	18	3	0.0
049-102	nervous (brain)	1	1	$2.06x10^{3}$
	digestive (liver)	1	1	$1.23x10^{4}$
	umbilical cord	1	1	$8.37x10^{3}$
	membranes	1	1	$4.87x10^{3}$
	primary placental disk	3	3	$4.96x10^{3a}$ ($\pm$ $4.00x10^{3}$)
	secondary placental disk	3	3	$3.61x10^{3a}$ ($\pm$ $1.16x10^{3}$)
	decidua	1	0	0.0
049-103	nervous (brain)	1	1	$1.74x10^{5}$
	digestive (liver)	1	1	$7.42x10^{4}$
	umbilical cord	1	1	$7.13x10^{4}$
	amnion	1	1	$7.08x10^{2}$
	chorionic jelly	1	1	$3.54x10^{3}$
	membranes (amnion and chorion)	1	1	$4.74x10^{3}$
	primary placental disk	3	3	$1.98x10^{3a}$ ($\pm$ $1.13x10^{3}$)
	secondary placental disk	3	3	$3.40x10^{3a}$ ($\pm$ $2.18x10^{3}$)
	decidua	1	0	0.0

[a]*mean vRNA load of multiple positive tissue samples.*

(COPLOW). Placental tissues from all dams and tissues for the fetus from dam 049-101 were assessed as described previously in Koenig et al. (44).

Tissue, Urine, and Amniotic Fluid vRNA Loads

Maternal-fetal interface (MFI) and fetal tissue vRNA loads were determined from approximately 20 mg of each specimen. ZIKV RNA was isolated from tissues using the Qiagen AllPrep DNA/RNA Mini Kit (cat# 80284, Qiagen, Germantown MD) using the QIAcube following the manufacturer's protocol. Viral RNA was isolated from 140 μl maternal urine or amniotic fluid using the QIAmp Viral RNA minikit (cat# 52904, Qiagen, Germantown MD) following the manufacturer's protocol. Following isolation, cDNA synthesis was performed using the Qiagen Sensiscript RT kit (cat# 205213, Qiagen, Germantown MD) according to the manufacturer's protocol. Quantification of vRNA load was performed by real-time PCR using the Taqman amplification system and the QuantStudio 12 K Flex Real-Time PCR System (ThermoFisher Scientific, Grand Island, NY) as described previously (43). The estimated limit of quantification of the assay is 50-100 ZIKV RNA copies/mg tissue (average = 75 copies/mg).

In Situ Hybridization (ISH)

ISH probes against the ZIKV genome were commercially purchased (cat# 468361, Advanced Cell Diagnostics, Newark, CA). ISH was performed using the RNAscope® Red 2.5 kit (cat# 322350, Advanced Cell Diagnostics, Newark, CA) according to the manufacturer's protocol. After deparaffinization with xylene, a series of ethanol washes, and peroxidase blocking, sections were heated with the antigen retrieval buffer and then digested by proteinase. Sections were then exposed to the ISH target probe and incubated at 40°C in a hybridization oven for two-hours. After rinsing, ISH signal was amplified using the provided pre-amplifier followed by the amplifier-containing labelled probe binding sites, and developed with a Fast Red chromogenic substrate for 10 minutes at room temperature. Sections were then stained with hematoxylin, air-dried, and mounted.

Plaque Reduction Neutralization Tests (PRNT)

Titers of ZIKV neutralizing antibodies were determined using plaque reduction neutralization tests (PRNT) on Vero cells (ATCC #CCL-81) with a cutoff value of 90% ($PRNT_{90}$) (45). Neutralization curves were generated in GraphPad Prism (San Diego, CA) and the resulting data were analyzed by nonlinear regression to estimate the dilution of serum required to inhibit 90% Vero cell culture infection (45, 46).

RESULTS

Repeated Intravaginal ZIKV Challenge Results in Infection In Pregnant Macaques

All three dams had detectable ZIKV RNA in plasma by 3 days post intravaginal ZIKV challenge (**Figure 2**). ZIKV RNA loads peaked on day 5 for dams 049-101 and 049-102, and on day 6 for dam 049-103. Peak vRNA loads ranged from $1.57x10^4$ copies/ml for 049-101 to $1.30x10^5$ copies/ml for 049-103 (**Figure 2**). The latest detectable plasma vRNA load for animal 049-101 was on day 24 post-challenge ($1.56x10^2$ copies/ml). Dam 049-103 had a detectable plasma vRNA load until day 14 ($2.46x10^3$ copies/ml) but was negative on day 17 (the next time point samples were collected). Dam 049-102 was consistently positive for ZIKV vRNA until day 14, was negative on day 17, and then positive again on days 21 and 24 post challenge. Dam 049-102 was positive for ZIKV RNA in blood plasma collected at hysterotomy, the last time point sampled for the study. Overall, maternal plasma vRNA loads for dams 049-101, 049-102, and 049-103 were somewhat delayed compared to animals subcutaneously inoculated with French Polynesian or Puerto Rican ZIKV isolates in our previous studies, but were consistent in magnitude with previous observations (42, 48, 49). In addition, maternal plasma vRNA loads peaked within a time period similar to subcutaneously inoculated animals infected with the same ZIKV isolate (ZIKV-DAK) (47) (**Figure 2**).

Embryonic Demise Following Intravaginal ZIKV Infection During Early Pregnancy

Ultrasound examinations indicated that the embryos of dams 049-102 and 049-103 were nonviable at approximately 17-18 days post-challenge. Hysterotomies were subsequently scheduled and performed and each dam's final blood and urine samples were collected (**Figure 3A**). Embryo and placental tissues from dams 049-102 and 049-103 were collected for vRNA analysis, histopathological assessment, and ISH. Dam 049-101's pregnancy progressed normally and sampling continued until the study endpoint and near-term hysterotomy at approximately 155 days gestational age (**Figure 3A**). All fetal and placental measurements for 049-101 were recorded and were considered within normal limits for gestational age (**Table 3**) (40).

MFI, Tissues, and Amniotic Fluid Are ZIKV RNA Positive in Nonviable Embryos

ZIKV RNA was detected in the amniotic fluid from the conceptus of both dams 049-102 and 049-103 at $3.87x10^3$ and $7.38x10^3$ copies/ml respectively at the time of hysterotomy (subsequent to embryonic death). In addition, ZIKV RNA was detected in the brain and liver of both non-viable embryos, as well as in MFI tissues including the primary and secondary placental disks and membranes (amnion and chorion) (**Figure 3B**). The highest tissue vRNA burden was detected in the brain of the embryo from dam 049-102 ($1.74x10^5$ copies/mg). ZIKV RNA was not detected in amniotic fluid collected from the fetus of dam 049-101 at hysterotomy. Although a large number of fetal and MFI tissues were assessed following hysterotomy, the presence of ZIKV RNA was only detected in a subset of sections of MFI tissues from 049-101 (**Table 2** and **Figure 3C**). The decidua from all three dams were negative for ZIKV RNA by qRT-PCR. Similarly, ZIKV RNA was not detected in the urine for any of the dams at any of the time points sampled. Overall, these results highlight the focal nature of ZIKV RNA detection in

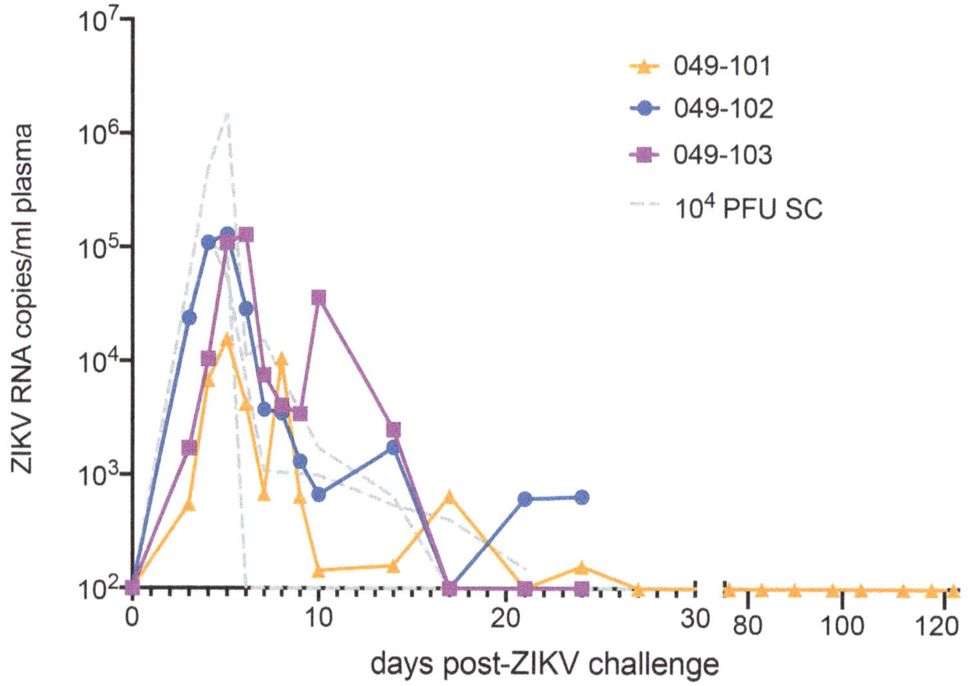

FIGURE 2 | Intravaginal ZIKV challenge resulted in detection of vRNA in plasma for all three dams. The x-axis shows days post-ZIKV challenge. The y-axis starts at the estimated limit of quantification of the qRT-PCR assay (1×10^2 copies/ml) and is shown as copies/ml plasma on the log scale. Plasma vRNA loads are displayed for dam 049-101 as orange triangles, for dam 049-102 as blue circles, and for dam 049-103 as magenta squares. For comparison, ZIKV plasma vRNA loads are also shown for three pregnant macaques subcutaneously (SC) inoculated with 1×10^4 PFU ZIKV-DAK and are displayed as gray dashed lines and noted as 10^4 PFU SC in the legend (47).

fetal and MFI tissues following infection during pregnancy. For a number of tissues, multiple samples were collected for vRNA analysis but ZIKV was only detected in a subset of those samples (**Table 2**).

Changes in Placental Tissues Following Intravaginal ZIKV Infection Are Non-Specific

Histopathological assessments of the placentas of dams 049-102 and 049-103 following embryonic demise showed generalized, non-specific mild necrosis (**Table 4** and **Supplemental Figures 1–3**). In particular, the secondary placental disk from dam 049-102 showed intervillous hemorrhage and parenchymal ischemia (**Supplemental Figures 2A, B**). In addition, the decidua from dam 049-102 showed some evidence of minimal focal necrosis (**Supplemental Figure 2C**). Placentas from both dam 049-102 and dam 049-103 had minimal to mild multifocal villous mineralization. The secondary placental disk of dam 049-103 showed acute neutrophilic inflammation, mild focal ischemia, and hemorrhage (**Supplemental Figure 3B**). Similar to the placentas from the other two dams, the placenta of dam 049-101 showed mild, multifocal villous mineralization, findings which have previously been observed in control placentas. Focal hemorrhage of the primary placental disk basal plate was also noted for dam 049-101 (**Supplemental Figure 1A**). In addition, decidual tissue from dam 049-101 showed mild, multifocal muscularization of the decidual arteries (**Supplemental Figure 1B**). Overall, changes in the placental tissues were mild and not associated with any specific pathological processes. Assessment of fetal tissues from dam 049-101 showed normal brain and eye morphology with no identified lesions.

ZIKV Genomic RNA Is Detected in MFI Tissues From Demise Cases but Not From the Near-Term Pregnancy

Tissue sections from decidua, primary placental disks, and secondary placental disks (bidiscoid placentas) were assessed by ZIKV ISH using RNAscope (see *Methods*). ZIKV genomic RNA was detected in both the primary and secondary placental disks from dams 049-102 and 049-103 (**Figure 4**). No ZIKV RNA was detected by RNAscope in the primary placental disk from dam 049-101, nor any of the decidua sections from any of the pregnancies. The lack of ZIKV RNA in the decidua sections by ISH was consistent with the tissue vRNA assessment by qRT-PCR.

Animals Infected Intravaginally With ZIKV During Pregnancy Develop Neutralizing Antibodies

Serum neutralizing antibody titers (nAbs) against ZIKV were evaluated for dams 049-102 and 049-103 on days 0, 14, and 24

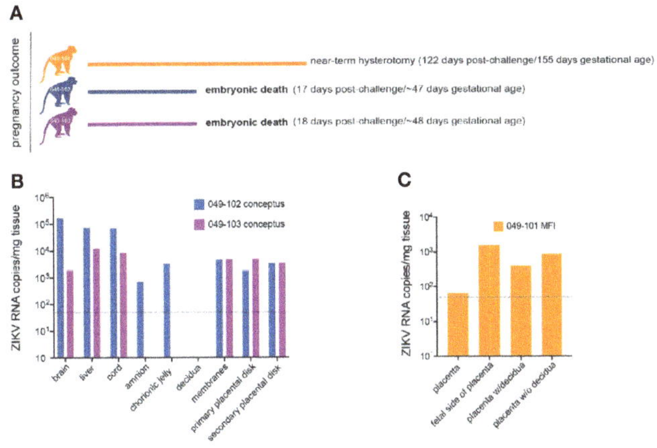

FIGURE 3 | Pregnancy outcomes and maternal-fetal interface (MFI) and fetal tissue vRNA loads. **(A)** Pregnancy outcomes for three dams intravaginally inoculated 3x with ZIKV at approximately 30 days gestation. Two dams (049-102 and 049-103) were determined by ultrasound to have nonviable embryos at approximately 17-18 days post-ZIKV challenge. Hysterotomies and embryo and MFI tissue collections were performed 3 days after detection. Dam 049-101's pregnancy continued until scheduled hysterotomy and extensive tissue collection at approximately 155 days gestational age. **(B)** Average ZIKV vRNA loads for positive embryo and MFI tissues collected at hysterotomy from dams 049-102 (blue) and 049-103 (magenta) following embryonic death at approximately 17-18 days post-ZIKV challenge. The dashed line represents the average of the estimated limit of detection (50-100 copies/mg, average: 75 copies/mg tissue) for the qRT-PCR assay. **(C)** Average ZIKV vRNA loads for positive MFI tissues collected at hysterotomy from dam 049-101 (orange) at approximately 122 days post-ZIKV infection. Fetal tissues were negative for ZIKV RNA by qRT-PCR. The dashed line represents the average of the estimated limit of detection (50-100 copies/mg, average: 75 copies/mg tissue) for the qRT-PCR assay.

TABLE 3 | 049-101 fetal and placental measurements (~155 days gestation, 122 days post challenge).

Tissue	Measure (mm)	Weight (g)
whole body	180.0	405.75
biparietal diameter	52.3	–
head circumference	186.0	–
r./l. femur	52.8/53.0	–
brain	–	54.42
cerebrum	–	50.2
cerebellum with midbrain	–	3.31
cerebellum without midbrain	–	2.47
r./l. eye	13.6/13.8	1.34/1.35
r./l. thyroid	–	0.07/0.07
thymus	–	1.42
spleen	–	0.58
liver	–	12.08
r./l. adrenal	–	0.12/0.17
r./l. kidney	–	1.00/0.99
lung lobes	–	8.76
r./l. testis	–	0.06/0.06
placenta	145.0 x 85.0	159.19

Measurements were considered to be within normal limits by ultrasound and gross assessment (40). R, right; L, left.

post-challenge by 90% plaque reduction neutralization tests ($PRNT_{90}$). Serum samples from 0, 14, 27, and 122 days post-challenge collected from dam 049-101 were similarly assessed. Samples collected on day 0 (pre-challenge) from all animals were negative for ZIKV nAbs. Neutralizing Ab titers above 1:10 are indicative of immunity against ZIKV. Serum collected on day 14 post-challenge from all animals neutralized ZIKV-DAK at levels considered protective by $PRNT_{90}$ (between 1:100 and 1:1000 for each animal). Serum collected on day 24 post-challenge from dams 049-102 and 049-103, and on day 27 post-challenge from dam 049-101 showed an increased neutralization response relative to baseline (day 0) and day 14 for each individual animal (**Figure 5**). By day 122 post-challenge, the ZIKV nAb response for animal 049-101 was lower than on days 14 or 27, but still demonstrated a strong protective response ($PRNT_{90}$ titer approximately 1:300) (**Figure 5**). These results suggest that all animals developed a nAb response against ZIKV following intravaginal ZIKV challenge consistent with findings previously noted for rhesus dams infected subcutaneously (42, 48, 49).

DISCUSSION

Here we describe a proof-of-concept study that indicates intravaginal challenge with ZIKV during early pregnancy results in productive maternal infection and suggests that infection by this route can result in embryonic demise. ZIKV RNA was detected at the MFI and in embryonic tissues, as well as in the amniotic fluid from the pregnancies of dams 049-102 and 049-103, supporting a role for ZIKV in the adverse pregnancy outcomes for these animals. Although ZIKV was detected by qRT-PCR in the MFI tissues from dam 049-101, no vRNA was detected in fetal tissues directly. Interestingly, although vRNA was detectable in the placenta of dam 049-101 by qRT-PCR, it was not detected by ISH. Given the focal nature of ZIKV RNA detected in the placental tissue samples collected from dam 049-101, it is likely that the samples evaluated by ISH were simply from areas without vRNA present (**Table 2**). In order to assess

TABLE 4 | Histopathological assessment of placental tissues from all animals and fetal tissues from 049-101.

Dam ID	Tissue	Findings
049-101	primary placental disk	focally extensive hemorrhage within the basal plate; mild multifocal villous mineralization
	decidua	mild multifocal persistent muscularization of decidual arteries
	fetal brain	no pathological changes
	fetal eye	no pathological changes
	fetal lung	mild bilateral diffuse intra-alveolar squamous cells, similar to control
049-102	primary placental disk	minimal multifocal villous mineralization
	secondary placental disk	intervillous hemorrhage and parenchymal ischemia with acute intervillous inflammation involving the lateral margin; not associated with specific pathologic process
	decidua	minimal focal necrosis
049-103	primary placental disk	mild multifocal mineralization of the anchoring villi
	secondary placental disk	mild focal parenchymal ischemia with coagulative necrosis and acute neutrophilic inflammation and mild multifocal villous mineralization
	decidua	minimal multifocal decidual necrosis with rare neutrophils

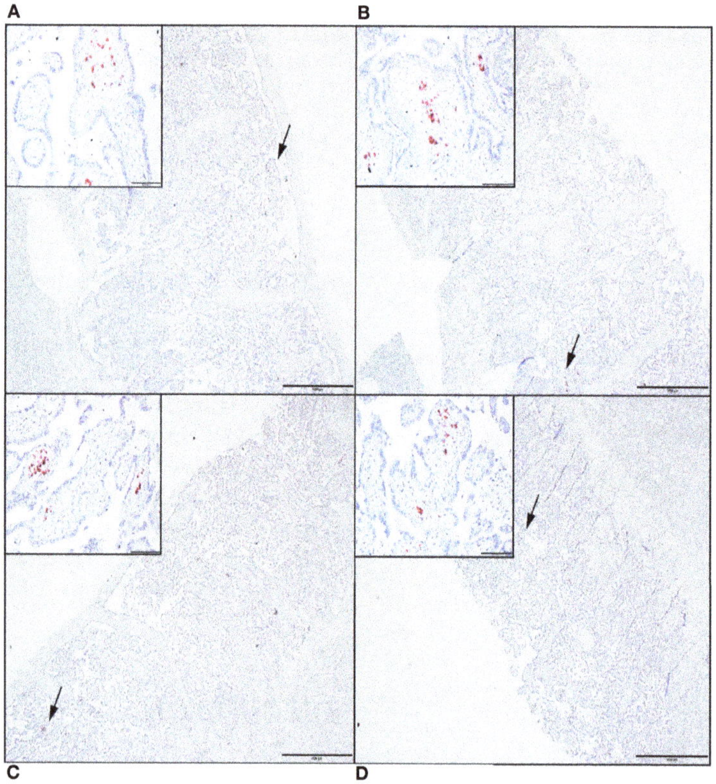

FIGURE 4 | ZIKV genomic RNA was detected by *in situ* hybridization (ISH) in placental tissues collected from dams 049-102 and 049-103, but not from dam 049-101. For all images, red coloration is indicative of positive staining for ZIKV genomic RNA. Overall, positive staining is focal but visible in multiple areas. Insets show high magnification of the areas denoted by the black arrows in each larger panel. Representative images are shown of **(A)** primary placental disk from 049-103, **(B)** secondary placental disk from 049-103, **(C)** primary placental disk from 049-102, and **(D)** secondary placental disk from 049-102. Scale bar = 1000 micrometers.

transmission in these studies we intentionally avoided any intrauterine sampling to ensure no confounding variables. Because vRNA was not detected in any fetal tissues, our results may suggest that vertical transmission did not occur between dam 049-101 and the developing fetus. Alternatively, the results may suggest immunologic elimination of virus at later gestational ages as previously suggested by a study using direct fetal ZIKV inoculation (43). Our decision to challenge the animals in this study early in pregnancy (~30 days gestation) was based on findings in humans suggesting that during the first trimester, ZIKV infection is associated with a higher risk of adverse fetal and pregnancy outcomes (27, 43, 50–53). In addition, we hypothesized that early pregnancy, possibly before a woman knows she is pregnant, may be a period of especially high risk for

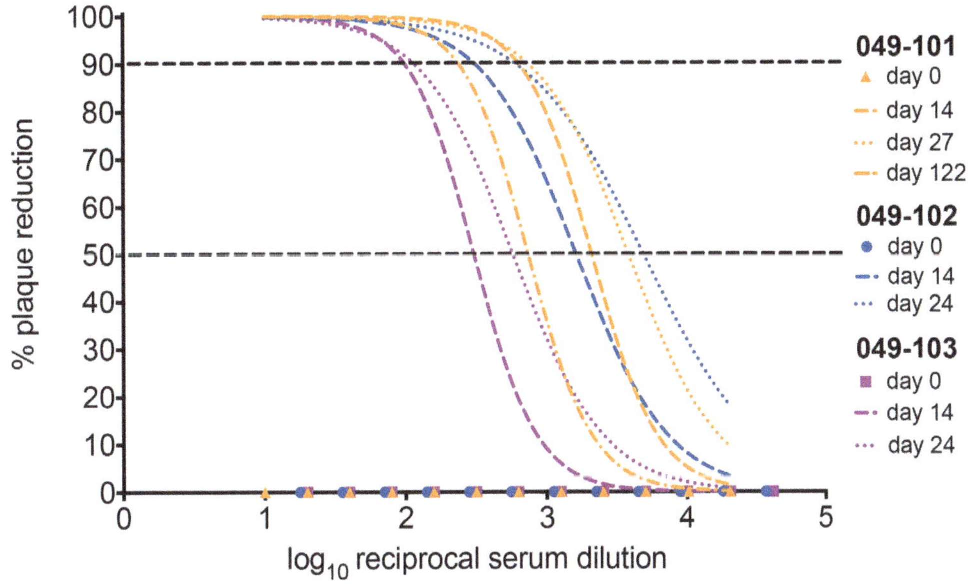

FIGURE 5 | All three dams developed neutralizing antibodies (nAbs) against ZIKV as detected by $PRNT_{90}$ following intravaginal ZIKV infection. The x-axis is the log10 reciprocal serum dilution and the y-axis is the percent plaque reduction for ZIKV-DAK. Day 0 for all animals is shown as symbols with 049-101 represented by orange triangles, 049-102 represented by blue circles, and 049-103 represented by magenta squares. Dashed gray horizontal lines indicate the $PRNT_{90}$ and $PRNT_{50}$ cut-offs, respectively. Neutralization curves were generated using non-linear regression to estimate the dilution of serum required to inhibit 90% of Vero cell culture infection. Neutralization curves are shown for days 14 (dashed lines) and 24 (dotted lines) for dams 049-102 (blue) and 049-103 (magenta), and for days 14, 27, and 122 (dashed and dotted line) for dam 049-101 (orange).

sexual transmission of ZIKV because precautions against this transmission route, such as condoms, may not be utilized (23, 24). Overall, our results suggest that sexual transmission of ZIKV during early pregnancy may represent a significant risk for adverse outcomes.

Our results indicating early demise as a result of ZIKV infection are consistent with those described previously in a cross-center, cross-NHP species study (29). Interestingly, our finding that 2 of 3 (~66%) pregnancies resulted in nonviable embryos following intravaginal ZIKV infection during early pregnancy represents a higher rate of loss than the ~26% previously reported for NHP (29). We acknowledge this loss rate is based on small animal numbers and could change as more animals are studied. Despite this higher rate compared to other NHP models reported to date, both early gestation and near term reflect periods of higher rates of spontaneous loss for macaques (54). While the loss rate reported in our study may be higher than the background rate of early loss in humans during the first trimester, data are very limited regarding the rate at which ZIKV-associated loss occurs in humans during the first trimester. A rate of approximately 11% was recently reported in a study during a period of epidemic transmission in Manaus, Brazil (55–58), although as noted, in many cases women may not be aware of an early pregnancy, thus the rate of loss could actually be higher. Additional studies with larger animal numbers will be necessary to determine the impact of the challenge dose, virus isolate, gestational age, and route of infection on pregnancy loss and how this relates to rates of spontaneous loss in early gestation.

Some limitations of this study include the use of a relatively high dose of ZIKV to inoculate the dams, the inclusion of multiple challenges over a short timeframe, and the small number of animals included in the study. The dose of inoculum chosen for this study is representative of the high end of the ZIKV vRNA range reportedly detected in human semen, which can be up to 100,000 times higher than that in blood (16–18). In part, this dose was chosen due to the small number of animals included, our interest in the impact of intravaginal ZIKV exposure early in pregnancy, and the need to maximize chances of successful infection during early gestation. Previous studies in nonpregnant NHP have shown that intravaginal ZIKV inoculation results in successful infection after a single challenge approximately 33-75 percent of the time (31, 37, 59). In pregnant olive baboons, a single intravaginal inoculation mid-gestation with semen containing ZIKV (originating from French Polynesia or Puerto Rico) resulted in 4 of 6 animals developing detectable vRNA in blood, with an additional animal having detectable vRNA in blood after a second inoculation (33). This was the rationale for the choice to perform repeat challenges at two-hour intervals in this study: in order to maximize the likelihood of establishing a productive infection in our small cohort within a single day. We acknowledge that it is difficult to determine whether the inoculation route played a significant role in our observed outcomes or whether the cumulative inoculum dose, virus isolate, timing of infection, or some combination of these factors played a role in the observed outcomes. Future studies modeling sexual transmission should aim to determine which of these factors significantly impact pregnancy outcome.

We chose to utilize a low passage African ZIKV isolate (ZIKV-DAK) rather than a more contemporary isolate such as the commonly utilized PRVABC59 because, although it is also low passage, recent studies have suggested that this virus may have an attenuated phenotype and is not as pathogenic as ZIKV-DAK in mice (41, 60). In addition, ZIKV was first isolated from a febrile rhesus macaque in the Zika Forest near Entebbe, Uganda in 1947 (61, 62). Since that time, serologic and molecular (RNA or virus isolation) evidence of continued circulation in Africa has been intermittently reported in humans, animals, and mosquitoes (63–67). Prior to a report from Guinea-Bissau from 2016, during which an outbreak and subsequent identification of infant microcephaly cases was attributed to an African lineage virus, there were no reports of ZIKV impacting pregnancies and infant development in Africa (63, 68). This has led to a number of hypotheses as to why, which includes, but is not limited to the following: widespread immunity in populations of childbearing age due to infection earlier in life; masking of ZIKV-associated adverse outcomes due to a high number of other, co-circulating pathogens in many populations, such as malaria; or embryonic loss during very early pregnancy simply unrecognized due to unknown status or inconsistent access to prenatal care (63, 64, 69). The data generated in this work supports the latter hypothesis of early loss. In reality, depending on the region, many of these factors could be playing an additive role in low and/or underreporting of ZIKV-associated pregnancy outcomes in Africa. Whether the early pregnancy losses observed in our study were due to increased pathogenicity of the African ZIKV isolate utilized relative to other isolates, the intravaginal route of infection, or both will require additional studies.

Many key questions remain with regard to understanding how different ZIKV geographic isolates may differentially impact pregnancy and fetal developmental outcomes. This study suggests that NHP models may be able to differentiate pregnancy outcomes between different isolates. Route of maternal infection may also play a role in pregnancy outcomes, at least in the case of NHP, as intravenous and intra-amniotic ZIKV infections in combination during pregnancy have been associated with a trend toward lower fetal survival rates across multiple studies compared to subcutaneous infections (29). However, both routes of ZIKV infection have been previously shown to result in early pregnancy loss in macaques, in particular when maternal infection occurred in the first trimester (29). Zika virus infection of common marmoset dams *via* an intramuscular route during the first or second trimesters has also been shown to result in spontaneous pregnancy loss (70). In the case of the marmosets, the timing of pregnancy loss (16-18 days post-infection) was very similar to that reported here for intravaginal inoculation (70). Overall, our study suggests that intravaginal infection during early pregnancy may also lower survival rates in macaques. Ultimately, our study was designed to balance all of the potential influential factors previously mentioned within the constraints of a proof-of-concept study and the requirement for challenge and infection to occur during early pregnancy in order to evaluate this question.

Our results suggest that low passage, African lineage virus (ZIKV-DAK) has the potential to result in embryonic demise in rhesus macaques when infection occurs intravaginally and in early pregnancy. To our knowledge, this is the first NHP study to show clear evidence of vertical transmission of ZIKV following intravaginal infection, which has only previously been observed in mice (20, 30, 36). NHP, due to susceptibility without immune modulation, as well as having significant similarities to human pregnancy, may provide better approximations for human infections than other animal models (71). Furthermore, this is the first NHP study to show that African lineage ZIKV infection during pregnancy has the potential to result in severe fetal outcomes. Taken together, our results suggest that additional attention should be given to ongoing perinatal surveillance in African communities and to promoting awareness regarding the risks of sexual transmission of ZIKV in endemic areas.

ETHICS STATEMENT

The animal study was reviewed and approved by University of California, Davis Institutional Animal Care and Use Committee.

AUTHOR CONTRIBUTIONS

CN, AT, CM, and DHO designed the study. AT provided animal oversight and monitoring, ultrasound imaging, and performed all sample collections. AT and CM performed animal infections. AT, MM, MB, XZ, HS, TM, MA, EB analyzed samples. CN, DD, and JR curated data. CN and JR prepared the figures. CN prepared the initial manuscript draft. All authors contributed to the article and approved the submitted version.

FUNDING

DHHS/PHS/NIH R01 A|1116382-01A1, NIH P51 OD011107 and NIH S10 OD016261.

ACKNOWLEDGMENTS

We thank the research, animal care, and veterinary staff at the California National Primate Research Center for caring for the animals and supporting this study amid the emerging SARS-CoV-2 pandemic. We also thank DHHS/PHS/NIH for providing the supplemental funding for R01 A1116382-01A1 that allowed this work to be completed. These studies were also supported by the California National Primate Research Center base operating grant #OD011107. *In vivo* imaging was performed with instrumentation funded by an NIH S10 grant #OD016261.

REFERENCES

1. *Zika Cumulative Cases.* PAHO. Available at: https://www.paho.org/hq/index.php?option=com_content&view=article&id=12390:zika-cumulative-cases&Itemid=42090&lang=en (Accessed March 22, 2021).
2. Moore CA, Staples JE, Dobyns WB, Pessoa A, Ventura CV, Fonseca EB da, et al. Characterizing the Pattern of Anomalies in Congenital Zika Syndrome for Pediatric Clinicians. *JAMA Pediatr* (2017) 171:288–95. doi: 10.1001/jamapediatrics.2016.3982
3. van der Eijk AA, van Genderen PJ, Verdijk RM, Reusken CB, Mögling R, van Kampen JJA, et al. Miscarriage Associated With Zika Virus Infection. *N Engl J Med* (2016) 375:1002–4. doi: 10.1056/NEJMc1605898
4. Azevedo RSS, Araujo MT, Oliveira CS, Filho AJM, Nunes BTD, Henriques DF, et al. Zika Virus Epidemic in Brazil. II. Post-Mortem Analyses of Neonates With Microcephaly, Stillbirths, and Miscarriage. *J Clin Med Res* (2018) 7:496–508. doi: 10.3390/jcm7120496
5. Tabata T, Petitt M, Puerta-Guardo H, Michlmayr D, Wang C, Fang-Hoover J, et al. Zika Virus Targets Different Primary Human Placental Cells, Suggesting Two Routes for Vertical Transmission. *Cell Host Microbe* (2016) 20:155–66. doi: 10.1016/j.chom.2016.07.002
6. Gregory CJ, Oduyebo T, Brault AC, Brooks JT, Chung K-W, Hills S, et al. Modes of Transmission of Zika Virus. *J Infect Dis* (2017) 216:S875–83. doi: 10.1093/infdis/jix396
7. Counotte MJ, Kim CR, Wang J, Bernstein K, Deal CD, Broutet NJN, et al. Sexual Transmission of Zika Virus and Other Flaviviruses: A Living Systematic Review. *PloS Med* (2018) 15:e1002611. doi: 10.1371/journal.pmed.1002611
8. de Barros ACWG, Santos KG, Massad E, Coelho FC. Sex-Specific Asymmetrical Attack Rates in Combined Sexual-Vectorial Transmission Epidemics. *Microorganisms* (2019) 7:112–25. doi: 10.3390/microorganisms7040112
9. Foy BD, Kobylinski KC, Chilson Foy JL, Blitvich BJ, Travassos da Rosa A, Haddow AD, et al. Probable Non-Vector-Borne Transmission of Zika Virus, Colorado, USA. *Emerg Infect Dis* (2011) 17:880–2. doi: 10.3201/eid1705.101939
10. McCarthy M. Zika Virus was Transmitted by Sexual Contact in Texas, Health Officials Report. *BMJ* (2016) 352:i720. doi: 10.1136/bmj.i720
11. D'Ortenzio E, Matheron S, Yazdanpanah Y, de Lamballerie X, Hubert B, Piorkowski G, et al. Evidence of Sexual Transmission of Zika Virus. *N Engl J Med* (2016) 374:2195–8. doi: 10.1056/NEJMc1604449
12. Deckard DT, Chung WM, Brooks JT, Smith JC, Woldai S, Hennessey M, et al. Male-to-Male Sexual Transmission of Zika Virus–Texas, January 2016. *MMWR Morb Mortal Wkly Rep* (2016) 65:372–4. doi: 10.15585/mmwr.mm6514a3
13. Davidson A, Slavinski S, Komoto K, Rakeman J, Weiss D. Suspected Female-to-Male Sexual Transmission of Zika Virus - New York City, 2016. *MMWR Morb Mortal Wkly Rep* (2016) 65:716–7. doi: 10.15585/mmwr.mm6528e2
14. Yarrington CD, Hamer DH, Kuohung W, Lee-Parritz A. Congenital Zika Syndrome Arising From Sexual Transmission of Zika Virus, a Case Report. *Fertil Res Pract* (2019) 5:1. doi: 10.1186/s40738-018-0053-5
15. Turmel JM, Abgueguen P, Hubert B, Vandamme YM, Maquart M, Le Guillou-Guillemette H, et al. Late Sexual Transmission of Zika Virus Related to Persistence in the Semen. *Lancet* (2016) 387:2501. doi: 10.1016/S0140-6736(16)30775-9
16. Musso D, Richard V, Teissier A, Stone M, Lanteri MC, Latoni G, et al. Recipient Epidemiology and Donor Evaluation Study (Reds-III) ZIKV Study Group. Detection of Zika Virus RNA in Semen of Asymptomatic Blood Donors. *Clin Microbiol Infect* (2017) 23:1001.e1–3. doi: 10.1016/j.cmi.2017.07.006
17. Mead PS, Duggal NK, Hook SA, Delorey M, Fischer M, Olzenak McGuire D, et al. Zika Virus Shedding in Semen of Symptomatic Infected Men. *N Engl J Med* (2018) 378:1377–85. doi: 10.1056/NEJMoa1711038
18. Mansuy JM, Dutertre M, Mengelle C, Fourcade C, Marchou B, Delobel P, et al. Zika Virus: High Infectious Viral Load in Semen, a New Sexually Transmitted Pathogen? *Lancet Infect Dis* (2016) 16:405. doi: 10.1016/S1473-3099(16)00138-9
19. McDonald EM, Duggal NK, Brault AC. Pathogenesis and Sexual Transmission of Spondweni and Zika Viruses. *PloS Negl Trop Dis* (2017) 11:e0005990. doi: 10.1371/journal.pntd.0005990
20. Duggal NK, Ritter JM, Pestorius SE, Zaki SR, Davis BS, Chang G-JJ, et al. Frequent Zika Virus Sexual Transmission and Prolonged Viral RNA Shedding in an Immunodeficient Mouse Model. *Cell Rep* (2017) 18:1751–60. doi: 10.1016/j.celrep.2017.01.056
21. Rosenberg ES, Doyle K, Munoz-Jordan JL, Klein L, Adams L, Lozier M, et al. Prevalence and Incidence of Zika Virus Infection Among Household Contacts of Patients With Zika Virus Disease, Puerto Rico, 2016-2017. *J Infect Dis* (2019) 220:932–9. doi: 10.1093/infdis/jiy689
22. Racicot K, Cardenas I, Wünsche V, Aldo P, Guller S, Means RE, et al. Viral Infection of the Pregnant Cervix Predisposes to Ascending Bacterial Infection. *J Immunol* (2013) 191:934–41. doi: 10.4049/jimmunol.1300661
23. Teasdale CA, Abrams EJ, Chiasson MA, Justman J, Blanchard K, Jones HE. Sexual Risk and Intravaginal Practice Behavior Changes During Pregnancy. *Arch Sex Behav* (2017) 46:539–48. doi: 10.1007/s10508-016-0818-z
24. Salvesen von Essen B, Kortsmit K, Warner L, D'Angelo DV, Shulman HB, Virella WH, et al. Preventing Sexual Transmission of Zika Virus Infection During Pregnancy, Puerto Rico, USA, 20161. *Emerg Infect Dis* (2019) 25:2115–9. doi: 10.3201/eid2511.190915
25. Hoen B, Schaub B, Funk AL, Ardillon V, Boullard M, Cabié A, et al. Pregnancy Outcomes After ZIKV Infection in French Territories in the Americas. *N Engl J Med* (2018) 378:985–94. doi: 10.1056/NEJMoa1709481
26. Lin HZ, Tambyah PA, Yong EL, Biswas A, Chan S-Y. A Review of Zika Virus Infections in Pregnancy and Implications for Antenatal Care in Singapore. *Singapore Med J* (2017) 58:171–8. doi: 10.11622/smedj.2017026
27. Kleber de Oliveira W, Cortez-Escalante J, De Oliveira WTGH, do Carmo GMI, Henriques CMP, Coelho GE, et al. Increase in Reported Prevalence of Microcephaly in Infants Born to Women Living in Areas With Confirmed Zika Virus Transmission During the First Trimester of Pregnancy - Brazil, 2015. *MMWR Morb Mortal Wkly Rep* (2016) 65:242–7. doi: 10.15585/mmwr.mm6509e2
28. Pomar L, Malinger G, Benoist G, Carles G, Ville Y, Rousset D, et al. Association Between Zika Virus and Fetopathy: A Prospective Cohort Study in French Guiana. *Ultrasound Obstet Gynecol* (2017) 49:729–36. doi: 10.1002/uog.17404
29. Dudley DM, Van Rompay KK, Coffey LL, Ardeshir A, Keesler RI, Bliss-Moreau E, et al. Miscarriage and Stillbirth Following Maternal Zika Virus Infection in Nonhuman Primates. *Nat Med* (2018) 24:1104–7. doi: 10.1038/s41591-018-0088-5
30. Duggal NK, McDonald EM, Ritter JM, Brault AC. Sexual Transmission of Zika Virus Enhances In Utero Transmission in a Mouse Model. *Sci Rep* (2018) 8:4510. doi: 10.1038/s41598-018-22840-6
31. Haddow AD, Perez-Sautu U, Wiley MR, Miller LJ, Kimmel AE, Principe LM, et al. Modeling Mosquito-Borne and Sexual Transmission of Zika Virus in an Enzootic Host, the African Green Monkey. *PloS Negl Trop Dis* (2020) 14: e0008107. doi: 10.1371/journal.pntd.0008107
32. Schmidt JK, Mean KD, Puntney RC, Alexander ES, Sullivan R, Simmons HA, et al. Zika Virus in Rhesus Macaque Semen and Reproductive Tract Tissues: A Pilot Study of Acute Infection†. *Biol Reprod* (2020) 103:1030–42. doi: 10.1093/biolre/ioaa137
33. Gurung S, Nadeau H, Maxted M, Peregrine J, Reuter D, Norris A, et al. Maternal Zika Virus (Zikv) Infection Following Vaginal Inoculation With ZIKV-Infected Semen in Timed-Pregnant Olive Baboons. *J Virol* (2020) 94:1–16. doi: 10.1128/JVI.00058-20
34. Peregrine J, Gurung S, Lindgren MC, Husain S, Zavy MT, Myers DA, et al. Zika Virus Infection, Reproductive Organ Targeting, and Semen Transmission in the Male Olive Baboon. *J Virol* (2019) 94:1–16. doi: 10.1128/JVI.01434-19
35. Woollard SM, Olwenyi OA, Dutta D, Dave RS, Mathews S, Gorantla S, et al. Preliminary Studies on Immune Response and Viral Pathogenesis of Zika Virus in Rhesus Macaques. *Pathogens* (2018) 7:70–81. doi: 10.3390/pathogens7030070
36. Winkler CW, Woods TA, Rosenke R, Scott DP, Best SM, Peterson KE. Sexual and Vertical Transmission of Zika Virus in Anti-Interferon Receptor-Treated Rag1-Deficient Mice. *Sci Rep* (2017) 7:7176. doi: 10.1038/s41598-017-07099-7
37. Carroll T, Lo M, Lanteri M, Dutra J, Zarbock K, Silveira P, et al. Zika Virus Preferentially Replicates in the Female Reproductive Tract After Vaginal Inoculation of Rhesus Macaques. *PloS Pathog* (2017) 13:e1006537. doi: 10.1371/journal.ppat.1006537
38. Tang WW, Young MP, Mamidi A, Regla-Nava JA, Kim K, Shresta S. A Mouse Model of Zika Virus Sexual Transmission and Vaginal Viral Replication. *Cell Rep* (2016) 17:3091–8. doi: 10.1016/j.celrep.2016.11.070

39. Yockey LJ, Varela L, Rakib T, Khoury-Hanold W, Fink SL, Stutz B, et al. Vaginal Exposure to Zika Virus During Pregnancy Leads to Fetal Brain Infection. *Cell* (2016) 166:1247–56.e4. doi: 10.1016/j.cell.2016.08.004
40. TA F. Ultrasound Imaging in Rhesus (*Macaca mulatta*) and Long-Tailed (*Macaca fascicularis*) Macaques: Reproductive and Research Applications. *Lab Primate* (2005), 317–52. doi: 10.1016/b978-012080261-6/50020-9
41. Jaeger AS, Murrieta RA, Goren LR, Crooks CM, Moriarty RV, Weiler AM, et al. Zika Viruses of African and Asian Lineages Cause Fetal Harm in a Mouse Model of Vertical Transmission. *PloS Negl Trop Dis* (2019) 13: e0007343. doi: 10.1371/journal.pntd.0007343
42. Dudley DM, Aliota MT, Mohr EL, Weiler AM, Lehrer-Brey G, Weisgrau KL, et al. A Rhesus Macaque Model of Asian-lineage Zika Virus Infection. *Nat Commun* (2016) 7:12204. doi: 10.1038/ncomms12204
43. Tarantal AF, Hartigan-O'Connor DJ, Penna E, Kreutz A, Martinez ML, Noctor SC. Fetal Rhesus Monkey First Trimester Zika Virus Infection Impacts Cortical Development in the Second and Third Trimesters. *Cereb Cortex* (2020) 31:2309–21. doi: 10.1093/cercor/bhaa336
44. Koenig MR, Razo E, Mitzey A, Newman CM, Dudley DM, Breitbach ME, et al. Quantitative Definition of Neurobehavior, Vision, Hearing and Brain Volumes in Macaques Congenitally Exposed to Zika Virus. *PloS One* (2020) 15:e0235877. doi: 10.1371/journal.pone.0235877
45. Breitbach ME, Newman CM, Dudley DM, Stewart LM, Aliota MT, Koenig MR, et al. Primary Infection With Dengue or Zika Virus Does Not Affect the Severity of Heterologous Secondary Infection in Macaques. *PloS Pathog* (2019) 15:e1007766. doi: 10.1371/journal.ppat.1007766
46. Lindsey HS, Calisher CH, Mathews JH. Serum Dilution Neutralization Test for California Group Virus Identification and Serology. *J Clin Microbiol* (1976) 4:503–10.
47. Crooks CM, Weiler AM, Rybarczyk SL, Bliss M, Jaeger AS, Murphy ME, et al. African-Lineage Zika Virus Replication Dynamics and Maternal-Fetal Interface Infection in Pregnant Rhesus Macaques. *Cold Spring Harbor Lab* (2020). doi: 10.1101/2020.11.30.405670
48. Nguyen SM, Antony KM, Dudley DM, Kohn S, Simmons HA, Wolfe B, et al. Highly Efficient Maternal-Fetal Zika Virus Transmission in Pregnant Rhesus Macaques. *PloS Pathog* (2017) 13:e1006378. doi: 10.1371/journal.ppat.1006378
49. Mohr EL, Block LN, Newman CM, Stewart LM, Koenig M, Semler M, et al. Ocular and Uteroplacental Pathology in a Macaque Pregnancy With Congenital Zika Virus Infection. *PloS One* (2018) 13:e0190617. doi: 10.1371/journal.pone.0190617
50. Honein MA, Dawson AL, Petersen EE, Jones AM, Lee EH, Yazdy MM, et al. Birth Defects Among Fetuses and Infants of US Women With Evidence of Possible Zika Virus Infection During Pregnancy. *JAMA* (2017) 317:59–68. doi: 10.1001/jama.2016.19006
51. Peña F, Pimentel R, Khosla S, Mehta SD, Brito MO. Zika Virus Epidemic in Pregnant Women, Dominican Republic, 2016-2017. *Emerg Infect Dis* (2019) 25:247–55. doi: 10.3201/eid2502.181054
52. Ospina ML, Tong VT, Gonzalez M, Valencia D, Mercado M, Gilboa SM, et al. Zika Virus Disease and Pregnancy Outcomes in Colombia. *N Engl J Med* (2020) 383:537–45. doi: 10.1056/NEJMoa1911023
53. Ades AE, Soriano-Arandes A, Alarcon A, Bonfante F, Thorne C, Peckham CS, et al. Vertical Transmission of Zika Virus and its Outcomes: A Bayesian Synthesis of Prospective Studies. *Lancet Infect Dis* (2020) 21:537–45. doi: 10.1016/S1473-3099(20)30432-1
54. Hendrie TA, Peterson PE, Short JJ, Tarantal AF, Rothgarn E, Hendrie MI, et al. Frequency of Prenatal Loss in a Macaque Breeding Colony. *Am J Primatol* (1996) 40:41–53. doi: 10.1002/(SICI)1098-2345(1996)40:1<41::AID-AJP3>3.0.CO;2-0
55. Brasil P, Pereira JP Jr, Moreira ME, Ribeiro Nogueira RM, Damasceno L, Wakimoto M, et al. Zika Virus Infection in Pregnant Women in Rio De Janeiro. *N Engl J Med* (2016) 375:2321–34. doi: 10.1056/NEJMoa1602412
56. Cohain JS, Buxbaum RE, Mankuta D. Spontaneous First Trimester Miscarriage Rates Per Woman Among Parous Women With 1 or More Pregnancies of 24 Weeks or More. *BMC Pregnancy Childbirth* (2017) 17:437. doi: 10.1186/s12884-017-1620-1
57. Redivo E de F, Bôtto Menezes C, da Costa Castilho M, Brock M, da Silva Magno E, Gomes Saraiva M das G, et al. Zika Virus Infection in a Cohort of Pregnant Women With Exanthematic Disease in Manaus, Brazilian Amazon. *Viruses* (2020) 12:1362–77. doi: 10.3390/v12121362
58. Oliver A, Overton C. Diagnosis and Management of Miscarriage. *Practitioner* (2014) 258:25–8.
59. Haddow AD, Nalca A, Rossi FD, Miller LJ, Wiley MR, Perez-Sautu U, et al. High Infection Rates for Adult Macaques After Intravaginal or Intrarectal Inoculation With Zika Virus. *Emerg Infect Dis* (2017) 23:1274–81. doi: 10.3201/eid2308.170036
60. Duggal NK, McDonald EM, Weger-Lucarelli J, Hawks SA, Ritter JM, Romo H, et al. Mutations Present in a Low-Passage Zika Virus Isolate Result in Attenuated Pathogenesis in Mice. *Virology* (2019) 530:19–26. doi: 10.1016/j.virol.2019.02.004
61. Dick GWA, Kitchen SF, Haddow AJ. Zika Virus. I. Isolations and Serological Specificity. *Trans R Soc Trop Med Hyg* (1952) 46:509–20. doi: 10.1016/0035-9203(52)90042-4
62. Dick GWA. Zika Virus. II. Pathogenicity and Physical Properties. *Trans R Soc Trop Med Hyg* (1952) 46:521–34. doi: 10.1016/0035-9203(52)90043-6
63. Nutt C, Adams P. Zika in Africa-the Invisible Epidemic? *Lancet* (2017) 389:1595–6. doi: 10.1016/S0140-6736(17)31051-6
64. Marchi S, Viviani S, Montomoli E, Tang Y, Boccuto A, Vicenti I, et al. Zika Virus in West Africa: A Seroepidemiological Study Between 2007 and 2012. *Viruses* (2020) 12:641–70. doi: 10.3390/v12060641
65. McCrae AW, Kirya BG. Yellow Fever and Zika Virus Epizootics and Enzootics in Uganda. *Trans R Soc Trop Med Hyg* (1982) 76:552–62. doi: 10.1016/0035-9203(82)90161-4
66. Dick GW. Epidemiological Notes on Some Viruses Isolated in Uganda; Yellow Fever, Rift Valley Fever, Bwamba Fever, West Nile, Mengo, Semliki Forest, Bunyamwera, Ntaya, Uganda S and Zika Viruses. *Trans R Soc Trop Med Hyg* (1953) 47:13–48. doi: 10.1016/0035-9203(53)90021-2
67. Kirya BG. A Yellow Fever Epizootic in Zika Forest, Uganda, During 1972: Part 1: Virus Isolation and Sentinel Monkeys. *Trans R Soc Trop Med Hyg* (1977) 71:254–60. doi: 10.1016/0035-9203(77)90020-7
68. Rosenstierne MW, Schaltz-Buchholzer F, Bruzadelli F, Có A, Cardoso P, Jørgensen CS, et al. Zika Virus Igg in Infants With Microcephaly, Guinea-Bissau, 2016. *Emerg Infect Dis* (2018) 24:948–50. doi: 10.3201/eid2405.180153
69. Sheridan MA, Yunusov D, Balaraman V, Alexenko AP, Yabe S, Verjovski-Almeida S, et al. Vulnerability of Primitive Human Placental Trophoblast to Zika Virus. *Proc Natl Acad Sci USA* (2017) 114:E1587–96. doi: 10.1073/pnas.1616097114
70. Seferovic M, Sánchez-San Martín C, Tardif SD, Rutherford J, Castro ECC, Li T, et al. Experimental Zika Virus Infection in the Pregnant Common Marmoset Induces Spontaneous Fetal Loss and Neurodevelopmental Abnormalities. *Sci Rep* (2018) 8:6851. doi: 10.1038/s41598-018-25205-1
71. Dudley DM, Aliota MT, Mohr EL, Newman CM, Golos TG, Friedrich TC, et al. Using Macaques to Address Critical Questions in Zika Virus Research. *Annu Rev Virol* (2019) 6:481–500. doi: 10.1146/annurev-virology-092818-015732

5

MicroRNA-Mediated Control of Inflammation and Tolerance in Pregnancy

Ranjith Kamity[1], *Surendra Sharma*[2*] *and Nazeeh Hanna*[1*]

[1] *Women and Children Research Laboratory, Division of Neonatology, Department of Pediatrics, NYU Winthrop Hospital, Mineola, NY, United States,* [2] *Department of Pediatrics, Women and Infants Hospital, Warren Alpert Medical School of Brown University, Providence, RI, United States*

Correspondence:
Surendra Sharma
ssharma@wihri.org
Nazeeh Hanna
nazeehhanna@gmail.com

Gestational age-dependent immune intolerance at the maternal-fetal interface might be a contributing factor to placental pathology and adverse pregnancy outcomes. Although the intrauterine setting is highly choreographed and considered to be a protective environment for the fetus, unscheduled inflammation might overwhelm the intrauterine milieu to cause a cascade of events leading to adverse pregnancy outcomes. The old paradigm of a sterile intrauterine microenvironment has been challenged, and altered microflora has been detected in gestational tissues and amniotic fluid in the absence of induction of significant inflammation. Is there a role for endotoxin tolerance at the maternal-fetal interface? Endotoxin tolerance is a phenomenon in which tissues or cells exposed to the bacterial product, particularly lipopolysaccharide, become less responsive to subsequent exposures accompanied by decreased expression of pro-inflammatory mediators. This could also be related to trained or experienced immunity that leads to the successful outcome of subsequent pregnancies. Adaptation to endotoxin tolerance or trained immunity might be critical in preventing rejection of the fetus by the maternal immune system and protecting the fetus from excessive maternal inflammatory responses to infectious agents; however, to date, the exact mechanisms contributing to the establishment and maintenance of tolerance at the maternal-fetal interface remain incompletely understood. There is now extensive evidence suggesting that microRNAs (miRNAs) play important roles in the maintenance of a healthy pregnancy. miRNAs not only circulate freely in extracellular fluids but are also packaged within extracellular vesicles (EVs) produced by various cells and tissues. The placenta is a known, abundant, and transient source of EVs; therefore, our proposed model suggests that repeated exposure to infectious agents induces a tolerant phenotype at the maternal-fetal interface mediated by specific miRNAs mostly contained within placental EVs. We hypothesize that impaired endotoxin tolerance or failed trained immunity at the maternal-fetal interface will result in a pathological inflammatory response contributing to early or late pregnancy maladies.

Keywords: microRNA, immune tolerance, endotoxin tolerance, extracellular vesicles, pregnancy, maternal-fetal interface, innate immunity

INTRODUCTION

Our current understanding of immunity at the maternal-fetal interface has been shaped by acceptance of periodic concepts and approaches formed based on tissue-allograft studies in non-pregnant individuals, male or female, and by the paradigm suggesting the uterus as a sterile organ (1, 2). However, our contemporary understanding of the role of the placenta, hormones, and novel cellular controls warrants re-evaluation of old paradigms associated with fetal immune-protection in both hostile and normal intrauterine microenvironments (3, 4). The decidua, the maternal tissue in pregnancy, is replete with immune cells that should intrinsically harm the fetus; however, normal pregnancy ensues, suggesting that the placenta transforms these cells into a specialized, pregnancy compatible milieu (5). What remains incompletely understood is why the placenta fails to counter challenges from intrauterine infections or sterile inflammation. This is further complicated by the observations that some women can experience a successful pregnancy despite repeated exposure to infectious agents, particularly endotoxins, and other environmental factors. This review discusses recent observations that might explain successful pregnancy outcomes despite repeated intrauterine infections and potentially provide important insights into the role of the placenta via secretion of extracellular vesicles (EVs).

Despite constant exposure to hygienic challenges and infection during pregnancy, most of the 4 million annual deliveries in the United States have a successful outcome without presenting any clinical evidence of intrauterine infection (6). In this regard, the onus can be placed on the placenta to counter inflammation and ensure trained immunity for a successful pregnancy (7–10); however, it remains unclear how the placenta programs these pregnancy compatible events. The placenta is a transient organ that supports fetal growth and development by ensuring respiratory gas exchange, regulates maternal-fetal nutrient transport, provides protection for the fetus against maternal immunity, and acts as a transient endocrine organ by producing hormones, such as estrogen, progesterone, human chorionic gonadotropin, and human placental lactogen, while protecting the fetus from external infectious and immune threats (11, 12). Increasing evidence suggests that molecular exchanges occur between maternal and fetal systems to enable adaptation of maternal physiology for growing fetal requirements during gestation, with the focus placed on placenta-derived EVs as a medium of placental communication with maternal physiology (13–15). An important question arises from these observations and concerns whether placental EVs play a role in protecting the fetus from infectious agents.

Among various models of immune tolerance, microRNAs (miRNAs) are implicated as mediators, as well as markers of immune tolerance in various tissues; however, the mechanisms associated with miRNA-mediated immune tolerance in gestational tissues are not well-understood. Because miRNAs are also included as cargo in EVs, do placental EVs and their embedded miRNA cargo play a role in immune tolerance at the maternal-fetal interface? This review focuses on immune tolerance at the maternal-fetal interface and reviews the role of miRNA in mediating immune tolerance via EVs in gestational tissues.

MATERNAL-FETAL INTERFACE IMMUNITY AND ITS ROLE IN ADVERSE PREGNANCY OUTCOMES

Pregnancy is a period of physiological stress accompanied by a vital balance between proinflammatory and anti-inflammatory stimuli. Disruption of this delicate balance at the maternal-fetal interface has been linked to various adverse pregnancy outcomes. Starting from exposure to seminal antigens at coitus, to implantation, an active inflammatory period facilitates implantation and initial pregnancy (16). The cytokines and chemokines in seminal fluid play a role in attracting regulatory T cells (Tregs) to the microenvironment (17). Female dendritic cells recognize fetal antigens and cross-present seminal-fluid antigens that transform effector $CD4^+$ T cells into Tregs, which are then recruited to the endometrium. Tregs and decidual natural killer (dNK) cells increase during early pregnancy and play a vital role in implantation and maintenance of pregnancy (17–19). Although *in vitro* fertilization (IVF) pregnancies involving fertilized eggs with washed semen do occur, Treg recruitment to the implantation site appears to be a physiologically helpful and critical event for implantation and pregnancy maintenance (20, 21). dNK cells and Tregs are integral cellular components that contribute to normal placentation and vascular support at the maternal-fetal interface, while playing an important role in preventing fetal rejection (22).

This period of inflammatory activity during implantation is subsequently followed by a period of relative inflammatory quiescence during mid-pregnancy to enable fetal growth and development (17, 23). Dysregulated immunity with excessive maternal inflammation further into pregnancy contributes to impaired angiogenesis, especially of the spiral arteries, resulting in gestational vascular disorders, such as preeclampsia (24–27). The concept of trained immunity and inflammation tolerance might be applicable in the case of preeclampsia, as subsequent pregnancy with the same partner within a few years of first pregnancy is not always associated with recurrence of the pregnancy complication (28, 29).

Pregnancy can be divided into three phases of inflammatory milieu: implantation (inflammatory), active gestation (anti-inflammatory), and parturition (inflammatory) (17, 23). At parturition, labor is induced by an inflammation-associated cascade of events that result in delivery. Premature activation of this process results in preterm labor and delivery. Why

Abbreviations: CD, cluster of differentiation; DAMP, damage associated molecular patterns; EV, extracellular vesicle; IL, interleukin; IRAK, interleukin-1 receptor associated kinase; miRNA, microRNA; MV, microvesicles; MVB, multivesicular body/late endosome; MyD88, myeloid differentiation primary response 88 protein; NF-κB, transcription factor nuclear factor kappa-light-chain-enhancer of activated B cells; PAMP, pathogen associated molecular patterns; PLAP, placental alkaline phosphatase; PRR, pattern recognition receptors; TLR, toll-like receptor; TNF, tumor necrosis factor; TRAF6, TNF-receptor associated factor 6.

are the placenta or its EVs and miRNAs unable to blunt this premature activation of inflammation? It is possible that inflammation tolerance (not necessarily immune tolerance) escapes the placenta due to detrimental activation of dNK cells and Tregs, or that EVs carry an inflammatory cargo that does not counter inflammation.

TYPES OF INFLAMMATION AT THE MATERNAL-FETAL INTERFACE: INFECTION-MEDIATED OR STERILE?

A fetus in the intrauterine environment is believed to be in a relatively protected state. Occasionally, microbes gain passage into the intrauterine milieu by ascending infection or transplacental routes, with the transplacental transmission of infection from mother to fetus capable of occurring antenatally or perinatally (12). Pregnant women with altered immunity secondary to various stressors, including infection, can potentially experience preterm delivery. Romero et al. showed that despite evidence of preterm birth being linked to infection, preterm birth without infection is more common (30). Furthermore, antibiotics alone are ineffective at preventing preterm birth related to infection, suggesting that preterm birth induced by infection is mediated by inflammation rather than the organism *per se* (31). One possible explanation for antibiotic failure is that inflammatory damage has already been established, and detrimental pathways have been initiated and cannot be controlled by poorly timed treatment with antibiotics (32). Our understanding of inflammatory signals also suffers from a poor definition of sterile inflammation and its role in programming preterm birth. Therefore, it is important to understand the mechanistic differences between sterile inflammation and infection-mediated inflammation.

Pro-inflammatory stimuli can arise from both host (self) and alien (non-self) sources, also described as "danger" and "stranger" stimuli (23), that include damage-associated molecular patterns (DAMPs; also known as alarmins) and pathogen-associated molecular patterns (PAMPs), which interact with a group of pattern-recognition receptors (PRRs) expressed on the cell surface. Sterile pathways that trigger inflammation include host factors (e.g., tissue injury, cell death, and environmental factors, such as low oxygen tension and elevated uric acid) that act via DAMPs (25). These differ from infectious triggers (e.g., bacteria or viruses) that act via PAMPs (23). However, pathological inflammatory processes can be triggered by either sterile or infection-mediated pathways.

DAMPs are a group of endogenous intracellular molecules released in the early stages of unplanned cell death to signal cell injury (33). The most common DAMPs include uric acid, high-mobility group box 1, interleukin (IL)-1α, and cell-free DNA. High-mobility group box 1 levels increase in multiple animal models along with sterile inflammation, as well as in human models of acute organ injury, autoimmune diseases, and cancer (34–37). High concentrations of uric acid, a byproduct of cell death, can form monosodium urate crystals in the presence of extracellular sodium and induce acute inflammation. Upon exposure to foreign antigens and as the non-specific first line of defense against foreign microorganisms, monocytes differentiate into macrophages capable of phagocytosing the offending agents. Monosodium urate crystals, upon phagocytosis by antigen-presenting cells, can interact with the NALP3 inflammasome to convert pro-IL-1β to IL-1β, thereby resulting in an inflammatory response (23) recognized as pyroptosis. Inflammasome activation has been shown in both intra-amniotic infections as well as sterile intra-amniotic inflammation with preterm labor (38). Furthermore, treating sterile inflammation by inhibiting inflammasome activation has also been shown to reduce preterm delivery in a mice model (39).

PRRs include Toll-like receptors (TLRs) 1 through TLR13, C-type lectins, scavenger receptors, and nucleotide-binding oligomerization-domain-like receptors, all of which operate transduction pathways resulting in cytokine-mediated inflammatory responses. PRRs are expressed in multiple human cells, including decidua, placenta, membranes, and myometrium, throughout pregnancy and in immune and non-immune cells (23, 40–42). The release of DAMPs secondary to tissue injury from hypoxia-ischemia, oxidative stress, vascular dysfunction, or other stressors is implicated in sterile inflammation that acts not only on the placenta but also on the uterus, cervix, fetal membranes, and the fetus. This inflammatory process needs to be tightly regulated since such inflammation left unchecked can cause extensive tissue injury, septic shock, and death. In the placenta, this resultant maternal-fetal inflammation is suggested to contribute to various adverse pregnancy outcomes, including placental dysfunction, preeclampsia, intrauterine growth restriction, and preterm labor (23). Therefore, attenuation of this inflammation at the maternal-fetal interface can play a key role in fetal health and survival.

INDUCTION OF INNATE IMMUNITY VIA microRNAs AND SHAPING OF IMMUNE TOLERANCE: FROM MICE TO HUMANS

The systemic immune system is regulated and dominated by T lymphocytes and adaptive immunity. On the other hand, the decidual leukocyte population in the pregnant uterus is replete with NK cells (65–70%) and antigen presenting cells (macrophages and dendritic cells 10–20%), both contributors to innate immunity (4, 5). Other cell types have also been described to a lesser extent at the maternal-fetal interface, in varying numbers at different stages of pregnancy, and in certain pathological conditions (43, 44), including innate lymphoid cells, other T cell subsets and B cells. Innate immunity at the maternal-fetal interface is of a specialized variety, wherein NK cells and macrophages are pregnancy compatible and support local vascular activity. Prolonged exposure to microbial products, such as lipopolysaccharide (LPS) induces a form of innate immunity that resembles trained immunity (memory) and blunts subsequent responses to unrelated pathogens [referred to as endotoxin tolerance] (45). What is the molecular basis of endotoxin tolerance, and does this occur in the female reproductive tract? Recent pioneering work by Seeley et al.

(45) suggests that repeated exposure to LPS induces tolerance-associated miRNAs (miR-221 and miR-222) in macrophages, with this tolerance phenotype achieved through silencing of inflammatory genes and chromatin remodeling. Most studies of endotoxin tolerance have been undertaken in mouse models, as well as human cell and tissue models, resulting in links between endotoxin tolerance and protection against tissue injury and death (46, 47). Seeley et al. (45) suggest that in humans with sepsis, increased expression of these miRNAs is associated with immunoparalysis and organ damage; therefore, it is possible that a threshold level of tolerance-associated miRNAs needs to be maintained for a longer period of time in order to influence a better outcome in humans.

The molecular mechanisms associated with endotoxin tolerance are believed to be multifactorial, with multiple levels of negative feedback to blunt the inflammatory response. Mice deficient in IL-10 are more susceptible to endotoxic shock following repeated exposure to LPS, suggesting a role for IL-10 in endotoxin tolerance (48). In gestational tissues, endotoxin tolerance has been identified in mouse models, whereas human studies are lacking. During pregnancy, this adaptation due to tolerance might be critical to preventing fetal rejection by the maternal immune system, as well as protecting the fetus from excessive maternal inflammatory responses to various infectious and inflammatory agents. An increase in proinflammatory cytokine responses to bacterial insult can trigger undesirable consequences, including preterm labor and delivery, as well as fetal mal-development and inflammatory injury. Although bacterial exposure during pregnancy is associated with preterm delivery and intra-amniotic infections (49, 50), a wide array of organisms have been described in the maternal-fetal compartments in healthy pregnancies. Interestingly, the presence of an organism in the uterine environment is not always pathological, as previously reported in gene-amplification studies using amniotic fluid from women who delivered healthy newborns following an uncomplicated pregnancy (32, 51, 52).

IMMUNE TOLERANCE MEDIATED BY microRNA

miRNAs are small (18–22 nucleotides), non-coding RNA sequences that play an important role in regulating multiple cellular processes critical for development, differentiation, and organ function and are associated with marked biological consequences in health and disease (53). miRNAs act as negative regulators at the post-transcriptional level by binding to the 3′ untranslated region on target mRNA to inhibit the translation of respective proteins. Thousands of genes are regulated by miRNAs, with the list continuing to grow (53, 54). It is estimated that ~60% of all protein-coding genes can be regulated by miRNA (54); therefore, it is now accepted that mutations that cause dysfunctional miRNA can potentially affect multiple disease conditions.

Multiple organs harbor specific miRNAs that play vital roles. miR-122 is associated with cholesterol and lipid metabolism in the liver (55), whereas the miR-1 and mir-133 families regulate heart development and play roles in cardiovascular disorders (56, 57). Additionally, numerous recently identified miRNAs have been implicated in a wide array of human diseases, including cardiovascular diseases, neoplasms, and liver and kidney disorders (58–60). Moreover, early gestational tissues, such as human blastocysts, express miRNA, which might be essential for successful implantation and subsequent survival by guiding processes that navigate the intrauterine environment. Euploid and aneuploid embryos exhibit differential expression of miRNAs, ultimately resulting in different eventual outcomes (61). Furthermore, the presence of miRNAs in breast milk and serum could represent markers or mediators of cell signaling. Maternal serum miR-191 is currently being investigated as a potential non-invasive candidate for aneuploidy, whereas other miRNAs, including miR-191, miR-372, and miR-645, have been implicated in IVF failure, and elevated levels of miR-25, miR-302c, miR-196a2, and miR-181a have been identified in degenerate embryos as compared with their levels in blastocyst embryos (62).

In addition to regulating multiple cellular processes, various miRNAs are also implicated in regulating the immune system, including the differentiation and function of innate immune cells (63, 64). miRNAs have also been shown to regulate immune responses to bacterial, viral and parasitic infections (65–67). For example, miR146a polymorphism has been linked to increased risk of malaria in pregnant women. Also, miR 221 negatively regulated innate antiviral response, while miR 34/449 family has been implicated in various viral infections [(66), review]. The role of miRNA in bacterial infections is being studied in various scenarios- from a suggested role in Helicobacter pylori and Epstein-Barr virus-induced cancers [(68), review], to pathogen triggered TLR pathway stimulation.

Multiple miRNAs are up-regulated via TLR-ligand stimulation in monocytes (69) and suggested to play a major role in mediating immune tolerance by regulating the TLR pathway through TLR-receptor transcription and/or creating feedback loops by suppressing key downstream molecules that in turn down-regulate TLR activation (70). Moreover, the pattern of miRNA expression is related to the type of TLR ligand involved in its stimulation, overall ligand concentration, and the type of cells being stimulated.

Increases in miR-146a levels in response to LPS stimulation was observed in THP1 cells (63, 69, 71, 72). Additionally, Nahid et al. (71) showed that exposure to high-dose LPS (1,000 ng/mL) increases levels of the inflammatory cytokines tumor necrosis factor (TNF)α, IL-1-receptor-associated kinase (IRAK)1, and TNF-receptor-associated factor (TRAF)6 along with a simultaneous increase in miR146a levels. On the other hand, when the same cells were primed with low-dose LPS (10 ng/mL), transient elevations in TNFα, IRAK1, and TRAF6 were observed along with upregulated miR146a levels, with subsequent exposure to high-dose LPS (1,000 ng/mL) resulting in a blunted TNFα response in the presence of upregulated miR146. Other studies suggested that elevated miR-146a levels are involved in regulating TLR signaling and cytokine production by downregulating the inflammatory response (73, 74). Furthermore, miR-146a induction is mediated by NF-κB via TLR-ligand stimulation (69). Conversely, miRNAs can directly target TLRs in order to create a feedback loop that regulates the inflammatory response, with previous studies reporting that miR-105 targets the mRNA encoding the TLR2 receptor in order to attenuate its translation (75, 76). Additionally, miR-146a targets TRAF6 and IRAK activities to inhibit TLR4 signaling and downregulate NF-κB activation (69). By contrast, miRNAs, such as miR-155, can be significantly downregulated after the induction of endotoxin tolerance, suggesting cross-talk between miRNAs in order to maintain immune homeostasis and suppress proinflammatory responses. In addition to miRNAs, long non-coding RNAs are also altered upon endotoxin challenge and negatively regulate TLR signaling, thereby contributing to immune tolerance.

miRNAs are also being studied as diagnostic and therapeutic tools (77). A recent study suggests that decidual tissue from patients with recurrent spontaneous abortions shows decreased expression of miR-146a-5p (78). Similarly, quantification of 30 miRNAs from peripheral blood taken during the first trimester was used to predict preeclampsia, a late pregnancy complication (79). These observations support further study of miRNAs from gestational tissues and peripheral blood to investigate their role(s) in both endotoxin tolerance and pregnancy complications.

PLACENTA AND microRNA

The human placenta produces numerous miRNAs. miRNAs play roles in various key steps in pregnancy, including implantation, maintenance, and labor (80–84). miRNAs have been identified in trophoblasts and mostly originated from the two largest clusters on chromosomes 14 and 19 (C14MC and C19MC, respectively). Most miRNAs identified in primary trophoblasts originate from C19MC, which gives rise to 46 intronic miRNAs that are converted to 54 mature miRNAs (85). miRNAs from C19MC are found in human embryonic stem cells and play an important role in cell proliferation, invasion, and differentiation. C19MC expression is reduced in extravillous trophoblasts and several malignancies while the increase in C19MC expression confers resistance to viral infections (85, 86).

Interestingly, abundant expression of miRNA does not always translate to functional significance. A previous study reported the deletion of the miR379/410 cluster (from C14MC) without consequence (84). Additionally, miR-675 exhibits anti-proliferative effects by silencing *insulin-like growth factor receptor-1*, whereas miR-675 deletion is associated with placental overgrowth (87). Moreover, miR-378a-5p and miR-376c are involved in trophoblast proliferation and invasion regulated by the nodal signaling pathway (88, 89), and the miR17-92 cluster regulates primary human trophoblast differentiation (90). Furthermore, recently identified miR-155 inhibits trophoblasts invasion and is implicated in the pathogenesis of preeclampsia, and increased levels of plasma and placental miR-210 have been reported in association with preeclampsia (91). Although additional miRNAs continue to be discovered their precise clinical implications and roles remain elusive; however, a non-invasive sampling of such placenta-derived miRNAs is potentially useful for diagnosing placental dysfunction.

The majority of miRNAs function in the cell of origin by regulating mRNA levels and translation; however, some miRNAs are selectively secreted by cells into the extracellular space (mainly packaged within EVs) to regulate intercellular signaling of distant "target" cells. Analyses of miRNA from EVs show that EVs' miRNAs content is distinct from that found in the cytoplasm of donor cells from which they were derived. This suggests active miRNA sorting into these vesicles (92–95), although the exact mechanism remains unclear. Our unpublished data confirm that placental miRNAs play an important role in placental endotoxin tolerance resulting in blunted immune response to repeated exposure to LPS. Specifically, placenta-derived miR519c (derived from C19MC) was shown to inhibit TNFα gene expression in our placental explant model. miR519c is placenta-specific and produced by trophoblasts and can be released as free miRNA or packaged into EVs.

EXTRACELLULAR VESICLES IN GESTATIONAL TISSUES

EVs are membrane vesicles of various sizes that are secreted by almost every cell type and multiple organisms ranging from bacteria to humans. EVs are broadly classified according to size and origin into two different categories: exosomes and microvesicles (MVs; including microparticles and apoptotic bodies) (14, 96). MVs are larger membrane-derived vesicles >150 nm in size and secreted directly from the cell membrane. Exosomes are cell-secreted, membrane-derived nanovesicles, which represent a subpopulation of EVs measuring from 40 to 120 nm and with a density of between 1.13 and 1.19 g/mL (14). Exosomes arise from the endosomal compartment as intraluminal vesicles and are secreted by the fusion of endosomes or multivesicular bodies (MVBs) with the cell membrane. Additionally, exosomes can be described according to morphological characteristics (spherical or cup-shaped) and surface markers (CD63, CD9, CD81, and Tsg101) (14, 97). Various gestational tissues, including pre-implantation embryos, oviduct epithelium, placental trophoblasts, and endometrium, secrete EVs, with their source determined according to cell-specific markers. Previous studies suggest that miRNAs are protected from RNase degradation in serum by encapsulation within EVs, which act as carriers of regulatory RNA (53, 98).

THE ROLE OF EXTRACELLULAR VESICLES IN NORMAL PREGNANCY AND GESTATIONAL VASCULAR DISORDERS

The placenta releases EVs as early as the sixth gestational week, with this activity implicated in regulating maternal pregnancy physiology and fetal development, including pregnancy-induced hypertension, gestational diabetes, preterm labor, and delivery (14, 15, 97, 99). EVs (especially exosomes) play a vital role in the preparatory cross-talk between endometrium and embryo at the onset of pregnancy (83, 100–102). Trophoblast-derived EVs harbor molecules specific to placental physiology and cell-cell communication and that exert diverse effects on maternal and embryonic compartments. These molecules include fibronectin, syncytin, galectin-3, human leukocyte antigen-G, and cytokines as well as bioactive lipids and/or miRNAs, capable of immunomodulation (103). Placental alkaline phosphatase (PLAP), a membrane protein of the placenta, is primarily produced by syncytiotrophoblasts and used as a marker to identify placenta-derived exosomes in maternal circulation (104). $PLAP^+$ exosomes have only been described in the peripheral circulation of pregnant women (13, 14), with the number of placental exosomes positively correlated with total exosomes concentrations during the first trimester in normal pregnancy (105). The total number of exosomes ($CD63^+$) and placental exosomes ($PLAP^+$) present in maternal plasma increases exponentially in the second and third trimesters (14). Although PLAP shows potential as a useful marker for measuring exosomes in normal pregnancy, its levels have not yet been quantified in pathological pregnancies. Furthermore, syncytiotrophoblast EVs are secreted into maternal circulation as early as the tenth gestational week, their numbers increasing by the third trimester; however, their excessive secretion has also been reported in association with preeclampsia (15).

EVs in pregnancy play a pro-coagulant role to a greater degree than that observed in non-pregnant women (103). Levels of EVs harboring the tissue factor antigen, which is involved in the first step of the coagulation cascade, increase during pregnancy, and a significant increase in EVs harboring tissue factor is related to gestational vascular disorders, suggesting a pro-coagulant immune profile in such situations. Moreover, EVs play a significant role in regulating the inflammatory milieu during pregnancy, as EVs from pregnant women show higher levels of inflammatory proteins. Furthermore, EVs from hypoxic trophoblasts exhibit a more intense inflammatory response to peripheral blood mononuclear cells than do EVs from normal trophoblasts. Additionally, placenta-derived EVs carry a functional Fas ligand and TNF-related apoptosis-inducing ligand molecules that convey signals for apoptosis, suggesting a role in establishing EV-mediated immune privilege on behalf of the fetus (106). It is also possible that placental EVs modulate the response to LPS in pregnant women. Unpublished data from our lab showed that exosomal miRNAs mediate endotoxin tolerance in the placenta after repeated LPS exposure. Cytochalasin-D, an inhibitor of exosomes release and uptake, blocked endotoxin tolerance and restored the proinflammatory response in placental explants treated with repeated doses of LPS, thereby suggesting that exosomes mediate endotoxin tolerance in the placenta.

EXTRACELLULAR VESICLE TARGETING OF SPECIFIC TISSUE AND CELLS

The process of EV formation is complex and aimed at secreting selectively prepared vesicles with their content and presenting surface markers geared toward specific target cells. Although the mechanisms of exosomes biogenesis and release continue to be investigated, little is known regarding how exosomes' content is

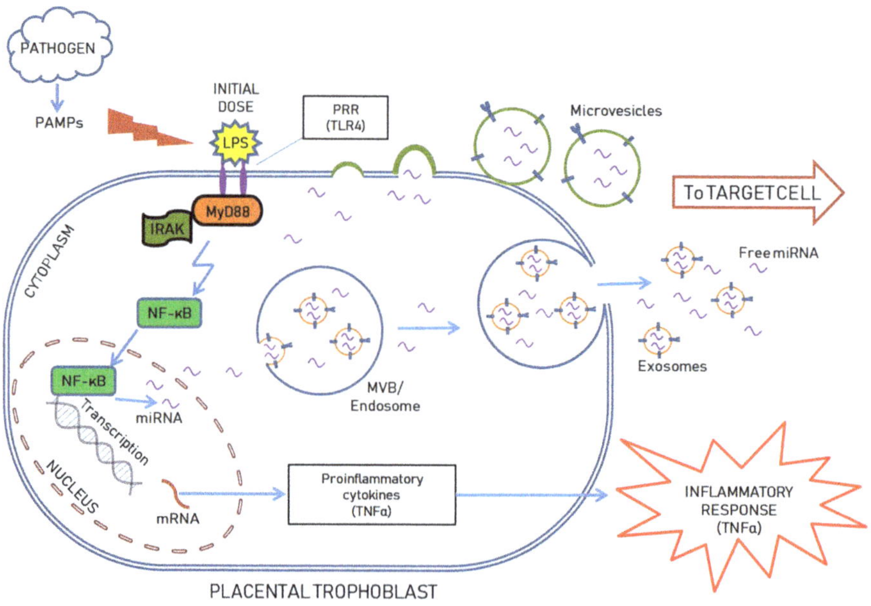

FIGURE 1 | Hypothetical illustration showing LPS mediated inflammatory response, possible mechanism of anti-inflammatory miRNAs mediated endotoxin tolerance as well as packaging within extracellular vesicles (EVs; including exosomes and microvesicles) in a placental trophoblast. The initial LPS dose stimulates TLR4 pathway in the placental trophoblast to prompt the initial inflammatory response, while also upregulating miRNA transcription. The miRNAs are either found freely in the cytoplasm and released outside the cells, or selectively packaged into extracellular vesicles by various mechanisms. Exosomes are formed intraluminally in the endosomal system within multivesicular bodies (MVB) while microvesicles are secreted by membrane derived vesicle formation. They are selectively packaged with nucleic acids (DNAs, mRNAs, miRNAs), proteins, lipids and carbohydrates, specific to the cell of origin and the intended target. The EVs and free miRNAs are transported to the target cell via the extracellular space.

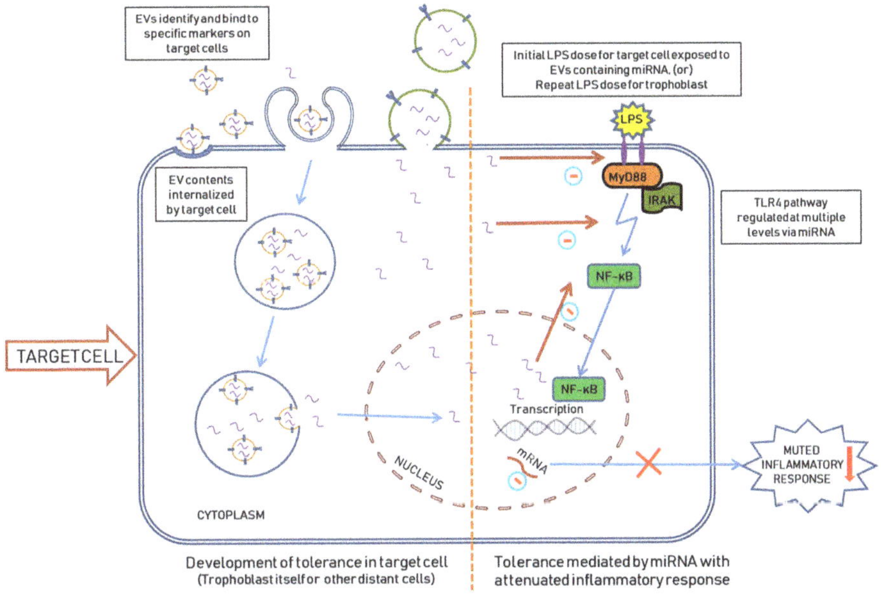

FIGURE 2 | Hypothetical illustration showing the development of endotoxin tolerance in a target cell mediated by miRNA packaged within the EVs. EVs carrying miRNAs (and other contents) are released from the original placental trophoblasts upon exposure to initial LPS dose as seen in **Figure 1**. The released EVs travel to the target cells where they are selectively internalized by different mechanisms as shown. Microvesicles are internalized into the cytoplasm by fusing with the cell membrane while exosomes are internalized into vesicular bodies, lipid rafts on cell surface or by directly binding with specific cell surface receptors (96). The target cell in this scenario can represent a distant cell (exposed to first dose of LPS) or the original trophoblast cell (exposed to a second dose of LPS). We hypothesize that the miRNAs within the EVs are released into the cytoplasm and enter the nucleus thereby negatively regulating the inflammatory pathway at multiple levels (including direct inhibition of TLR4, downregulating mRNA translation of TLR and negative feedback for NF-κB mediated TLR4 pathway). Upon exposure to a second dose of LPS, the original tolerized cell generates an attenuated inflammatory response (since it has high levels of anti-inflammatory miRNAs as a result form the first LPS exposure).

regulated as well as which cells they target. Cell-specific markers presented by exosomes are proposed to play a role in target-cell identification and interaction. Adaptor proteins reportedly recruit an exosome-associated helicase (MTR4) to unique RNA substrates, and exosome cofactors, such as the TRAMP-like protein complex, localize to the cytoplasm and recruit exosomes to specific viral RNA for degradation (107). Other examples of EV targets include cancer cells, which subsequently use EVs to target other organs, such as the lung and liver, to identify pre-metastatic niches based on specific integrin composition (108).

A PLACENTAL MODEL FOR microRNA-MEDIATED ENDOTOXIN TOLERANCE via EVs

Our lab demonstrated that endotoxin tolerance exists in placental tissues (109) and we proposed a model of miRNA-mediated placental immune tolerance packaged within EVs. An LPS stimulus primes placental trophoblasts to exhibit a proinflammatory response through the TLR4 pathway, which activates NF-κB to increase pro-inflammatory cytokine expression and release (such as TNFα) (**Figure 1**). Additionally, TLR4 activation increases the production of placenta-specific miRNAs (either free or packaged in EVs; **Figure 1**) likely also mediated by NF-κB (110, 111). Free miRNAs induce a feedback loop to down-regulate TLR4 signaling and alter related downstream processes, including the inflammatory response, as well as inhibiting mRNA translation of TLR receptors and directly attenuate TLR-receptor levels (**Figure 2**). The secreted EVs translocate to specific target cells/sites, such as placental trophoblasts (autocrine mechanisms), local gestational tissues (paracrine mechanisms), or other maternal and fetal compartments, via circulating peripheral blood or other extracellular fluid, according to specific chemo-attractants or cell-surface markers. EVs then interact with target tissue using cognate surface markers and release their contents, thereby potentially affecting several biological mechanisms, including protein biosynthesis and/or post-transcriptional regulation. The miRNAs within the EVs will reduce the ability of the target cells to produce TNFα in response to LPS exposure. The anti-inflammatory miRNAs implicated in endotoxin tolerance likely act using similar mechanisms, including negative feedback loop at the TLR receptor, to inhibit downstream regulators of the TLR pathway as well as decrease the transcription of pro-inflammatory molecules, such as TNFα (**Figure 2**).

Therefore, LPS insult of target cells/tissue harboring these anti-inflammatory miRNAs increases the readiness for subsequent LPS doses by attenuating the TLR response, thereby tipping the balance against a proinflammatory environment at the maternal-fetal interface (immune tolerance to repeated LPS dose). **Figure 3A**, shows a hypothetical response involving suppressed TNFα levels in the presence of miRNA-induced endotoxin tolerance. Unprimed cells challenged with LPS

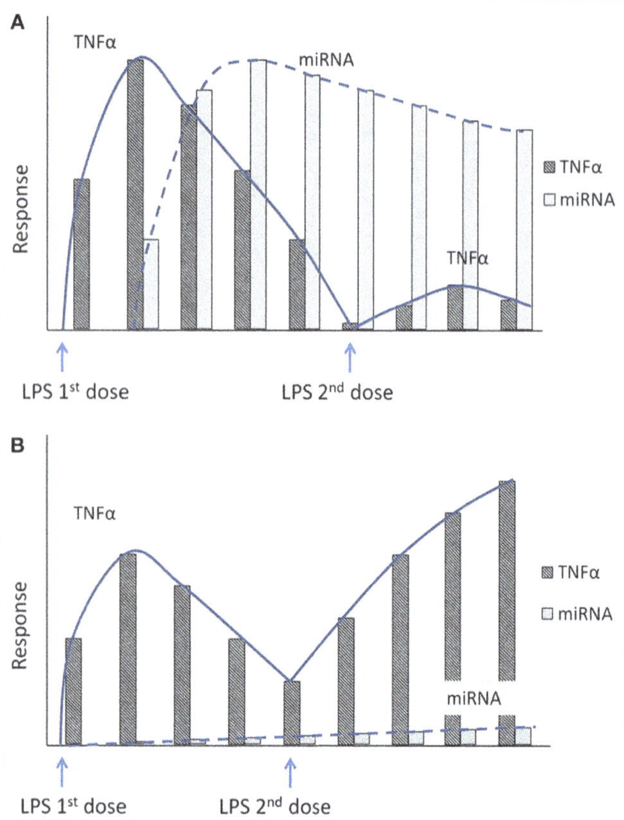

FIGURE 3 | (A) Hypothetical figure illustrates the inflammatory response to repeated LPS exposure. Exposure to the first dose of LPS increases the proinflammatory marker TNFα. Shortly following the initial dose of LPS, the cells also secrete specific anti-inflammatory miRNAs that accumulate in the cytoplasm. Upon exposure to second dose of LPS, the sustained high levels of the anti-inflammatory miRNAs will blunt the inflammatory response with decreased TNFα levels (endotoxin tolerance). **(B)** Hypothetical figure illustrates the inflammatory response in the absence of the anti-inflammatory miRNAs mediated endotoxin tolerance. In a knockout model of specific miRNA, the miRNA levels do not increase after initial exposure to LPS. A subsequent exposure to a second dose of LPS thus produces an unchecked inflammatory response with an exaggerated increase in proinflammatory cytokines (TNFα).

produced a prominent TNFα response followed by an increase in anti-inflammatory miRNA production, which corresponds to later down-regulation of TNFα (**Figure 3A**). As shown in **Figure 3A**, in the presence of sustained high anti-inflammatory miRNA expression, a second dose of LPS will lead to a muted TNFα production by the cells (*tolerized cells*). However, in the absence of these specific miRNAs, subsequent exposure to LPS would result in failure of immune tolerance to repeated infection resulting in exaggerated inflammation at the maternal-fetal interface (**Figure 3B**). We speculate that placentas from women with infection-induced preterm births will have reduced expression of specific placental anti-inflammatory miRNAs. This will lead to endotoxin tolerance failure and exaggerated inflammatory response to repeated infections that result in preterm births or other inflammatory diseases of pregnancy.

CONCLUDING REMARKS

In summary, we propose that miRNAs play a vital role in mediating immune tolerance at the maternal-fetal interface by attenuating immune responses following repeated exposure to inflammatory insult. Packaging and transport of miRNAs by EVs is suggested as a "smart" process specifically intended to address the potential requirements of the target cell/tissue. The success of this activity is dependent upon the homeostasis of the origin cell (placenta, in this case). Therefore, normal or pathologic conditions in the placenta might affect EVs composition and number, resulting in an altered response to endotoxins or other inflammatory stimuli. Additionally, we suggest that the target cells are not randomly selected and are, in fact, pre-identified according to specific markers presented on the EV surface to allow specific identification of target cell/tissue. Perturbations in this process can result in the failure of miRNA-mediated endotoxin tolerance and an imbalanced proinflammatory state leading to adverse pregnancy outcomes, including preterm labor or preeclampsia. The identification of placenta-specific miRNAs and EV markers will promote identification of novel molecules as potential biomarkers for further study of endotoxin tolerance, as well as possible molecular targets for controlling injury from failed immune tolerance.

AUTHOR CONTRIBUTIONS

All authors listed have made a substantial, direct and intellectual contribution to the work, and approved it for publication.

ACKNOWLEDGMENTS

This work was supported in part by the NIH grant, 1P20 GM121298-01 (SS, COBRE for Reproductive Health).

REFERENCES

1. Medawar PB. Some immunological and endocrinological problems raised by the evolution of viviparity in vertebrates. *Symp Soc Exp Biol.* (1952) 7:320–38.
2. Moffett-King A. Natural killer cells and pregnancy. *Nat Rev Immunol.* (2002) 2:656–63. doi: 10.1038/nri886
3. Abelius MS, Janefjord C, Ernerudh J, Berg G, Matthiesen L, Duchen K, et al. The placental immune milieu is characterized by a Th2- and anti-inflammatory transcription profile, regardless of maternal allergy, and associates with neonatal immunity. *Am J Reprod Immunol.* (2015) 73:445–59. doi: 10.1111/aji.12350
4. Mor G, Aldo P, Alvero AB. The unique immunological and microbial aspects of pregnancy. *Nat Rev Immunol.* (2017) 17:469–82. doi: 10.1038/nri.2017.64
5. Bulmer JN, Pace D, Ritson A. Immunoregulatory cells in human decidua: morphology, immunohistochemistry and function. *Reprod Nutr Dev.* (1988) 28:1599–613. doi: 10.1051/rnd:19881006

6. Martin JA, Hamilton BE, Osterman MJK, Driscoll AK, Drake P. *Births: Final data for 2017. National Vital Statistics Reports, Vol 67*, no 8. Hyattsville, MD: National Center for Health Statistics (2018).
7. Romero R, Espinoza J, Goncalves LF, Kusanovic JP, Friel L, Hassan S. The role of inflammation and infection in preterm birth. *Semin Reprod Med.* (2007) 25:21–39. doi: 10.1055/s-2006-956773
8. Bastek JA, Gomez LM, Elovitz MA. The role of inflammation and infection in preterm birth. *Clin Perinatol.* (2011) 38:385–406. doi: 10.1016/j.clp.2011.06.003
9. Anders AP, Gaddy JA, Doster RS, Aronoff DM. Current concepts in maternal-fetal immunology: recognition and response to microbial pathogens by decidual stromal cells. *Am J Reprod Immunol.* (2017) 77:e12623. doi: 10.1111/aji.12623
10. Strauss JF III, Romero R, Gomez-Lopez N, Haymond-Thornburg H, Modi BP, Teves ME, et al. Spontaneous preterm birth: advances toward the discovery of genetic predisposition. *Am J Obstet Gynecol.* (2018) 218:294–314.e292. doi: 10.1016/j.ajog.2017.12.009
11. Burton GJ, Jauniaux E. What is the placenta? *Am J Obstet Gynecol.* (2015) 213:S6.e1, S6–8. doi: 10.1016/j.ajog.2015.07.050
12. Arora N, Sadovsky Y, Dermody TS, Coyne CB. Microbial vertical transmission during human pregnancy. *Cell Host Microbe.* (2017) 21:561–7. doi: 10.1016/j.chom.2017.04.007
13. Salomon C, Torres MJ, Kobayashi M, Scholz-Romero K, Sobrevia L, Dobierzewska A, et al. A gestational profile of placental exosomes in maternal plasma and their effects on endothelial cell migration. *PLoS ONE.* (2014) 9:e98667. doi: 10.1371/journal.pone.0098667
14. Mitchell MD, Peiris HN, Kobayashi M, Koh YQ, Duncombe G, Illanes SE, et al. Placental exosomes in normal and complicated pregnancy. *Am J Obstet Gynecol.* (2015) 213:S173–81. doi: 10.1016/j.ajog.2015.07.001
15. Tannetta D, Masliukaite I, Vatish M, Redman C, Sargent I. Update of syncytiotrophoblast derived extracellular vesicles in normal pregnancy and preeclampsia. *J Reprod Immunol.* (2017) 119:98–106. doi: 10.1016/j.jri.2016.08.008
16. Sharma S. Natural killer cells and regulatory T cells in early pregnancy loss. *Int J Dev Biol.* (2014) 58:219–29. doi: 10.1387/ijdb.140109ss
17. Schjenken JE, Zhang B, Chan HY, Sharkey DJ, Fullston T, Robertson SA. miRNA regulation of immune tolerance in early pregnancy. *Am J Reprod Immunol.* (2016) 75:272–80. doi: 10.1111/aji.12490
18. Aluvihare VR, Kallikourdis M, Betz AG. Regulatory T cells mediate maternal tolerance to the fetus. *Nat Immunol.* (2004) 5:266–71. doi: 10.1038/ni1037
19. Rowe JH, Ertelt JM, Xin L, Way SS. Pregnancy imprints regulatory memory that sustains anergy to fetal antigen. *Nature.* (2012) 490:102–6. doi: 10.1038/nature11462
20. Samstein RM, Josefowicz SZ, Arvey A, Treuting PM, Rudensky AY. Extrathymic generation of regulatory T cells in placental mammals mitigates maternal-fetal conflict. *Cell.* (2012) 150:29–38. doi: 10.1016/j.cell.2012.05.031
21. Robertson SA, Moldenhauer LM. Immunological determinants of implantation success. *Int J Dev Biol.* (2014) 58:205–17. doi: 10.1387/ijdb.140096sr
22. Kahn DA, Baltimore D. Pregnancy induces a fetal antigen-specific maternal T regulatory cell response that contributes to tolerance. *Proc Natl Acad Sci USA.* (2010) 107:9299–304. doi: 10.1073/pnas.1003909107
23. Nadeau-Vallee M, Obari D, Palacios J, Brien ME, Duval C, Chemtob S, et al. Sterile inflammation and pregnancy complications: a review. *Reproduction.* (2016) 152:R277–92. doi: 10.1530/REP-16-0453
24. Cotechini T, Komisarenko M, Sperou A, Macdonald-Goodfellow S, Adams MA, Graham CH. Inflammation in rat pregnancy inhibits spiral artery remodeling leading to fetal growth restriction and features of preeclampsia. *J Exp Med.* (2014) 211:165–79. doi: 10.1084/jem.20130295
25. Cheng SB, Sharma S. Preeclampsia and health risks later in life: an immunological link. *Semin Immunopathol.* (2016) 38:699–708. doi: 10.1007/s00281-016-0579-8
26. Ferguson KK, Meeker JD, Mcelrath TF, Mukherjee B, Cantonwine DE. Repeated measures of inflammation and oxidative stress biomarkers in preeclamptic and normotensive pregnancies. *Am J Obstet Gynecol.* (2017) 216:527.e1–e9. doi: 10.1016/j.ajog.2016.12.174
27. Gill N, Leng Y, Romero R, Xu Y, Panaitescu B, Miller D, et al. The immunophenotype of decidual macrophages in acute atherosis. *Am J Reprod Immunol.* (2019). doi: 10.1111/aji.13098. [Epub ahead of print].
28. Saito S, Sakai M, Sasaki Y, Nakashima A, Shiozaki A. Inadequate tolerance induction may induce pre-eclampsia. *J Reprod Immunol.* (2007) 76:30–9. doi: 10.1016/j.jri.2007.08.002
29. Saftlas AF, Rubenstein L, Prater K, Harland KK, Field E, Triche EW. Cumulative exposure to paternal seminal fluid prior to conception and subsequent risk of preeclampsia. *J Reprod Immunol.* (2014) 101–2:104–10. doi: 10.1016/j.jri.2013.07.006
30. Romero R, Gomez R, Chaiworapongsa T, Conoscenti G, Kim JC, Kim YM. The role of infection in preterm labour and delivery. *Paediatr Perinat Epidemiol.* (2001) 15(Suppl. 2):41–56. doi: 10.1046/j.1365-3016.2001.00007.x
31. Olson DM, Christiaens I, Gracie S, Yamamoto Y, Mitchell BF. Emerging tocolytics: challenges in designing and testing drugs to delay preterm delivery and prolong pregnancy. *Expert Opin Emerg Drugs.* (2008) 13:695–707. doi: 10.1517/14728210802568764
32. Romero R, Miranda J, Chaiworapongsa T, Korzeniewski SJ, Chaemsaithong P, Gotsch F, et al. Prevalence and clinical significance of sterile intra-amniotic inflammation in patients with preterm labor and intact membranes. *Am J Reprod Immunol.* (2014) 72:458–74. doi: 10.1111/aji.12296
33. Matzinger P. Tolerance, danger, and the extended family. *Annu Rev Immunol.* (1994) 12:991–1045. doi: 10.1146/annurev.iy.12.040194.005015
34. Petrovski G, Ayna G, Majai G, Hodrea J, Benko S, Madi A, et al. Phagocytosis of cells dying through autophagy induces inflammasome activation and IL-1beta release in human macrophages. *Autophagy.* (2011) 7:321–30. doi: 10.4161/auto.7.3.14583
35. Wang XW, Karki A, Zhao XJ, Xiang XY, Lu ZQ. High plasma levels of high mobility group box 1 is associated with the risk of sepsis in severe blunt chest trauma patients: a prospective cohort study. *J Cardiothorac Surg.* (2014) 9:133. doi: 10.1186/s13019-014-0133-5
36. Gomez-Lopez N, Romero R, Plazyo O, Panaitescu B, Furcron AE, Miller D, et al. Intra-amniotic administration of HMGB1 induces spontaneous preterm labor and birth. *Am J Reprod Immunol.* (2016) 75:3–7. doi: 10.1111/aji.12443
37. Plazyo O, Romero R, Unkel R, Balancio A, Mial TN, Xu Y, et al. HMGB1 induces an inflammatory response in the chorioamniotic membranes that is partially mediated by the inflammasome. *Biol Reprod.* (2016) 95:130. doi: 10.1095/biolreprod.116.144139
38. Gomez-Lopez N, Romero R, Panaitescu B, Leng Y, Xu Y, Tarca AL, et al. Inflammasome activation during spontaneous preterm labor with intra-amniotic infection or sterile intra-amniotic inflammation. *Am J Reprod Immunol.* (2018) 80:e13049. doi: 10.1111/aji.13049
39. Gomez-Lopez N, Romero R, Garcia-Flores V, Leng Y, Miller D, Hassan SS, et al. Inhibition of the NLRP3 inflammasome can prevent sterile intra-amniotic inflammation, preterm labor/birth and adverse neonatal outcomes. *Biol Reprod.* (2018). doi: 10.1093/biolre/ioy264. [Epub ahead of print].
40. Koga K, Mor G. Toll-like receptors at the maternal-fetal interface in normal pregnancy and pregnancy disorders. *Am J Reprod Immunol.* (2010) 63:587–600. doi: 10.1111/j.1600-0897.2010.00848.x
41. Lappas M. NOD1 and NOD2 regulate proinflammatory and prolabor mediators in human fetal membranes and myometrium via nuclear factor-kappa B. *Biol Reprod.* (2013) 89:14. doi: 10.1095/biolreprod.113.110056
42. Zhang YY, Chen H, Sun C, Wang HZ, Liu ML, Li YY, et al. Expression and functional characterization of NOD2 in decidual stromal cells isolated during the first trimester of pregnancy. *PLoS ONE.* (2014) 9:e99612. doi: 10.1371/journal.pone.0099612
43. Rieger L, Segerer S, Bernar T, Kapp M, Majic M, Morr AK, et al. Specific subsets of immune cells in human decidua differ between normal pregnancy and preeclampsia–a prospective observational study. *Reprod Biol Endocrinol.* (2009) 7:132. doi: 10.1186/1477-7827-7-132
44. Milosevic-Stevanovic J, Krstic M, Stefanovic M, Zivadinovic R, Vukomanovic P, Trajkovic-Dinic SP, et al. T lymphocytes in the third trimester decidua in preeclampsia. *Hypertens Pregnancy.* (2019) 38:52–7. doi: 10.1080/10641955.2019.1575393
45. Seeley JJ, Baker RG, Mohamed G, Bruns T, Hayden MS, Deshmukh SD, et al. Induction of innate immune memory via microRNA

targeting of chromatin remodelling factors. *Nature.* (2018) 559:114–9. doi: 10.1038/s41586-018-0253-5
46. Wheeler DS, Lahni PM, Denenberg AG, Poynter SE, Wong HR, Cook JA, et al. Induction of endotoxin tolerance enhances bacterial clearance and survival in murine polymicrobial sepsis. *Shock.* (2008) 30:267–73. doi: 10.1097/shk.0b013e318162c190
47. Landoni VI, Chiarella P, Martire-Greco D, Schierloh P, Van-Rooijen N, Rearte B, et al. Tolerance to lipopolysaccharide promotes an enhanced neutrophil extracellular traps formation leading to a more efficient bacterial clearance in mice. *Clin Exp Immunol.* (2012) 168:153–63. doi: 10.1111/j.1365-2249.2012.04560.x
48. Varma TK, Durham M, Murphey ED, Cui W, Huang Z, Lin CY, et al. Endotoxin priming improves clearance of *Pseudomonas aeruginosa* in wild-type and interleukin-10 knockout mice. *Infect Immun.* (2005) 73:7340–7. doi: 10.1128/IAI.73.11.7340-7347.2005
49. Han YW, Shen T, Chung P, Buhimschi IA, Buhimschi CS. Uncultivated bacteria as etiologic agents of intra-amniotic inflammation leading to preterm birth. *J Clin Microbiol.* (2009) 47:38–47. doi: 10.1128/JCM.01206-08
50. Combs CA, Gravett M, Garite TJ, Hickok DE, Lapidus J, Porreco R, et al. Amniotic fluid infection, inflammation, and colonization in preterm labor with intact membranes. *Am J Obstet Gynecol.* (2014) 210:125.e1–e15. doi: 10.1016/j.ajog.2013.11.032
51. Wenstrom KD, Andrews WW, Bowles NE, Towbin JA, Hauth JC, Goldenberg RL. Intrauterine viral infection at the time of second trimester genetic amniocentesis. *Obstet Gynecol.* (1998) 92:420–4. doi: 10.1016/S0029-7844(98)00210-5
52. Ramos Bde A, Kanninen TT, Sisti G, Witkin SS. Microorganisms in the female genital tract during pregnancy: tolerance versus pathogenesis. *Am J Reprod Immunol.* (2015) 73:383–9. doi: 10.1111/aji.12326
53. Valadi H, Ekstrom K, Bossios A, Sjostrand M, Lee JJ, Lotvall JO. Exosome-mediated transfer of mRNAs and microRNAs is a novel mechanism of genetic exchange between cells. *Nat Cell Biol.* (2007) 9:654–9. doi: 10.1038/ncb1596
54. Friedman RC, Farh KK, Burge CB, Bartel DP. Most mammalian mRNAs are conserved targets of microRNAs. *Genome Res.* (2009) 19:92–105. doi: 10.1101/gr.082701.108
55. Szabo G, Bala S. MicroRNAs in liver disease. *Nat Rev Gastroenterol Hepatol.* (2013) 10:542–52. doi: 10.1038/nrgastro.2013.87
56. Romaine SP, Tomaszewski M, Condorelli G, Samani NJ. MicroRNAs in cardiovascular disease: an introduction for clinicians. *Heart.* (2015) 101:921–8. doi: 10.1136/heartjnl-2013-305402
57. Liu Y, Liang Y, Zhang JF, Fu WM. MicroRNA-133 mediates cardiac diseases: mechanisms and clinical implications. *Exp Cell Res.* (2017) 354:65–70. doi: 10.1016/j.yexcr.2017.03.037
58. Dangwal S, Thum T. microRNA therapeutics in cardiovascular disease models. *Annu Rev Pharmacol Toxicol.* (2014) 54:185–203. doi: 10.1146/annurev-pharmtox-011613-135957
59. Dai Y, Jia P, Fang Y, Liu H, Jiao X, He JC, et al. miR-146a is essential for lipopolysaccharide (LPS)-induced cross-tolerance against kidney ischemia/reperfusion injury in mice. *Sci Rep.* (2016) 6:27091. doi: 10.1038/srep27091
60. Hayes CN, Chayama K. MicroRNAs as biomarkers for liver disease and hepatocellular carcinoma. *Int J Mol Sci.* (2016) 17:280. doi: 10.3390/ijms17030280
61. Rosenbluth EM, Shelton DN, Sparks AE, Devor E, Christenson L, Van Voorhis BJ. MicroRNA expression in the human blastocyst. *Fertil Steril.* (2013) 99:855–61.e3. doi: 10.1016/j.fertnstert.2012.11.001
62. Kropp J, Salih SM, Khatib H. Expression of microRNAs in bovine and human pre-implantation embryo culture media. *Front Genet.* (2014) 5:91. doi: 10.3389/fgene.2014.00091
63. Nahid MA, Satoh M, Chan EK. MicroRNA in TLR signaling and endotoxin tolerance. *Cell Mol Immunol.* (2011) 8:388–403. doi: 10.1038/cmi.2011.26
64. Kumar Kingsley SM, Vishnu Bhat B. Role of MicroRNAs in the development and function of innate immune cells. *Int Rev Immunol.* (2017) 36:154–75. doi: 10.1080/08830185.2017.1284212
65. Du H, Cui S, Li Y, Yang G, Wang P, Fikrig E, et al. MiR-221 negatively regulates innate anti-viral response. *PLoS ONE.* (2018) 13:e0200385. doi: 10.1371/journal.pone.0200385
66. Lv J, Zhang Z, Pan L, Zhang Y. MicroRNA-34/449 family and viral infections. *Virus Res.* (2019) 260:1–6. doi: 10.1016/j.virusres.2018.11.001
67. Van Loon W, Gai PP, Hamann L, Bedu-Addo G, Mockenhaupt FP. MiRNA-146a polymorphism increases the odds of malaria in pregnancy. *Malar J.* (2019) 18:7. doi: 10.1186/s12936-019-2643-z
68. Polakovicova I, Jerez S, Wichmann IA, Sandoval-Borquez A, Carrasco-Veliz N, Corvalan AH. Role of microRNAs and exosomes in *Helicobacter pylori* and epstein-barr virus associated gastric cancers. *Front Microbiol.* (2018) 9:636. doi: 10.3389/fmicb.2018.00636
69. Taganov KD, Boldin MP, Chang KJ, Baltimore D. NF-kappaB-dependent induction of microRNA miR-146, an inhibitor targeted to signaling proteins of innate immune responses. *Proc Natl Acad Sci USA.* (2006) 103:12481–6. doi: 10.1073/pnas.0605298103
70. Vergadi E, Vaporidi K, Tsatsanis C. Regulation of endotoxin tolerance and compensatory anti-inflammatory response syndrome by non-coding RNAs. *Front Immunol.* (2018) 9:2705. doi: 10.3389/fimmu.2018.02705
71. Nahid MA, Pauley KM, Satoh M, Chan EK. miR-146a is critical for endotoxin-induced tolerance: implication in innate immunity. *J Biol Chem.* (2009) 284:34590–9. doi: 10.1074/jbc.M109.056317
72. Pauley KM, Satoh M, Pauley BA, Dominguez-Gutierrez PR, Wallet SM, Holliday LS, et al. Formation of GW/P bodies as marker for microRNA-mediated regulation of innate immune signaling in THP-1 cells. *Immunol Cell Biol.* (2010) 88:205–12. doi: 10.1038/icb.2009.84
73. Yang K, He YS, Wang XQ, Lu L, Chen QJ, Liu J, et al. MiR-146a inhibits oxidized low-density lipoprotein-induced lipid accumulation and inflammatory response via targeting toll-like receptor 4. *FEBS Lett.* (2011) 585:854–60. doi: 10.1016/j.febslet.2011.02.009
74. Doxaki C, Kampranis SC, Eliopoulos AG, Spilianakis C, Tsatsanis C. Coordinated regulation of miR-155 and miR-146a genes during induction of endotoxin tolerance in macrophages. *J Immunol.* (2015) 195:5750–61. doi: 10.4049/jimmunol.1500615
75. Chen XM, Splinter PL, O'hara SP, Larusso NF. A cellular micro-RNA, let-7i, regulates toll-like receptor 4 expression and contributes to cholangiocyte immune responses against *Cryptosporidium parvum* infection. *J Biol Chem.* (2007) 282:28929–38. doi: 10.1074/jbc.M702633200
76. Benakanakere MR, Li Q, Eskan MA, Singh AV, Zhao J, Galicia JC, et al. Modulation of TLR2 protein expression by miR-105 in human oral keratinocytes. *J Biol Chem.* (2009) 284:23107–15. doi: 10.1074/jbc.M109.013862
77. Martinez B, Peplow PV. MicroRNAs as diagnostic and therapeutic tools for Alzheimer's disease: advances and limitations. *Neural Regen Res.* (2019) 14:242–55. doi: 10.4103/1673-5374.244784
78. Zhao L, Li J, Huang S. Patients with unexplained recurrent spontaneous abortion show decreased levels of microrna-146a-5p in the deciduae. *Ann Clin Lab Sci.* (2018) 48:177–82.
79. Winger EE, Reed JL, Ji X, Nicolaides K. Peripheral blood cell microRNA quantification during the first trimester predicts preeclampsia: proof of concept. *PLoS ONE.* (2018) 13:e0190654. doi: 10.1371/journal.pone.0190654
80. Chakrabarty A, Tranguch S, Daikoku T, Jensen K, Furneaux H, Dey SK. MicroRNA regulation of cyclooxygenase-2 during embryo implantation. *Proc Natl Acad Sci USA.* (2007) 104:15144–9. doi: 10.1073/pnas.0705917104
81. Chen CZ, Schaffert S, Fragoso R, Loh C. Regulation of immune responses and tolerance: the microRNA perspective. *Immunol Rev.* (2013) 253:112–28. doi: 10.1111/imr.12060
82. Bidarimath M, Khalaj K, Wessels JM, Tayade C. MicroRNAs, immune cells and pregnancy. *Cell Mol Immunol.* (2014) 11:538–47. doi: 10.1038/cmi.2014.45
83. Ouyang Y, Mouillet JF, Coyne CB, Sadovsky Y. Review: placenta-specific microRNAs in exosomes–good things come in nano-packages. *Placenta.* (2014) 35:S69–73. doi: 10.1016/j.placenta.2013.11.002
84. Mouillet JF, Ouyang Y, Coyne CB, Sadovsky Y. MicroRNAs in placental health and disease. *Am J Obstet Gynecol.* (2015) 213:S163–72. doi: 10.1016/j.ajog.2015.05.057
85. Donker RB, Mouillet JF, Chu T, Hubel CA, Stolz DB, Morelli AE, et al. The expression profile of C19MC microRNAs in primary human trophoblast cells and exosomes. *Mol Hum Reprod.* (2012) 18:417–24. doi: 10.1093/molehr/gas013

86. Delorme-Axford E, Donker RB, Mouillet JF, Chu T, Bayer A, Ouyang Y, et al. Human placental trophoblasts confer viral resistance to recipient cells. *Proc Natl Acad Sci USA.* (2013) 110:12048–53. doi: 10.1073/pnas.1304718110
87. Keniry A, Oxley D, Monnier P, Kyba M, Dandolo L, Smits G, et al. The H19 lincRNA is a developmental reservoir of miR-675 that suppresses growth and Igf1r. *Nat Cell Biol.* (2012) 14:659–65. doi: 10.1038/ncb2521
88. Luo L, Ye G, Nadeem L, Fu G, Yang BB, Honarparvar E, et al. MicroRNA-378a-5p promotes trophoblast cell survival, migration and invasion by targeting Nodal. *J Cell Sci.* (2012) 125:3124–32. doi: 10.1242/jcs.096412
89. Fu G, Ye G, Nadeem L, Ji L, Manchanda T, Wang Y, et al. MicroRNA-376c impairs transforming growth factor-beta and nodal signaling to promote trophoblast cell proliferation and invasion. *Hypertension.* (2013) 61:864–72. doi: 10.1161/HYPERTENSIONAHA.111.203489
90. Kumar P, Luo Y, Tudela C, Alexander JM, Mendelson CR. The c-Myc-regulated microRNA-17~92 (miR-17~92) and miR-106a~363 clusters target hCYP19A1 and hGCM1 to inhibit human trophoblast differentiation. *Mol Cell Biol.* (2013) 33:1782–96. doi: 10.1128/MCB.01228-12
91. Gan L, Liu Z, Wei M, Chen Y, Yang X, Chen L, et al. MiR-210 and miR-155 as potential diagnostic markers for pre-eclampsia pregnancies. *Medicine (Baltimore).* (2017) 96:e7515. doi: 10.1097/MD.0000000000007515
92. Mittelbrunn M, Gutierrez-Vazquez C, Villarroya-Beltri C, Gonzalez S, Sanchez-Cabo F, Gonzalez MA, et al. Unidirectional transfer of microRNA-loaded exosomes from T cells to antigen-presenting cells. *Nat Commun.* (2011) 2:282. doi: 10.1038/ncomms1285
93. Hessvik NP, Phuyal S, Brech A, Sandvig K, Llorente A. Profiling of microRNAs in exosomes released from PC-3 prostate cancer cells. *Biochim Biophys Acta.* (2012) 1819:1154–63. doi: 10.1016/j.bbagrm.2012.08.016
94. Nolte-'t Hoen EN, Buermans HP, Waasdorp M, Stoorvogel W, Wauben MH, 't Hoen PA. Deep sequencing of RNA from immune cell-derived vesicles uncovers the selective incorporation of small non-coding RNA biotypes with potential regulatory functions. *Nucleic Acids Res.* (2012) 40:9272–85. doi: 10.1093/nar/gks658
95. Hessvik NP, Llorente A. Current knowledge on exosome biogenesis and release. *Cell Mol Life Sci.* (2018) 75:193–208. doi: 10.1007/s00018-017-2595-9
96. Van Niel G, D'angelo G, Raposo G. Shedding light on the cell biology of extracellular vesicles. *Nat Rev Mol Cell Biol.* (2018) 19:213–28. doi: 10.1038/nrm.2017.125
97. Jin J, Menon R. Placental exosomes: a proxy to understand pregnancy complications. *Am J Reprod Immunol.* (2018) 79:e12788. doi: 10.1111/aji.12788
98. Hunter MP, Ismail N, Zhang X, Aguda BD, Lee EJ, Yu L, et al. Detection of microRNA expression in human peripheral blood microvesicles. *PLoS ONE.* (2008) 3:e3694. doi: 10.1371/journal.pone.0003694
99. Adam S, Elfeky O, Kinhal V, Dutta S, Lai A, Jayabalan N, et al. Review: fetal-maternal communication via extracellular vesicles–implications for complications of pregnancies. *Placenta.* (2017) 54:83–8. doi: 10.1016/j.placenta.2016.12.001
100. Ng YH, Rome S, Jalabert A, Forterre A, Singh H, Hincks CL, et al. Endometrial exosomes/microvesicles in the uterine microenvironment: a new paradigm for embryo-endometrial cross talk at implantation. *PLoS ONE.* (2013) 8:e58502. doi: 10.1371/journal.pone.0058502
101. Saadeldin IM, Oh HJ, Lee BC. Embryonic-maternal cross-talk via exosomes: potential implications. *Stem Cells Cloning.* (2015) 8:103–7. doi: 10.2147/SCCAA.S84991
102. Tong M, Abrahams VM, Chamley LW. Immunological effects of placental extracellular vesicles. *Immunol Cell Biol.* (2018) 96:714–22. doi: 10.1111/imcb.12049
103. Orozco AF, Jorgez CJ, Ramos-Perez WD, Popek EJ, Yu X, Kozinetz CA, et al. Placental release of distinct DNA-associated micro-particles into maternal circulation: reflective of gestation time and preeclampsia. *Placenta.* (2009) 30:891–7. doi: 10.1016/j.placenta.2009.06.012
104. Vongthavaravat V, Nurnberger MM, Balodimos N, Blanchette H, Koff RS. Isolated elevation of serum alkaline phosphatase level in an uncomplicated pregnancy: a case report. *Am J Obstet Gynecol.* (2000) 183:505–6. doi: 10.1067/mob.2000.105841
105. Sarker S, Scholz-Romero K, Perez A, Illanes SE, Mitchell MD, Rice GE, et al. Placenta-derived exosomes continuously increase in maternal circulation over the first trimester of pregnancy. *J Transl Med.* (2014) 12:204. doi: 10.1186/1479-5876-12-204
106. Stenqvist AC, Nagaeva O, Baranov V, Mincheva-Nilsson L. Exosomes secreted by human placenta carry functional Fas ligand and TRAIL molecules and convey apoptosis in activated immune cells, suggesting exosome-mediated immune privilege of the fetus. *J Immunol.* (2013) 191:5515–23. doi: 10.4049/jimmunol.1301885
107. Thoms M, Thomson E, Bassler J, Gnadig M, Griesel S, Hurt E. The exosome is recruited to RNA substrates through specific adaptor proteins. *Cell.* (2015) 162:1029–38. doi: 10.1016/j.cell.2015.07.060
108. Hoshino A, Costa-Silva B, Shen TL, Rodrigues G, Hashimoto A, Tesic Mark M, et al. Tumour exosome integrins determine organotropic metastasis. *Nature.* (2015) 527:329–35. doi: 10.1038/nature15756
109. Kim ML, Maloney C, Klimova N, Gurzenda E, Lin X, Arita Y, et al. Repeated lipopolysaccharide exposure leads to placental endotoxin tolerance. *Am J Reprod Immunol.* (2018) 81:e13080. doi: 10.1111/aji.13080
110. El Gazzar M, Church A, Liu T, Mccall CE. MicroRNA-146a regulates both transcription silencing and translation disruption of TNF-α during TLR4-induced gene reprogramming. *J Leukoc Biol.* (2011) 90:509–19. doi: 10.1189/jlb.0211074
111. Wendlandt EB, Graff JW, Gioannini TL, Mccaffrey AP, Wilson ME. The role of microRNAs miR-200b and miR-200c in TLR4 signaling and NF-kappaB activation. *Innate Immun.* (2012) 18:846–55. doi: 10.1177/1753425912443903

6

Understanding Viral and Immune Interplay During Vertical Transmission of HIV: Implications for Cure

Omayma Amin[1], *Jenna Powers*[1], *Katherine M. Bricker*[1] *and Ann Chahroudi*[1,2*]

[1] *Department of Pediatrics, Emory University School of Medicine, Atlanta, GA, United States,* [2] *Center for Childhood Infections and Vaccines of Children's Healthcare of Atlanta and Emory University, Atlanta, GA, United States*

Correspondence:
Ann Chahroudi
ann.m.chahroudi@emory.edu

Despite the significant progress that has been made to eliminate vertical HIV infection, more than 150,000 children were infected with HIV in 2019, emphasizing the continued need for sustainable HIV treatment strategies and ideally a cure for children. Mother-to-child-transmission (MTCT) remains the most important route of pediatric HIV acquisition and, in absence of prevention measures, transmission rates range from 15% to 45% *via* three distinct routes: *in utero*, intrapartum, and in the postnatal period through breastfeeding. The exact mechanisms and biological basis of these different routes of transmission are not yet fully understood. Some infants escape infection despite significant virus exposure, while others do not, suggesting possible maternal or fetal immune protective factors including the presence of HIV-specific antibodies. Here we summarize the unique aspects of HIV MTCT including the immunopathogenesis of the different routes of transmission, and how transmission in the antenatal or postnatal periods may affect early life immune responses and HIV persistence. A more refined understanding of the complex interaction between viral, maternal, and fetal/infant factors may enhance the pursuit of strategies to achieve an HIV cure for pediatric populations.

Keywords: HIV, MTCT, cure, pediatric, shock and kill, antiretroviral, breast milk, reservoir

INTRODUCTION

Pediatric AIDS was first described in 1982, shortly after the first adult cases were reported (1). Of the estimated 37.5 million people currently living with HIV-1 as of 2020, 1.7 million of those individuals are children (2). While heterosexual transmission is the major transmission mode in adults, the majority of pediatric infections occur through mother-to-child transmission (MTCT) during pregnancy, labor and delivery, and postpartum through breastfeeding. Tremendous progress has been made in both prevention and treatment of HIV in children. However, despite the implementation of prevention of mother-to-child transmission (PMTCT) measures that decrease the risk of vertical HIV transmission to less than 5% (3, 4), approximately 150,000 children were newly infected with HIV in 2020, the majority of whom live in sub-Saharan Africa (5). As with HIV infection in adults, the primary targets for infection are activated CD4+ T cells expressing the

CCR5 co-receptor. Risk of MTCT transmission is influenced by geography, maternal viral load, co-infections, delivery mode, and breast-feeding (6), among other factors. The precise mechanisms of MTCT and how its timing influences establishment of HIV infection and persistence have not been fully elucidated. In this review, we aim to summarize what is known about HIV MTCT, the immunologic and virologic factors involved in HIV transmission in the fetal and neonatal/infant periods, and provide implications for HIV cure strategies targeting perinatally infected children.

ROUTES AND MECHANISMS OF VERTICAL TRANSMISSION

Mother-to-child transmission (MTCT) remains the most important route of pediatric HIV acquisition and, in the absence of preventative measures, transmission rates range from 15% to 45% *via* three distinct routes: *in utero*, intrapartum, and in the postnatal period through breastfeeding. Overall, it is estimated that 20-25%, 35-50% and 25-45% of perinatal HIV transmissions occur *in utero*, intrapartum, and through breastfeeding, respectively (7–9). It is important to note that despite the prolonged exposure to HIV during fetal development, delivery, and breastfeeding, MTCT of HIV is relatively inefficient, and many children born to women with HIV do not become infected, even in absence of preventative services. Here, we will discuss the biological mechanisms of HIV MTCT and with emphasis on the factors influencing transmission. While this is still an active area of research, further elucidating these mechanisms of transmission is likely to inform cure approaches that should be considered for the almost 2 million children living with HIV.

In Utero Transmission

Transmission of HIV *in utero* is the least efficient route of MTCT, accounting for an estimated absolute rate of 5-10% of MTCT for women not receiving antiretroviral therapy (ART) (7, 8). The major risk factors for *in utero* transmission are high maternal viral loads and placental inflammation (8, 10, 11). The mechanisms of *in utero* HIV transmission are incompletely understood, but some have been proposed. Early studies suggested that *in utero* transmission may occur though HIV in the amniotic fluid coming into contact with fetal mucosal surfaces (12). Although the fetal gastrointestinal tract is populated with targets for HIV infection (e.g., CD4+CCR5+ T cells) (13), more recent studies have found that even in women with detectable virus in the plasma, HIV is not detected in the amniotic fluid (14–16). Another study found that amniotic fluid has innate inhibitory activity against the replication of HIV (17). Consequently, it is more likely that *in utero* transmission occurs primarily through the placenta. The placenta is a highly effective barrier that successfully inhibits most pathogens from reaching fetal circulation through various protective mechanisms. The placenta is composed of fetal-derived trophoblast progenitor cells that differentiate into specialized cell layers. These specialized trophoblasts have broad antiviral activity in addition to acting as a physical barrier to pathogens (18). Maternal blood comes into direct contact with the placenta by 10-12 weeks of gestation when trophoblasts form the placental villi and mediate the exchange of gases, nutrients, and waste products between maternal and fetal tissue (18).

While *in utero* transmission of HIV has been documented to occur as early as 8 weeks gestation (19), the vast majority of transmissions *via* this mode occur in the third trimester (20, 21). There are two mechanisms of transplacental transmission: infection of the trophoblasts and transcytosis across the trophoblastic layer. Although trophoblasts have low to no expression of CD4 receptors, multiple studies have detected HIV in these cells (22–24). More recent evidence suggests that transmission occurs primarily through cell-associated virus, as trophoblasts appear to be naturally nonpermissive to cell-free HIV (25). In a study designed to mimic the complex cellular architecture of the placenta, transcytosis and infection of the trophoblastic layer were only accomplished by cell-associated virus (26). New evidence suggests that cell-associated HIV enters trophoblasts *via* fusion with maternal lymphocytes (27). This cell-fusion mediated spread of HIV may be less sensitive to ART than cell-free infection, causing the placenta to become a potential reservoir for the virus during pregnancy (27). It is important to note that even when HIV successfully traverses the placenta, transmission to the fetus is not guaranteed. Studies have shown that both infected and uninfected infants had maternal cells with HIV DNA in their dried cord blood, and there was no significant difference between the rate of infection and the presence of HIV-infected cells in cord blood (28, 29). These findings suggest that there are likely more factors, some of which we will discuss in later sections of this paper, governing *in utero* transmission of HIV.

Intrapartum Transmission

The most common route of HIV MTCT occurs during labor and delivery, accounting for an absolute rate of 10-20% of infections in children born to women not receiving ART (7, 8). A major risk factor for intrapartum transmission is again maternal viral load (30–32), and while in the United States the current standard of care is delivery by Caesarian section unless women are on ART with low viral loads, most women deliver vaginally elsewhere in the world (33). Although multiple mechanisms of intrapartum transmission have been proposed, most of the evidence supports infection *via* exposure of infant mucosal surfaces to maternal secretions and blood during birth. The fetal intestines are populated with high levels CD4+CCR5+ T cells (13), and evidence suggests that higher viral loads in the birth canal correlate with increased transmission rates (10). Additionally, factors that would increase contact of fetal mucosal surfaces with maternal viral secretions also increase transmission rates. For example, genital ulcers have been shown to cause an increase in intrapartum transmission rates (34). This association remained significant even after adjusting for plasma HIV viral load. Several possible mechanisms are thought to explain this association including increased recruitment of HIV-infected CD4+ T cells to the mucosal surface of the genital lesions resulting in increased viral load in the genital tract (35, 36). Finally, the protective effect of elective Caesarian section against MTCT of HIV is attributed to the reduction of fetal contact with the birth canal (37–39).

Another proposed mechanism of intrapartum transmission is maternal-fetal microtransfusion (also called placental microtransfusion) causing fetal exposure to maternal blood containing both cell-free HIV RNA and cell-associated HIV DNA. Although the cause is unknown, microtransfusions occur at or near time of delivery when there is a disruption of the placental barrier and are thought to increase when uterine contractions intensify causing membranes to rupture. One study done using placental alkaline phosphatase (PLAP) as a marker for microtransfusions found that in women who had vaginal deliveries, high levels of PLAP were associated with higher intrapartum transmission risk (40). However, there was no significant association between PLAP (microtransfusion) levels and perinatal transmission as a whole. As described above, further studies designed to detect maternal cells in dried fetal cord blood as a proxy for microtransfusion also found no correlation (28, 29). Maternal-fetal microtransfusions are still relatively understudied, however.

Postpartum Transmission

Breastfeeding contributes to a considerable proportion of pediatric HIV infections accounting for an estimated absolute rate of 5-15% of MTCT for women not receiving ART (8). Premastication, where an adult chews foods before feeding it to the child, is also a risk factor for MTCT and this risk is associated with predisposing oral conditions that lead to the presence of blood in the mouth (41). It was recognized early on that breastfeeding was a potential mechanism for HIV transmission; however, the World Health Organization recommends that women in sub-Saharan Africa (with high HIV prevalence) breastfeed their children due to lack of consistent access to a safe water supply (42). Other factors such as the cost of formula and the stigma associated with not breastfeeding play into this decision (7). In order for MTCT to occur during breast feeding, the virus must first pass through the mammary epithelium, remain infectious within breast milk, traverse the infant mucosal barriers and establish infection. Studies in *ex vivo* organ tissue model systems and *in vivo* animal models have provided evidence that transmission can occur *via* the oral route (43, 44). Oral inoculations of simian immunodeficiency virus (SIV) have been shown to cause infection in infant rhesus macaques, providing proof of concept, although often these experimental inoculums contained higher doses of virus than would be seen in normal levels in breast milk (45–47). Cord blood and neonatal blood contain low levels of CD4+ T cells expressing CCR5, but, as described above, CD4+CCR5+ T cells populating the fetal intestines are abundant (13), a finding that has also been described in infant rhesus macaques (48–50). The mammary epithelium, like the placenta, however, successfully inhibits many pathogens from entering the breast milk through various protective mechanisms. Additionally, there is evidence that breast milk and saliva have innate inhibitory activity that restricts HIV transmission (51–54). The protective mechanisms of the maternal and fetal immune responses that limit breast milk transmission will be discussed in more detail below.

One major risk factor for MTCT during breastfeeding is viral load in the breast milk (10), and both cell-free and cell-associated HIV are thought to contribute to transmission. HIV RNA levels in breast milk correlate with plasma levels but are generally 100-fold lower (8, 55). Conditions that increase breast milk viral shedding are associated with higher transmission rates. Nonexclusive breastfeeding and infrequent emptying of the breast can lead to breast inflammation secondary to milk stasis, which in turn increases the viral load and has a strong association with increased MTCT (56–61). However, conflicting research found that nonexclusive breast feeding and mastitis do not significantly increase viral loads in breast milk (56). Still, HIV transmission was increased in breastfed infants who also received solid foods when compared to exclusively breastfed children (58). This mixed feeding is thought to cause disruption of the infant's gut mucosal lining secondary to the introduction of non-breast-milk foods and early introduction of pathogens or foreign antigens, leading to immune activation and increased susceptibility to infection (62–64). Microbiome differences between mixed fed and exclusively breastfed infants may also impact transmission (65). Multiple studies suggested that cell-associated viruses also have a role in transmission during breastfeeding (66, 67). Understanding these biological mechanisms of breast milk viral spread is an important first step in characterizing the establishment of HIV reservoirs during this period. Further, it should be recognized that breastfeeding transmission can occur outside of the neonatal period and infants may be diagnosed after more time has elapsed since infection than occurs with *in utero* and intrapartum transmission. This later diagnosis, coupled with rapid immune system changes in early life, likely leads to a unique immunovirologic environment defining HIV persistence in children infected through the breastfeeding route.

FACTORS INFLUENCING VERTICAL TRANSMISSION

MTCT is multifactorial, with different viral, maternal, and fetal/infant factors at play that influence the risk of HIV transmission (**Figure 1**). Knowledge of these risk factors and understanding of their roles in MTCT have been crucial to develop preventative measures and here we postulate that their consideration should also inform the investigation into curative approaches.

Viral Factors Impacting MTCT

Viral Burden

Maternal viral load has been shown to be the strongest predictor of perinatal HIV transmission. Many studies have demonstrated increased risk of transmission with high levels of maternal viremia and high p24 antigenemia (68–71). Acute infection during pregnancy is associated with increased risk of perinatal transmission and is likely related to the high viral loads in plasma

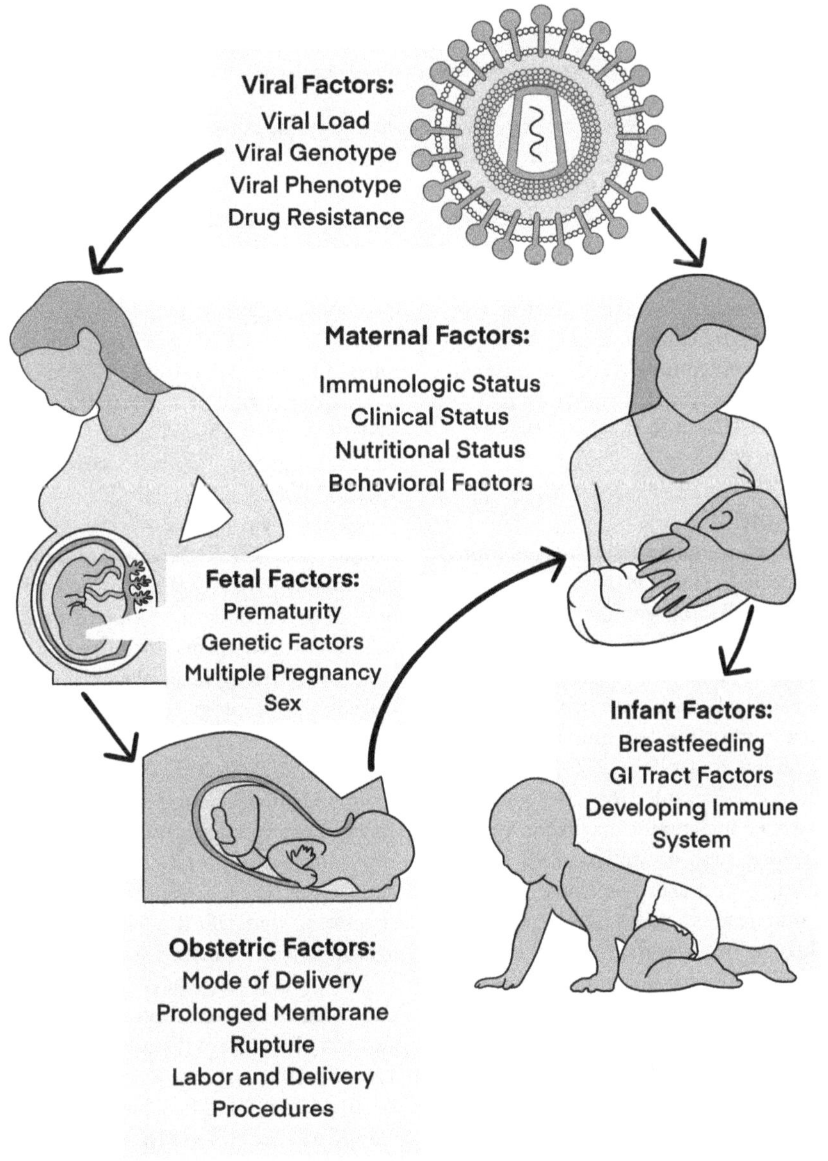

FIGURE 1 | Factors influencing vertical transmission.

and the genital tract (72). Consequently, maternal viral suppression *via* use of ART during pregnancy has been proven to lower the risk of perinatal transmission. This was first supported by the 076 trial which showed that administration of zidovudine during pregnancy, delivery, and to the newborn for the first 6 months of life reduced transmission by nearly 70% in women with HIV who did not breast-feed (73). Subsequent studies have indicated that transmission is reduced even further with triple-drug regimens (74). Several studies have tried to establish a threshold of maternal viral load below which transmission does not occur (75); however, it has been demonstrated that transmission can occur in some cases where women have low levels of HIV RNA in the blood, indicating the presence of other factors influencing the transmission process. In one study that included 320 women from 18 different centers in France showed that perinatal transmission occurred in 12% of the women at less than 1000 copies/ml compared to 29% in women with more than 10,000 copies/ml (76). In contrast, in Bangkok 281 pregnant women were followed and no transmission occurred in those with virus load less than 2,000 copies/ml (77).

Several behavioral practices have been associated with increased risk of maternal to infant HIV transmission due to resultant increases in viral load. These behavioral factors include illicit drug use (IDU), cigarette smoking, and alcohol use. IDU is associated with increased risk of MTCT (78–81). Alcohol and drug use like heroin, amphetamine and cocaine, may be associated with failure to control viral load in the presence of

ART, hence increased transmission rate (82–85). Additionally, transmission may be increased through drug interactions with ART and placental injury (86). Some have demonstrated an association between IDU and lack of adherence to ART which can lead to increased viral load (83, 85–87).

In addition to plasma viral load, viral levels in cervicovaginal fluid and breast milk are also thought to influence transmission risk in the intrapartum and postnatal periods (56, 88–90). As referenced above, levels of HIV DNA in breast milk cells (ie, CD4+ T cells) are positively correlated with postnatal transmission, and this intracellular HIV DNA is not significantly reduced by maternal ART. Risk of transmission is higher during early lactation due to the increased cellular content of colostrum (91). Both maternal ART and extended infant prophylaxis (at least with a single agent) during breastfeeding significantly reduces but does not eliminate MTCT, an observation that likely reflects virus persistence in CD4+ T cells (92–97).

Viral Genotype and Phenotype

Several studies of viral variants in mothers and infants attempted to characterize HIV quasispecies associated with MTCT and have yielded conflicting results. Major, minor, and multiple variant transmission events have been described (98–100). Most evidence suggests that a single or restricted subset of maternal viral variants establish infection in the infant suggesting selective pressure during the transmission process. However, the basis and the factors controlling MTCT bottleneck are not yet fully understood. Different properties of virus populations have been reported in studies analyzing vertical transmission stratified by timing, with transmission during the intrapartum period found to be primarily associated with the transmission of minor maternal variants while *in utero* transmission was more likely to occur with single or multiple HIV variants (100–104). Maternal antiretroviral drug resistance is associated with transmission during breastfeeding, but not during the *in utero*/intrapartum periods (105).

Phylogenetic analyses of HIV *env* in infected infants showed that they have a more homogenous virus population when compared to their mothers (106, 107). Studies have also shown that macrophage-tropic and non-syncytium-inducing (NSI) or CCR5-utilizing HIV viral strains are selectively transmitted (108). Another characteristic found in transmitted viruses was shorter variable loops and fewer putative N-linked glycosylation (PNG) sites encoded in *env* (70, 109–111). Different HIV subtypes may also have distinct MTCT rates. Work conducted in Tanzania showed that subtype C is preferentially transmitted from mother to child compared to subtype A and D (100). In another study from Kenya, the MTCT rate appeared to be higher among mothers infected with subtype D compared with subtype A (112). However, no such differences have been observed in other cohorts (100, 112–115).

Host Factors Impacting MTCT

Genetic Factors

Genetic polymorphisms in the coding and regulatory regions of HIV receptors and their ligands influence the risk of HIV acquisition. Infants with a single nucleotide polymorphism (SNP) in the CD4 gene at position C868T that may modify the tertiary structure of CD4 were more likely to acquire HIV compared to infants with wild type CD4 (116). In the setting of MTCT, most of the transmitted viruses use CCR5 as a coreceptor (117). As has been shown for horizontal infection in adults, the presence of a 32-bp deletion in the coding region of the *CCR5* gene (*CCR5*-Δ32) in the homozygous state in infants results in non-functional coreceptors and confers protection from vertical infection (118, 119). Heterozygosity also exerts a protective effect when carried by mothers due to lower maternal viral burden (107). Conversely, polymorphisms in the CCR5 promoter region at positions 59029 and 59353T increase the expression of CCR5 leading to increased risk of MTCT when carried by infants (120–123).

Increased risk of vertical transmission was also seen with genetic polymorphisms resulting in decreased expression of the natural ligands for HIV coreceptors (CCL3, CCL4, and CCL5) (124).

Genetic variations affecting innate immunity may also influence MTCT. Defensins are antimicrobial peptides that are expressed by epithelial cells, known for innate mucosal defense and antiviral activities. Defensins inhibit HIV infection *via* different mechanisms including direct binding to virions as well as disturbing intracellular signaling by modulation of host cell surface receptors. Three SNPs in the 5′ untranslated region of β-defensin-1 (*DEFB1*) gene were reported to modulate risk of MTCT: –52G/A, -20(G/A) and –44C/G (125–127). Braida et al. described an association between -44(C/G) and HIV infection in Italian pediatric population (125). Another study found a lower copy number of *DEFB104* among HIV-infected children when compared to HIV-exposed children and healthy controls, suggesting that *DEFB104* may have a potential protective role against vertical transmission (128).

Multiple studies have investigated the influence of HLA concordance between mother and infant on vertical transmission and as well as risk of disease progression in infected infants (129–131). Specific maternal HLA polymorphisms, including B4901, B5301, A2/6802 and B18, have also been associated with decreased risk of MTCT (132–134). HLA-G, a non-classical class I MHC gene highly expressed in placental trophoblasts, has several SNPs found to be associated with decreased risk of vertical transmission (135, 136). Certain class II MHC alleles have also been reported to influence MTCT among certain ethnicities such as *DQB1*0604, DR3, DR13, DRB1*1501* (137–139).

Gender specific differences in MTCT have been reported in several cohorts (140, 141). Female infants are reported to have two- to three-fold increased risk of infection at birth compared to male infants (7, 140, 141). This increased susceptibility has been linked to subversion of innate immunity, with female fetuses acquiring maternal variants resistant to type I interferons (142). Sex-specific differences in *in utero* infection have also been attributed to the fact that *in utero* mortality rates of HIV-infected male infants are disproportionately higher and thus more HIV-infected female infants are liveborn. It is also proposed that a minor histocompatibility reaction between infant male Y chromosome-derived antigens and maternal lymphocytes reduce the risk of MTCT to boys (140).

Maternal Co-Infections

Several coexisting maternal infections have been found to be associated with increased MTCT of HIV. Multiple studies demonstrated an increased risk of vertical transmission in the setting of chorioamnionitis (143–145), primarily related to disruption of the placental barrier and entrance of HIV-infected cells into the amniotic fluid (143, 144, 146). Chorioamnionitis complications including preterm labor and premature rupture of membranes can also lead to increased risk of MTCT related to immaturity of the skin and mucosal membranes as well as the premature fetal immune system. In a multicenter prospective cohort, clinical and biologic factors that contributed to MTCT were studied. Histologic chorioamnionitis was found to be a major risk factor for transmitting HIV (147).

Adachi and colleagues evaluated the effect of sexually transmitted infections (STIs) on risk of MTCT in a large cohort of HIV-infected pregnant women and found increased rates of HIV transmission in the presence of a another sexually transmitted disease (148). In general, inflammation of the maternal genital tract mucosa has been shown to increase rate of vertical transmission independent of maternal plasma HIV load (59). Infections resulting in genital ulcer disease such as HSV-2 are also associated with increased genital shedding of HIV (35, 149, 150). Conflicting data exist regarding maternal syphilis infection and MTCT of HIV. A study in Zimbabwe showed that active maternal syphilis at the time of delivery was not associated with intra-partum MTCT risk while several other groups have demonstrated an increased risk of vertical HIV acquisition in the setting of maternal syphilis (146, 151). HIV and Hepatitis B virus (HBV) co-infection are associated with increased HBV, but not HIV transmission to the infant. Maternal Hepatitis C virus (HCV) co-infection has been linked to higher rates of vertical HIV transmission (152–160).

Unprotected sexual intercourse during pregnancy itself is thought to be associated with increased risk of MTCT (161, 162). Bulterys et al. conducted a prospective cohort study in Rwanda that showed that unprotected sexual intercourse with multiple partners before and during pregnancy in a population with high HIV-1 seroprevalence may increase risk of transmission from infected mother to infants (161). Another study by Burns and colleagues also found higher frequency of intercourse during pregnancy among women transmitting HIV to their infants (163). Potential mechanisms include increased HIV strain diversity (i.e., superinfection) (164, 165) and vaginal or cervical inflammation due to microabrasions or STIs that result in chorioamnionitis and/or increased viral shedding in genital fluids (164).

Tuberculosis (TB) is one of the most important causes of mortality and morbidity in HIV infection, especially in women residing in TB endemic areas. Active TB infection increases HIV viral load which is a known risk factor for perinatal transmission (166–168). Gupta et al., found a 2.5-fold increase in the odds of MTCT of HIV in pregnant women with TB/HIV coinfection, after adjusting for maternal and infant factors (169). Similarly, malaria and HIV coinfection is associated with an increased risk of adverse outcomes in pregnant women (170) as well as increased HIV viral load (171). As such, a few studies have suggested an increased risk of perinatal transmission with maternal malaria (172–174), yet others failed to demonstrate this relationship (144, 175, 176). Finally, other common viral infections, such as Cytomegalovirus (CMV), may play a critical role in influencing MTCT. One described mechanism has been through enhancement of placental susceptibility to HIV infection (177).

Maternal Immunological Factors

There are multiple maternal immunological factors associated with increased risk of perinatal transmission, including low CD4+ T cell count, CD4+ T cell percentage, and CD4/CD8 ratio (178). Shivakoti et al. showed that high maternal soluble CD14 concentration during the peripartum period was associated with increased risk of MTCT, independent of maternal viral load, CD4+ T cell count and ART exposure (179), implicating immune activation in transmission.

Adaptive immune responses play an important role in transmission from mother to infant. MTCT is a unique setting where HIV-1 acquisition occurs in the presence of naturally elicited HIV-specific antibodies that are passively transferred prior to birth. Several studies have examined the impact of maternal antibodies on MTCT; however, there have been conflicting results and their role in protecting infants against HIV-1 transmission remains unclear. These contradicting results may be explained by small cohort sizes, lack of control for the other known risk factors for HIV transmission, timing, and methods used in infant diagnosis, and potential clade-specific differences in virus–antibody interactions. Initial studies demonstrated that higher levels of maternal HIV-1 envelope (Env)-specific IgG antibody responses were associated with reduced transmission risk (180, 181).This association was not observed in subsequent studies and research focus was shifted to examine the effect of neutralizing antibodies (nAbs) and their role in modulating the risk of transmission (182, 183). Work conducted in nonhuman primates showed that passive immunization of infants with a cocktail of HIV-1-neutralizing antibodies provided partial protection against oral simian-human immunodeficiency virus transmission (184). Subsequent human studies showed that high levels of maternal nAbs were correlated with reduced MTCT rates while others failed to confirm this association (185–188). However, founder viruses in infants are generally more resistant to neutralization by maternal antibodies (189, 190), suggesting that the transmitted variants are able to escape nAbs and supportive of the idea that maternal antibodies may confer partial protection.

In a large cohort of non-breastfeeding HIV-1 infected women enrolled in the pre-ART era Women and Infant Transmission Study (WITS), Permar and her group found that maternal V3-specific IgG binding responses and CD4 binding site-blocking responses correlated and were independently predictive of reduced MTCT risk (191). They also found that both binding and neutralizing responses targeting the C-terminal region of HIV envelope (Env) were associated with decreased risk of transmission (191). Antibody effector functions beyond neutralization have also been examined for their contribution to MTCT. Maternal antibody-dependent cellular cytotoxicity (ADCC) is thought to have a role in protection against HIV-1 transmission. In one such investigation, plasma and breast milk obtained soon after delivery from 9 transmitting and 10 non-transmitting women in Kenya demonstrated that breast milk Env-specific IgG responses with ADCC activity were associated with decreased MTCT risk (192). However, Pollara et al. found no association of ADCC-mediating responses and MTCT risk in HIV clade C breastfeeding women in Malawi (193). In addition to antibodies and antibody effector functions, Lohman-Payne et al. also reported breast milk HIV gag-specific IFNg responses to be associated with protection from MTCT *via* breastfeeding in a Kenyan cohort (194).

Infant Immunological Factors

Most infants born to HIV-1 infected mothers do not become infected despite having an immature immune system and repeated exposures to HIV-1 throughout the peripartum and breastfeeding periods. To survive to term, the developing fetus must avoid generating an inflammatory response to the many foreign maternal antigens to which it is exposed during development resulting in a predominantly tolerogenic immune system in the fetus and newborn (195). The tolerogenic environment is facilitated by high levels of anti-inflammatory cytokines such as TGFb and IL-10 (196), which likely subvert immune activation and establishment of infection upon HIV exposure. TGFb also directs naïve CD4+ T cell to differentiate to Tregs resulting in a larger Treg pool in infants, representing 15% of fetal blood T cells compared to 5% of adult blood T cells. These Tregs promote immune tolerance and are long-lived (196, 197). Much of these regulatory cells reside in intestinal tissue and are critical for mucosal immune homeostasis. In addition to higher levels of Tregs, the CD4+ effector cells of infants are predominantly of the Th17 and Th2 phenotype (rather than Th1 as in adults) (198, 199). Th17 cells are critical to maintaining the integrity of the intestinal mucosal barrier and may thus restrict dissemination of infection. Conversely, Tugizov and colleagues have reported lower levels of innate proteins that restrict infection, such as defensins, in infant compared to adult oral epithelia (43).

In the mother-child transmission pair, the infant may be disadvantaged in that the transmitted virus in has already adapted to evade a genetically similar immune system. Anti-HIV-1 antibodies and T cells transferred to the child either *in utero* or through breastmilk have pre-adapted to the transmitted virus and may be ineffective. Additionally, because of shared HLA alleles the transmitted virus may be preadapted to escape CD8+ T cells targeting HIV epitopes restricted by HLA alleles inherited from the mother further complicating pediatric HIV-1 infection (200, 201). HIV-specific cellular immune responses are detected in exposed uninfected infants, but their role in influencing virus acquisition is uncertain (202, 203).

IMPLICATIONS FOR CURE APPROACHES

The World Health Organization recommendations state that all infants and children under two years of age with confirmed HIV-1 begin ART immediately at the time of diagnosis irrespective of CD4+ T cell counts (204). Despite this recommendation, HIV-1-infected children are one third less likely to receive ART than infected adults (205). Reasons for this include fewer drugs available for use by children, higher treatment cost, and dependence on a caregiver to provide ART (206). These factors can complicate the design and implementation of cure studies in children.

A major barrier to HIV cure is the establishment of a reservoir of HIV-infected cells that persists despite suppressive ART and can give rise to rebound viremia if ART is interrupted. In adults, it is well documented that viral reservoirs are established during early stages of HIV infection (207) and this finding is supported by the SIV/macaque model in which rapid seeding of the viral reservoir within 3 days of infection has been described (208). Furthermore, rebound of viremia is almost always seen after ART discontinuation in both horizontally infected adults and perinatally-infected children (209–211). However, little is known about the exact timing of reservoir seeding in different MTCT settings and whether there are differences in reservoir establishment in relation to time of infection and mode of transmission. Increased understanding of these factors may aid in the development of approaches to eradicate viral reservoirs and/or induce viral remission (sustained viral suppression in absence of ART) in children.

The uniqueness of the in-utero transmission window allows for rapid detection and treatment as children born to women with HIV can be screened at birth. Such early detection is not generally feasible in adult transmissions. Infants diagnosed at birth *via* rapid point-of-care testing can begin ART within the first few hours of life (212). Infections arising from intra- or post-partum transmission will not be detected at the time of birth, so follow-up care and repeated testing are required to monitor these transmission modes. In these instances, early ART initiation is not as practical in resource limited settings, although current United States guidelines recommend triple drug prophylaxis (given at therapeutic dosing) for neonates with high risk of acquiring HIV infection.

Contemporary studies of HIV reservoirs in perinatally infected infants and children have focused on *in utero* transmission, following the description of the 'Mississippi child'. This child received ART between 30 hours and 18 months of age, and then remained persistently aviremic for 27 months after discontinuation of ART before rebound (209, 213). *In utero* infection was documented, but the child did not develop HIV-specific antibody or T cell responses, thought due to the very early initiation of ART. Despite the eventual rebound, this partial remission led to several clinical trials of very early ART (typically considered to be within 48 hours) to limit the size of the HIV reservoir and investigate the possibility of achieving post-treatment control after ART interruption. Results from the Early Infant Treatment (EIT) study in Botswana have demonstrated that very early ART leads to an exceptionally small reservoir of intact proviral HIV DNA as well as an improved innate and adaptive antiviral immune response compared to delayed ART (214). As of this writing, results from the ART interruption phase of the very early ART trials, including EIT and IMPAACT P1115 (215), have not been published. Kuhn and colleagues describe challenges in meeting predetermined virologic and immunologic criteria for ART interruption in the LEOPARD trial of very early/early ART conducted in South Africa (216).

The South African Children with HIV Early antiRetroviral therapy (CHER) trial (217), that included children with *in utero* and intrapartum HIV infection, has led to a number of key findings regarding persistent HIV reservoirs. One report demonstrated rare intact proviral sequences in children after 6-9 years of ART initiated after 2 months of age but within the first year of life using near full-length proviral amplification and sequencing (218). This group further identified clones of infected cells shortly after birth that could also be detected after almost a decade on ART, suggesting that clonal expansion of reservoir cells maintains HIV persistence in children as it does for adults (219). Two additional case reports of long-term HIV remission have emerged, one from the CHER trial, with unknown timing of infection (*in utero vs* intrapartum) (220) and the other from a French cohort, with presumed intrapartum transmission (221), both of whom started ART at 2-3 months of life.

There have been relatively fewer studies of reservoir characteristics in children infected postpartum through breastfeeding. However, presently over half of new infections occur postnatally through breast milk (9). As this route has become predominant in perinatal HIV infection, a nonhuman primate model has been established to better understand virologic and immunologic features of lentivirus infection following postpartum transmission, more precisely define anatomic sites of virus persistence, and test strategies to promote reservoir eradication or remission (46, 47, 222–224). These and other ongoing studies may inform the design of future cure-directed clinical trials in children with HIV infection acquired through breast milk.

Regardless of the mode of transmission earlier ART is generally associated with a smaller reservoir during viremia suppression (210, 214, 225–237), although starting ART within 14 days of life may not lead to significantly greater HIV DNA persistence compared to within 48 hours of life (238). ART initiation within 8 days has also been associated with a faster HIV DNA decay compared to ART started at 5 months (239). Female sex and maternal acute HIV infection during pregnancy have been associated with higher levels of persistent HIV DNA (240).

While protocol-specified ART interruption has not occurred in recent clinical trials, studies of intermittent viremia *vs.* sustained viral suppression can be informative to identify biomarkers that may be predictive of viral rebound dynamics. These findings are by nature complicated by behavioral factors, including adherence to ART regimens. Millar and colleagues assessed factors associated with intermittent viremia in *in utero* infected infants started on early ART (in the first 3 weeks of life) (240). A smaller reservoir size as measured by total HIV DNA in PBMCs was not correlated with maintained viral suppression whereas a longer time to initial viral suppression was, implicating immunologic contributions to aviremia, although this finding may have been influenced by ART nonadherence. In children in the EIT study who started on ART at < 7 days of life, sustained HIV RNA suppression was associated with negative HIV serostatus and negative qualitative HIV DNA PCR at ~20 months (225). HIV seronegativity has also been described in other studies of early or very early ART and has been proposed as an estimate for reservoir size (227, 228, 241–244).

Identification of cure strategies that target latently infected cells, allow immune recognition and clearance of the reservoir, and/or promote viral remission are currently considered extremely high priority for the field. Unlike in adults, few cure strategies have been tested in children to date, with the exception of very early ART that it is now understood is insufficient to lead to cure in the majority of individuals. However, there are several approaches that may provide benefit in the setting of perinatal HIV transmission, and their study should be carefully considered for certain populations (**Figure 2**). The design of such studies should take into consideration not only the timing of ART initiation, but also the duration of ART (and therefore age of the trial participant), as well as the known or presumed mode of HIV transmission (*in utero*, intrapartum, or postpartum). For example, a neonate infected *in utero* and initiating very early ART is likely to be vastly different both virologically and immunologically from an adolescent who acquired HIV through breastfeeding with delayed ART initiation and periods of unsuppressed viremia over years. In the former case, adding the cure directed therapy at the time of early ART initiation may lead to an extremely small reservoir size (or even prevent reservoir establishment in the best-case scenario). This cure-directed therapy might include one or multiple broadly neutralizing antibodies delivered by passive (as is being tested in IMPAACT 2008 (215) or active immunization along with ART. A novel proposed strategy, termed "surge and purge," combines very early ART, passive antibody administration, and immune stimulation to destabilize reservoir establishment (245). Infants and children with very small reservoirs may also be good candidates for approaches designed to silence HIV expression ("block and lock"). For the school aged or adolescent child with a larger reservoir size, the "kick and kill" approach may be more effective, with a latency reversal agent used to reactivate virus expression followed by immune-based clearance of infected cells. Studies in nonhuman primates support the notion that pre-existing reservoir size as well as age-related factors may influence susceptibility to latency reversal (246, 247). Therapeutic HIV vaccines designed to boost antiviral T cell responses may have benefit in kick and kick strategies targeting established infection (223, 248) and possibly in limiting reservoir size early in infection, although in both settings the impact may depend on the child's age at vaccination, the timing of ART, and the degree of immune exhaustion present. Results from the HVRRICANE trial are forthcoming, in which a prime-boost vaccine strategy will be tested in combination with a TLR4 adjuvant (hypothesized to reverse latency) in HIV-1-infected children with history of early ART or previous immunization with one of the vaccine components (215).

In summary, HIV MTCT is promoted by distinct immunopathogenesis for the three different routes of transmission that may also affect HIV persistence. Consideration of the complex interaction between viral, maternal, and fetal/infant factors may enhance the pursuit of strategies to achieve an

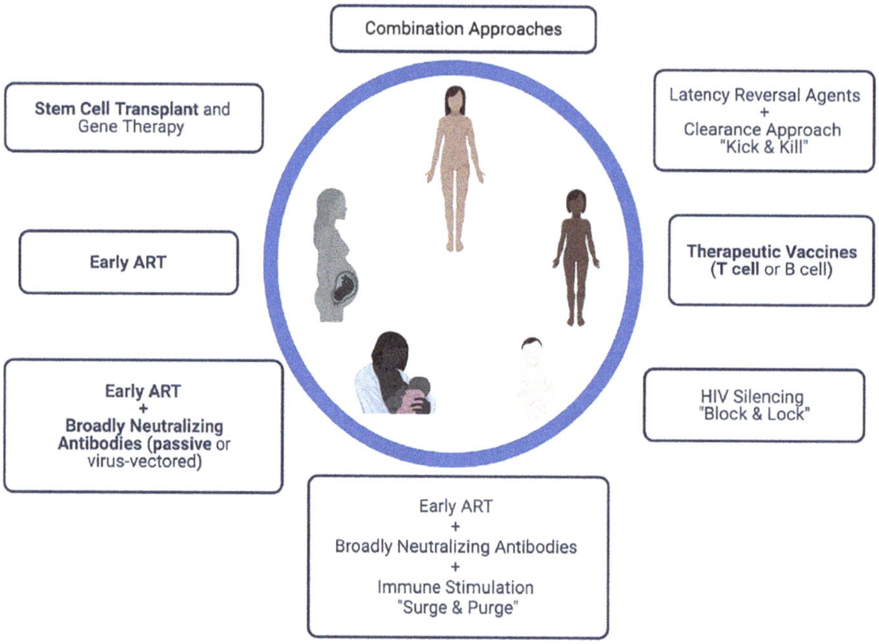

FIGURE 2 | Possible HIV cure approaches for perinatally infected infants, children and adolescents. Strategies in bold have been or are being studied in pediatric clinical trials.

HIV cure for pediatric populations. Future preclinical and clinical trials from the neonatal period through adolescence will further elucidate how MTCT influences the potential for HIV cure.

AUTHOR CONTRIBUTIONS

OA is the first author, the rest of the coauthors AC, KB, JP contributed to the manuscript. All authors reviewed the final manuscript. All authors contributed to the article and approved the submitted version.

FUNDING

AC would like to acknowledge funding support from the NIH (R01 AI133706, P01 AI131276, R37 AI157862, and UM1 AI164566).

REFERENCES

1. Centers for Disease C. Unexplained Immunodeficiency and Opportunistic Infections in Infants–New York, New Jersey, California. *MMWR Morb Mortal Wkly Rep* (1982) 31(49):665–7.
2. UNAIDS. *Global HIV & AIDS Statistics - Fact Sheet*. UNAIDS (2011). Available at: https://www.unaids.org/en/resources/fact-sheet (Accessed 10/06/2020).
3. WHO. *Antiretroviral Drugs for Treatment Pregnant Women and Preventing HIV Infection in Infants: Recommendations for a Public Health Approach*. Geneva: WHO (2010).
4. HIV/AIDS) UJUNPo. *Press Release: "World Leaders Launch Plan to Eliminate New HIV Infections Among Children by 2015"*. Geneva: UNAIDS (2011).
5. UNAIDS. *Global HIV & AIDS Statistics*. UNAIDS (2020).
6. Goulder PJ, Lewin SR, Leitman EM. Paediatric HIV Infection: The Potential for Cure. *Nat Rev Immunol* (2016) 16(4):259–71. doi: 10.1038/nri.2016.19
7. Lehman DA, Farquhar C. Biological Mechanisms of Vertical Human Immunodeficiency Virus (HIV-1) Transmission. *Rev Med Virol* (2007) 17 (6):381–403. doi: 10.1002/rmv.543
8. Tobin NH, Aldrovandi GM. Immunology of Pediatric HIV Infection. *Immunol Rev* (2013) 254(1):143–69. doi: 10.1111/imr.12074
9. Luzuriaga K, Mofenson LM. Challenges in the Elimination of Pediatric HIV-1 Infection. *N Engl J Med* (2016) 374(8):761–70. doi: 10.1056/NEJMra1505256
10. John GC, Nduati RW, Mbori-Ngacha DA, Richardson BA, Panteleeff D, Mwatha A, et al. Correlates of Mother-to-Child Human Immunodeficiency Virus Type 1 (HIV-1) Transmission: Association With Maternal Plasma HIV-1 RNA Load, Genital HIV-1 DNA Shedding, and Breast Infections. *J Infect Dis* (2001) 183(2):206–12. doi: 10.1086/317918
11. Kumar SB, Rice CE, Milner DA Jr., Ramirez NC, Ackerman WE 4th, Mwapasa V, et al. Elevated Cytokine and Chemokine Levels in the Placenta Are Associated With in-Utero HIV-1 Mother-to-Child Transmission. *AIDS* (2012) 26(6):685–94. doi: 10.1097/QAD.0b013e3283519b00
12. Fazely F, Sharma PL, Fratazzi C, Greene MF, Wyand MS, Memon MA, et al. Simian Immunodeficiency Virus Infection *via* Amniotic Fluid: A Model to Study Fetal Immunopathogenesis and Prophylaxis. *J Acquir Immune Defic Syndr (1988)* (1993) 6(2):107–14.
13. Bunders MJ, van der Loos CM, Klarenbeek PL, van Hamme JL, Boer K, Wilde JCH, et al. Memory CD4(+)CCR5(+) T Cells Are Abundantly Present in the Gut of Newborn Infants to Facilitate Mother-to-Child Transmission of HIV-1. *Blood* (2012) 120(22):4383–90. doi: 10.1182/blood-2012-06-437566

14. Lobato AC, Aguiar RA, Aleixo AW, Andrade BA, Cavallo IK, Kakehasi FM, et al. HIV-1 RNA Detection in the Amniotic Fluid of HIV-Infected Pregnant Women. *Mem Inst Oswaldo Cruz* (2010) 105(5):720–1. doi: 10.1590/S0074-02762010000500021
15. Maiques V, García-Tejedor A, Perales A, Córdoba J, Esteban RJ. HIV Detection in Amniotic Fluid Samples. Amniocentesis Can Be Performed in HIV Pregnant Women? *Eur J Obstet Gynecol Reprod Biol* (2003) 108 (2):137–41. doi: 10.1016/S0301-2115(02)00405-0
16. Mohlala BK, Tucker TJ, Besser MJ, Williamson C, Yeats J, Smit L, et al. Investigation of HIV in Amniotic Fluid From HIV-Infected Pregnant Women at Full Term. *J Infect Dis* (2005) 192(3):488–91. doi: 10.1086/431604
17. Farzin A, Boyer P, Ank B, Nielsen-Saines K, Bryson Y. Amniotic Fluid Exhibits an Innate Inhibitory Activity Against HIV Type 1 Replication *In Vitro*. *AIDS Res Hum Retroviruses* (2013) 29(1):77–83. doi: 10.1089/aid.2011.0355
18. Arora N, Sadovsky Y, Dermody TS, Coyne CB. Microbial Vertical Transmission During Human Pregnancy. *Cell Host Microbe* (2017) 21 (5):561–7. doi: 10.1016/j.chom.2017.04.007
19. Lewis SH, Reynolds-Kohler C, Fox HE, Nelson JA. HIV-1 in Trophoblastic and Villous Hofbauer Cells, and Haematological Precursors in Eight-Week Fetuses. *Lancet* (1990) 335(8689):565–8. doi: 10.1016/0140-6736(90)90349-A
20. Rouzioux C, Costagliola D, Burgard M, Blanche S, Mayaux MJ, Griscelli C, et al. Estimated Timing of Mother-To-Child Human Immunodeficiency Virus Type 1 (HIV-1) Transmission by Use of a Markov Model. *Am J Epidemiol* (1995) 142(12):1330–7. doi: 10.1093/oxfordjournals.aje.a117601
21. Chouquet C, Richardson S, Burgard M, Blanche S, Mayaux MJ, Rouzioux C, et al. Timing of Human Immunodeficiency Virus Type 1 (HIV-1) Transmission From Mother to Child: Bayesian Estimation Using a Mixture. *Stat Med* (1999) 18 (7):815–33. doi: 10.1002/(SICI)1097-0258(19990415)18:7<815::AID-SIM74>3.0.CO;2-G
22. Menu E, Mbopi-Keou FX, Lagaye S, Pissard S, Mauclère P, Scarlatti G, et al. Selection of Maternal Human Immunodeficiency Virus Type 1 Variants in Human Placenta. European Network for *In Utero* Transmission of HIV-1. *J Infect Dis* (1999) 179(1):44–51. doi: 10.1086/314542
23. Zachar V, Zacharova V, Fink T, Thomas RA, King BR, Ebbesen P, et al. Genetic Analysis Reveals Ongoing HIV Type 1 Evolution in Infected Human Placental Trophoblast. *AIDS Res Hum Retroviruses* (1999) 15(18):1673–83. doi: 10.1089/088922299309711
24. De Andreis C, Simoni G, Rossella F, Castagna C, Pesenti E, Porta G, et al. HIV-1 Proviral DNA Polymerase Chain Reaction Detection in Chorionic Villi After Exclusion of Maternal Contamination by Variable Number of Tandem Repeats Analysis. *AIDS* (1996) 10(7):711–5. doi: 10.1097/00002030-199606001-00004
25. Ross AL, Cannou C, Barré-Sinoussi F, Menu E. Proteasome-Independent Degradation of HIV-1 in Naturally Non-Permissive Human Placental Trophoblast Cells. *Retrovirology* (2009) 6:46. doi: 10.1186/1742-4690-6-46
26. Lagaye S, Derrien M, Menu E, Coïto C, Tresoldi E, Mauclère P, et al. Cell-To-Cell Contact Results in a Selective Translocation of Maternal Human Immunodeficiency Virus Type 1 Quasispecies Across a Trophoblastic Barrier by Both Transcytosis and Infection. *J Virol* (2001) 75(10):4780–91. doi: 10.1128/JVI.75.10.4780-4791.2001
27. Tang Y, Woodward BO, Pastor L, George AM, Petrechko O, Nouvet FJ, et al. Endogenous Retroviral Envelope Syncytin Induces HIV-1 Spreading and Establishes HIV Reservoirs in Placenta. *Cell Rep* (2020) 30(13):4528–39.e4. doi: 10.1016/j.celrep.2020.03.016
28. Biggar RJ, Lee TH, Wen L, Broadhead R, Kumwenda N, Taha TE, et al. The Role of Transplacental Microtransfusions of Maternal Lymphocytes in HIV Transmission to Newborns. *AIDS* (2008) 22(17):2251–6. doi: 10.1097/QAD.0b013e328314e36b
29. Lee TH, Chafets DM, Biggar RJ, McCune JM, Busch MP. The Role of Transplacental Microtransfusions of Maternal Lymphocytes in *In Utero* HIV Transmission. *J Acquir Immune Defic Syndr* (2010) 55(2):143–7. doi: 10.1097/QAI.0b013e3181eb301e
30. Magder LS, Mofenson L, Paul ME, Zorrilla CD, Blattner WA, Tuomala RE, et al. Risk Factors for *In Utero* and Intrapartum Transmission of HIV. *J Acquir Immune Defic Syndr* (2005) 38(1):87–95. doi: 10.1097/00126334-200501010-00016
31. Fawzi W, Msamanga G, Renjifo B, Spiegelman D, Urassa E, Hashemi L, et al. Predictors of Intrauterine and Intrapartum Transmission of HIV-1 Among Tanzanian Women. *AIDS* (2001) 15(9):1157–65. doi: 10.1097/00002030-200106150-00011
32. Mofenson LM, Lambert JS, Stiehm ER, Bethel J, Meyer WA, Whitehouse J, et al. Risk Factors for Perinatal Transmission of Human Immunodeficiency Virus Type 1 in Women Treated With Zidovudine. Pediatric AIDS Clinical Trials Group Study 185 Team. *N Engl J Med* (1999) 341(6):385–93. doi: 10.1056/NEJM199908053410601
33. Briand N, Jasseron C, Sibiude J, Azria E, Pollet J, Hammou Y, et al. Cesarean Section for HIV-Infected Women in the Combination Antiretroviral Therapies Era, 2000-2010. *Am J Obstet Gynecol* (2013) 209(4):335.e1–12. doi: 10.1016/j.ajog.2013.06.021
34. Drake AL, John-Stewart GC, Wald A, Mbori-Ngacha DA, Bosire R, Wamalwa DC, et al. Herpes Simplex Virus Type 2 and Risk of Intrapartum Human Immunodeficiency Virus Transmission. *Obstet Gynecol* (2007) 109(2 Pt 1):403–9. doi: 10.1097/01.AOG.0000251511.27725.5c
35. Mbopi-Kéou FX, Legoff J, Grésenguet G, Si-Mohamed A, Matta M, Mayaud P, et al. Genital Shedding of Herpes Simplex Virus-2 DNA and HIV-1 RNA and Proviral DNA in HIV-1- and Herpes Simplex Virus-2-Coinfected African Women. *J Acquir Immune Defic Syndr* (2003) 33(2):121–4. doi: 10.1097/00126334-200306010-00001
36. McClelland RS, Wang CC, Overbaugh J, Richardson BA, Corey L, Ashley RL, et al. Association Between Cervical Shedding of Herpes Simplex Virus and HIV-1. *AIDS* (2002) 16(18):2425–30. doi: 10.1097/00002030-200212060-00007
37. Parazzini F, Ricci E, Chiaffarino F, Di Cintio E, Di Cintio E, Pardi G, et al.Elective Caesarean-Section *Versus* Vaginal Delivery in Prevention of Vertical HIV-1 Transmission: A Randomised Clinical Trial. *Lancet* (1999) 353(9158):1035–9. doi: 10.1016/s0140-6736(98)08084-2
38. Andiman W, Bryson Y, de Martino M, Bryson Y, Farley J, Fowler H, et al. The Mode of Delivery and the Risk of Vertical Transmission of Human Immunodeficiency Virus Type 1–A Meta-Analysis of 15 Prospective Cohort Studies. *N Engl J Med* (1999) 340(13):977–87. doi: 10.1056/NEJM199904013401301
39. Kennedy CE, Yeh PT, Pandey S, Betran AP, Narasimhan M. Elective Cesarean Section for Women Living With HIV: A Systematic Review of Risks and Benefits. *AIDS* (2017) 31(11):1579–91. doi: 10.1097/QAD.0000000000001535
40. Kwiek JJ, Mwapasa V, Milner DA Jr, Alker AP, Miller WC, Tadesse E, et al. Maternal-Fetal Microtransfusions and HIV-1 Mother-to-Child Transmission in Malawi. *PloS Med* (2006) 3(1):e10. doi: 10.1371/journal.pmed.0030010
41. Ivy WI, Dominguez KL, Rakhmanina NY, Iuliano AD, Danner SP, Borkowf CB, et al. Premastication as a Route of Pediatric HIV Transmission: Case-Control and Cross-Sectional Investigations. *JAIDS J Acquired Immune Defic Syndr* (2012) 59(2):207–12. doi: 10.1097/QAI.0b013e31823b4554
42. Organization WH. *Breastfeeding and HIV*. World Health Organization (2016).
43. Tugizov SM, Herrera R, Veluppillai P, Greenspan D, Soros V, Greene WC, et al. Differential Transmission of HIV Traversing Fetal Oral/Intestinal Epithelia and Adult Oral Epithelia. *J Virol* (2012) 86(5):2556–70. doi: 10.1128/JVI.06578-11
44. Milush JM, Kosub D, Marthas M, Schmidt K, Scott F, Wozniakowski A, et al. Rapid Dissemination of SIV Following Oral Inoculation. *AIDS* (2004) 18 (18):2371–80.
45. Van Rompay KK, Abel K, Lawson JR, Singh RP, Schmidt KA, Evans T, et al. Attenuated Poxvirus-Based Simian Immunodeficiency Virus (SIV) Vaccines Given in Infancy Partially Protect Infant and Juvenile Macaques Against Repeated Oral Challenge With Virulent SIV. *J Acquir Immune Defic Syndr* (2005) 38(2):124–34. doi: 10.1097/00126334-200502010-00002
46. Obregon-Perko V, Bricker KM, Mensah G, Uddin F, Kumar MR, Fray EJ, et al. Simian-Human Immunodeficiency Virus SHIV.C.CH505 Persistence in ART-Suppressed Infant Macaques Is Characterized by Elevated SHIV RNA in the Gut and a High Abundance of Intact SHIV DNA in Naive CD4+ T Cells. *J Virol* (2020) 95(2):e01669-20. doi: 10.1128/JVI.01669-20
47. Mavigner M, Habib J, Deleage C, Rosen E, Mattingly C, Bricker K, et al. Simian Immunodeficiency Virus Persistence in Cellular and Anatomic Reservoirs in Antiretroviral Therapy-Suppressed Infant Rhesus Macaques. *J Virol* (2018) 92(18):e00562–18. doi: 10.1128/JVI.00562-18

48. Chahroudi A, Cartwright E, Lee ST, Mavigner M, Carnathan DG, Lawson B, et al. Target Cell Availability, Rather Than Breast Milk Factors, Dictates Mother-To-Infant Transmission of SIV in Sooty Mangabeys and Rhesus Macaques. *PloS Pathog* (2014) 10(3):e1003958. doi: 10.1371/journal.ppat.1003958
49. Veazey RS, Lifson JD, Pandrea I, Purcell J, Piatak M, Lackner AA. Simian Immunodeficiency Virus Infection in Neonatal Macaques. *J Virol* (2003) 77 (16):8783–92. doi: 10.1128/jvi.77.16.8783-8792.2003
50. Wang X, Xu H, Pahar B, Alvarez X, Green LC, Dufour J, et al. Simian Immunodeficiency Virus Selectively Infects Proliferating CD4+ T Cells in Neonatal Rhesus Macaques. *Blood* (2010) 116(20):4168–74. doi: 10.1182/blood-2010-03-273482
51. Lyimo MA, Howell AL, Balandya E, Eszterhas SK, Connor RI. Innate Factors in Human Breast Milk Inhibit Cell-Free HIV-1 But Not Cell-Associated HIV-1 Infection of CD4+ Cells. *J Acquir Immune Defic Syndr* (2009) 51 (2):117–24. doi: 10.1097/QAI.0b013e3181a3908d
52. Fouda GG, Jaeger FH, Amos JD, Ho C, Kunz EL, Anasti K, et al. Tenascin-C Is an Innate Broad-Spectrum, HIV-1-Neutralizing Protein in Breast Milk. *Proc Natl Acad Sci USA* (2013) 110(45):18220–5. doi: 10.1073/pnas.1307336110
53. Mall AS, Habte H, Mthembu Y, Peacocke J, de Beer C. Mucus and Mucins: Do They Have a Role in the Inhibition of the Human Immunodeficiency Virus? *Virol J* (2017) 14(1):192. doi: 10.1186/s12985-017-0855-9
54. Kazmi SH, Naglik JR, Sweet SP, Evans RW, O'Shea S, Banatvala JE, et al. Comparison of Human Immunodeficiency Virus Type 1-Specific Inhibitory Activities in Saliva and Other Human Mucosal Fluids. *Clin Vaccine Immunol* (2006) 13(10):1111–8. doi: 10.1128/CDLI.00426-05
55. Milligan C, Overbaugh J. The Role of Cell-Associated Virus in Mother-To-Child HIV Transmission. *J Infect Dis* (2014) 210(suppl_3):S631–40. doi: 10.1093/infdis/jiu344
56. Lunney KM, Iliff P, Mutasa K, Ntozini R, Magder LS, Moulton LH, et al. Associations Between Breast Milk Viral Load, Mastitis, Exclusive Breast-Feeding, and Postnatal Transmission of HIV. *Clin Infect Dis* (2010) 50 (5):762–9. doi: 10.1086/650535
57. Kuhn L, Sinkala M, Kankasa C, Semrau K, Kasonde P, Scott N, et al. High Uptake of Exclusive Breastfeeding and Reduced Early Post-Natal HIV Transmission. *PloS One* (2007) 2(12):e1363. doi: 10.1371/journal.pone.0001363
58. Coovadia HM, Rollins NC, Bland RM, Little K, Coutsoudis A, Bennish ML, et al. Mother-To-Child Transmission of HIV-1 Infection During Exclusive Breastfeeding in the First 6 Months of Life: An Intervention Cohort Study. *Lancet* (2007) 369(9567):1107–16. doi: 10.1016/S0140-6736(07)60283-9
59. Coutsoudis A, Dabis F, Fawzi W, Gaillard P, Haverkamp G, Harris DR, et al. Late Postnatal Transmission of HIV-1 in Breast-Fed Children: An Individual Patient Data Meta-Analysis. *J Infect Dis* (2004) 189(12):2154–66. doi: 10.1086/420834
60. Gejo NG, Weldearegay HG, W/tinsaie KT, Mekango DE, Woldemichael ES, Buda AS, et al. Exclusive Breastfeeding and Associated Factors Among HIV Positive Mothers in Northern Ethiopia. *PloS One* (2019) 14(1):e0210782. doi: 10.1371/journal.pone.0210782
61. Coutsoudis A, Pillay K, Spooner E, Kuhn L, Coovadia HM. Influence of Infant-Feeding Patterns on Early Mother-to-Child Transmission of HIV-1 in Durban, South Africa: A Prospective Cohort Study. South African Vitamin A Study Group. *Lancet* (1999) 354(9177):471–6. doi: 10.1016/S0140-6736(99)01101-0
62. Semrau K, Kuhn L, Brooks DR, Cabral H, Sinkala M, Kankasa C, et al. Exclusive Breastfeeding, Maternal HIV Disease, and the Risk of Clinical Breast Pathology in HIV-Infected, Breastfeeding Women. *Am J Obstet Gynecol* (2011) 205(4):344.e1–8. doi: 10.1016/j.ajog.2011.06.021
63. Semba RD, Kumwenda N, Hoover DR, Taha TE, Quinn TC, Mtimavalye L, et al. Human Immunodeficiency Virus Load in Breast Milk, Mastitis, and Mother-to-Child Transmission of Human Immunodeficiency Virus Type 1. *J Infect Dis* (1999) 180(1):93–8. doi: 10.1086/314854
64. Embree JE, Njenga S, Datta P, Nagelkerke NJD, Ndinya-Achola JO, Mohammed Z, et al. Risk Factors for Postnatal Mother-Child Transmission of HIV-1. *AIDS* (2000) 14(16):2535–41. doi: 10.1097/00002030-200011100-00016
65. Wood LF, Brown BP, Lennard K, Karaoz U, Havyarimana E, Passmore J-AS, et al. Feeding-Related Gut Microbial Composition Associates With Peripheral T-Cell Activation and Mucosal Gene Expression in African Infants. *Clin Infect Dis* (2018) 67(8):1237–46. doi: 10.1093/cid/ciy265
66. Rousseau CM, Nduati RM, Richardson BA, John-Stewart GC, Mbori-Ngacha DA, Kreiss JK, et al. Association of Levels of HIV-1–Infected Breast Milk Cells and Risk of Mother-To-Child Transmission. *J Infect Dis* (2004) 190(10):1880–8. doi: 10.1086/425076
67. Ndirangu J, Viljoen J, Bland RM, Danaviah S, Thorne C, Vande Perre P, et al. Cell-Free (RNA) and Cell-Associated (DNA) HIV-1 and Postnatal Transmission Through Breastfeeding. *PloS One* (2012) 7(12):e51493. doi: 10.1371/journal.pone.0051493
68. Thea DM, Steketee RW, Pliner V, Bornschlegel K, Brown T, Orloff S, et al. The Effect of Maternal Viral Load on the Risk of Perinatal Transmission of HIV-1. *AIDS* (1997) 11(4):437–44. doi: 10.1097/00002030-199704000-00006
69. Cao Y, Krogstad P, Korber BT, Koup RA, Muldoon M, Macken C, et al. Maternal HIV-1 Viral Load and Vertical Transmission of Infection: The Ariel Project for the Prevention of HIV Transmission From Mother to Infant. *Nat Med* (1997) 3(5):549–52. doi: 10.1038/nm0597-549
70. Scarlatti G, Hodara V, Rossi P, Muggiasca L, Bucceri A, Albert J, et al. Transmission of Human Immunodeficiency Virus Type 1 (HIV-1) From Mother to Child Correlates With Viral Phenotype. *Virology* (1993) 197 (2):624–9. doi: 10.1006/viro.1993.1637
71. O'Shea S, Newell M-L, Dunn DT, Garcia-Rodriguez M-C, Bates I, Mullen J, et al. Maternal Viral Load, CD4 Cell Count and Vertical Transmission of HIV-1. *J Med Virol* (1998) 54(2):113–7. doi: 10.1002/(SICI)1096-9071 (199802)54:2<113::AID-JMV8>3.0.CO;2-9
72. Morrison CS, Demers K, Kwok C, Bulime S, Rinaldi A, Munjoma M, et al. Plasma and Cervical Viral Loads Among Ugandan and Zimbabwean Women During Acute and Early HIV-1 Infection. *AIDS* (2010) 24(4):573–82. doi: 10.1097/QAD.0b013e32833433df
73. Connor EM, Sperling RS, Gelber R, Kiselev P, Scott G, O'Sullivan MJ, et al. Reduction of Maternal-Infant Transmission of Human Immunodeficiency Virus Type 1 With Zidovudine Treatment. Pediatric AIDS Clinical Trials Group Protocol 076 Study Group. *N Engl J Med* (1994) 331(18):1173–80. doi: 10.1056/NEJM199411033311801
74. Cooper ER, Charurat M, Mofenson L, Hanson CI, Pitt J, Diaz C, et al. Combination Antiretroviral Strategies for the Treatment of Pregnant HIV-1-Infected Women and Prevention of Perinatal HIV-1 Transmission. *J Acquir Immune Defic Syndr* (2002) 29(5):484–94. doi: 10.1097/00042560-200204150-00009
75. Dickover RE, Garratty EM, Herman SA, Sim MS, Plaeger S, Boyer PJ, et al. Identification of Levels of Maternal HIV-1 RNA Associated With Risk of Perinatal Transmission: Effect of Maternal Zidovudine Treatment on Viral Load. *JAMA* (1996) 275(8):599–605. doi: 10.1001/jama.1996.03530320023029
76. Mayaux MJ, Dussaix E, Isopet J, Rekacewicz C, Mandelbrot L, Ciraru-Vigneron N, et al. Maternal Virus Load During Pregnancy and Mother-To-Child Transmission of Human Immunodeficiency Virus Type 1: The French Perinatal Cohort Studies. *J Infect Dis* (1997) 175(1):172–5. doi: 10.1093/infdis/175.1.172
77. Shaffer N, Roongpisuthipong A, Siriwasin W, Chotpitayasunondh T, Chearskul S, Young NL, et al. Maternal Virus Load and Perinatal Human Immunodeficiency Virus Type 1 Subtype E Transmission, Thailand. *J Infect Dis* (1999) 179(3):590–9. doi: 10.1086/314641
78. Burns DN, Landesman S, Muenz LR, Nugent RP, Goedert JJ, Minkoff H, et al. Cigarette Smoking, Premature Rupture of Membranes, and Vertical Transmission of HIV-1 Among Women With Low CD4+ Levels. *J Acquir Immune Defic Syndr (1988)* (1994) 7(7):718–26.
79. Turner BJ, Hauck WW, Fanning TR, Markson LE. Cigarette Smoking and Maternal-Child HIV Transmission. *J Acquir Immune Defic Syndr Hum Retrovirol* (1997) 14(4):327–37. doi: 10.1097/00042560-199704010-00004
80. Matheson PB, Schoenbaum E, Greenberg B, Pliner V. Association of Maternal Drug Use During Pregnancy With Mother-to-Child HIV Transmission. New York City Perinatal HIV Transmission Collaborative Study. *AIDS* (1997) 11(7):941–2.
81. Rodriguez EM, Mofenson LM, Chang BH, Rich KC, Fowler MG, Smeriglio V, et al. Association of Maternal Drug Use During Pregnancy With Maternal HIV Culture Positivity and Perinatal HIV Transmission. *AIDS* (1996) 10 (3):273–82. doi: 10.1097/00002030-199603000-00006

82. Carrico AW, Johnson MO, Moskowitz JT, Neilands TB, Morin SF, Charlebois ED, et al. Affect Regulation, Stimulant Use, and Viral Load Among HIV-Positive Persons on Anti-Retroviral Therapy. *Psychosom Med* (2007) 69(8):785–92. doi: 10.1097/PSY.0b013e318157b142
83. Baum MK, Rafie C, Lai S, Sales S, Page B, Campa A. Crack-Cocaine Use Accelerates HIV Disease Progression in a Cohort of HIV-Positive Drug Users. *J Acquir Immune Defic Syndr* (2009) 50(1):93–9. doi: 10.1097/QAI.0b013e3181900129
84. Ellis RJ, Childers ME, Cherner M, Lazzaretto D, Letendre S, Grant I. Increased Human Immunodeficiency Virus Loads in Active Methamphetamine Users Are Explained by Reduced Effectiveness of Antiretroviral Therapy. *J Infect Dis* (2003) 188(12):1820–6. doi: 10.1086/379894
85. Chander G, Lau B, Moore RD. Hazardous Alcohol Use: A Risk Factor for Non-Adherence and Lack of Suppression in HIV Infection. *J Acquir Immune Defic Syndr* (2006) 43(4):411–7. doi: 10.1097/01.qai.0000243121.44659.a4
86. Purohit V, Rapaka RS, Schnur P, Shurtleff D. Potential Impact of Drugs of Abuse on Mother-to-Child Transmission (MTCT) of HIV in the Era of Highly Active Antiretroviral Therapy (HAART). *Life Sci* (2011) 88(21-22):909–16. doi: 10.1016/j.lfs.2011.03.022
87. Arnsten JH, Demas PA, Grant RW, Gourevitch MN, Farzadegan H, Howard AA. Impact of Active Drug Use on Antiretroviral Therapy Adherence and Viral Suppression in HIV-Infected Drug Users. *J Gen Intern Med* (2002) 17(5):377–81. doi: 10.1007/s11606-002-0044-3
88. John GC, Nduati RW, Mbori-Ngacha D, Overbaugh J, Welch M, Richardson BA, et al. Genital Shedding of Human Immunodeficiency Virus Type 1 DNA During Pregnancy: Association With Immunosuppression, Abnormal Cervical or Vaginal Discharge, and Severe Vitamin A Deficiency. *J Infect Dis* (1997) 175(1):57–62. doi: 10.1093/infdis/175.1.57
89. Clemetson DBA. Detection of HIV DNA in Cervical and Vaginal Secretions. *JAMA* (1993) 269(22):2860. doi: 10.1001/jama.1993.03500220046024
90. Loussert-Ajaka I, Mandelbrot L, Delmas MC, Bastian H, Benifla JL, Farfara I, et al. HIV-1 Detection in Cervicovaginal Secretions During Pregnancy. *AIDS* (1997) 11(13):1575–81. doi: 10.1097/00002030-199713000-00005
91. Rousseau CM, Nduati RM, Richardson BA, Steele MS, John-Stewart GC, Mbori-Ngacha DA, et al. Longitudinal Analysis of Human Immunodeficiency Virus Type 1 RNA in Breast Milk and of Its Relationship to Infant Infection and Maternal Disease. *J Infect Dis* (2003) 187(5):741–7. doi: 10.1086/374273
92. Nagot N, Kankasa C, Tumwine JK, Meda N, Hofmeyr GJ, Vallo R, et al. Extended Pre-Exposure Prophylaxis With Lopinavir–Ritonavir *Versus* Lamivudine to Prevent HIV-1 Transmission Through Breastfeeding Up to 50 Weeks in Infants in Africa (ANRS 12174): A Randomised Controlled Trial. *Lancet* (2016) 387(10018):566–73. doi: 10.1016/S0140-6736(15)00984-8
93. Flynn PM, Taha TE, Cababasay M, Fowler MG, Mofenson LM, Owor M, et al. Prevention of HIV-1 Transmission Through Breastfeeding: Efficacy and Safety of Maternal Antiretroviral Therapy *Versus* Infant Nevirapine Prophylaxis for Duration of Breastfeeding in HIV-1-Infected Women With High CD4 Cell Count (IMPAACT PROMISE): A Randomi. *JAIDS J Acquir Immune Defic Syndr* (2018) 77(4):383–92. doi: 10.1097/QAI.0000000000001612
94. Flynn PM, Taha TE, Cababasay M, Butler K, Fowler MG, Mofenson LM, et al. Association of Maternal Viral Load and CD4 Count With Perinatal HIV-1 Transmission Risk During Breastfeeding in the PROMISE Postpartum Component. *JAIDS J Acquired Immune Deficiency Syndromes* (2021) 88(2):206–13. doi: 10.1097/QAI.0000000000002744
95. Shapiro RL, Hughes MD, Ogwu A, Kitch D, Lockman S, Moffat C, et al. Antiretroviral Regimens in Pregnancy and Breast-Feeding in Botswana. *New Engl J Med* (2010) 362(24):2282–94. doi: 10.1056/NEJMoa0907736
96. Luoga E, Vanobberghen F, Bircher R, Nyuri A, Ntamatungiro AJ, Mnzava D, et al. Brief Report: No HIV Transmission From Virally Suppressed Mothers During Breastfeeding in Rural Tanzania. *J Acquir Immune Defic Syndr* (2018) 79(1):e17–20. doi: 10.1097/QAI.0000000000001758
97. Giuliano M, Andreotti M, Liotta G, Jere H, Sagno J-B, Maulidi M, et al. Maternal Antiretroviral Therapy for the Prevention of Mother-To-Child Transmission of HIV in Malawi: Maternal and Infant Outcomes Two Years After Delivery. *PloS One* (2013) 8(7):e68950. doi: 10.1371/journal.pone.0068950
98. Kliks S, Contag CH, Corliss H, Learn G, Rodrigo A, Wara D, et al. Genetic Analysis of Viral Variants Selected in Transmission of Human Immunodeficiency Viruses to Newborns. *AIDS Res Hum Retroviruses* (2000) 16(13):1223–33. doi: 10.1089/08892220050116998
99. Zhang H, Tully DC, Hoffmann FG, He J, Kankasa C, Wood C. Phylogenetic and Phenotypic Analysis of HIV Type 1 Env Gp120 in Cases of Subtype C Mother-to-Child Transmission. *AIDS Res Hum Retroviruses* (2002) 18 (18):1415–23. doi: 10.1089/088922202320935492
100. Renjifo B, Chung M, Gilbert P, Mwakagile D, Msamanga G, Fawzi W, et al. In-Utero Transmission of Quasispecies Among Human Immunodeficiency Virus Type 1 Genotypes. *Virology* (2003) 307(2):278–82. doi: 10.1016/S0042-6822(02)00066-1
101. Dickover RE, Garratty EM, Plaeger S, Bryson YJ. Perinatal Transmission of Major, Minor, and Multiple Maternal Human Immunodeficiency Virus Type 1 Variants *In Utero* and Intrapartum. *J Virol* (2001) 75(5):2194–203. doi: 10.1128/JVI.75.5.2194-2203.2001
102. Kwiek JJ, Russell ES, Dang KK, Burch CL, Mwapasa V, Meshnick SR, et al. The Molecular Epidemiology of HIV-1 Envelope Diversity During HIV-1 Subtype C Vertical Transmission in Malawian Mother–Infant Pairs. *AIDS* (2008) 22(7):863–71. doi: 10.1097/QAD.0b013e3282f51ea0
103. Ahmad N, Baroudy BM, Baker RC, Chappey C. Genetic Analysis of Human Immunodeficiency Virus Type 1 Envelope V3 Region Isolates From Mothers and Infants After Perinatal Transmission. *J Virol* (1995) 69(2):1001–12. doi: 10.1128/jvi.69.2.1001-1012.1995
104. Wolinsky S, Wike C, Korber B, Hutto C, Parks WP, Rosenblum L, et al. Selective Transmission of Human Immunodeficiency Virus Type-1 Variants From Mothers to Infants. *Science* (1992) 255(5048):1134–7. doi: 10.1126/science.1546316
105. Boyce CL, Sils T, Ko D, Wong-On-Wing A, Beck IA, Styrchak SM, et al. Maternal HIV Drug Resistance Is Associated With Vertical Transmission and Is Prevalent in Infected Infants. *Clin Infect Dis* (2021). doi: 10.1093/cid/ciab744
106. Baan E, de Ronde A, Luchters S, Vyankandondera J, Lange JM, Pollakis G, et al. HIV Type 1 Mother-to-Child Transmission Facilitated by Distinctive Glycosylation Sites in the Gp120 Envelope Glycoprotein. *AIDS Res Hum Retroviruses* (2012) 28(7):715–24. doi: 10.1089/aid.2011.0023
107. Ometto L, Zanchetta M, Mainardi M, De Salvo GL, Garcia-Rodriguez MC, Gray L, et al. Co-Receptor Usage of HIV-1 Primary Isolates, Viral Burden, and CCR5 Genotype in Mother-to-Child HIV-1 Transmission. *AIDS* (2000) 14(12):1721–9. doi: 10.1097/00002030-200008180-00006
108. Derdeyn CA, Hunter E. Viral Characteristics of Transmitted HIV. *Curr Opin HIV AIDS* (2008) 3(1):16–21. doi: 10.1097/COH.0b013e3282f2982c
109. John GC, Kreiss J. Mother-To-Child Transmission of Human Immunodeficiency Virus Type 1. *Epidemiologic Rev* (1996) 18(2):149–57. doi: 10.1093/oxfordjournals.epirev.a017922
110. Bryson YJ. Perinatal HIV-1 Transmission: Recent Advances and Therapeutic Interventions. *AIDS* (1996) 10 Suppl 3:S33–42.
111. Van'T Wout AB, Kootstra NA, Mulder-Kampinga GA, Albrecht-van Lent N, Scherpbier HJ, Veenstra J, et al. Macrophage-Tropic Variants Initiate Human Immunodeficiency Virus Type 1 Infection After Sexual, Parenteral, and Vertical Transmission. *J Clin Invest* (1994) 94(5):2060–7. doi: 10.1172/JCI117560
112. Yang C, Li M, Newman RD, Shi Y-P, Ayisi J, van Eijk AM, et al. Genetic Diversity of HIV-1 in Western Kenya: Subtype-Specific Differences in Mother-to-Child Transmission. *AIDS* (2003) 17(11):1667–74. doi: 10.1097/00002030-200307250-00011
113. Walter J, Kuhn L, Aldrovandi GM. Advances in Basic Science Understanding of Mother-to-Child HIV-1 Transmission. *Curr Opin HIV AIDS* (2008) 3 (2):146–50. doi: 10.1097/COH.0b013e3282f50bb2
114. Koulinska IN, Villamor E, Chaplin B, Msamanga G, Fawzi W, Renjifo B, et al. Transmission of Cell-Free and Cell-Associated HIV-1 Through Breast-Feeding. *J Acquir Immune Defic Syndr (1999)* (2006) 41(1):93–9. doi: 10.1097/01.qai.0000179424.19413.24
115. Eshleman SH, Church JD, Chen S, Guay LA, Mwatha A, Fiscus SA, et al. Comparison of HIV-1 Mother-to-Child Transmission After Single-Dose Nevirapine Prophylaxis Among African Women With Subtypes A, C and D. *J Acquir Immune Defic Syndr* (2006) 42(4):518–21. doi: 10.1097/01.qai.0000221676.22069.b8
116. Choi RY, Farquhar C, Juno J, Mbori-Ngacha D, Lohman-Payne B, Vouriot F, et al. Infant CD4 C868T Polymorphism Is Associated With Increased

Human Immunodeficiency Virus (HIV-1) Acquisition. *Clin Exp Immunol* (2010) 160(3):461–5. doi: 10.1111/j.1365-2249.2010.04096.x

117. Shearer WT, Kalish LA, Zimmerman PA. CCR5 HIV-1 Vertical Transmission. Women and Infants Transmission Study Group. *J Acquir Immune Defic Syndr Hum Retrovirol* (1998) 17(2):180–1. doi: 10.1097/00042560-199802010-00014
118. Mandl CW, Aberle SW, Henkel JH, Puchhammer-Stöckl E, Heinz FX. Possible Influence of the Mutant CCR5 Allele on Vertical Transmission of HIV-1. *J Med Virol* (1998) 55(1):51–5. doi: 10.1002/(SICI)1096-9071(199805)55:1<51::AID-JMV9>3.0.CO;2-N
119. Philpott S, Burger H, Charbonneau T, Grimson R, Vermund SH, Visosky A, et al. CCR5 Genotype and Resistance to Vertical Transmission of HIV-1. *J Acquir Immune Defic Syndr* (1999) 21(3):189–93. doi: 10.1097/00126334-199907010-00002
120. Kostrikis LG, Neumann AU, Thomson B, Korber BT, McHardy P, Karanicolas R, et al. A Polymorphism in the Regulatory Region of the CC-Chemokine Receptor 5 Gene Influences Perinatal Transmission of Human Immunodeficiency Virus Type 1 to African-American Infants. *J Virol* (1999) 73(12):10264–71. doi: 10.1128/JVI.73.12.10264-10271.1999
121. Pedersen BR, Kamwendo D, Blood M, Mwapasa V, Molyneux M, North K, et al. CCR5 Haplotypes and Mother-to-Child HIV Transmission in Malawi. *PloS One* (2007) 2(9):e838. doi: 10.1371/journal.pone.0000838
122. Singh KK, Hughes MD, Chen J, Phiri K, Rousseau C, Kuhn L, et al. Associations of Chemokine Receptor Polymorphisms With HIV-1 Mother-to-Child Transmission in Sub-Saharan Africa: Possible Modulation of Genetic Effects by Antiretrovirals. *J Acquir Immune Defic Syndr* (2008) 49(3):259–65. doi: 10.1097/QAI.0b013e318186eaa4
123. Salkowitz JR, Bruse SE, Meyerson H, Valdez H, Mosier DE, Harding CV, et al. CCR5 Promoter Polymorphism Determines Macrophage CCR5 Density and Magnitude of HIV-1 Propagation *in vitro*. *Clin Immunol* (2003) 108(3):234–40. doi: 10.1016/S1521-6616(03)00147-5
124. De Rossi A. Virus-Host Interactions in Paediatric HIV-1 Infection. *Curr Opin HIV AIDS* (2007) 2(5):399–404. doi: 10.1097/COH.0b013e3282ced163
125. Braida L, Boniotto M, Pontillo A, Tovo PA, Amoroso A, Crovella S. A Single-Nucleotide Polymorphism in the Human Beta-Defensin 1 Gene Is Associated With HIV-1 Infection in Italian Children. *AIDS* (2004) 18 (11):1598–600. doi: 10.1097/01.aids.0000131363.82951.fb
126. Ricci E, Malacrida S, Zanchetta M, Montagna M, Giaquinto C, De Rossi A. Role of Beta-Defensin-1 Polymorphisms in Mother-to-Child Transmission of HIV-1. *J Acquir Immune Defic Syndr* (2009) 51(1):13–9. doi: 10.1097/QAI.0b013e31819df249
127. Milanese M, Segat L, Pontillo A, Arraes LC, de Lima Filho JL, Crovella S. DEFB1 Gene Polymorphisms and Increased Risk of HIV-1 Infection in Brazilian Children. *AIDS* (2006) 20(12):1673–5. doi: 10.1097/01.aids.0000238417.05819.40
128. Milanese M, Segat L, Arraes LC, Garzino-Demo A, Crovella S. Copy Number Variation of Defensin Genes and HIV Infection in Brazilian Children. *J Acquir Immune Defic Syndr* (2009) 50(3):331–3. doi: 10.1097/QAI.0b013e3181945f39
129. Polycarpou A, Ntais C, Korber BT, Elrich HA, Winchester R, Krogstad P, et al. Association Between Maternal and Infant Class I and II HLA Alleles and of Their Concordance With the Risk of Perinatal HIV Type 1 Transmission. *AIDS Res Hum Retroviruses* (2002) 18(11):741–6. doi: 10.1089/08892220260139477
130. Aikhionbare FO, Hodge T, Kuhn L, Bulterys M, Abrams EJ, Bond VC. Mother-To-Child Discordance in HLA-G Exon 2 Is Associated With a Reduced Risk of Perinatal HIV-1 Transmission. *AIDS* (2001) 15(16):2196–8. doi: 10.1097/00002030-200111090-00019
131. MacDonald KS, Embree J, Njenga S, Nagelkerke NJD, Ngatia I, Mohammed Z, et al. Mother-Child Class I HLA Concordance Increases Perinatal Human Immunodeficiency Virus Type 1 Transmission. *J Infect Dis* (1998) 177 (3):551–6. doi: 10.1086/514243
132. MacDonald KS, Embree JE, Nagelkerke NJ, Castillo J, Ramhadin S, Njenga S, et al. The HLA A2/6802 Supertype Is Associated With Reduced Risk of Perinatal Human Immunodeficiency Virus Type 1 Transmission. *J Infect Dis* (2001) 183(3):503–6. doi: 10.1086/318092
133. Farquhar C, Rowland-Jones S, Mbori-Ngacha D, Redman M, Lohman B, Slyker J, et al. Human Leukocyte Antigen (HLA) B*18 and Protection Against Mother-to-Child HIV Type 1 Transmission. *AIDS Res Hum Retroviruses* (2004) 20(7):692–7. doi: 10.1089/0889222041524616
134. Mackelprang RD, John-Stewart G, Carrington M, Richardson B, Rowland-Jones S, Gao X, et al. Maternal HLA Homozygosity and Mother-Child HLA Concordance Increase the Risk of Vertical Transmission of HIV-1. *J Infect Dis* (2008) 197(8):1156–61. doi: 10.1086/529528
135. Fabris A, Catamo E, Segat L, Morgutti M, Arraes LC, de Lima-Filho JL, et al. Association Between HLA-G 3'UTR 14-Bp Polymorphism and HIV Vertical Transmission in Brazilian Children. *AIDS* (2009) 23(2):177–82. doi: 10.1097/QAD.0b013e32832027bf
136. Aikhionbare FO, Kumaresan K, Shamsa F, Bond VC. HLA-G DNA Sequence Variants and Risk of Perinatal HIV-1 Transmission. *AIDS Res Ther* (2006) 3:28. doi: 10.1186/1742-6405-3-28
137. Kilpatrick DC, Hague RA, Yap PL, Mok JY. HLA Antigen Frequencies in Children Born to HIV-Infected Mothers. *Dis Markers* (1991) 9(1):21–6.
138. Winchester R, Chen Y, Rose S, Selby J, Borkowsky W. Major Histocompatibility Complex Class II DR Alleles DRB1*1501 and Those Encoding HLA-DR13 Are Preferentially Associated With a Diminution in Maternally Transmitted Human Immunodeficiency Virus 1 Infection in Different Ethnic Groups: Determination by an Automated Sequence-Based Typing Method. *Proc Natl Acad Sci USA* (1995) 92(26):12374–8. doi: 10.1073/pnas.92.26.12374
139. Just JJ, Abrams E, Louie LG, Urbano R, Wara D, Nicholas SW, et al. Influence of Host Genotype on Progression to Acquired Immunodeficiency Syndrome Among Children Infected With Human Immunodeficiency Virus Type 1. *J Pediatr* (1995) 127(4):544–9. doi: 10.1016/S0022-3476(95)70110-9
140. Biggar RJ, Taha TE, Hoover DR, Yellin F, Kumwenda N, Broadhead R. Higher *In Utero* and Perinatal HIV Infection Risk in Girls Than Boys. *J Acquir Immune Defic Syndr* (2006) 41(4):509–13. doi: 10.1097/01.qai.0000191283.85578.46
141. Taha TE, Nour S, Kumwenda NI, Broadhead RL, Fiscus SA, Kafulafula G, et al. Gender Differences in Perinatal HIV Acquisition Among African Infants. *Pediatrics* (2005) 115(2):e167–72. doi: 10.1542/peds.2004-1590
142. Adland E, Millar J, Bengu N, Muenchhoff M, Fillis R, Sprenger K, et al. Author Correction: Sex-Specific Innate Immune Selection of HIV-1 In Utero Is Associated With Increased Female Susceptibility to Infection. *Nat Commun* (2020) 11(1). doi: 10.1038/s41467-020-16215-7
143. St Louis ME, Kamenga M, Brown C, Tarande Manzila AMNM, Batter V, Behets F, et al. Risk for Perinatal HIV-1 Transmission According to Maternal Immunologic, Virologic, and Placental Factors. *Jama* (1993) 269(22):2853–9. doi: 10.1001/jama.1993.03500220039023
144. Mwanyumba F, Gaillard P, Inion I, Verhofstede C, Claeys P, Chohan V, et al. Placental Inflammation and Perinatal Transmission of HIV-1. *J Acquir Immune Defic Syndr* (2002) 29(3):262–9. doi: 10.1097/00042560-200203010-00006
145. Temmerman M, Nyong'o AO, Bwayo J, Fransen K, Coppens M, Piot P. Risk Factors for Mother-to-Child Transmission of Human Immunodeficiency Virus-1 Infection. *Am J Obstet Gynecol* (1995) 172(2 Pt 1):700–5. doi: 10.1016/0002-9378(95)90597-9
146. Wabwire-Mangen F, Gray RH, Mmiro FA, Ndugwa C, Abramowsky C, Wabinga H, et al. Placental Membrane Inflammation and Risks of Maternal-to-Child Transmission of HIV-1 in Uganda. *J Acquir Immune Defic Syndr* (1999) 22(4):379–85. doi: 10.1097/00126334-199912010-00009
147. Van Dyke RB, Korber BT, Popek E, Macken C, Widmayer SM, Bardeguez A, et al. The Ariel Project: A Prospective Cohort Study of Maternal-Child Transmission of Human Immunodeficiency Virus Type 1 in the Era of Maternal Antiretroviral Therapy. *J Infect Dis* (1999) 179(2):319–28. doi: 10.1086/314580
148. Adachi K, Xu J, Yeganeh N, Camarca M, Morgado MG, Watts D, et al. Combined Evaluation of Sexually Transmitted Infections in HIV-Infected Pregnant Women and Infant HIV Transmission. *PloS One* (2018) 13(1): e0189851. doi: 10.1371/journal.pone.0189851
149. Hitti J, Watts DH, Burchett SK, Schacker T, Selke S, Brown ZA, et al. Herpes Simplex Virus Seropositivity and Reactivation at Delivery Among Pregnant Women Infected With Human Immunodeficiency Virus-1. *Am J Obstet Gynecol* (1997) 177(2):450–4. doi: 10.1016/S0002-9378(97)70214-X
150. McClelland RS, Wang CC, Richardson BA, Corey L, Ashley RL, Mandaliya K, et al. A Prospective Study of Hormonal Contraceptive Use and Cervical

Shedding of Herpes Simplex Virus in Human Immunodeficiency Virus Type 1-Seropositive Women. *J Infect Dis* (2002) 185(12):1822–5. doi: 10.1086/340639

151. Gray RH, Wabwire-Mangen F, Kigozi G, Sewankambo NK, Serwadda D, Moulton LH, et al. Randomized Trial of Presumptive Sexually Transmitted Disease Therapy During Pregnancy in Rakai, Uganda. *Am J Obstet Gynecol* (2001) 185(5):1209–17. doi: 10.1067/mob.2001.118158
152. Menendez C, Sanchez-Tapias JM, Kahigwa E, Mshinda H, Costa J, Vidal J, et al. Prevalence and Mother-to-Infant Transmission of Hepatitis Viruses B, C, and E in Southern Tanzania. *J Med Virol* (1999) 58(3):215–20. doi: 10.1002/(SICI)1096-9071(199907)58:3<215::AID-JMV5>3.0.CO;2-K
153. Tess BH, Rodrigues LC, Newell ML, Dunn DT, Lago TD. Breastfeeding, Genetic, Obstetric and Other Risk Factors Associated With Mother-to-Child Transmission of HIV-1 in Sao Paulo State, Brazil. Sao Paulo Collaborative Study for Vertical Transmission of HIV-1. *AIDS* (1998) 12(5):513–20. doi: 10.1097/00002030-199805000-00013
154. England K, Thorne C, Newell ML. Vertically Acquired Paediatric Coinfection With HIV and Hepatitis C Virus. *Lancet Infect Dis* (2006) 6 (2):83–90. doi: 10.1016/S1473-3099(06)70381-4
155. Giovannini M, Tagger A, Ribero ML, Zuccotti G, Pogliani L, Grossi A, et al. Maternal-Infant Transmission of Hepatitis C Virus and HIV Infections: A Possible Interaction. *Lancet* (1990) 335(8698):1166. doi: 10.1016/0140-6736 (90)91174-9
156. Hershow RC, Riester KA, Lew J, Quinn TC, Mofenson LM, Davenny K, et al. Increased Vertical Transmission of Human Immunodeficiency Virus From Hepatitis C Virus-Coinfected Mothers. Women and Infants Transmission Study. *J Infect Dis* (1997) 176(2):414–20. doi: 10.1086/514058
157. Paccagnini S, Principi N, Massironi E, Tanzi E, Romanò L, Muggiasca ML, et al. Perinatal Transmission and Manifestation of Hepatitis C Virus Infection in a High Risk Population. *Pediatr Infect Dis J* (1995) 14(3):195–9. doi: 10.1097/00006454-199503000-00005
158. Papaevangelou V, Pollack H, Rochford G, Kokka R, Hou Z, Chernoff D, et al. Increased Transmission of Vertical Hepatitis C Virus (HCV) Infection to Human Immunodeficiency Virus (HIV)-Infected Infants of HIV- and HCV-Coinfected Women. *J Infect Dis* (1998) 178(4):1047–52. doi: 10.1086/515668
159. Thomas DL, Villano SA, Riester KA, Hershow R, Mofenson LM, Landesman SH, et al. Perinatal Transmission of Hepatitis C Virus From Human Immunodeficiency Virus Type 1-Infected Mothers. Women and Infants Transmission Study. *J Infect Dis* (1998) 177(6):1480–8. doi: 10.1086/515315
160. Tovo PA, Palomba E, Ferraris G, Principi N, Ruga E, Dallacasa P, et al. Increased Risk of Maternal-Infant Hepatitis C Virus Transmission for Women Coinfected With Human Immunodeficiency Virus Type 1. Italian Study Group for HCV Infection in Children. *Clin Infect Dis* (1997) 25 (5):1121–4. doi: 10.1086/516102
161. Bulterys M, Landesman S, Burns DN, Rubinstein A, Goedert JJ. Sexual Behavior and Injection Drug Use During Pregnancy and Vertical Transmission of HIV-1. *JAIDS J Acquired Immune Deficiency Syndromes* (1997) 15(1):76–82. doi: 10.1097/00042560-199705010-00012
162. Matheson PB, Thomas PA, Abrams EJ, Pliner V, Lambert G, Bamji M, et al. Heterosexual Behavior During Pregnancy and Perinatal Transmission of HIV-1. New York City Perinatal HIV Transmission Collaborative Study Group. *AIDS* (1996) 10(11):1249–56. doi: 10.1097/00002030-199609000-00011
163. Burns DN, Landesman S, Wright DJ, Waters D, Mitchell RM, Rubinstein A, et al. Influence of Other Maternal Variables on the Relationship Between Maternal Virus Load and Mother-to-Infant Transmission of Human Immunodeficiency Virus Type 1. *J Infect Dis* (1997) 175(5):1206–10. doi: 10.1086/593569
164. Taha TE, Gray RH. Genital Tract Infections and Perinatal Transmission of HIV. *Ann N Y Acad Sci* (2000) 918:84–98. doi: 10.1111/j.1749-6632.2000.tb05477.x
165. Bulterys M, Chao A, Dushimimana A, Phocas NP, Kurawige J-B, Musanganire F, et al. Multiple Sexual Partners and Mother-to-Child Transmission of HIV-1. *AIDS* (1993) 7(12):1639–45. doi: 10.1097/00002030-199312000-00015
166. Day JH, Grant AD, Fielding KL, Morris L, Moloi V, Charalambous S, et al. Does Tuberculosis Increase HIV Load? *J Infect Dis* (2004) 190(9):1677–84. doi: 10.1086/424851
167. Goletti D, Weissman D, Jackson RW, Graham NM, Vlahov D, Klein RS, et al. Effect of Mycobacterium Tuberculosis on HIV Replication. Role of Immune Activation. *J Immunol* (1996) 157(3):1271–8.
168. Toossi Z, Mayanja-Kizza H, Hirsch CS, Edmonds KL, Spahlinger T, Hom DL, et al. Impact of Tuberculosis (TB) on HIV-1 Activity in Dually Infected Patients. *Clin Exp Immunol* (2001) 123(2):233–8. doi: 10.1046/j.1365-2249.2001.01401.x
169. Gupta A, Bhosale R, Kinikar A, Gupte N, Bharadwaj R, Kagal A, et al. Maternal Tuberculosis: A Risk Factor for Mother-to-Child Transmission of Human Immunodeficiency Virus. *J Infect Dis* (2011) 203(3):358–63. doi: 10.1093/jinfdis/jiq064
170. Taha TE, Canner JK, Dallabetta GA, Chiphangwi JD, Liomba G, Wangel AM, et al. Childhood Malaria Parasitaemia and Human Immunodeficiency Virus Infection in Malawi. *Trans R Soc Trop Med Hyg* (1994) 88(2):164–5. doi: 10.1016/0035-9203(94)90277-1
171. Hoffman IF, Jere CS, Taylor TE, Munthali P, Dyer JR, Wirima JJ, et al. The Effect of Plasmodium Falciparum Malaria on HIV-1 RNA Blood Plasma Concentration. *AIDS* (1999) 13(4):487–94. doi: 10.1097/00002030-199903110-00007
172. Brahmbhatt H, Sullivan D, Kigozi G, Askin F, Wabwire-Mangenm F, Serwadda D, et al. Association of HIV and Malaria With Mother-to-Child Transmission, Birth Outcomes, and Child Mortality. *J Acquir Immune Defic Syndr* (2008) 47(4):472–6. doi: 10.1097/QAI.0b013e318162afe0
173. Brahmbhatt H, Kigozi G, Wabwire-Mangen F, Serwadda D, Sewankambo N, Lutalo T, et al. The Effects of Placental Malaria on Mother-to-Child HIV Transmission in Rakai, Uganda. *AIDS* (2003) 17(17):2539–41. doi: 10.1097/00002030-200311210-00020
174. Ayouba A, Badaut C, Kfutwah A, Cannou C, Juillerat A, Gangnard S, et al. Specific Stimulation of HIV-1 Replication in Human Placental Trophoblasts by an Antigen of Plasmodium Falciparum. *AIDS* (2008) 22(6):785–7. doi: 10.1097/QAD.0b013e3282f560ee
175. Mwapasa V, Rogerson SJ, Molyneux ME, Abrams ET, Kamwendo DD, Lema VM, et al. The Effect of Plasmodium Falciparum Malaria on Peripheral and Placental HIV-1 RNA Concentrations in Pregnant Malawian Women. *AIDS* (2004) 18(7):1051–9. doi: 10.1097/00002030-200404300-00014
176. Msamanga GI, Taha TE, Young AM, Brown ER, Hoffman IF, Read JS, et al. Placental Malaria and Mother-to-Child Transmission of Human Immunodeficiency Virus-1. *Am J Trop Med Hyg* (2009) 80(4):508–15. doi: 10.4269/ajtmh.2009.80.508
177. Johnson EL, Chakraborty R. HIV-1 at the Placenta: Immune Correlates of Protection and Infection. *Curr Opin Infect Dis* (2016) 29(3):248–55. doi: 10.1097/QCO.0000000000000267
178. Fowler MG, Rogers MF. Overview of Perinatal HIV Infection. *J Nutr* (1996) 126(suppl_10):2602S–7S. doi: 10.1093/jn/126.suppl_10.2602S
179. Shivakoti R, Gupta A, Ray JC, Uprety P, Gupte N, Bhosale R, et al. Soluble CD14: An Independent Biomarker for the Risk of Mother-To-Child Transmission of HIV in a Setting of Preexposure and Postexposure Antiretroviral Prophylaxis. *J Infect Dis* (2016) 213(5):762–5. doi: 10.1093/infdis/jiv479
180. Rossi P, Moschese V, Broliden PA, Fundaró C, Quinti I, Plebani A, et al. Presence of Maternal Antibodies to Human Immunodeficiency Virus 1 Envelope Glycoprotein Gp120 Epitopes Correlates With the Uninfected Status of Children Born to Seropositive Mothers. *Proc Natl Acad Sci* (1989) 86(20):8055–8. doi: 10.1073/pnas.86.20.8055
181. Broliden PA, Moschese V, Ljunggren K, Rosen J, Fundaro C, Plebani A, et al. Diagnostic Implication of Specific Immunoglobulin G Patterns of Children Born to HIV-Infected Mothers. *AIDS (London England)* (1989) 3(9):577–82. doi: 10.1097/00002030-198909000-00004
182. Pancino G, Leste-Lasserre T, Burgard M, Costagliola D, Ivanoff S, Blanche S, et al. Apparent Enhancement of Perinatal Transmission of Human Immunodeficiency Virus Type 1 by High Maternal Anti-Gp160 Antibody Titer. *J Infect Dis* (1998) 177(6):1737–41. doi: 10.1086/517435
183. Guevara H, Casseb J, Zijenah LS, Mbizvo M, Oceguera LF 3rd, Hanson CV, et al. Maternal HIV-1 Antibody and Vertical Transmission in Subtype C Virus Infection. *J Acquir Immune Defic Syndr* (2002) 29(5):435–40. doi: 10.1097/00042560-200204150-00002
184. Hofmann-Lehmann R, Vlasak J, Rasmussen RA, Smith BA, Baba TW, Liska V, et al. Postnatal Passive Immunization of Neonatal Macaques With a Triple Combination of Human Monoclonal Antibodies Against Oral Simian-Human Immunodeficiency Virus Challenge. *J Virol* (2001) 75 (16):7470–80. doi: 10.1128/JVI.75.16.7470-7480.2001
185. Dickover R, Garratty E, Yusim K, Miller C, Korber B, Bryson Y. Role of Maternal Autologous Neutralizing Antibody in Selective Perinatal

Transmission of Human Immunodeficiency Virus Type 1 Escape Variants. *J Virol* (2006) 80(13):6525–33. doi: 10.1128/JVI.02658-05
186. Ugen KE, Goedert JJ, Boyer J, Refaeli Y, Frank I, Williams WV, et al. Vertical Transmission of Human Immunodeficiency Virus (HIV) Infection. Reactivity of Maternal Sera With Glycoprotein 120 and 41 Peptides From HIV Type 1. *J Clin Invest* (1992) 89(6):1923–30. doi: 10.1172/JCI115798
187. Broliden K, Sievers E, Tovo PA, Moschese V, Scarlatti G, Broliden PA, et al. Antibody-Dependent Cellular Cytotoxicity and Neutralizing Activity in Sera of HIV-1-Infected Mothers and Their Children. *Clin Exp Immunol* (2008) 93 (1):56–64. doi: 10.1111/j.1365-2249.1993.tb06497.x
188. Omenda MM, Milligan C, Odem-Davis K, Nduati R, Richardson BA, Lynch J, et al. Evidence for Efficient Vertical Transfer of Maternal HIV-1 Envelope–Specific Neutralizing Antibodies But No Association of Such Antibodies With Reduced Infant Infection. *JAIDS J Acquired Immune Deficiency Syndromes* (2013) 64(2):163–6. doi: 10.1097/QAI.0b013e31829f6e41
189. Kliks SC. Features of HIV-1 That Could Influence Maternal-Child Transmission. *JAMA: J Am Med Assoc* (1994) 272(6):467.
190. Wu X, Parast AB, Richardson BA, Nduati R, John-Stewart G, Mbori-Ngacha D, et al. Neutralization Escape Variants of Human Immunodeficiency Virus Type 1 Are Transmitted From Mother to Infant. *J Virol* (2006) 80(2):835–44. doi: 10.1128/JVI.80.2.835-844.2006
191. Martinez DR, Vandergrift N, Douglas AO, McGuire E, Bainbridge J, Nicely NI, et al. Maternal Binding and Neutralizing IgG Responses Targeting the C-Terminal Region of the V3 Loop Are Predictive of Reduced Peripartum HIV-1 Transmission Risk. *J Virol* (2017) 91(9): e02422–16. doi: 10.1128/JVI.02422-16
192. Mabuka J, Nduati R, Odem-Davis K, Peterson D, Overbaugh J. HIV-Specific Antibodies Capable of ADCC Are Common in Breastmilk and Are Associated With Reduced Risk of Transmission in Women With High Viral Loads. *PloS Pathog* (2012) 8(6):e1002739. doi: 10.1371/journal.ppat.1002739
193. Pollara J, McGuire E, Fouda GG, Rountree W, Eudailey J, Overman RG, et al. Association of HIV-1 Envelope-Specific Breast Milk IgA Responses With Reduced Risk of Postnatal Mother-To-Child Transmission of HIV-1. *J Virol* (2015) 89(19):9952–61. doi: 10.1128/JVI.01560-15
194. Lohman-Payne B, Slyker JA, Moore S, Maleche-Obimboe E, Wamalwae DC, Richardson BA, et al. Breast Milk Cellular HIV-Specific Interferon γ Responses Are Associated With Protection From Peripartum HIV Transmission. *AIDS* (2012) 26(16):2007–16. doi: 10.1097/QAD.0b013e328359b7e0
195. Mor G, Aldo P, Alvero AB. The Unique Immunological and Microbial Aspects of Pregnancy. *Nat Rev Immunol* (2017) 17(8):469–82. doi: 10.1038/nri.2017.64
196. Mold JE, Michaelsson J, Burt TD, Muench MO, Beckerman KP, Busch MP, et al. Maternal Alloantigens Promote the Development of Tolerogenic Fetal Regulatory T Cells *In Utero*. *Science* (2008) 322(5907):1562–5. doi: 10.1126/science.1164511
197. Takahata Y, Nomura A, Takada H, Ohga S, Furuno K, Hikino S, et al. CD25+CD4+ T Cells in Human Cord Blood: An Immunoregulatory Subset With Naive Phenotype and Specific Expression of Forkhead Box P3 (Foxp3) Gene. *Exp Hematol* (2004) 32(7):622–9. doi: 10.1016/j.exphem.2004.03.012
198. Hebel K, Weinert S, Kuropka B, Knolle J, Kosak B, Jorch G, et al. CD4+ T Cells From Human Neonates and Infants Are Poised Spontaneously to Run a Nonclassical IL-4 Program. *J Immunol* (2014) 192(11):5160–70. doi: 10.4049/jimmunol.1302539
199. Siegrist CA. Neonatal and Early Life Vaccinology. *Vaccine* (2001) 19(25-26):3331–46. doi: 10.1016/S0264-410X(01)00028-7
200. Goulder PJ, Brander C, Tang Y, Tremblay C, Colbert RA, Addo MM, et al. Evolution and Transmission of Stable CTL Escape Mutations in HIV Infection. *Nature* (2001) 412(6844):334–8. doi: 10.1038/35085576
201. Wilson CC, Brown RC, Korber BT, Wilkes BM, Ruhl DJ, Sakamoto D, et al. Frequent Detection of Escape From Cytotoxic T-Lymphocyte Recognition in Perinatal Human Immunodeficiency Virus (HIV) Type 1 Transmission: The Ariel Project for the Prevention of Transmission of HIV From Mother to Infant. *J Virol* (1999) 73(5):3975–85. doi: 10.1128/JVI.73.5.3975-3985.1999
202. Liu AY, Lohman-Payne B, Chung MH, Kiarie J, Kinuthia J, Slyker J, et al. Maternal Plasma and Breastmilk Viral Loads Are Associated With HIV-1-Specific Cellular Immune Responses Among HIV-1-Exposed, Uninfected Infants in Kenya. *Clin Exp Immunol* (2015) 180(3):509–19. doi: 10.1111/cei.12599
203. Lohman-Payne B, Sandifer T, Ohainle M, et al. In-Uteroinfection With HIV-1 Associated With Suppressed Lymphoproliferative Responses at Birth. *Clin Exp Immunol* (2014) 178(1):86–93. doi: 10.1111/cei.12386
204. *The Use of Antiretroviral Drugs for Treating and Preventing HIV Infection.* Available at: http://apps.who.int/iris/bitstream/handle/10665/85321/9789241505727_eng.pdf?sequence=1 (Accessed 11/23/2018).
205. UNAIDS. *The Gap Report.* Available at: http://www.unaids.org/sites/default/files/media_asset/UNAIDS_Gap_report_en.pdf (Accessed 11/26/2018).
206. Organization GWH. *WHO Recommendations on the Diagnosis of HIV Infection in Infants and Children* (2010). Available at: http://whqlibdoc.who.int/publications/2010/9789241599085_eng.pdf?ua=1 (Accessed 11/26/2018).
207. Takata H, Buranapraditkun S, Kessing C, Fletcher JLK, Muir R, Tardif V, et al. Delayed Differentiation of Potent Effector CD8+T Cells Reducing Viremia and Reservoir Seeding in Acute HIV Infection. *Sci Trans Med* (2017) 9(377):eaag1809. doi: 10.1126/scitranslmed.aag1809
208. Whitney JB, Hill AL, Sanisetty S, Penaloza-MacMaster P, Liu J, Shetty M, et al. Rapid Seeding of the Viral Reservoir Prior to SIV Viraemia in Rhesus Monkeys. *Nature* (2014) 512(7512):74–7. doi: 10.1038/nature13594
209. Luzuriaga K, Gay H, Ziemniak C, Sanborn KB, Somasundaran M, Rainwater-Lovett K, et al. Viremic Relapse After HIV-1 Remission in a Perinatally Infected Child. *New Engl J Med* (2015) 372(8):786–8. doi: 10.1056/NEJMc1413931
210. Bitnun A, Samson L, Chun TW, Kakkar F, Brophy J, Murray D, et al. Early Initiation of Combination Antiretroviral Therapy in HIV-1-Infected Newborns Can Achieve Sustained Virologic Suppression With Low Frequency of CD4+ T Cells Carrying HIV in Peripheral Blood. *Clin Infect Dis* (2014) 59(7):1012–9. doi: 10.1093/cid/ciu432
211. Giacomet V, Trabattoni D, Zanchetta N, Biasin M, Gismondo M, Clerici M, et al. No Cure of HIV Infection in a Child Despite Early Treatment and Apparent Viral Clearance. *Lancet* (2014) 384(950):1320. doi: 10.1016/S0140-6736(14)61405-7
212. Jani IV, Meggi B, Mabunda N, Vubil A, Sitoe NE, Tobaiwa O, et al. Accurate Early Infant HIV Diagnosis in Primary Health Clinics Using a Point-of-Care Nucleic Acid Test. *J Acquir Immune Defic Syndr* (2014) 67(1):e1–4. doi: 10.1097/QAI.0000000000000250
213. Persaud D, Gay H, Ziemniak C, Chen YH, Piatak M Jr, Chun T-W, et al. Absence of Detectable HIV-1 Viremia After Treatment Cessation in an Infant. *N Engl J Med* (2013) 369(19):1828–35. doi: 10.1056/NEJMoa1302976
214. Garcia-Broncano P, Maddali S, Einkauf KB, Jiang C, Gao C, Chevalier J, et al. Early Antiretroviral Therapy in Neonates With HIV-1 Infection Restricts Viral Reservoir Size and Induces a Distinct Innate Immune Profile. *Sci Trans Med* (2019) 11(520):eaax7350. doi: 10.1126/scitranslmed.aax7350
215. Safety and Effects of Using Prime-boost HIVIS DNA and MVA-CMDR Vaccine Regimens With or Without Toll-like Receptor 4 Agonist on HIV Reservoirs in Perinatally HIV Infected Children and Youth (HVRRICANE). Available at: https://clinicaltrials.gov/ct2/show/NCT04301154.
216. Kuhn L, Strehlau R, Shiau S, Patelc F, Shena Y, Technauc K-G, et al. Early Antiretroviral Treatment of Infants to Attain HIV Remission. *EClinicalMedicine* (2020) 18:100241. doi: 10.1016/j.eclinm.2019.100241
217. Violari A, Cotton MF, Gibb DM, Babiker AG, Steyn J, Madhi SA, et al. Early Antiretroviral Therapy and Mortality Among HIV-Infected Infants. *New Engl J Med* (2008) 359(21):2233–44. doi: 10.1056/NEJMoa0800971
218. Katusiime MG, Halvas EK, Wright I, Joseph K, Bale MJ, Kirby-McCullough B, et al. Intact HIV Proviruses Persist in Children Seven to Nine Years After Initiation of Antiretroviral Therapy in the First Year of Life. *J Virol* (2020) 94 (4):e01519-19. doi: 10.1128/JVI.01519-19
219. Bale M, Katusiime M-G, Wells D, Wu X, Spindler J, Halvas EK, et al. Early Emergence and Long-Term Persistence of HIV-Infected T-Cell Clones in Children. *mBio* (2021) 12:e00568-21. doi: 10.1128/mBio.00568-21
220. Violari A, Cotton MF, Kuhn L, Schramm DB, Paximadis M, Loubser S, et al. A Child With Perinatal HIV Infection and Long-Term Sustained Virological Control Following Antiretroviral Treatment Cessation. *Nat Commun* (2019) 10(1):412–23. doi: 10.1038/s41467-019-08311-0
221. Frange P, Faye A, Avettand-Fenoël V, Bellaton E, Descamps D, Angin M, et al. HIV-1 Virological Remission Lasting More Than 12 Years After Interruption of Early Antiretroviral Therapy in a Perinatally Infected Teenager Enrolled in

the French ANRS EPF-CO10 Paediatric Cohort: A Case Report. *Lancet HIV* (2016) 3(1):e49–54. doi: 10.1016/S2352-3018(15)00232-5

222. Goswami R, Nelson AN, Tu JJ, Dennis M, Feng L, Kumar A, et al. Analytical Treatment Interruption After Short-Term Antiretroviral Therapy in a Postnatally Simian-Human Immunodeficiency Virus-Infected Infant Rhesus Macaque Model. *mBio* (2019) 10(5):e01971-19. doi: 10.1128/mBio.01971-19
223. Bricker KM, Obregon-Perko V, Uddin F, Williams B, Uffman E, Garrido C, et al. Therapeutic Vaccination of SIV-Infected, ART-Treated Infant Rhesus Macaques Using Ad48/MVA in Combination With TLR-7 Stimulation. *PloS Pathog* (2020) 16(10):e1008954. doi: 10.1371/journal.ppat.1008954
224. Obregon-Perko V, Bricker K, Chahroudi A. The Brain Retains: Nonhuman Primate Models for Pediatric HIV-1 in the CNS. *Curr HIV/AIDS Rep* (2020) 17(4):343–53. doi: 10.1007/s11904-020-00503-4
225. Ajibola G, Garcia-Broncano P, Maswabi K, Bennett K, Hughes MD, Moyo S, et al. Viral Reservoir in Early-Treated Human Immunodeficiency Virus-Infected Children and Markers for Sustained Viral Suppression. *Clin Infect Dis* (2021) 22:e997–1003. doi: 10.1093/cid/ciab143
226. Martínez-Bonet M, Puertas MC, Fortuny C, Ouchi D, Mellado MJ, Rojo P, et al. Establishment and Replenishment of the Viral Reservoir in Perinatally HIV-1-Infected Children Initiating Very Early Antiretroviral Therapy. *Clin Infect Dis* (2015) 61(7):1169–78. doi: 10.1093/cid/civ456
227. Persaud D, Patel K, Karalius B, Rainwater-Lovett K, Ziemniak C, Ellis A, et al. Influence of Age at Virologic Control on Peripheral Blood Human Immunodeficiency Virus Reservoir Size and Serostatus in Perinatally Infected Adolescents. *JAMA Pediatr* (2014) 168(12):1138. doi: 10.1001/jamapediatrics.2014.1560
228. Rocca S, Zangari P, Cotugno N, Ferns B, Foster C, De Rossi A, et al. Human Immunodeficiency Virus (HIV)-Antibody Repertoire Estimates Reservoir Size and Time of Antiretroviral Therapy Initiation in Virally Suppressed Perinatally HIV-Infected Children. *J Pediatr Infect Dis Soc* (2019) 8(5):433–8. doi: 10.1093/jpids/piy080
229. Tagarro A, Chan M, Zangari P, Ferns B, Foster C, De Rossi A, et al. Early and Highly Suppressive Antiretroviral Therapy Are Main Factors Associated With Low Viral Reservoir in European Perinatally HIV-Infected Children. *J Acquired Immune Deficiency Syndromes (1999)* (2018) 79(2):269–76. doi: 10.1097/QAI.0000000000001789
230. Kuhn L, Paximadis M, Da Costa Dias B, Loubser S, Strehlau R, Patel F, et al. Age at Antiretroviral Therapy Initiation and Cell-Associated HIV-1 DNA Levels in HIV-1-Infected Children. *PloS One* (2018) 13(4):e0195514. doi: 10.1371/journal.pone.0195514
231. Ananworanich J, Avihingsanon A. HIV and Noncommunicable Diseases: The Asian Perspective. *J Acquir Immune Defic Syndr* (2014) 67 Suppl 1:S99–103. doi: 10.1097/QAI.0000000000000262
232. Uprety P, Chadwick EG, Rainwater-Lovett K, Ziemniak C, Luzuriaga K, Capparelli EV, et al. Cell-Associated HIV-1 DNA and RNA Decay Dynamics During Early Combination Antiretroviral Therapy in HIV-1-Infected Infants. *Clin Infect Dis* (2015) 61(12):1862–70. doi: 10.1093/cid/civ688
233. Luzuriaga K, Tabak B, Garber M, Chen YH, Ziemniak C, McManus MM, et al. HIV Type 1 (HIV-1) Proviral Reservoirs Decay Continuously Under Sustained Virologic Control in HIV-1–Infected Children Who Received Early Treatment. *J Infect Dis* (2014) 210(10):1529–38. doi: 10.1093/infdis/jiu297
234. Massanella M, Puthanakit T, Leyre L, Jupimai T, Sawangsinth P, de Souza M, et al. Continuous Prophylactic ARV/ART Since Birth Reduces Seeding and Persistence of the Viral Reservoir in Vertically HIV-Infected Children. *Clin Infect Dis* (2020) 73:427–38. doi: 10.1093/cid/ciaa718
235. Foster C, Domínguez-Rodríguez S, Tagarro A, Gkouleli T, Heaney J, Watters S, et al. The CARMA Study: Early Infant Antiretroviral Therapy—Timing Impacts on Total HIV-1 DNA Quantitation 12 Years Later. *J Pediatr Infect Dis Soc* (2021) 10(3):295–301. doi: 10.1093/jpids/piaa071
236. Van Zyl GU, Bedison MA, Van Rensburg AJ, Laughton B, Cotton MF, Mellors JW. Early Antiretroviral Therapy in South African Children Reduces HIV-1-Infected Cells and Cell-Associated HIV-1 RNA in Blood Mononuclear Cells. *J Infect Dis* (2015) 212(1):39–43. doi: 10.1093/infdis/jiu827
237. Avettand-Fenoel V, Lechenadec J, Diallo MS, Fillion M, Melard A, Samri A, et al. Initiating Antiretroviral Treatment Early in Infancy Has Long-Term Benefits on the Human Immunodeficiency Virus Reservoir in Late Childhood and Adolescence. *Clin Infect Dis* (2021). doi: 10.1093/cid/ciaa1931
238. Kuhn L. Early Infant Treatment: Still a Long Way to Go to Reach Human Immunodeficiency Virus Remission. *Clin Infect Dis* (2021) 72(3):394–5. doi: 10.1093/cid/ciaa033
239. Veldsman KA, Rensburg A, Isaacs S, Naidoo S, Laughton B, Lombard C, et al. HIV-1 DNA Decay Is Faster in Children Who Initiate ART Shortly After Birth Than Later. *J Int AIDS Soc* (2019) 22(8):e25368. doi: 10.1002/jia2.25368
240. Millar JR, Bengu N, Vieira VA, Adland E, Roider J, Muenchhoff M, et al. Early Initiation of Antiretroviral Therapy Following In Utero HIV Infection Is Associated With Low Viral Reservoirs But Other Factors Determine Subsequent Plasma Viral Rebound. *J Infect Dis* (2021). doi: 10.1093/infdis/jiab223
241. Veldsman KA, Laughton B, Janse van Rensburg A, Zuidewind P, Dobbels E, Barnabas S, et al. Viral Suppression Is Associated With HIV-Antibody Level and HIV-1 DNA Detectability in Early Treated Children at 2 Years of Age. *AIDS* (2021) 35(8):1247–52. doi: 10.1097/QAD.0000000000002861.
242. McManus WR, Bale MJ, Spindler J, Wiegand A, Musick A, Patro SC, et al. HIV-1 in Lymph Nodes Is Maintained by Cellular Proliferation During Antiretroviral Therapy. *J Clin Invest* (2019) 129(11):4629–42. doi: 10.1172/JCI126714
243. Bitnun A, Ransy DG, Brophy J, Kakkar F, Hawkes M, Samson L, et al. Clinical Correlates of Human Immunodeficiency Virus–1 (HIV-1) DNA and Inducible HIV-1 RNA Reservoirs in Peripheral Blood in Children With Perinatally Acquired HIV-1 Infection With Sustained Virologic Suppression for at Least 5 Years. *Clin Infect Dis* (2020) 70(5):859–66. doi: 10.1093/cid/ciz251
244. Palma P, McManus M, Cotugno N, Rocca S, Rossi P, Luzuriaga K. The HIV-1 Antibody Response: A Footprint of the Viral Reservoir in Children Vertically Infected With HIV. *Lancet HIV* (2020) 7(5):e359–65. doi: 10.1016/S2352-3018(20)30100-4
245. Singh V, Dashti A, Mavigner M, Chahroudi A. Latency Reversal 2.0: Giving the Immune System a Seat at the Table. *Curr HIV/AIDS Rep* (2021) 18 (2):117–27. doi: 10.1007/s11904-020-00540-z
246. Nixon CC, Mavigner M, Sampey GC, Brooks AD, Spagnuolo RA, Irlbeck DM, et al. Systemic HIV and SIV Latency Reversal *via* Non-Canonical NF-κb Signalling *In Vivo*. *Nature* (2020) 578(7793):160–5. doi: 10.1038/s41586-020-1951-3
247. Dashti A, Waller C, Mavigner M, Schoof N, Bar KJ, Shaw GM, et al. SMAC Mimetic Plus Triple-Combination Bispecific HIVxCD3 Retargeting Molecules in SHIV.C.CH505-Infected, Antiretroviral Therapy-Suppressed Rhesus Macaques. *J Virol* (2020) 94(21):e00793-20. doi: 10.1128/JVI.00793-20
248. Palma P, Romiti ML, Montesano C, Santilli V, Mora N, Aquilani A, et al. Therapeutic DNA Vaccination of Vertically HIV-Infected Children: Report of the First Pediatric Randomised Trial (PEDVAC). *PloS One* (2013) 8(11): e79957. doi: 10.1371/journal.pone.0079957

7

Immune Checkpoint Molecules in Reproductive Immunology

Eva Miko [1,2], Matyas Meggyes [1,2], Katalin Doba [1], Aliz Barakonyi [1,2] and Laszlo Szereday [1,2]*

[1] Department of Medical Microbiology and Immunology, Medical School, University of Pécs, Pécs, Hungary, [2] Janos Szentagothai Research Centre, Pécs, Hungary

***Correspondence:**
Eva Miko
miko.eva@pte.hu

Immune checkpoint molecules, like CTLA-4, TIM-3, PD-1, are negative regulators of immune responses to avoid immune injury. Checkpoint regulators are thought to actively participate in the immune defense of infections, prevention of autoimmunity, transplantation, and tumor immune evasion. Maternal-fetal immunotolerance represents a real immunological challenge for the immune system of the mother: beside acceptance of the semiallogeneic fetus, the maternal immune system has to be prepared for immune defense mostly against infections. In this particular situation, the role of immune checkpoint molecules could be of special interest. In this review, we describe current knowledge on the role of immune checkpoint molecules in reproductive immunology.

Keywords: immune checkpoint molecule, reproductive immunology, pregnancy, immunotolerance, CTLA-4, TIM-3, PD-1

INTRODUCTION

The activation of the immune system to eliminate harmful agents is usually followed by tissue damage at the site of the exposure. In order to keep this side effect of the immune response limited and localized, efficient immunoactivation of immune cells requires multiple incoming signals. Beside antigen recognition, co-stimulatory, survival, and proliferative signals, even environmental factors can determine the outcome of the immune response (1–4).

Immune checkpoint molecules are co-stimulatory receptors, occurring on the surface of several immune cells. After ligand binding, these regulators are capable of transducing inhibitory signals (5). CTLA-4, TIM-3, PD-1 are the most studied members from this group of cell surface receptors (5). The physiological role of immune checkpoints is to prevent a harmful immune attack against self-antigens during an immune response by negatively regulating the effector immune cells, e.g., by inducing T cell exhaustion (5, 6). Recent studies suggest that each checkpoint decreases immunoactivation through different intracellular signaling mechanisms (5, 7). Immune checkpoint regulators are thought to actively participate in the immune defense of infections, prevention of autoimmunity, transplantation, and tumor immune evasion (5, 7).

Pregnancy is a natural model of active immunotolerance, where maternal immune system simultaneously faces two challenges: beside acceptance of the semiallogeneic fetus, the maternal immune system has to be prepared for immune defense mostly against infections. In this particular situation, the role of immune checkpoint molecules could be of special interest. Therefore, this paper aims to review the literature presenting current knowledge about the role of immune checkpoint molecules in reproductive immunology.

CTLA-4

The first described inhibitory receptor CTLA-4 (Cytotoxic T-lymphocyte-associated protein 4) is predominantly and constitutively expressed intracellularly in regulatory T cells, and it is missing in naive conventional T cells (8, 9). Following activation, CTLA-4 is expressed on the cell surface of Tregs, but it can also be found on the cell surface of activated CD8+ or CD4+ T cells (10). The inhibitory effect of CTLA-4 results from the competition with the T cell activatory CD28 receptor to bind the B7 ligands CD80/CD86 present on the cell surface of antigen presenting cells (11). The ability of Treg cells to induce IDO expression in APCs through the CTLA-4-B7 binding was thought to be one of the major mechanism of immune suppression by these cells (12, 13). Interestingly, current thinking suggests, that the main function of CTLA-4 is not delivering negative signals through ligand binding but the removal of its ligands CD80/CD86 from the cell surface of APCs preventing thereby their binding to the costimulatory CD28 present on T cells (8, 14).

CTLA-4 in Murine Pregnancy

The significance of the CD80/86-CD28 activation pathway in T cells during fetal rejection was shown by blocking both ligands with mAb during the pregnancy of the abortion-prone murine model. The blockade resulted in the improvement of fetal survival with an increase of Th2 type cytokines at the maternal-fetal interface (MFI) and in the peripheral expansion of the CD4+ CD25+ T cell population. Furthermore, CTLA-4 expression by T cells increased as well which was found to be significantly reduced at the MFI in abortion-prone matings (15, 16). Preventing binding of CD80/CD86 to CD28 is thought to be the way of action of CTLA-4 with similar beneficial effects in maternal-fetal tolerance. Blocking only CD86 using the same experimental setting resulted in the same observations (17). These findings support previous theories about CD80 might be the most functional ligand for CTLA-4. Blockade of the CD86 could turn off the co-stimulatory CD86/CD28 pathway while allowing a prolonged CD80/CTLA-4 interaction with all of the benefits (17–19).

Further evidence for the immunosuppressive capacity of CTLA-4 was delivered from experiments with the CTLA4Ig fusion protein. Using an adenoviral vector, CTLA4Ig was shown to be heavily expressed at the MFI. CTLA4Ig therapy of abortion-prone CBA/DBA matings could effectively improve pregnancy outcome by shifting serum cytokine levels toward Th2 bias and expanding regulatory T cell population at the periphery (20). Furthermore, the CTLA4Ig fusion protein significantly inhibited splenic lymphocyte proliferation and apoptosis of the fetoplacental unit (21). Interestingly, adoptive transfer of Treg with CTLA-4 blockade from normal pregnant mouse to CBA/DBA pregnancy didn't abolish the protective effect of Treg treatment without a blockade resulting in decreased abortion rates (22).

In another abortion-prone setting, in sonic stressed pregnant mice, decidual lymphocytes expressed decreased levels of CTLA-4, without any changes in CD28 expression suggesting the failure of the control of local immunoactivation. CTLA-4 expression by decidual lymphocytes of stressed animals could be enhanced by injections of the dipeptidyl peptidase IV inhibitor, a well-known terminator of T-cell activation (23, 24).

CTLA-4 in Human Pregnancy (Figure 1)

CTLA-4 at the Periphery

Although regulatory T cells increase in number in the periphery during early pregnancy, the enhanced CTLA-4 expression on the cell surface was not observed (10, 25). In contrast to these findings, the expression of one of the ligands of CTLA-4, namely CD86 showed an increased expression by peripheral DCs and monocytes in healthy pregnancy while CD80 expression patterns did not change (26).

CTLA-4Ig treatment of peripheral blood mononuclear cells resulted in a significantly higher IFN-γ secretion in normal

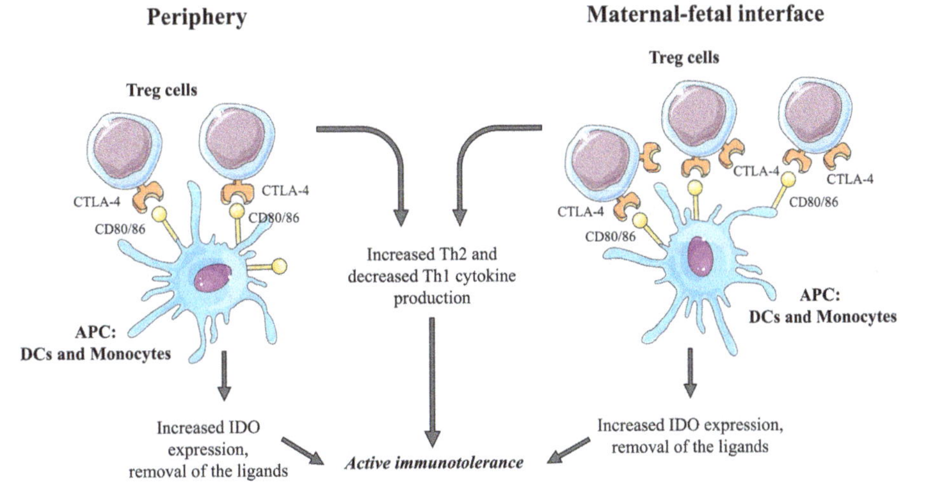

FIGURE 1 | Summarizing the possible role of the CTLA-4/CD80, CD86 pathway during human pregnancy.

pregnancy compared to non-pregnant condition (26). Despite the fact, that CTLA-4 is capable of inducing indoleamine 2,3 dioxygenase (IDO) expression in dendritic cells and monocytes through the induction of IFN-γ, there are conflicting data about whether CTLA-4Ig treatment could enhance IDO expression in DCs and monocytes in normal pregnancy (13, 26, 27).

CTLA-4 at the Maternal-Fetal Interface

Compared to the periphery, decidual Treg cells further increase in number, and the frequency of Treg expressing intracellular or surface CTLA-4 was also found to be elevated in the decidua (10, 27, 28). Interestingly, placental fibroblasts also express CTLA-4, but it is supposed to have non-immunological functions since fibroblasts are not directly in contact with maternal tissues (29). The CTLA-4 ligands, CD80, and CD86, are also present on decidual DCs and monocytes, and they show the same expression profile as in the periphery in normal pregnancy (26, 30). The decidual CTLA-4 expression is in a significantly positive correlation with decidual Th2 cytokine production and a negative correlation with decidual Th1 cytokine production suggesting remarkable immunosuppressive effects locally (30).

CTLA-4Ig treatment of decidual lymphocytes resulted in enhanced IFN-γ and IDO expression (10).

CTLA-4 in Pregnancy Complications

In the case of spontaneous abortion/miscarriage peripheral and decidual Tregs fail to increase to the levels observed in normal pregnancy (10). Data about CTLA-4 expression in these conditions are conflicting. In one hand, the overall ratio of CTLA-4+ peripheral and decidual lymphocytes as wells as the ratio of CTLA-4+ Tregs was found to be significantly reduced. Moreover, the ratios of CTLA-4+/CD28+ in regulatory T cells from miscarriage were significantly lower than that of normal pregnancy (30, 31). On the other hand, there was no significant difference in intracellular and cell surface expression of CTLA-4 on both peripheral and decidual Tregs when compared to non-pregnant and healthy pregnant controls (10). These controversy data may result from different patient inclusion criteria. From the two possible CTLA-4 ligands, only CD86 expression was found to be affected in miscarriage: peripheral monocytes, decidual monocytes, and DC showed significantly lower expression rates compared to those in normal pregnancy (26, 30). Response levels of IDO expression by both peripheral and decidual monocytes and DCs in spontaneous abortion with CTLA-4 treatments were lower compared to a healthy pregnancy (26).

Extensive research focused on the role of *CTLA-4* gene polymorphism with different conclusions (32–37). The A/G polymorphism at position 49 in exon 1 of cytotoxic T lymphocyte antigen-4 (*CTLA-4*) gene may result in abnormal protein modification in the rough endoplasmic reticulum leading to reduced expression (38, 39). Further studies confirmed, that the 49 GG genotype was associated with a reduced inhibitory function of CTLA-4 whereas individuals with AA genotype had more expression of CTLA-4 both intracellular as on the cell surface of activated T cells (33, 40, 41). Further studies with larger sample sizes are needed to prove increased frequencies of G allele and GG genotype among patients with recurrent miscarriage.

Although preeclampsia is characterized by a diminished Treg frequency, a well-known alteration (42–46), little information is available about the possible role of CTLA-4 in the pathogenesis of the disease. CD80 and CD86 ligand expression levels on monocytes decrease in preeclampsia, while data about CTLA-4 expression of Treg are not conclusive, increased and unchanged expression patterns were reported as well. Therefore, it is difficult to determine the significance of the CTLA-4 pathway in preeclampsia (47–49). Two gene polymorphism studies of the exon-1 A49G region of the *CTLA-4* gene revealed an increased frequency of the heterozygosity and GG phenotype in preeclamptic women (38, 50).

In women with successful IVF treatment, there is an increase in the peripheral Treg population compared to failed IVF attempts. Investigating CTLA-4 expression at the mRNA level, no differences could be observed in the two IVF patient group (51).

Heterozygous mutations in the immune checkpoint protein CTLA-4 leading to CTLA-4 deficiency results in different autoimmune clinical features, but no further information is available about pregnancy proceeding in these patients (52, 53).

TIM-3

Extensive research has established that Tim-3/gal-9 pathway plays a significant role in the regulation of immune responses and induction of tolerance (54–58). TIM-3 was shown to be expressed by many types of immune cells, including Th1, Th17, NK and NKT-like cells, Tregs, and also on antigen-presenting immune cells (59). Interestingly, TIM-3 activity is thought to participate in both activation and inhibition of immune response (60, 61). In the case of a healthy pregnancy, expression of TIM-3 on Th1 cells may be a key element for reducing proinflammatory Th1-dependent T-cell response (57).

The ligand of TIM-3 receptor is galectin-9 (Gal-9), a β-galactose binding protein (62). Among other identified receptors of Gal-9, TIM-3 has been studied most intensively (54). Both in mice and humans, binding of TIM-3 to its ligand Gal-9 leads to the apoptosis of Th1 and Th17 cells and induce immunotolerance (63–65). Thus, the TIM-3/Gal-9 pathway may serve as a checkpoint regulator limiting the Th1- and Th17-driven immune response and modulating the Th1/Th2 cytokine balance (54).

TIM-3 in Murine Pregnancy

TIM-3 has been studied in detail in murine pregnancy models by several groups (66–71). First, immunofluorescence stainings revealed the presence of TIM-3 in midgestational uterus and flow cytometric analysis proved that this inhibitory molecule is expressed by a variety of immune cells residing locally in the uterus/decidua: uterine NK cells, γ/δ T cells, NKT-like cells, macrophages, dendritic cells (DC), and even by myeloid-derived (66–68). TIM-3 expression by these cells was shown to be dominant but variable throughout pregnancy, in the case of the most prevalent decidual immune cell type, NK cells upregulate TIM-3 during the first half of murine gestation (66, 67). Although TIM-3 expression of decidual NK cells and γ/δ T cells is similar to that in the periphery, their upregulated relative TIM-3 expression locally suggest that these cells are more mature and entirely functional (68, 72). However, the cytotoxic capacity of TIM-3+ decidual NK cells and γ/δ T cells was shown to be reduced when compared to the periphery; this might be due to the special local microenvironment at the MFI (68). In contrast to these findings, there is a smaller TIM-3+ NKT-like cell subset in the decidua with stronger lytic capacity. Therefore, separate action of TIM-3 on different immune cell types with varying functional outcomes could be concluded (68).

The TIM-3 ligand, galectin-9 is also present at the MFI at different sites. Both murine placental spongiotrophoblast and decidual regulatory T cells express galectin-9 and decidual Gal-9+ Th cells are the main source of the secreted, soluble form of Gal-9 (68). Since the presence of both the ligand, Gal-9 and its receptor, TIM-3 side by side, their binding interaction could be hypothesized, and the inhibitory signal derived from TIM-3 might contribute to maternal immunotolerance observed in murine pregnancy. This hypothesis is supported by the observation that TIM-3 blockade of allogeneic murine pregnancy resulted in litter size reduction, reduced live births, and an increased rate of resorption *in vivo* (66, 71).

Blocking TIM-3 with monoclonal antibodies (mAbs) provided further information about the possible function of this molecule at the MFI. Following inhibition, both apoptotic cells and macrophages accumulate locally, suggesting a deficiency of phagocytic clearance via failed recognition of phosphatidylserine through TIM-3 and enhanced pro-inflammatory cytokine production (66). Uterine granulocytes were also shown to increase in number and to enhance Th1 cytokine expression. These observations are in line with previous studies of experimental autoimmune/ischemic murine models where increased inflammation was due to macrophage and granulocyte activation following TIM-3 blockade (73, 74). Blocking TIM-3 on uterinal NK (uNK) cells affect both physiologic phenotype and function of these dominant cell population at the MFI (67). Although local accumulation and cytotoxic capacity of TIM-3+ uNK cells did not change, uNK cells upregulated the activation marker CD69, and their expression pattern of activating and inhibitory cell surface receptors was notably altered. Secretion of both proangiogenic (VEGF, IFN-γ) and immunosuppressive (IL-10) cytokines by TIM-3+ uNK cells were decreased. Additionally, TIM-3 inhibition resulted in reduced placental expression of the cytokines IL-15 and IL-9, which are important factors for NK cell survival and development (67, 75).

In abortion-prone mouse models, a reduced number of TIM-3+ dNK and CD4+ Th cells can be observed with predominantly Th1 cytokine profiles (69, 70).

All these data from murine pregnancy models suggest a protective role of TIM-3 present at the MFI.

TIM-3 in Human Pregnancy (Figure 2)

TIM-3 at the Periphery

In pregnant women, upregulation of TIM-3 expression by peripheral leukocytes throughout pregnancy was mainly observed on monocytes and NK cells (59, 76). The percentage of TIM-3+ Th, Tc, and NKT-like cells remained relatively constant (57). In the third trimester of a healthy pregnancy, among lymphocytes, ~80% of NK cells, 15% of CD8+ T cells express TIM-3, in the case of CD4+ T, and NKT-like cells, the ratio of TIM3+ cells was below 5% (77).

TIM-3+ CD8+ T and NK cells show increased cytotoxicity in the third trimester of pregnancy suggesting altered functional capacities toward the end of pregnancy. The increasing levels of soluble Gal-9 throughout pregnancy might have a counter-regulatory function to control enhanced cytotoxicity of TIM-3+ CD8+ T and NK cells (57, 78). These data are inconsistent with other findings where TIM-3+ NK cells were found to have a high capacity to secrete Th2 type cytokines and reduced cytotoxicity toward trophoblast cells as a possible consequence of galectin-9/TIM-3 interaction (76).

TIM-3 expression on monocytes is regulated by IL-4 (upregulation) and IFN-γ (downregulation) cytokines, and it is involved in the effective anti-microbial immune defense by synergizing with TLR signaling (59).

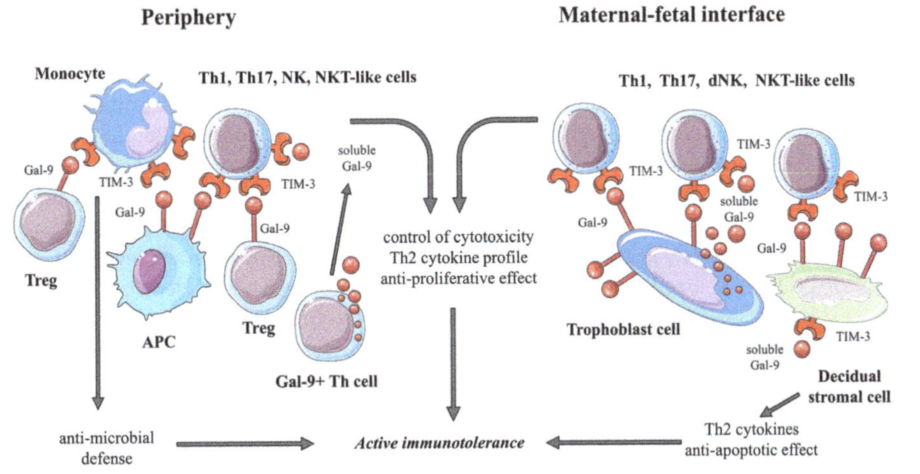

FIGURE 2 | Summarizing the possible role of the TIM-3/Gal-9 pathway during human pregnancy.

It has been demonstrated, that TGF-β1 can induce peripheral NK cells to form decidual NK-like phenotype (79, 80). TGF-β1 treatment upregulated TIM-3 expression on peripheral NK cells proposing an important function of this co-receptor at the MFI (81).

TIM-3 at the Maternal-Fetal Interface

Although TIM-3 expression at the MFI was shown on different decidual lymphocyte subsets, like CD8+, CD4+ T cells, NK cells (69–71, 81), little is known about their role in successful implantation and placentation. The majority of decidual NK (dNK) cells express TIM-3 (60–90%) (69, 81). According to CD117/CD94 expression, TIM-3+ dNK cells have a mature phenotype with Th2 cytokine profile (69, 81). Secretion of IL-4 could be further increased and secretion of TNF-α could be decreased by recombinant human Gal-9 treatment of LPS stimulated dNK cells suggesting regulatory function of TIM-3+ dNK cells on the exaggerated inflammatory response since trophoblast is capable of secreting a large amount of Gal-9, as well as decidual tissue showed high galectin-9 expression (69, 81). Interestingly, blocking TIM-3 signal with TIM-3 fusion protein resulted in the reduction of IFN-γ and TNF-α production of dNK cells (81). Immunohistochemical studies demonstrated, that the fetal part of the MFI, trophoblast cells of term placenta highly express galectin-9 as well (78).

Beside decidual immune cells, decidual stromal cells (DSCs) also express TIM-3, and TIM-3+ DSCs produce higher levels of Th2 cytokines suggesting immune activities of the decidual tissue itself (82). Furthermore, TIM-3 activation seems to be anti-apoptotic when DSCs were stressed through Toll-like receptor activation which is a new potential of this molecule since it acts pro-apoptotic on CD4+ T cells (64, 82, 83).

TIM-3 in Pregnancy Complications

The possible involvement of the TIM-3/Galectin-9 pathway in the pathogenesis of unexplained miscarriages, recurrent spontaneous abortion (RSA), and preeclampsia (PE) has been studied by several groups, both in the periphery as well as at the MFI. However, data should be interpreted cautiously since the inclusion and exclusion criteria for these clinical syndromes and recruitment of the patients involved may vary.

In RSA patient, reduced TIM-3 expression level of peripheral NK cells was observed which could be the result of lower serum TGF-β1 levels, a lack of stimulus for upregulation of TIM-3 (76, 81). Besides TIM-3 surface expression changes, there is an increase of soluble TIM-3 (sTIM-3) and a decrease of soluble galectin-9 in the sera of these patients assuming enhanced competitive binding of galectin-9 by sTIM-3 leading to failed inhibitory signals controlling inflammation (76, 84). Furthermore, TIM-3+ NK cells of RSA patients produce more pro-inflammatory and less anti-inflammatory cytokines suggesting functional deficiencies (76). The only genetic polymorphism analysis of the TIM-3 gene was carried out in RSA patients. TIM-3 polymorphism can affect ligand binding properties and may be involved in some immune-mediated diseases (85). However, analyzing polymorphism of the promoter region of the TIM-3 gene, no differences between the different genotype frequencies could be observed in healthy pregnant women and RSA patients (86). At the MFI, immunohistochemical studies revealed reduced expression of TIM-3 by decidual tissue of women with RSA. Furthermore, same findings were confirmed in the case of DSCs by flow cytometry (82). A decreased percentage of TIM-3 by dNK cells was also demonstrated, although in patients with unexplained miscarriage not with RSA (69). Conflicting data exist according to decidual TIM-3 expression, one study found upregulated TIM-3 and galectin-9 expression in decidua and chorionic villi, both at mRNA and at the protein level in patients with RSA. The authors interpret these findings as being reactive to downregulate Th1 responses observed in RSA (87).

There are few inconsistent data about the possible role of the TIM-3/Gal-9 pathway in the pathogenesis of preeclampsia. On the one hand, in preeclampsia, both TIM-3 and Gal-9 were found to be upregulated in decidual tissue, and TIM-3 expression of peripheral blood monocytes was shown to increase (4). On the other hand, a decreased ratio of TIM+3+ Th, NK, and Vdelta2+ T cells could be confirmed in the peripheral blood of preeclamptic patients (48, 77). Both findings suggest disturbed immune regulation of Th1 responses due to altered Gal-9 and TIM-3 interactions.

PD-1

PD-1 is a transmembrane receptor expressed by e.g., T cells, B cells, natural killer (NK) cells, antigen presenting cells (5, 88). PD-1 generates a strong inhibitory signal upon binding to its ligands PD-L1 and PD-L2, resulting in down-regulation of pro-inflammatory T-cell activity (89). PD-L1 can be found on several immune cells (resting T cells, B cells, dendritic cells, macrophages), in various tissues, like placenta, heart, spleen (5, 90, 91). In contrast to that, PD-L2 expression is limited to dendritic cells and macrophages (92). Furthermore, ligand expression of PD-1 can be regulated, e.g., through the local cytokine environment. PD-L1 expression is increased by many pro-inflammatory factors (LPS, GM-CSF, VEGF) and cytokines (IFN-γ, TNF-α) (5, 93, 94).

PD-1 in Murine Pregnancy

In the allogeneic murine pregnancy model, surface expression of PD-1 on peripheral CD4+ and CD8+ T cells was not altered after conception and during gestation (1). PD-1 blockade *in vivo* was shown to enhance the proliferation of CD4+ and CD8+ T cells in unmated and pregnant mice and to erase the protective effect of Treg cells in Treg treated abortion-prone animals (1, 22).

There are only a few but very informative data about the local presence of PD-1 in murine pregnancy showing PD-1 expression by a broad spectrum of decidual lymphocyte subsets including CD4+ T cells, CD8+ T cells, T follicular helper cells, γδ T cells, NK, and NKT-like cells (1, 68, 95, 96). Furthermore, increased PD-1 expression by decidual NK, NKT-like, and γδ T cells was associated with the reduced cytolytic activity of these cells when compared to the periphery suggesting PD-1 dependent regulation of innate effector functions at the MFI (68).

Concerning the tissue distribution profile of the two ligands for PD-1, PD-L1, and PD-L2 at the MFI, both fetal and maternal compartments are involved: PD-L2 is expressed throughout the murine decidua, whereas PD-L1 expression is limited to the decidua basalis (97). Insufficient data exist about PD-L expression by the trophoblast suggesting PD-L1 expression by the syncytiotrophoblast but not by trophoblastic giant cells, which are next to the decidua basalis (97, 98). Therefore, PD-1 interaction with its ligands may occur in the decidua itself and is not affected by the fetal part. *In vivo* blockade of PD-1 ligands in allogenic murine pregnancy highlighted the functional role of the PD-1/PD-L1 pathway since anti-PD-L1 treatment resulted in increased fetal resorption rate and a reduction in the litter size, whereas PD-L2 blockade had no effect on fetal resorption (97). At the MFI, PD-L1 blockade resulted in infiltration of T cells, complement deposits, and higher levels of IFN-γ suggesting T cell-mediated rejection mechanisms locally. Another supportive report on the protective role of the PD-1/PD-L1 interaction in maternal-fetal tolerance was revealed by observations of the PD-L1 deficient pregnant mice, which showed similar results in fetal resorption rate, litter size, and a shift toward Th17 emphasizing the role of PD-L1 expressing regulatory T cells controlling fetal antigen-specific maternal T cell (99, 100). Yet, data are conflicting since in another experimental setting neither PD-L1 nor PD-1 deficient mice had significant alterations in gestational or in neonatal offspring parameters (101). These findings indicate doubt about the role of the PD-1/PD-L1 pathway in the survival of the fetal allograft in mice and further studies are needed to reconcile previous controversial results.

PD-1 in Human Pregnancy (Figure 3)

PD-1 at the Periphery

Although immunological acceptance of the fetus is primarily based on maternal tolerance mechanisms at the MFI locally, it exerts a significant impact on systemic immunity as well (102). Despite the fact that syncytiotrophoblast cells—which are bathed in maternal blood—express PD-L1 and PD-L2, data about possible changes in the PD-1 mediated systemic immune response during human pregnancy compared to healthy, non-pregnant controls are lacking (90, 103). The only information regarding this topic is that the frequency of PD-1 expressing T lymphocytes is elevated in the blood of healthy pregnant women compared to non-pregnant counterparts and soluble PD-L1 levels increase throughout gestation (78).

PD-1 at the Maternal-Fetal Interface

Immunofluorescent studies revealed a significantly higher PD-1 expression by decidual T lymphocytes similarly to non-pregnant endometrial T cells. This increase in PD-1 expression was demonstrated more in detail when compared to the periphery during pregnancy: decidual CD8+, CD4+, and regulatory T cells were shown to enhance PD-1 expression (104).

As already mentioned before, PD-L1 and PD-L2 are present in the placenta throughout pregnancy (90, 103, 105). In the first trimester, the major fetal source of PD-L1 is the villous syncytiotrophoblast and extravillous cytotrophoblast, while PD-L2 expression is much more restricted to villous cytotrophoblast (103, 105). On the maternal side, decidual stromal cells constitutively express both PD-L1 and PD-L2, but Th1 cytokines can further enhance their surface expression. PD-L1 expression by decidual macrophages is evident as well (104, 106).

PD-1 interaction with its ligand PD-L1 in different co-culture experiments resulted in reduced Th1 cytokine production by CD4+ T cells (104, 106). These findings suggest the contribution of the PD-1 mediated pathway to the establishment of a favorable Th2 type immune balance at the FMI in healthy human pregnancy.

PD-1 in Pregnancy Complications

Limited information is available about the involvement of the PD-1/PD-L pathway in pregnancy disorders. In preeclampsia, the percentage of PD-1 positive regulatory T cells was significantly higher than in healthy pregnancy with no difference in their PD-L1 expression. While the ratio of PD-1+ Th17 cells was not altered, the PDL1 expression by Th17 cells increased. PD-1 expression by CD3+, and CD4+ T cells did not significantly differ suggesting dysregulated PD-1/PD-L1 axis within the Treg/Th17 imbalance in the clinical phase of preeclampsia (47, 107).

In the case of RSA, decidual PD-L1 expression was significantly reduced on both mRNA as well as on protein

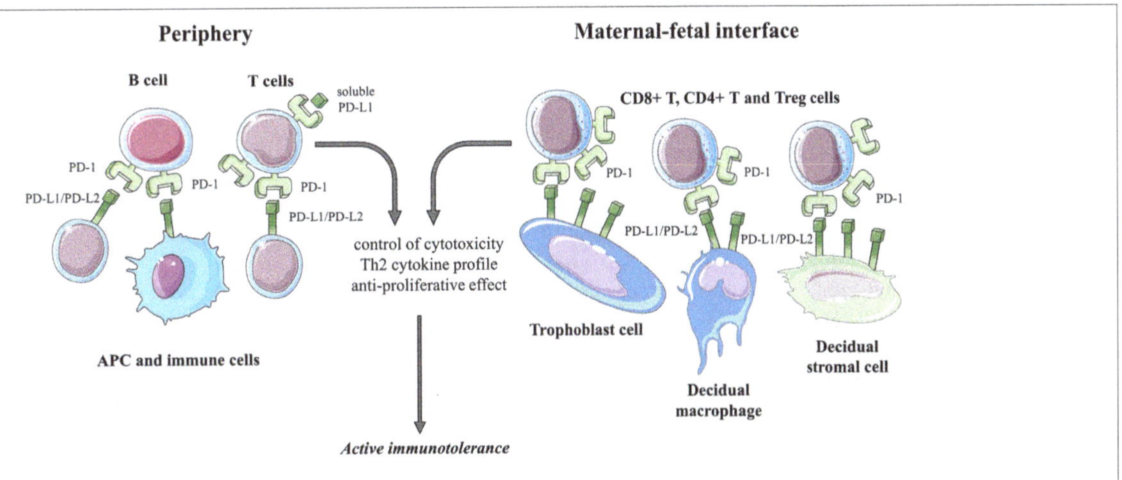

FIGURE 3 | Summarizing the possible role of the PD-1/PD-L1, PD-L2 pathway during human pregnancy.

TABLE 1 | Type of mouse models used in the experiments.

Type of mouse models used in the experiments	References
NORMAL ALLOGENEIC PREGNANCY MATINGS	
CBA/J × BALB/c	(16, 17, 20–22, 69–71)
CBA/J × C57BL/6	(66, 67, 97, 99, 100)
BALB/c × C57BL/6	(95, 96, 101)
NORMAL SYNGENEIC PREGNANCY MATINGS	
CBA/J × CBA/J	(67, 96)
BALB/c × BALB/c	(68)
C57BL/6 × C57BL/6	(1, 96, 101)
ABORTION-PRONE ALLOGENEIC MATING	
CBA/J × DBA/2	(15–17, 20–23, 69, 70)
NON-PREGNANT MICE	
BALB/c	(18, 19, 73, 98)
C57BL/6	(18, 19, 74, 75, 98)

level compared to healthy first-trimester decidua, while PD-1 expression by decidual lymphocytes showed no difference (108).

TIM-3 /PD-1 Co-expression

Effector cells of the immune system can be characterized by co-expression of different co-inhibitory molecules (109). In human pregnancy, TIM-3+PD-1+ CD8+ T cells preferentially accumulate in the decidua (71). Upregulation of both TIM-3 and PD-1 by decidual CD8+ T cells might be induced by embryonic trophoblast in an HLA-C dependent manner (71). These double positive cells display higher proliferative activity and produce more Th2 type cytokines than their TIM-3/PD-1 double negative CD8+ counterparts (71). Blocking both co-receptors increased cytotoxicity and decreased Th2 type cytokine production of TIM-3+PD-1+ CD8+ T cells suggesting a protective, anti-inflammatory role of TIM-3 and PD-1 co-expressing decidual CD8+ T lymphocytes at the MFI (71). This hypothesis is strengthened by further observations both in human as well as in mice. In murine pregnancy systemic blockade of both TIM-3 and PD-1 *in vivo* resulted in further reduction of fetal growth and litter size when compared to the blockade of either TIM-3 or PD-1 alone (71). In line with these findings, in patients with RSA, dual expression of TIM-3 and PD-1 by decidual CD8+ T cells was found to be significantly reduced and to be less proliferative in contrast to a healthy pregnancy (71).

SUMMARY

Immune checkpoint molecules have a major impact on cellular immunity by limiting inflammatory immune response and thereby maintaining physiologic tissue conditions. From this point of view, maternal-fetal immunotolerance represents a real immunological challenge for the immune system of the mother where accurate, tight, and dynamic immune control is required for healthy pregnancy proceeding from the time of implantation on.

As presented in this review in detail, the possible role of immune checkpoint molecules in the establishment of maternal-fetal immunotolerance has been extensively studied. In the case of CTLA-4, TIM-3, and PD-1, the participation and possible role of these molecules in maternal immune response have been confirmed by different approaches, e.g., animal and human experiments, *in vitro* and *in vivo* studies. **Table 1** shows the different mice strains used in animal experiments. However, data are sometimes conflicting and not comprehensive, which may be due to experimental setting differences, small sample size, and the highly complex and multilevel characteristics of immune cell activation. When considering the involvement of co-activatory molecules in maternofetal immune interactions, the co-signaling network is far more complicated (110).

Although there are no current clinical trials aiming at immune checkpoint molecules and interactions in pregnancy complications, some results of the studies discussed in this paper indicate the possible role of TIM-3 cell surface expression rate and serum levels of the soluble ligands PD-L1 and galectin-9 as potential biomarkers for screening during pregnancy (57, 76, 78).

Immune checkpoint inhibitors targeting the PD-1/PD-L1 and CTLA-4 pathways are revolutionary therapeutics in advanced malignancies and could be used in the treatment of chronic viral infections (HIV, HCV) as well in the future. Because of lacking a (68) adequate and well-controlled studies and based on the findings in mouse models, where blockade of the PD-1/PD-L1 pathway resulted in the adverse effect on pregnancy, checkpoint inhibitors are relatively contraindicated for the treatment of metastatic cancer in pregnant women requiring an individualized decision in each case (22, 97, 100, 111, 112).

Although intensive research and a large amount of information regarding the involvement of immune checkpoint molecules in reproductive immunology, the puzzle is not complete. Our current knowledge is quite deficient since there are several other immune checkpoint molecules described recently: Lymphocyte-activated gene-3 (LAG-3), T cell immunoreceptor with Ig and ITIM domains (TIGIT), B and T lymphocytes attenuator (BTLA), V-domain Ig suppressor of T cell activation (VISTA) are novel members of immune checkpoint molecules with proven immune regulatory activity (113). Until today, studies regarding this new generation of negative checkpoint regulators in the field of reproductive immunology are missing and urgently needed.

AUTHOR CONTRIBUTIONS

EM writing, original draft preparation. MM and AB original draft preparation. KD table and figure preparation and editing. LS writing, review, and editing.

FUNDING

This work was supported by National Research, Development, and Innovation Office (NKFIH K119529 and PD112465), by the PTE ÁOK KA Research Grant (KA-2018-07 and KA-2018-18), by grants of GINOP-2.3.2-15-201600021, EFOP-3.6.3-VEKOP-16-2017-00009, and 20765-3/2018/FEKUTSTRAT.

REFERENCES

1. Shepard MT, Bonney EA. PD-1 Regulates T cell proliferation in a tissue and subset-specific manner during normal mouse pregnancy. *Immunol Invest.* (2013) 42:385–408. doi: 10.3109/08820139.2013.782317
2. Matzinger P. Friendly and dangerous signals: is the tissue in control? *Nat Immunol.* (2007) 8:11–3. doi: 10.1038/ni0107-11
3. Haskins K, Kappler J, Marrack P. The major histocompatibility complex-restricted antigen receptor on T cells. *Annu Rev Immunol.* (1984) 2:51–66. doi: 10.1146/annurev.iy.02.040184.000411
4. Hao H, He M, Li J, Zhou Y, Dang J, Li F, et al. Upregulation of the Tim-3/Gal-9 pathway and correlation with the development of preeclampsia. *Eur J Obstet Gynecol Reprod Biol.* (2015) 194:85–91. doi: 10.1016/j.ejogrb.2015.08.022
5. Meggyes M, Szanto J, Lajko A, Farkas B, Varnagy A, Tamas P, et al. The possible role of CD8+/Vα7.2+/CD161++ T (MAIT) and CD8+/Vα7.2+/CD161 ^{lo} T (MAIT-like) cells in the pathogenesis of early-onset pre-eclampsia. *Am J Reprod Immunol.* (2018) 79:e12805. doi: 10.1111/aji.12805
6. Jiang Y, Li Y, Zhu B. T-cell exhaustion in the tumor microenvironment. *Cell Death Dis.* (2015) 6:e1792. doi: 10.1038/cddis.2015.162
7. Dai S, Jia R, Zhang X, Fang Q, Huang L. The PD-1/PD-Ls pathway and autoimmune diseases. *Cell Immunol.* (2014) 290:72–9. doi: 10.1016/j.cellimm.2014.05.006
8. Walker LSK. EFIS lecture: understanding the CTLA-4 checkpoint in the maintenance of immune homeostasis. *Immunol Lett.* (2017) 184:43–50. doi: 10.1016/j.imlet.2017.02.007
9. Saito S, Sasaki Y, Sakai M. CD4+CD25high regulatory T cells in human pregnancy. *J Reprod Immunol.* (2005) 65:111–20. doi: 10.1016/j.jri.2005.01.004
10. Sasaki Y. Decidual and peripheral blood CD4+CD25+ regulatory T cells in early pregnancy subjects and spontaneous abortion cases. *Mol Hum Reprod.* (2004) 10:347–53. doi: 10.1093/molehr/gah044
11. Chambers CA, Kuhns MS, Egen JG, Allison JP. C TLA−4-M ediated inhibition in regulation of T cell r esponses : mechanisms and manipulation in tumor immunotherapy. *Annu Rev Immunol.* (2001) 19:565–94. doi: 10.1146/annurev.immunol.19.1.565
12. Finger EB, Bluestone JA. When ligand becomes receptor—tolerance via B7 signaling on DCs. *Nat Immunol.* (2002) 3:1056–7. doi: 10.1038/ni1102-1056
13. Grohmann U, Orabona C, Fallarino F, Vacca C, Calcinaro F, Falorni A, et al. CTLA-4-Ig regulates tryptophan catabolism *in vivo*. *Nat Immunol.* (2002) 3:1097–101. doi: 10.1038/ni846
14. Walker LSK, Sansom DM. Confusing signals: recent progress in CTLA-4 biology. *Trends Immunol.* (2015) 36:63–70. doi: 10.1016/j.it.2014.12.001
15. Jin L-P, Zhou Y-H, Wang M-Y, Zhu X-Y, Li D-J. Blockade of CD80 and CD86 at the time of implantation inhibits maternal rejection to the allogeneic fetus in abortion-prone matings. *J Reprod Immunol.* (2005) 65:133–46. doi: 10.1016/j.jri.2004.08.009
16. Zhou WH, Dong L, Du MR, Zhu XY, Li DJ. Cyclosporin A improves murine pregnancy outcome in abortion-prone matings: involvement of CD80/86 and CD28/CTLA-44. *Reproduction.* (2008) 135:385–95. doi: 10.1530/REP-07-0063
17. Zhu X-Y, Zhou Y-H, Wang M-Y, Jin L-P, Yuan M-M, Li D-J. Blockade of CD86 signaling facilitates a Th2 bias at the maternal-fetal interface and expands peripheral CD4+CD25+ regulatory T cells to rescue abortion-prone fetuses1. *Biol Reprod.* (2005) 72:338–45. doi: 10.1095/biolreprod.104.034108
18. Judge TA, Wu Z, Zheng XG, Sharpe AH, Sayegh MH, Turka LA. The role of CD80, CD86, and CTLA4 in alloimmune responses and the induction of long-term allograft survival. *J Immunol.* (1999) 162:1947–51.
19. Yamada A, Kishimoto K, Dong VM, Sho M, Salama AD, Anosova NG, et al. CD28-independent costimulation of T cells in alloimmune responses. *J Immunol.* (2001) 167:140–6. doi: 10.4049/jimmunol.167.1.140
20. Li W, Li B, Fan W, Geng L, Li X, Li L, et al. CTLA4Ig gene transfer alleviates abortion in mice by expanding CD4+CD25+regulatory T cells and inducing indoleamine 2,3-dioxygenase. *J Reprod Immunol.* (2009) 80:1–11. doi: 10.1016/j.jri.2008.11.006
21. Li W, Li B, Li S. Adenovirus mediated CTLA4Ig transgene therapy alleviates abortion by inhibiting spleen lymphocyte proliferation and regulating apoptosis in the feto-placental unit. *J Reprod Immunol.* (2013) 97:167–74. doi: 10.1016/j.jri.2013.01.002
22. Wafula PO, Teles A, Schumacher A, Pohl K, Yagita H, Volk HD, et al. PD-1 but not CTLA-4 blockage abrogates the protective effect of regulatory T cells in a pregnancy murine model. *Am J Reprod Immunol.* (2009) 62:283–92. doi: 10.1111/j.1600-0897.2009.00737.x
23. Rüter J, Hoffmann T, Heiser U, Demuth HU, Arck PC, Klapp BF, et al. The expression of T-cell surface antigens CTLA-4, CD26, and CD28 is modulated by inhibition of dipeptidylpeptidase IV (DPP IV, CD26) activity in murine stress-induced abortions. *Cell Immunol.* (2002) 220:150–6. doi: 10.1016/S0008-8749(03)00028-5
24. Rüter J, Demuth H, Arck PC, Hofmann T, Klapp BF. Inhibition of dipeptidylpeptidase IV (DPP IV, CD26) activity modulates surface expression of CTLA-4 in stress-induced abortions. (2003)155–163.
25. Somerset DA, Zheng Y, Kilby MD, Sansom DM, Drayson MT. Normal human pregnancy is associated with an elevation in the immune suppressive CD25+ CD4+ regulatory T-cell subset. *Immunology.* (2004) 112:38–43. doi: 10.1111/j.1365-2567.2004.01869.x
26. Miwa N, Hayakawa S, Miyazaki S, Myojo S, Sasaki Y, Sakai M, et al. IDO expression on decidual and peripheral blood dendritic cells and monocytes/macrophages after treatment with CTLA-4 or interferon-γ increase in normal pregnancy but decrease in spontaneous abortion. *Mol Hum Reprod.* (2006) 11:865–70. doi: 10.1093/molehr/gah246
27. Heikkinen J, Möttönen M, Alanen A, Lassila O. Phenotypic characterization of regulatory T cells in the human decidua. *Clin Exp Immunol.* (2004) 136:373–8. doi: 10.1111/j.1365-2249.2004.02441.x
28. Dimova T, Nagaeva O, Stenqvist AC, Hedlund M, Kjellberg L, Strand M, et al. Maternal foxp3 expressing CD4+CD25+and CD4+CD25-regulatory T-cell populations are enriched in human early normal pregnancy decidua: a phenotypic study of paired decidual and peripheral blood samples. *Am J Reprod Immunol.* (2011) 66:44–56. doi: 10.1111/j.1600-0897.2011.01046.x
29. Kaufman KA, Bowen JA, Tsai AF, Bluestone JA, Hunt JS, Ober C. The CTLA-4 gene is expressed in placental fibroblasts. *Mol Hum Reprod.* (1999) 5:84–7. Available at: http://www.ncbi.nlm.nih.gov/pubmed/10050667 [Accessed January 9, 2019]
30. Jin LP, Fan DX, Zhang T, Guo PF, Li DJ. The costimulatory signal upregulation is associated with Thl bias at the maternal-fetal interface in human miscarriage. *Am J Reprod Immunol.* (2011) 66:270–8. doi: 10.1111/j.1600-0897.2011.00997.x
31. Jin LP, Chen QY, Zhang T, Guo PF, Li DJ. The CD4+CD25brightregulatory T cells and CTLA-4 expression in peripheral and decidual lymphocytes are down-regulated in human miscarriage. *Clin Immunol.* (2009) 133:402–10. doi: 10.1016/j.clim.2009.08.009
32. Fan Q, Zhang J, Cui Y, Wang C, Xie Y, Wang Q, et al. The synergic effects of CTLA-4/Foxp3-related genotypes and chromosomal aberrations on the risk of recurrent spontaneous abortion among a Chinese Han population. *J Hum Genet.* (2018) 63:579–87. doi: 10.1038/s10038-018-0414-2
33. Gupta R, Prakash S, Parveen F, Agrawal S. Association of CTLA-4 and TNF-α polymorphism with recurrent miscarriage among North Indian women. *Cytokine.* (2012) 60:456–62. doi: 10.1016/j.cyto.2012.05.018
34. Misra MK, Mishra A, Phadke SR, Agrawal S. Association of functional genetic variants of CTLA4 with reduced serum CTLA4 protein levels and increased risk of idiopathic recurrent miscarriages. *Fertil Steril.* (2016) 106:1115–23.e6. doi: 10.1016/j.fertnstert.2016.06.011
35. Nasiri M, Rasti Z. CTLA-4 and IL-6 gene polymorphisms: risk factors for recurrent pregnancy loss. *Hum Immunol.* (2016) 77:1271–4. doi: 10.1016/j.humimm.2016.07.236
36. Wang X, Lin Q, Ma Z, Hong Y, Zhao A, Di W, et al. Association of the A/G polymorphism at position 49 in exon 1 of CTLA-4 with the susceptibility to unexplained recurrent spontaneous abortion in the Chinese population. *Am J Reprod Immunol.* (2005) 53:100–5. doi: 10.1111/j.1600-0897.2004.00251.x
37. Wang X, Ma Z, Hong Y, Lu P, Lin Q. Expression of CD28 and cytotoxic T lymphocyte antigen 4 at the maternal-fetal interface in women with unexplained pregnancy loss. *Int J Gynecol Obstet.* (2006) 93:123–9. doi: 10.1016/j.ijgo.2006.01.027

38. Jääskeläinen E, Toivonen S, Keski-Nisula L, Paattiniemi EL, Helisalmi S, Punnonen K, et al. CTLA-4 polymorphism 49A-G is associated with placental abruption and preeclampsia in Finnish women. *Clin Chem Lab Med.* (2008) 46:169–73. doi: 10.1515/CCLM.2008.034
39. Anjos S, Nguyen A, Ounissi-Benkalha H, Tessier M-C, Polychronakos C. A common autoimmunity predisposing signal peptide variant of the cytotoxic T-lymphocyte antigen 4 results in inefficient glycosylation of the susceptibility allele. *J Biol Chem.* (2002) 277:46478–86. doi: 10.1074/jbc.M206894200
40. Ligers A, Teleshova N, Masterman T, Huang W-X, Hillert J. CTLA-4 gene expression is influenced by promoter and exon 1 polymorphisms. *Genes Immun.* (2001) 2:145–152. doi: 10.1038/sj.gene.6363752
41. Chistiakov DA, Turakulov RI. CTLA-4 and its role in autoimmune thyroid disease. *J Mol Endocrinol.* (2003) 31:21–36. doi: 10.1677/jme.0.0310021
42. Toldi G, Švec P, Vásárhelyi B, Mészáros G, Rigó J, Tulassay T, et al. Decreased number of FoxP3+ regulatory T cells in preeclampsia. *Acta Obstet Gynecol Scand.* (2008) 87:1229–33. doi: 10.1080/00016340802389470
43. Steinborn A, Haensch GM, Mahnke K, Schmitt E, Toermer A, Meuer S, et al. Distinct subsets of regulatory T cells during pregnancy: is the imbalance of these subsets involved in the pathogenesis of preeclampsia? *Clin Immunol.* (2008) 129:401–12. doi: 10.1016/j.clim.2008.07.032
44. Prins JR, Boelens HM, Heimweg J, Van der Heide S, Dubois AE, Van Oosterhout AJ, et al. Preeclampsia is associated with lower percentages of regulatory T cells in maternal blood. *Hypertens Pregnancy.* (2009) 28:300–11. doi: 10.1080/10641950802601237
45. Darmochwal-Kolarz D, Saito S, Rolinski J, Tabarkiewicz J, Kolarz B, Leszczynska-Gorzelak B, et al. Activated T lymphocytes in pre-eclampsia. *Am J Reprod Immunol.* (2007) 58:39–45. doi: 10.1111/j.1600-0897.2007.00489.x
46. Sasaki Y, Darmochwal-Kolarz D, Suzuki D, Sakai M, Ito M, Shima T, et al. Proportion of peripheral blood and decidual CD4+ CD25bright regulatory T cells in pre-eclampsia. *Clin Exp Immunol.* (2007) 149:139–45. doi: 10.1111/j.1365-2249.2007.03397.x
47. Toldi G, Vásárhelyi B, Biró E, Fügedi G, Rigó J, Molvarec A. B7 costimulation and intracellular indoleamine-2,3-dioxygenase expression in peripheral blood of healthy pregnant and pre-eclamptic women. *Am J Reprod Immunol.* (2013) 69:264–71. doi: 10.1111/aji.12069
48. Miko E, Szereday L, Barakonyi A, Jarkovich A, Varga P, Szekeres-Bartho J. Immunoactivation in preeclampsia: Vδ2+ and regulatory T cells during the inflammatory stage of disease. *J Reprod Immunol.* (2009) 80:100–8. doi: 10.1016/j.jri.2009.01.003
49. Boij R, Mjösberg J, Svensson-Arvelund J, Hjorth M, Berg G, Matthiesen L, et al. Regulatory T-cell subpopulations in severe or early-onset preeclampsia. *Am J Reprod Immunol.* (2015) 74:368–78. doi: 10.1111/aji.12410
50. Samsami Dehaghani A, Doroudchi M, Kalantari T, Pezeshki AM, Ghaderi A. Heterozygosity in CTLA-4 gene and severe preeclampsia. *Int J Gynecol Obstet.* (2005) 88:19–24. doi: 10.1016/j.ijgo.2004.09.007
51. Zhou J, Wang Z, Zhao X, Wang J, Sun H, Hu Y. An increase of treg cells in the peripheral blood is associated with a better *in vitro* fertilization treatment outcome. *Am J Reprod Immunol.* (2012) 68:100–6. doi: 10.1111/j.1600-0897.2012.01153.x
52. Verma N, Burns SO, Walker LSK, Sansom DM. Immune deficiency and autoimmunity in patients with CTLA-4 (CD152) mutations. *Clin Exp Immunol.* (2017) 190:1–7. doi: 10.1111/cei.12997
53. Lo B, Abdel-Motal UM. Lessons from CTLA-4 deficiency and checkpoint inhibition. *Curr Opin Immunol.* (2017) 49:14–9. doi: 10.1016/j.coi.2017.07.014
54. Lajko A, Meggyes M, Polgar B, Szereday L. The immunological effect of Galectin-9/TIM-3 pathway after low dose Mifepristone treatment in mice at 14.5 day of pregnancy. *PLoS ONE.* (2018) 13:e0194870. doi: 10.1371/journal.pone.0194870
55. Chabtini L, Mfarrej B, Mounayar M, Zhu B, Batal I, Dakle PJ, et al. TIM-3 regulates innate immune cells to induce fetomaternal tolerance. *J Immunol.* (2013) 190:88–96. doi: 10.4049/jimmunol.1202176
56. Sánchez-Fueyo A, Tian J, Picarella D, Domenig C, Zheng XX, Sabatos CA, et al. Tim-3 inhibits T helper type 1–mediated auto- and alloimmune responses and promotes immunological tolerance. *Nat Immunol.* (2003) 4:1093–101. doi: 10.1038/ni987
57. Meggyes M, Miko E, Polgar B, Bogar B, Farkas B, Illes Z, et al. Peripheral blood TIM-3 positive NK and CD8+ T cells throughout pregnancy: TIM-3/galectin-9 interaction and its possible role during pregnancy. *PLoS ONE.* (2014) 9:e92371. doi: 10.1371/journal.pone.0092371
58. Hastings WD, Anderson DE, Kassam N, Koguchi K, Greenfield EA, Kent SC, et al. TIM-3 is expressed on activated human CD4+ T cells and regulates Th1 and Th17 cytokines. *Eur J Immunol.* (2009) 39:2492–501. doi: 10.1002/eji.200939274
59. Zhao J, Lei Z, Liu Y, Li B, Zhang L, Fang H, et al. Human pregnancy up-regulates Tim-3 in innate immune cells for systemic immunity. *J Immunol.* (2009) 182:6618–24. doi: 10.4049/jimmunol.0803876
60. van de Weyer PS, Muehlfeit M, Klose C, Bonventre JV, Walz G, Kuehn EW. A highly conserved tyrosine of Tim-3 is phosphorylated upon stimulation by its ligand galectin-9. *Biochem Biophys Res Commun.* (2006) 351:571–6. doi: 10.1016/j.bbrc.2006.10.079
61. Lee J, Su EW, Zhu C, Hainline S, Phuah J, Moroco JA, et al. Phosphotyrosine-dependent coupling of Tim-3 to T-cell receptor signaling pathways. *Mol Cell Biol.* (2011) 31:3963–74. doi: 10.1128/MCB.05297-11
62. von Wolff M, Wang X, Gabius H-J, Strowitzki T. Galectin fingerprinting in human endometrium and decidua during the menstrual cycle and in early gestation. *MHR Basic Sci Reprod Med.* (2004) 11:189–94. doi: 10.1093/molehr/gah144
63. Seki M, Oomizu S, Sakata K, Sakata A, Arikawa T, Watanabe K, et al. Galectin-9 suppresses the generation of Th17, promotes the induction of regulatory T cells, and regulates experimental autoimmune arthritis. *Clin Immunol.* (2008) 127:78–88. doi: 10.1016/j.clim.2008.01.006
64. Zhu C, Anderson AC, Schubart A, Xiong H, Imitola J, Khoury SJ, et al. The Tim-3 ligand galectin-9 negatively regulates T helper type 1 immunity. *Nat Immunol.* (2005) 6:1245–52. doi: 10.1038/ni1271
65. Sabatos CA, Chakravarti S, Cha E, Schubart A, Sánchez-Fueyo A, Zheng XX, et al. Interaction of Tim-3 and Tim-3 ligand regulates T helper type 1 responses and induction of peripheral tolerance. *Nat Immunol.* (2003) 4:1102–10. doi: 10.1038/ni988
66. Chabtini L, Mfarrej B, Mounayar M, Zhu B, Batal I, Dakle PJ, et al. TIM-3 regulates innate immune cells to induce fetomaternal tolerance. *J Immunol.* (2013) 190:88–96. doi: 10.4049/jimmunol.1202176
67. Tripathi S, Chabtini L, Dakle PJ, Smith B, Akiba H, Yagita H, et al. Effect of TIM-3 blockade on the immunophenotype and cytokine profile of murine uterine NK cells. *PLoS ONE.* (2015) 10:e0123439. doi: 10.1371/journal.pone.0123439
68. Meggyes M, Lajko A, Palkovics T, Totsimon A, Illes Z, Szereday L, et al. Feto-maternal immune regulation by TIM-3/galectin-9 pathway and PD-1 molecule in mice at day 14.5 of pregnancy. *Placenta.* (2015) 36:1153–60. doi: 10.1016/j.placenta.2015.07.124
69. Li Y-H, Zhou W-H, Tao Y, Wang S-C, Jiang Y-L, Zhang D, et al. The galectin-9/Tim-3 pathway is involved in the regulation of NK cell function at the maternal–fetal interface in early pregnancy. *Cell Mol Immunol.* (2016) 13:73–81. doi: 10.1038/cmi.2014.126
70. Wang S, Zhu X, Xu Y, Zhang D, Li Y, Tao Y, et al. Programmed cell death-1 (PD-1) and T-cell immunoglobulin mucin-3 (Tim-3) regulate CD4+ T cells to induce Type 2 helper T cell (Th2) bias at the maternal-fetal interface. *Hum Reprod.* (2016) 31:700–11. doi: 10.1093/humrep/dew019
71. Wang S-C, Li Y-H, Piao H-L, Hong X-W, Zhang D, Xu Y-Y, et al. PD-1 and Tim-3 pathways are associated with regulatory CD8+ T-cell function in decidua and maintenance of normal pregnancy. *Cell Death Dis.* (2015) 6:e1738. doi: 10.1038/cddis.2015.112
72. Ndhlovu LC, Lopez-Verges S, Barbour JD, Jones RB, Jha AR, Long BR, et al. Tim-3 marks human natural killer cell maturation and suppresses cell-mediated cytotoxicity. *Blood.* (2012) 119:3734–43. doi: 10.1182/blood-2011-11-392951
73. Monney L, Sabatos CA, Gaglia JL, Ryu A, Waldner H, Chernova T, et al. Th1-specific cell surface protein Tim-3 regulates macrophage activation and severity of an autoimmune disease. *Nature.* (2002) 415:536–41. doi: 10.1038/415536a

74. Uchida Y, Ke B, Freitas MCS, Yagita H, Akiba H, Busuttil RW, et al. T-Cell immunoglobulin mucin-3 determines severity of liver ischemia/reperfusion injury in mice in a TLR4-dependent manner. *Gastroenterology.* (2010) 139:2195–206. doi: 10.1053/j.gastro.2010.07.003
75. Ashkar AA, Black GP, Wei Q, He H, Liang L, Head JR, et al. Assessment of requirements for IL-15 and IFN regulatory factors in uterine NK cell differentiation and function during pregnancy. *J Immunol.* (2003) 171:2937–44. doi: 10.4049/jimmunol.171.6.2937
76. Li Y, Zhang J, Zhang D, Hong X, Tao Y, Wang S, et al. Tim-3 signaling in peripheral NK cells promotes maternal-fetal immune tolerance and alleviates pregnancy loss. *Sci Signal.* (2017) 10:eaah4323. doi: 10.1126/scisignal.aah4323
77. Miko E, Meggyes M, Bogar B, Schmitz N, Barakonyi A, Varnagy A, et al. Involvement of galectin-9/TIM-3 pathway in the systemic inflammatory response in early-onset preeclampsia. *PLoS ONE.* (2013) 8:e71811. doi: 10.1371/journal.pone.0071811
78. Enninga EAL, Harrington SM, Creedon DJ, Ruano R, Markovic SN, Dong H, et al. Immune checkpoint molecules soluble program death ligand 1 and galectin-9 are increased in pregnancy. *Am J Reprod Immunol.* (2018) 79:e12795. doi: 10.1111/aji.12795
79. Keskin DB, Allan DSJ, Rybalov B, Andzelm MM, Stern JNH, Kopcow HD, et al. TGFbeta promotes conversion of CD16+ peripheral blood NK cells into CD16- NK cells with similarities to decidual NK cells. *Proc Natl Acad Sci USA.* (2007) 104:3378–83. doi: 10.1073/pnas.0611098104
80. Eriksson M, Meadows SK, Wira CR, Sentman CL. Unique phenotype of human uterine NK cells and their regulation by endogenous TGF-β. *J Leukoc Biol.* (2004) 76:667–75. doi: 10.1189/jlb.0204090
81. Sun J, Yang M, Ban Y, Gao W, Song B, Wang Y, et al. Tim-3 is upregulated in NK cells during early pregnancy and inhibits NK cytotoxicity toward trophoblast in galectin-9 dependent pathway. *PLoS ONE.* (2016) 11:e0147186. doi: 10.1371/journal.pone.0147186
82. Wang S, Cao C, Piao H, Li Y, Tao Y, Zhang X, et al. Tim-3 protects decidual stromal cells from toll-like receptor-mediated apoptosis and inflammatory reactions and promotes Th2 bias at the maternal-fetal interface. *Sci Rep.* (2015) 5:9013. doi: 10.1038/srep09013
83. Kuchroo VK, Meyers JH, Umetsu DT, DeKruyff RH. TIM family of genes in immunity and tolerance. in Frederick W. Alt, editor. *Advances in Immunology.* (2006) Academic press. p. 227–249. doi: 10.1016/S0065-2776(06)91006-2
84. Wu M, Zhu Y, Zhao J, Ai H, Gong Q, Zhang J, et al. Soluble costimulatory molecule sTim3 regulates the differentiation of Th1 and Th2 in patients with unexplained recurrent spontaneous abortion. *Int J Clin Exp Med.* (2015) 8:8812–9.
85. Xu J, Yang Y, Liu X, Wang Y. The −1541 C>T and +4259 G>T of TIM-3 polymorphisms are associated with rheumatoid arthritis susceptibility in a Chinese Hui population. *Int J Immunogenet.* (2011) 38:513–8. doi: 10.1111/j.1744-313X.2011.01046.x
86. Shen Y, Wang C, Hong D, Zeng B, Fang C, Yuan C, et al. The relationship between polymorphisms in the promoter region of Tim-3 and unexplained recurrent spontaneous abortion in Han Chinese women. *Reprod Biol Endocrinol.* (2013) 11:104. doi: 10.1186/1477-7827-11-104
87. Li J, Li F, Zuo W, Zhou Y, Hao H, Dang J, et al. Up-regulated expression of Tim-3/Gal-9 at maternal-fetal interface in pregnant woman with recurrent spontaneous abortion. *J Huazhong Univ Sci Technol.* (2014) 34:586–90. doi: 10.1007/s11596-014-1320-2
88. Keir ME, Butte MJ, Freeman GJ, Sharpe AH. PD-1 and its ligands in tolerance and immunity. *Annu Rev Immunol.* (2008) 26:677–704. doi: 10.1146/annurev.immunol.26.021607.090331
89. Chikuma S. Basics of PD-1 in self-tolerance, infection, and cancer immunity. *Int J Clin Oncol.* (2016) 21:448–55. doi: 10.1007/s10147-016-0958-0
90. Petroff MG, Chen L, Phillips TA, Azzola D, Sedlmayr P, Hunt JS. B7 family molecules are favorably positioned at the human maternal-fetal interfacel. *Biol Reprod.* (2003) 68:1496–504. doi: 10.1095/biolreprod.102.010058
91. Veras E, Kurman RJ, Wang T-L, Shih I-M. PD-L1 Expression in human placentas and gestational trophoblastic diseases. *Int J Gynecol Pathol.* (2016) 36:146–53. doi: 10.1097/PGP.0000000000000305
92. Lewkowich IP, Lajoie S, Stoffers SL, Suzuki Y, Richgels PK, Dienger K, et al. PD-L2 modulates asthma severity by directly decreasing dendritic cell IL-12 production. *Mucosal Immunol.* (2013) 6:728–39. doi: 10.1038/mi.2012.111
93. Radvanyi L, Pilon-Thomas S, Peng W, Sarnaik A, Mulé JJ, Weber J, et al. Antagonist antibodies to PD-1 and B7-H1 (PD-L1) in the treatment of advanced human cancer–letter. *Clin Cancer Res.* (2013) 19:5541. doi: 10.1158/1078-0432.CCR-13-1054
94. Kondo A, Yamashita T, Tamura H, Zhao W, Tsuji T, Shimizu M, et al. Interferon-gamma and tumor necrosis factor-alpha induce an immunoinhibitory molecule, B7-H1, via nuclear factor-kappaB activation in blasts in myelodysplastic syndromes. *Blood.* (2010) 116:1124–31. doi: 10.1182/blood-2009-12-255125
95. Zeng W, Liu Z, Zhang S, Ren J, Ma X, Qin C, et al. Characterization of T follicular helper cells in allogeneic normal pregnancy and PDL1 blockage-induced abortion. *Sci Rep.* (2016) 6:36560. doi: 10.1038/srep36560
96. Barton BM, Xu R, Wherry EJ, Porrett PM. Pregnancy promotes tolerance to future offspring by programming selective dysfunction in long-lived maternal T cells. *J Leukoc Biol.* (2017) 101:975–87. doi: 10.1189/jlb.1A0316-135R
97. Guleria I, Khosroshahi A, Ansari MJ, Habicht A, Azuma M, Yagita H, et al. A critical role for the programmed death ligand 1 in fetomaternal tolerance. *J Exp Med.* (2005) 202:231–7. doi: 10.1084/jem.20050019
98. Liang SC, Latchman YE, Buhlmann JE, Tomczak MF, Horwitz BH, Freeman GJ, et al. Regulation of PD-1, PD-L1, and PD-L2 expression during normal and autoimmune responses. *Eur J Immunol.* (2003) 33:2706–16. doi: 10.1002/eji.200324228
99. D'Addio F, Riella LV, Mfarrej BG, Chabtini L, Adams LT, Yeung M, et al. The link between the PDL1 costimulatory pathway and Th17 in fetomaternal tolerance. *J Immunol.* (2011) 187:4530–41. doi: 10.4049/jimmunol.1002031
100. Habicht A, Dada S, Jurewicz M, Fife BT, Yagita H, Azuma M, et al. A link between PDL1 and T regulatory cells in fetomaternal tolerance. *J Immunol.* (2007) 179:5211–9. doi: 10.4049/jimmunol.179.8.5211
101. Taglauer ES, Yankee TM, Petroff MG. Maternal PD-1 regulates accumulation of fetal antigen-specific CD8+ T cells in pregnancy. *J Reprod Immunol.* (2009) 80:12–21. doi: 10.1016/j.jri.2008.12.001
102. Borzychowski AM, Croy BA, Chan WL, Redman CWG, Sargent IL. Changes in systemic type 1 and type 2 immunity in normal pregnancy and pre-eclampsia may be mediated by natural killer cells. *Eur J Immunol.* (2005) 35:3054–63. doi: 10.1002/eji.200425929
103. Petroff MG, Kharatyan E, Torry DS, Holets L. The immunomodulatory proteins B7-DC, B7-H2, and B7-H3 are differentially expressed across gestation in the human placenta. *Am J Pathol.* (2005) 167:465–73. doi: 10.1016/S0002-9440(10)62990-2
104. Taglauer ES, Trikhacheva AS, Slusser JG, Petroff MG. Expression and function of PDCD1 at the human maternal-fetal interface. *Biol Reprod.* (2008) 79:562–9. doi: 10.1095/biolreprod.107.066324
105. Petroff MG, Chen L, Phillips TA, Hunt JS. B7 family molecules: novel immunomodulators at the maternal-fetal interface. *Placenta.* (2002) 23:S95–101. doi: 10.1053/plac.2002.0813
106. Nagamatsu T, Schust DJ, Sugimoto J, Barrier BF. Human decidual stromal cells suppress cytokine secretion by allogenic CD4+ T cells via PD-1 ligand interactions. *Hum Reprod.* (2009) 24:3160–71. doi: 10.1093/humrep/dep308
107. Tian M, Zhang Y, Liu Z, Sun G, Mor G, Liao A. The PD-1/PD-L1 inhibitory pathway is altered in pre-eclampsia and regulates T cell responses in pre-eclamptic rats. *Sci Rep.* (2016) 6:27683. doi: 10.1038/srep27683
108. Li G, Lu C, Gao J, Wang X, Wu H, Lee C, et al. Association between PD-1/PD-L1 and T regulate cells in early recurrent miscarriage. *Int J Clin Exp Pathol.* (2015) 8:6512–8.
109. Blackburn SD, Shin H, Haining WN, Zou T, Workman CJ, Polley A, et al. Coregulation of CD8+ T cell exhaustion by multiple inhibitory receptors during chronic viral infection. *Nat Immunol.* (2009) 10:29–37. doi: 10.1038/ni.1679
110. Xu Y-Y, Wang S-C, Li D-J, Du M-R. Co-signaling molecules in maternal-fetal immunity. *Trends Mol Med.* (2017) 23:46–58. doi: 10.1016/j.molmed.2016.11.001

111. Poulet FM, Wolf JJ, Herzyk DJ, DeGeorge JJ. An evaluation of the impact of PD-1 pathway blockade on reproductive safety of therapeutic PD-1 inhibitors. *Birth Defects Res Part B Dev Reprod Toxicol.* (2016) 107:108–19. doi: 10.1002/bdrb.21176
112. Johnson DB, Sullivan RJ, Menzies AM. Immune checkpoint inhibitors in challenging populations. *Cancer.* (2017) 123:1904–11. doi: 10.1002/cncr.30642
113. Le Mercier I, Lines JL, Noelle RJ. Beyond CTLA-4 and PD-1, the generation Z of negative checkpoint regulators. *Front Immunol.* (2015) 6:418. doi: 10.3389/fimmu.2015.00418

8

Association Between COVID-19 Pregnant Women Symptoms Severity and Placental Morphologic Features

Patricia Zadorosnei Rebutini[1], Aline Cristina Zanchettin[2], Emanuele Therezinha Schueda Stonoga[3], Daniele Margarita Marani Prá[1], André Luiz Parmegiani de Oliveira[1], Felipe da Silva Dezidério[1], Aline Simoneti Fonseca[2], Júlio César Honório Dagostini[3], Elisa Carolina Hlatchuk[3], Isabella Naomi Furuie[4], Jessica da Silva Longo[4], Bárbara Maria Cavalli[5], Carolina Lumi Tanaka Dino[5], Viviane Maria de Carvalho Hessel Dias[1], Ana Paula Percicote[3], Meri Bordignon Nogueira[5,6], Sonia Mara Raboni[7], Newton Sergio de Carvalho[5], Cleber Machado-Souza[2*] and Lucia de Noronha[1]*

[1] Postgraduate Program of Health Sciences, School of Medicine, Pontifícia Universidade Católica do Paraná-PUCPR, Curitiba, Brazil, [2] Postgraduate Program in Biotechnology Applied in Health of Children and Adolescent, Pelé Pequeno Príncipe, Research Institute, Faculdades Pequeno Príncipe, Curitiba, Brazil, [3] Department of Medical Pathology, Clinical Hospital, Universidade Federal do Paraná-UFPR, Curitiba, Brazil, [4] Department of Tocogynecology, Clinical Hospital, Universidade Federal do Paraná, UFPR, Curitiba, Brazil, [5] Postgraduate Program of Tocogynecology and Women's Health, Clinical Hospital, Universidade Federal do Paraná-UFPR, Curitiba, Brazil, [6] Virology Laboratory, Clinical Hospital, Universidade Federal do Paraná-UFPR, Curitiba, Brazil, [7] Department of Infectious Disease, Clinical Hospital, Universidade Federal do Paraná-UFPR, Curitiba, Brazil

***Correspondence:**
Cleber Machado-Souza
Cleberius@gmail.com
Patricia Zadorosnei Rebutini
rebutini@gmail.com

Since the beginning of the pandemic, few papers describe the placenta's morphological and morphometrical features in SARS-CoV-2–positive pregnant women. Alterations, such as low placental weight, accelerated villous maturation, decidual vasculopathy, infarcts, thrombosis of fetal placental vessels, and chronic histiocytic intervillositis (CHI), have been described.

Objective: To analyze clinical data and the placental morphological and morphometric changes of pregnant women infected with SARS-CoV-2 (COVID-19 group) in comparison with the placentas of non-infected pregnant women, matched for maternal age and comorbidities, besides gestational age of delivery (Control group).

Method: The patients in the COVID-19 and the Control group were matched for maternal age, gestational age, and comorbidities. The morphological analysis of placentas was performed using Amsterdam Placental Workshop Group Consensus Statement. The quantitative morphometric evaluation included perimeter diameter and number of tertiary villi, number of sprouts and knots, evaluation of deposition of villous fibrin, and deposition of intra-villous collagen I and III by Sirius Red. Additionally, Hofbauer cells (HC) were counted within villi by immunohistochemistry with CD68 marker.

Results: Compared to controls, symptomatic women in the COVID-19 group were more likely to have at least one comorbidity, to evolve to preterm labor and infant death, and to have positive SARS-CoV-2 RNA testing in their concepts. Compared to controls, placentas in the COVID-19 group were more likely to show features of maternal and fetal vascular malperfusion. In the COVID-19 group, placentas of symptomatic women were more likely to show CHI. No significant results were found after morphometric analysis.

Conclusion: Pregnant women with symptomatic SARS-CoV-2 infection, particularly with the severe course, are more likely to exhibit an adverse fetal outcome, with slightly more frequent histopathologic findings of maternal and fetal vascular malperfusion, and CHI. The morphometric changes found in the placentas of the COVID-19 group do not seem to be different from those observed in the Control group, as far as maternal age, gestational age, and comorbidities are paired. Only the deposition of villous fibrin could be more accentuated in the COVID-19 group (p = 0.08 borderline). The number of HC/villous evaluated with CD68 immunohistochemistry did not show a difference between both groups.

Keywords: SARS-CoV-2, COVID-19, vertical transmission, placenta, morphometric analysis, placental histopathology

INTRODUCTION

One year after the recognition of the outbreak of the severe acute respiratory distress syndrome coronavirus 2 (SARS-CoV-2), it has spread all over the world, thus developing into a global pandemic with nearly 150 million confirmed infections and more than 3.1 million deaths worldwide so far (1). Fatalities and severe courses were primarily seen in elderly patients with relevant comorbidities, but soon there were reports of younger patients showing adverse outcomes (2, 3).

No longer after its first documented appearance, SARS-CoV-2 was suspected to be perinatally transmitted (4–8). This enveloped single-stranded RNA virus infects target cells by binding to angiotensin-converting enzyme 2 (ACE2) and entry into cells after spike protein cleavage by the transmembrane serine protease 2 (TMPRSS2). Since both proteins have been detected in the placenta and fetal tissues, a possible mechanism of intrauterine transmission and neonatal infection emerged (9–14), and the coronavirus disease 2019 (COVID-19) impact on pregnant women became of particular interest.

Along with the worldwide dissemination of COVID-19, reports of adverse pregnancy outcomes have emerged in the literature, such as preeclampsia, preterm delivery, miscarriage, intrauterine fetal demise, and neonatal death (15–18). Congenital infection can be challenging to characterize since pathogen detection usually requires specific methods, not always available, applied in a myriad of maternal and fetal samples. Despite that, antepartum or peripartum vertical transmission is now substantially documented. Almost 30% of neonatal infections reported to date occurred due to transplacental transmission, and the remaining due to environmental exposure. Additionally, Raschetti et al. observed that 55% of infected neonates developed COVID-19 (19–25).

It is well recognized that analysis of the placental histopathological changes can provide valuable information, considering that a variety of pathological agents, including infectious ones, are associated with characteristic morphological findings (26–29). Regardless, few papers describe the placenta's morphological and morphometrical features in SARS-CoV-2–positive pregnant women (30–34), and the association between maternal infection and abnormal placental findings is still to be determined.

Accordingly, the purpose of this study was to analyze clinical data and the morphological and morphometric changes in placentas of pregnant women infected with SARS-CoV-2 (COVID-19 group) and to compare the placentas of non-infected pregnant women (Control group) matched in a 1:1 fashion by gestational age at delivery, maternal age, and comorbidities.

MATERIALS AND METHODS

Ethical Approvals

The Brazilian National Ethics Committee approved the presented study of Human Experimentation under the protocol number CAAE: 35129820.6.0000.0096. Families signed the informed consent forms. The authors followed all relevant guidelines, regulations, and ethics and safety protocols during this study execution at all stages. The data that support the findings of this study are available from the corresponding author.

Study Design

A prospective observational case-control study.

Study Patients and Control Group Selection

For the COVID-19 group (study group), pregnant women with laboratory-confirmed infection, whose respective placenta specimens have been sent for histologic examination, were eligible for inclusion. This group comprises 19 women who had SARS-CoV-2 infection confirmed either in the second (n = 3) or in the third gestational trimester (n = 16). Initially, we included women who spontaneously sought treatment at Complexo Hospital de Clínicas, Universidade Federal do Paraná

(CHC-UFPR) or at Hospital Nossa Senhora das Graças (HNSG), Curitiba, Brazil, for symptoms of COVID-19 varying from mild to severe (n = 9). After the implementation of universal testing for SARS-CoV-2 infection for all obstetrical patients admitted to labor and delivery in both institutions, asymptomatic pregnant women were added thereafter (n=10).

For the Control group (n = 19), placentas of pregnant women who gave birth at CHC-UFPR in years prior to the SARS-CoV-2 outbreak were selected (from 2016 to 2018) and matched in a 1:1 fashion by gestational age at delivery, maternal age, and maternal comorbidities.

Historical controls were selected to ensure that women with false-negative test results for SARS-CoV-2 infection were excluded. Gestational age at delivery is a universally used matching variable since there is a correlation between placental development and the advancing gestation, which could interfere in the analysis. Maternal age and maternal comorbidities were also incorporated as matching variables, given their possible role as confounders when analyzing placental abnormalities.

Samples

Submission criteria for placental examination included maternal or fetal conditions previously diagnosed during prenatal care or gross abnormalities noted during delivery, as routinely implemented in both institutions. Therefore, the maternal-positive SARS-CoV-2 testing result was considered an abnormal maternal condition and a placental evaluation criterion.

All placentas were examined according to a standardized protocol that consisted of immediate fixation after delivery in 10 % buffered formalin for 72 h, gross examination with measurement of placental dimensions and chord length, weight evaluation of the placental disc after trimming of the fetal membranes and umbilical cord, followed by serial sectioning through 1.5-cm interval and cut surface examination. Macroscopic alterations were recorded and sampled. Additional representative samples of the umbilical cord (two sections), the membranes (one fetal membrane roll), and the chorionic plate (at least two full-thickness, non-peripheral sections including maternal and fetal surface) were submitted to paraffin embedding.

Clinical Information

Clinical and laboratory data were obtained from medical records during hospitalization; the mother and the newborn were followed up until discharge from the hospital.

Maternal information sought from each medical record for both groups comprised maternal age and comorbidities, parity, gestational age at delivery, mode of delivery, neonatal birth weight, and APGAR score. All pregnant women in both groups were tested for congenital intrauterine infections (TORCH) during prenatal care; only one (Patient code—PC 20-3744) tested positive for syphilis in the first trimester and received the preconized treatment.

For the study group, it was also retrieved the gestational age at and method used for SARS-CoV-2 infection diagnosis, presence or absence of symptoms typically attributed to COVID-19 (body temperature over 38°C, dyspnea, cough, myalgias, nausea and vomiting, diarrhea, headache, anosmia), disease severity (ranging from mild symptoms to critical organ dysfunction), and maternal outcome.

SARS-CoV-2 Testing

Maternal nasopharyngeal swabs specimens (n = 17) were tested for SARS-CoV-2 infection by real-time reverse transcriptase-polymerase chain reaction (RT-PCR). In the remaining two cases, the diagnosis was achieved by serologic testing (n = 2).

Detection of SARS-CoV-2 RNA in infants was performed in 13 case samples (n = 13), including umbilical cord blood (n = 13), amniotic fluid (n = 3), and infants' nasopharyngeal swabs specimens (n = 6), all of them collected immediately after birth. The mothers' milk was also tested in three cases.

Samples from formalin-fixed paraffin-embedded (FFPE) tissue were also tested to verify the presence of SARS-CoV-2 RNA in the placenta (n=11). Viral RNA extraction was performed with a commercially available paraffin extraction kit (Qiagen®) in Pelé Pequeno Príncipe Research Institute.

SARS-CoV-2 RNA identification tests were performed at CHC-UFPR and HNSG using XGEN MASTER COVID-19 Kit (Mobius Life Science, Inc, Brazil). Quantitative anti-SARS-CoV-2 IgM and IgG dosage was done in peripheral blood samples in both institutions.

Morphologic Analysis

All representative placental samples taken for microscopic assessment underwent routine processing, embedding, sectioning at 5 μm, and staining with hematoxylin and eosin (H&E).

The qualitative morphological analysis was performed in all placentas from the COVID-19 and Control groups (n = 38) using the Amsterdam Placental Workshop Group Consensus Statement (35). Histological sections containing at least one sample of the umbilical cord, membrane roll, and chorionic plate of every case from both groups were randomly selected and renamed by one research team member (blinding step). Two experienced perinatal pathologists systematically evaluated the slides.

Selected parameters were computed simply as "present" (yes) or "absent" (no). The extension and intensity of specific alterations were graded following Amsterdam protocol recommendations. The remaining parameters were subdivided into three quantitative categories: <30%, 30% to 70%, and > 70%, to record both the presence and extension of most alterations.

Assessed parameters included features of maternal vascular malperfusion (villous infarction, distal villous hypoplasia, accelerated villous maturation/increase in syncytial knots, decidual acute atherosis, decidual vascular fibrinoid necrosis with or without foam cells, decidual vascular mural hypertrophy, decidual chronic perivasculitis, absence of spiral artery remodeling, decidual arterial thrombosis, persistence of intramural endovascular trophoblast), features of fetal vascular malperfusion (fetal vascular thrombosis, fetal vascular intramural fibrin deposition, avascular villi, stem vessel obliteration/ fibromuscular sclerosis, villous stromal-vascular karyorrhexis, vascular ectasia), delayed villous maturation, features of maternal inflammatory response (chorionitis, chorioamnionitis), features of fetal inflammatory response (umbilical vasculitis, funisitis), features of chronic inflammation (chronic deciduous, villitis, intervillositis), intervillous thrombi, microcalcification foci, chorangiosis, and membrane meconium and hemosiderin staining.

Morphometric Analysis

The morphometric analysis included measurement of the perimeter and diameter of the villi, counting the number of tertiary villi, sprouts and knots of tertiary villi, quantifying the villous fibrin and the intra-villous collagen I and III depositions. It was performed in 11 cases of the COVID-19 group and eleven Control group cases (n = 22), matched for gestational age, maternal age, and maternal comorbidities.

One histological section stained with H&E containing at least one sample of the chorionic plate was randomly selected from every case in both groups (n = 22). Samples of grossly identified lesions were previously excluded. Each section was subsequently photographed at a magnification of 200× (medium power field—MPF) using the Scanner Axion Scan.Z1 (Zeiss AG, Oberkochen, Germany), resulting in about 5,000 high-resolution images for each case (ZEN Blue Edition, Zeiss, Germany). Following the exclusion of unfocused images, with artifacts, with non-villous tissue, or less than 100% of the field occupied with placental villi, the remaining images were randomized to obtain about 100 images for each case of both groups. The villi's perimeter and diameter were measured using Image-Pro Plus® 4 software, based on freehand drawing on 100 villi in consecutive images. At the end of each villus' contour, the program provided perimeter and minor diameter in micrometers (μm).

The variables number of tertiary villi, number of sprouts, and knots of tertiary villi were assessed by simply counting these microscopic structures by an experienced perinatal pathologist, in 30 of those 100 images, after a new cycle of randomization.

Histological sections were also stained with phosphotungstic hematoxylin (n = 22) and Sirius Red (n = 22), aiming to evaluate villous fibrin and intra-villous collagen I and III depositions, respectively. As previously described for H&E, the slides were photographed at MPF using the Scanner Axion Scan.Z1, and the resulting images were randomized to obtain about 200 images for every case of the COVID-19 and Control group for each stain. Positive control was chosen as a "mask," which contained adequate levels of specific pigment precipitation. The mask was then superimposed on the sample images, and Image-Pro Plus 4 software identified the positive areas, expressing the results as positive pigment deposition areas per μm^2. The values obtained for the collagen analysis were further divided by the observed field's total area, generating a percentage value for each image (36).

The morphometric analysis was also blind since each case was previously renamed by one member of the research team not involved in the data acquisition, and the images were also randomly generated by the software afterward, with no investigator's interference.

Immunohistochemistry

Histological sections of the placentas from both groups (n = 22) were fixed on electrically charged glass slides and subsequently dewaxed with heated xylol (37°C), dehydrated by successive baths of absolute ethyl alcohol with decreasing solution concentrations and rehydrated with water. Methyl alcohol and hydrogen peroxide were used to block endogenous peroxidase and distilled water and hydrogen peroxide for the second block. Next, incubation with anti-CD68 primary antibody (KP1 clone, monoclonal mouse, Biocare, California, USA) for 1 h and secondary antibody associated with the dextran polymer (Spring Bioscience, Pleasanton, USA) for 30 min. For development, DAB/substrate complex (DAB, DakoCytomation) was added onto the slides, followed by counterstaining with Mayer's hematoxylin, dehydration with ethyl alcohol baths in increasing concentrations, clarification with xylol, and blending with Canada balsam. The protocol developed and described above is already standardized and routinely used in CHC-UFPR. To quantify Hofbauer cells (HC), the number of villi and CD68+ cells in those villi were counted in 30 high-power random fields (HPF= 400×). Only positive cells morphologically compatible with histocytes, with visible nuclei, and located within villi were considered suitable for counting. Unspecific staining, staining of any other cells, and cells without visible nuclei were excluded.

All immunohistochemistry assays included a negative control (missing a primary antibody) and positive control (human lymph node).

Statistical Analysis

Means, standard deviations, medians, minimum, maximum values, frequencies, or percentages were used to describe the findings. The nominal variables are expressed as actual values and frequency and analyzed by Pearson chi-square test and or by Fisher exact test. Most of the quantitative variables exhibited normal distribution, as verified by the Shapiro–Wilk test, and were compared with the t-test. The Kruskal–Wallis non-parametric test was performed to compare the remaining quantitative variable between groups (fibrin deposition). For both tests, statistical significance was defined as a p-value of <0.05. The data were analyzed using the IBM SPSS Statistics v.20.0 software. Armonk, NY: IBM Corp.

RESULTS

Relevant clinical information about each case in both groups is summarized in **Tables 1** and **2**. Comparison between groups regarding clinical data and morphologic findings are resumed in **Table 3** (n = 38). In **Table 4**, morphometric data are presented along with clinical information of the cases evaluated from both groups (n = 22). **Figure 1** exemplifies morphometric and morphological parameters evaluated.

Maternal Clinical Profile and SARS-CoV-2 Testing Results

Among the nineteen patients testing positive for SARS-CoV-2 infection, almost half (9/19, 47.4%) were symptomatic. Three had COVID-19 symptoms varying from mild (fever, cough, among others, but without dyspnea) to moderate (with dyspnea, but without the necessity of complementary life

TABLE 1 | Clinical information of the COVID-19 group.

Patient code	Maternal age (yr)	Maternal Comorbidities	COVID-19 Symptoms/ Severe Disease	SARS-CoV-2 testing			Outcome			
				RT-PCR Maternal NS swab/ Trimester	Maternal Serology	RT-PCR placenta/ RT-PCR fetal samples	Gestational age at delivery	APGAR (1 min/5 min)/ Fetal-Maternal Outcome	Fetal weight (g)	Placental weight (g)/ Macroscopic alterations
20–3594	26	Hypertensive disorder in pregnancy and hypothyroidism	+/+	+/3rd	IgM+/IgG+	–/–	33	(5/9) Preterm newborn	2450	448/Infarcts (<5%)
20–3561	38	Hypothyroidism	+/+	*/2nd	IgM+/IgG+	–/–	28+2	(na) Preterm newborn	na	245
20–3282	40	*Situs inversus totalis* with metallic stent	+/+	+/3rd	na	–/+**	33+5	(0/0) Neonatal death/ Maternal death	2300	416
20–5379	38	Gestational diabetes	+/+	+/2nd	na	–/+**	23+6	(1/5) Neonatal death/ Maternal death	610	168/Placental hypoplasia
20–3744	29	Gestational diabetes, hypothyroidism, obesity, bipolar disorder, and syphilis (treated)	+/–	+/3rd	IgM+/IgG+	–/+**	34+1	(na) Preterm newborn	na	412/Infarcts (<5%)
20–5105	29	None	–	+/3rd	na	–/na	38+6	(9/10) Term newborn	2960	462
20–3369	29	Gestational diabetes and Hyperthyroidism	+/–	+/3rd	na	–/na	37+4	(8/9) Term newborn	2600	358/Infarcts (<5%)
20–3364	42	Hypertensive disorder in pregnancy	+/+	+/2nd	IgM+/IgG+	+/+§	28+3	Intrauterine death	1020	135/Placental hypoplasia and infarcts (30–40%)
20–5776	42	None	–	+/3rd	na	–/+**	36+5	(9/10) Preterm newborn	2605	382
20–5869	27	None	+/–	+/3rd	na	–/na	37+2	(9/10) Term newborn	2345	370
20–3916	24	None	–	+/3rd	IgM+/IgG+	–/na	38+6	(9/10) Term newborn	3030	650
20–4850	25	Obesity	+/+	+/3rd	na	na/–	30+2	(na) Preterm newborn	na	410
20–5006	22	Obesity	–	+/3rd	na	na/–	41+0	(4/9) Term newborn	3110	670
20–5009	23	Hypothyroidism	–	*/3rd	IgM+/IgG+	na/–	38+4	(5/9) Term newborn	3925	775/Hydropic placenta
20–5031	35	Gestational diabetes, obesity	–	+/3rd	na	na/–	36+4	(8/9) Preterm newborn	2720	450
20–6551	32	None	–	+/3rd	na	na/na	38+5	(8/9) Term newborn	3070	448
20–6680	38	None	–	+/3rd	na	na/na	37	(9/10) Term newborn	2875	318
20–7035	34	None	–	+/3rd	na	na/–	39	(9/9) Term newborn	3115	438
20–6071	34	Hypertensive disorder in pregnancy	–	+/3rd	na	na/–	34+6	(7/8) Preterm newborn	2370	384

**rt-PCR not available—diagnostic by serology.*
*RT-PCR positive in fetal samples: **Nasofaringeal swab and §Umbilical cord blood.*
na, not available.

Patient code	Maternal age (yr)	Maternal Comorbidities	Outcome			
			Gestational age at delivery	APGAR (1 min/5 min)/ Fetal Outcome	Fetal weight (g)	Placental weight (g) Macroscopic alterations
16–7859	20	Hypothyroidism	32+3	(3/7) Preterm newborn	1180	270/Placental hypoplasia
18–13016	23	Chronic hypertension and hypothyroidism	35+2	(4/8) Preterm newborn	2223	498/none
16–8315	18	Obesity	40+4	(7/9) Term newborn	3810	514 none
18–4906	20	None	28	(7/8) Preterm newborn	1205	248/none
18–14057	42	Diabetes, chronic hypertension, bipolar disorder	33+4	(2/8) Preterm newborn	1650	243/Placental hypoplasia
16–7599	25	Gestational diabetes	39	(8/10) Term newborn	3460	480/none
16–3340	39	None	38+3	(7/9) Term newborn	3005	395/none
18–9951	24	None	37+2	(8/9) Term newborn	3690	574/none
16–6144	29	None	39	(9/10) Term newborn	3345	394/none
17–2491	35	None	32+4	(8/9) Preterm newborn	2900	416/none
16–7667	36	None	36+4	(9/9) Preterm newborn	2315	319/none
18–5040	24	None	32+4	(1/6/8) Preterm newborn	1555	297/Infarcts (5%)
16–7155	25	Obesity	40	(7/9) Term newborn	2830	375/none
16–5762	39	Hypothyroidism	39+3	(8/9) Term newborn	3490	465/Infarcts (10%)
18–11859	38	Gestational diabetes, obesity	36+1	(6/9) Preterm newborn	2925	450/none
18–5502	27	None	37+2	(7/9) Term newborn	2500	552/none
16–3787	24	None	37+4	(9/10) Term newborn	2945	461/none
18–4510	19	None	40+2	(7/8) Term newborn	1990	413/none
18–6601	16	Hypertensive disorder in pregnancy	24+5	(8/9) Preterm newborn	2235	368/none

support) (3/9, 33.3%). Six developed severe courses, requiring orotracheal intubation and hemodynamic support within less than seven days after admission (6/9, 66.6%). Two of them died due to COVID-19 associated complications (2/6, 33.3%).

Twelve patients of the COVID-19 group had at least one comorbidity (12/19, 63.2%), such as hypertension (3/19, 15.8%), diabetes (4/19, 21%), obesity (4/19, 21%), and hypothyroidism (4/19, 21%). One patient had a diagnosis of Kartagener syndrome (chronic sinusitis, bronchiectasis, and situs inversus with dextrocardia) and had a cardiac valvar replacement (metallic) for 10 years (Patient code—PC 20-3282).

Most pregnant women tested positive for SARS-CoV-2 in the third gestational trimester (16/19, 84.2%), either immediately before delivery in asymptomatic patients or within less than 15 days from delivery in symptomatic ones.

Only three patients had a positive result in the second trimester, all of them with severe COVID-19 symptoms and equally close to delivery. In this subgroup, one woman died due to COVID-19 complications along with her infant (PC 20-5379). One had an intrauterine demise (PC 20-3364) and recovered utterly afterward. The third evolved to preterm labor (PC 20-3561).

Newborns Clinical Outcome and SARS-CoV-2 Testing Results

The mode of delivery, APGAR score, placental weight, fetal weight, fetal/placental weight ratio were similar between both groups (p=NS).

Among the 19 infants in the COVID-19 group, sixteen were born alive (16/19, 84.2%). We observed three infant deaths, being one intrauterine demise and two neonatal deaths within hours of delivery (3/19, 15.8%). All infant deaths occurred in women with severe COVID-19 symptoms, including the two who died due to COVID-19 complications (PC 20-3282 and 20-5379). In the Control group, all infants were born alive.

Preterm delivery was recorded in ten cases (10/19, 52.6%), including those with infant deaths mentioned above. In the Control group, nine pregnancies ended prematurely (9/19, 47.4%), a similarity that was expected due to methodological design. However, there were no recorded infant or maternal deaths.

SARS-CoV-2 RNA was detected in samples from five infants among thirteen tested (5/13, 38.4%). It was positive in one cord blood sample (PC 20-3364) and four newborns nasopharyngeal swabs specimens (PC 20-3282, 20-5379, 20-3744, and 20-5776). All amniotic fluid and mother's milk samples tests returned negative.

From all FFPE placental tissue tested (n = 11), only one case was positive for SARS-CoV-2 RNA, being the case of intrauterine demise (PC 20-3364).

Morphologic Alterations

All parameters enumerated in *Materials and Methods* were sought systematically. Many of them were not identified in any sample. The histopathological alterations identified in both groups are listed in **Table 3** and discussed below.

Morphometric Alterations and Immunohistochemistry Evaluation

The average number of sprouts and knots (per villous) of the COVID-19 group tertiary villi was 0.19 and 0.81, respectively, compared to 0.16 and 0.81 of the Control group (p=NS). The average perimeter of the COVID-19 group tertiary villi was 271.93 µm compared to 288.42 µm in the Control group (p=0.37).

TABLE 3 | Clinical and morphological comparisons between COVID-19 group (n=19) and Control group (n=19) placentas.

		Variable	Control	COVID-19	*p*-value
Clinical data	**Maternal**	Maternal age (years)	25 (16–42)	32 (22–42)	0.21
		Gestational age (weeks)	36 (23–40)	36 (23–41)	0.97
		Comorbidities	Hypertensive disorder (3) Gestational diabetes (3) Obesity (3) Hypothyroidism (3) None (11)	Hypertensive disorder (3) Gestational diabetes (4) Obesity (4) Hypothyroidism (4) None (7)	1
	Fetal	APGAR 1 min/5 min	7 (1–9)/9 (6–10)	8(0–9)/9 (0–10)	0.41/0.33
		Fetal weight (grams)	2865 (1,180–3,810)	2663 (610–3,925)	0,94
		Placental Weight (grams)	406 (243–573)	412 (135–775)	0,79
		Placental diameter (centimeters)	17 (12–19)	16 (12–22)	0,87
		Infant death	0	3	**0.09**
		Preterm delivery	9	10	0.74
		Term delivery	10	9	0.74
Morphological variables	**MVM**	Villous infarction	5	2	0.21
		Distal villous hypoplasia	6	4	0.46
		Accelerated villous maturation/increase in syncytial knots	5	8	0.30
		Decidual vascular mural hypertrophy	5	10	**0.09**
		Absence of spiral artery remodeling	1	6	**0.03**
		Decidual vascular fibrinoid necrosis without foam cells	1	3	0.29
		Decidual vascular fibrinoid necrosis with foam cells	0	2	0.14
		Decidual arterial thrombosis	0	1	0.31
	FVM	Avascular villi small foci	1	1	1.0
		Avascular villi intermediate foci	1	0	0.31
		Fetal vascular thrombosis	1	6	**0.03**
		Fetal vascular thrombosis—umbilical cord	0	5	**0.02**
		Fetal vascular intramural fibrin deposition (non-occlusive)	0	2	0.14
		Vascular ectasia	2	1	0.54
	DVM	Delayed villous maturation (focal - <30%)	1	4	0.15
		Delayed villous maturation (extensive - >70%)	2	2	1.0
	CI	Chronic deciduitis—non-intense	17	16	0.31
		Chronic deciduitis—intense	1	0	0.29
		Villitis—low grade	1	1	1.0
		Chronic intervillositis—low grade	3	2	0.63
		Chronic intervillositis—high grade	1	2	0.54
	MIR	Subchorionitis/chorionitis	5	6	0.72
		Chorioamnionitis—non-intense	2	0	0.14
		Chorioamnionitis (necrosis)—intense	0	1	0.31
	FIR	Umbilical vasculitis	2	1	0.63
	Others	Intervillous thrombi	3	1	0.29
		Villous fibrin (focal—<30%)	15	14	0.70
		Villous fibrin (multifocal 30–70%)	3	5	0.42
		Villous fibrin (extensive—>70%)	1	0	0.31
		Villous edema	3	4	0.70
		Chorangiosis	4	3	0.42

p-value refers to the comparison between COVID-19 vs. the Control group; relevant values are highlighted (bold). p-value < 0.05. MVM, maternal vascular malperfusion; FVM, fetal vascular malperfusion; DVM, delayed vilous maturation; CI, chronic inflammation; MIR, maternal inflammatory response; FIR, fetal inflammatory response.

The mean diameter of the COVID-19 group tertiary villi was 51.78 μm than 50.52 μm in the Control group (p=0.57).

The quantitative morphometric analysis of deposition of villous fibrin revealed an average area of 686.64 μm^2 in the COVID-19 group compared to 485.36 μm^2 in the Control group (p=0.08 - borderline).

The quantitative morphometric analysis of deposition of intra-villous collagen I and III revealed that COVID-19 group average areas were 36.40% and 63.60%, respectively, compared to 41.01% and 58.99% of the Control group (p=0.45).

HC counting revealed an average number of 1,7 CD68+ cell/villous in the COVID-19 group and 1,2 CD68+ cell/villous in the Control group (p=0.12).

DISCUSSION

New insights are being acquired on SARS-CoV-2 infection pathophysiology. COVID-19 is associated with an exaggerated inflammatory response, usually proportional to the disease's

TABLE 4 | Clinical and morphometrical comparisons between COVID-19 group (n=11) and Control group (n=11) placentas.

		Variable	Control	COVID-19	*p*-value
Clinical data	**Maternal**	Maternal age (years)	28.3 (18–42)	33 (26–42)	0.41
		Gestational age (weeks)	33.9 (23–39)	33.6 (23–38)	0.78
		Comorbidities	Hypertensive disorder (2) Gestational diabetes (2) Hypothyroidism (2) None (7)	Hypertensive disorder (2) Gestational diabetes (2) Hypothyroidism (2) None (4)	1
	Fetal	APGAR 1 min/5 min	6.5 (2–9)/8.7 (7–10)	6.6(0–9)/7 (0–10)	0.59/0.48
		Fetal weight (grams)	2656 (1,180–3,810)	2213 (610–3,030)	0.94
		Placental Weight (grams)	395 (243–573)	367 (135–650)	0.87
		Fetal/Placental ratio	6.74 (4.3–8.4)	5.96(3.63–7.55)	0.61
		Placental diameter (centimeters)	16.45 (13–19)	16.2 (12–20)	0.88
		Infant death	0	3	0.11
		Preterm newborn	7	6	0.66
		Term newborn	4	4	0.66
Morphometric variables	**HE**	Villi number	9.0 (5.3–14.5)	8.3 (4.7–10.9)	0.62
		Knots/villus	0.81 (0.6–1.0)	0.81 (0.6–1.0)	0.97
		Sprouts/villus	0.16 (0.1–0.3)	0.19 (0.1–0.5)	0.92
		Villus diameter	50.52 (43.4–58.8)	51.4 (45.5–63.0)	0.57
		Villus perimeter	288.42 (202.7–368.5)	271.93(213.8–358.4)	0.37
	HPt	Fibrin area (μm^2)	485.36(61.9–1749.6)	686.64 (170.3–2053.0)	**0.08**
	SiriusRed	Collagen I percentage	41.01(10.1–66.1)	36.40(13.8–68.6)	0.45
		Collagen III percentage	58.99(33.9–89.9)	63.60 (31.4–86.2)	0.45
Immunohistochemistry		CD68+ Hofbauer cell/villous	1.2	1.7	0.12

p-value refers to the comparison between COVID-19 vs. the Control group; relevant values are highlighted (bold). p-value < 0.05. HPt, phosphotungstic hematoxylin.

severity, recognized as a cytokine storm (37). Such inflammatory alterations cause endothelial damage and disruption in the coagulation system, which may play a direct pathogenic role in the disease (38). Reports of hypercoagulability, with d-dimer elevation, development of ischemic changes as gangrene of extremities, and even disseminated intravascular coagulopathy, are not uncommon. There is emerging evidence that at least part of COVID-19 manifestations is associated with a systemic thrombotic and microvascular injury (39–45). In pregnant women, when coagulation is already altered by pregnancy itself, the impact of COVID-19 is still the object of study.

In this context, placental findings are invaluable. To date, histopathological alterations described encompass maternal vascular malperfusion (MVM) features, including low placental weight, accelerated villous maturation, decidual vasculopathy, and infarcts. The MVM findings are frequently observed in placentas from pregnant women with hypertensive disorders, such as gestational hypertension and preeclampsia, and have been associated with oligohydramnios, preterm birth, and stillbirth. Fetal vascular malperfusion (FVM) alterations have been described as well, such as focal thrombosis of fetal placental vessels (30–34, 46). However, various authors did not identify a correlation between placental lesions and maternal infection, notably when the samples analyzed were obtained from uninfected placentas and infants (47).

Interestingly, in cases with confirmed transplacental infection, inflammatory alterations were more frequently observed, particularly chronic histiocytic intervillositis with trophoblast necrosis. In these cases, SARS-CoV-2 was detected in the syncytiotrophoblast by immunohistochemistry and or RNA *in situ* hybridization (48, 49). It is not yet clear if the syncytiotrophoblast destruction is caused by a direct viral effect or is secondary to inflammatory or ischemic injury. Whichever mechanism is involved, the damage of this protective villous layer can facilitate fetal infection.

Recognition of the disease's impact on the placenta, and the maternal-fetal response's nature, may help understand the processes involved in pathogenesis, and ultimately, it may lead to an explanation for an adverse outcome.

Maternal Clinical Profile and SARS-CoV-2 Testing Results

There were no significant differences in maternal age, gestational age at delivery, and maternal comorbidities profile between groups, thus corroborating that matching variables were adequately paired (p=NS).

In our COVID-19 group, the proportion of symptomatic patients is elevated (9/19, 47.4%). Since patients' recruitment was done at the beginning of the pandemic, almost half of our cases correspond to symptomatic patients. After the universal screening was adopted, asymptomatic patients were also incorporated into the study.

In the literature, pregnant women's outcomes have not been worse when compared to non-pregnant adult individuals. The severity of the COVID-19 seems to be related to existing comorbidities, like hypertension, obesity, among others (50–53), similarly to the general population. Most symptomatic patients in our study group had at least one comorbidity (8/9, 89%), including all the severely ill ones. In comparison, less than half of asymptomatic women had one comorbidity (4/10, 40%), and only one patient without comorbidities presented with mild symptoms (1/7, 15%—PC 20-5869).

Two women died from COVID-19 complications (PC 20-3282 and PC 20-5379). Both died shortly after hospitalization (three and one days after admission, respectively).

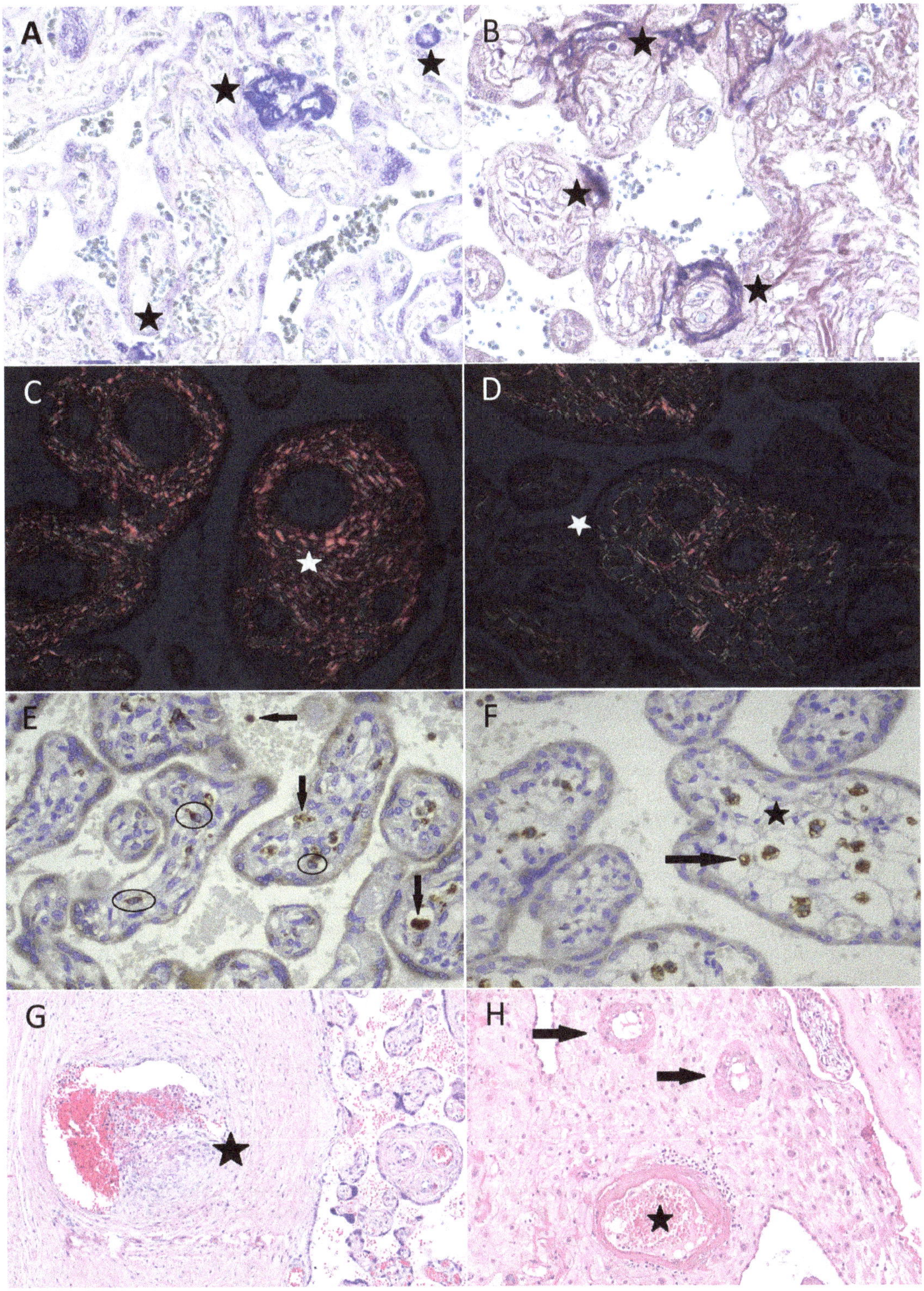

FIGURE 1 | Morphometric and morphological analysis of placental specimens from women infected with SARS-CoV-2 (COVID-19 group) and the Control Group. Fibrin deposition evaluation in COVID-19 group **(A)** and Control group **(B)** in phosphotungstic hematoxylin (star—deep blue amorphous material); both perivillous and intravillous deposition were included. Sirius Red: bright red collagen I **(C)** and green collagen III fibers **(D)** under polarized light. Photomicrography of immunostaining with CD68 (KP1 Clone, Biocare) in COVID-19 group **(E)** and in Control group **(F)**; eligible Hofbauer cells to counting (circled cells and those near the star). Macrophages outside villi and unspecific marking were excluded (arrows). Fetal vascular thrombosis **(G)** and decidual vasculopathy **(H)** in COVID-19 cases.

Newborns Clinical Outcome and SARS-CoV-2 Testing Results

The newborn outcome was directly related to the mother's health status among women with COVID-19. In patients with severe disease, the conceptus health deteriorated after Intensive Care Unit admission in all cases. Thus, not surprisingly, an adverse fetal outcome was more likely to occur in symptomatic patients (7/9, 77.7%) when compared to asymptomatic ones (3/10, 30%). Most of the asymptomatic patients had term deliveries (7/10, 70%) without recorded complications.

When considering patients with comorbidities (12/19, 63.2%), eight gestations ended prematurely (8/12, 66.6%). This proportion is slightly higher than what was observed in the Control group (5/9, 55.5%), even though clinical variables were adequately paired. Compared to the Control group, COVID-19 was also more frequently associated with maternal and infant deaths (although not statistically significant, p = 0.09).

Pertaining perinatal transmission of SARS-CoV-2, published reports to date suggest that it occurs, but is considered rare, with less than 2% of neonates with positive results until 24 h of life (54, 55).

Schwartz et al. proposed that positive samples for SARS-CoV-2 RNA collected within the initial 72 h of life can be considered diagnostic of early-onset COVID-19 infection. The probability that the infection resulted from the vertical transmission is even greater if the test is performed until 24 h of life (very early-onset COVID-19 infection). The authors also proposed that in cases where pregnant women and their neonates both tested positive for SARS-CoV-2, transplacental transmission could be confirmed by demonstrating the virus in fetal-derived placental tissue using immunohistochemistry to demonstrate SARS-CoV-2 antigens or RNA *in situ* hybridization to demonstrate viral nucleic acid (56). The World Health Organization recently published a manual with a definition and categorization of the timing of mother-to-child transmission of the SARS-CoV-2. Since various fetal samples are prone to cross-contamination, it preconizes rigorous methodology for sample gathering and strict criteria for establishing congenital transmission. Viral detection should be preferably performed in sterile samples, collected at birth, using nucleic acid detection techniques to confirm transplacental transmission (54).

From newborns' nasopharyngeal swabs and umbilical cord blood specimens tested, five resulted positive and were considered a possible congenital infection, or very early-onset COVID-19 infection, by the criteria above.

In two cases, the newborns were healthy until hospital discharge (PC 20-3744 and 20-5776). Two cases resulted in short-term neonatal deaths (PC 20-3282 and 20-5379); the families did not authorize postmortem evaluation in both cases. None of them exhibited symptoms attributable to SARS-CoV-2 disease.

In the fifth positive infant, a stillborn, SARS-CoV-2 RNA was detected in the umbilical cord blood sample collected immediately after delivery and in the placental FFPE tissue (PC 20-3364). An autopsy was performed, and evaluation of fetal tissues showed mild microglial hyperplasia, mild lymphocytic infiltrate, and edema in skeletal muscle. Other findings were unspecific and probably caused by intrauterine asphyxia. All fetal tissue samples tested negative for viral RNA. The authors (57) previously reported those results.

Morphologic Alterations

Our samples exhibited alterations spanning all major Amsterdam Placental Workshop Group Consensus Statement categories (MVM, FVM, delayed villous maturation, and inflammatory features). Most of them exhibited similar distribution between the two groups, which was expected due to the matching process. However, some results were unexpected.

Although maternal age and comorbidities were adequately matched, COVID-19 group placentas were more likely to show some MVM features when compared to controls, particularly signs of decidual vasculopathy. Decidual vascular mural hypertrophy was more frequently observed in the COVID-19 group (but did not reach statistical significance, p = 0.09). Ten patients exhibited this alteration (10/19, 56.6%), the majority without a recorded hypertensive disorder (7/10, 70%). In contrast, three of the five women with decidual vascular mural hypertrophy in the Control group had a hypertensive disorder.

The absence of spiral artery remodeling was significantly more frequent in the COVID-19 group (p=0,03). Six patients (6/19, 31.6%) exhibited this alteration combined with decidual vascular fibrinoid necrosis, mainly in women without the hypertensive disorder (5/6, 83.3%). In the Control group, those findings were noticed in only two cases, both in women with hypertension. Decidual arterial thrombosis was observed in only one case that ended with maternal and fetal death (PC 20-5379).

Accelerated villous maturation or increase in syncytial knots was similar in both groups, and those findings are supported by the morphometric analysis results discussed below. On the other hand, villous infarction and distal villous hypoplasia were less frequent in the study group.

Those findings are in consonance with previous reports describing higher decidual arteriopathy rates as a maternal vascular malperfusion feature in SARS-CoV-2 infected women. According to Shanes et al., though at least some of those alterations are thought to be chronic, its precise time of development is not precisely known, and as decidual arteriopathy appears to be more strongly related to COVID-19, it may be originating from a different mechanism (30).

Fetal vascular thrombosis was the FVM feature more frequently observed in our COVID-19 group. It was present in six cases (6/19, 31,5%), a significantly higher rate than in the Control group (p = 0.03). Of note, one case corresponded to the mother with Kartagener syndrome that evolved to maternal and neonatal death (PC 20-3282). In the Control group, this finding was detected only in one case, the mother showing no comorbidity (PC 20-5502). The distal lesions in villi indicative of fetal malperfusion were similar between both groups.

The frequency of inflammatory changes was similar between groups. Chronic histiocytic intervillositis, characterized by the accumulation of histocytes in the intervillous space, belongs to this category. In the context of COVID-19, such alteration is not frequently reported, and when present, was associated with adverse fetal outcomes and or with documented newborn infection by SARS-CoV-2 (30–33, 48, 49).

We identified chronic histiocytic intervillositis in four of our cases (PC 20-3282, PC 20-5379, PC 20-3364, and PC 20-4850). All four mothers with placentas having this finding had a severe COVID-19 course; two of them died. Their infants were prematurely born; three of them were positive for SARS-CoV-2 RNA in nasopharyngeal swab or umbilical cord blood samples. Those three died as well.

In the three cases that resulted in maternal and or infant death (PC 20-3282, PC 20-5379, PC 20-3364), features of MVM, FVM, and inflammatory changes were identified in various combinations. However, only in one case (PC 20-3364), MVM and FVM features were more intense and exhibited a broader distribution throughout the placenta than other specimens from both groups. This patient had a hypertensive disorder as well; because of that, those alterations cannot be attributed entirely to viral injury, even though COVID-19 may have a contributory role in the pathophysiology. Of note, chronic histiocytic intervillositis was observed in all three, two of them categorized as high grade (PC 20-5379, PC 20-3364).

Considering only the two cases that resulted in maternal deaths, placental findings were similar to those observed in the COVID-19 group, except for the presence of chronic histiocytic intervillositis.

Although the frequency of chronic histiocytic intervillositis was similar in COVID-19 and Control groups, this finding was not associated with adverse outcomes in the Control group. Interestingly, in the COVID-19 group, this finding was more frequently observed in placentas of severely ill patients, including those that died from COVID-19 complications, those associated with infant deaths, and with a positive SARS-CoV-2 RNA test in fetal tissues.

Morphometric Alterations and Immunohistochemistry Evaluation

Measurements of villi, such as diameter and perimeter, and counting of sprouts and knots in tertiary villi, aimed to evaluate villi maturity objectively (58, 59). Changes found in the placentas of the COVID-19 group do not seem to be different from those observed in the Control group, as far as maternal age, gestational age, and comorbidities are paired. Those data corroborate the morphological impression that villous maturity retardation or acceleration was not different between our COVID-19 and Control groups.

Fibrosis can be the final event after villi damage, following inflammatory, infectious, or vascular insults, such as described in FVM physiopathology (60). The relative amount of villous fibrosis estimated by evaluation of collagen I and III depositions with Sirius Red histochemical stain showed no difference between groups. There was no difference between groups for global collagen deposition analysis as well, meaning that there was no relative increase in the amount of villous fibrosis in the COVID-19 group.

The amount of fibrin deposited in the villi evaluated by the phosphotungstic hematoxylin histochemical stain could be more accentuated in the COVID-19 group since the difference between groups was borderline. However, such borderline difference between COVID-19 and Control groups was not perceived at the morphological analysis. In the qualitative evaluation, fibrin deposition seemed to be similarly increased in both groups, both in perivillous and intravillous topography.

The number of HC per tertiary villi was also similar between groups. This finding suggests that, at least in perinatally infected women, villous histocytes did not proliferate, and HC hyperplasia may not be as involved in the physiopathology of COVID-19 in the placenta as described for other viruses like Zika virus or HIV (28, 61–63).

In conclusion, pregnant women with symptomatic SARS-CoV-2 infection, particularly with the severe course, are more likely to exhibit an adverse fetal outcome, with slightly more frequent histopathologic findings of maternal and fetal vascular malperfusion, and chronic histiocytic intervillositis. The morphometric changes found in the placentas of the COVID-19 group do not seem to be different from those observed in the Control group, as far as maternal age, gestational age, and comorbidities are paired. Only the deposition of villous fibrin could be more accentuated in the COVID-19 group ($p = 0.08$ borderline). The number of HC/villous evaluated with CD68 immunohistochemistry did not show a difference between both groups.

ETHICS STATEMENT

The studies involving human participants were reviewed and approved by Comitê de Ética em Pesquisa em Seres Humanos do Hospital de Clínicas da Universidade Federal do Paraná. The patients/participants provided their written informed consent to participate in this study.

AUTHOR CONTRIBUTIONS

DP, AO, and VD contributed to collecting SARS-CoV-2 patients' samples and medical records in HNSG. IF and JL contributed to the collection of SARS-CoV-2 patients' samples and medical records in CHC-UFPR. AZ and AF contributed to the RNA extraction and RT-PCR reactions in HNSG. MN, BC, and CD were responsible for the RT-PCR reactions in CHC-UFPR. ES was responsible for selecting the controls and contributed to the immunohistochemistry analysis. PR was responsible for morphological and morphometrical analysis, interpretation of data, and drafted the manuscript. JD and EH contributed to the literature review and morphometrical analysis (Phosphotungstic hematoxylin). FD contributed with morphometrical analysis (Sirius

Red). AP contributed with morphological analysis. SR supported the experiments and contributed to the RT-PCR reactions in CHC-UFPR. CM-S supported the experiments and was responsible for the statistical analysis. NC contributed to the manuscript revision. LN supported the experiments, supervised the project, and was a significant contributor to the manuscript review. All authors contributed to the article and approved the submitted version.

FUNDING

This research was funded by productivity research level 2 of the National Council for Scientific and Technological Development (CNPq) and by Pontifícia Universidade Católica do Paraná with resources from BRDE, Banco Regional de Desenvolvimento do Extremo Sul.

ACKNOWLEDGMENTS

The authors express their gratitude to Seigo Nakashima for performing the image acquisition from slides and support with software usage (ZEN Blue Edition and Image-Pro Plus 4) and Maurício de Oliveira and Katiucia Thiara Fantinel Picolli for histochemical and immunohistochemical techniques. Also, to CAPES, CNPq, and BRDE/PUC-PR for financial support.

REFERENCES

1. World Health Organization. *Coronavirus (COVID-19) Dashboard* (2021). Available at: https://covid19.who.int/ (Accessed April 26, 2021).
2. Petrilli CM, Jones SA, Yang J, Rajagopalan H, O'Donnell L, Chernyak Y, et al. Factors Associated With Hospital Admission and Critical Illness Among 5279 People With Coronavirus Disease 2019 in New York City: Prospective Cohort Study. *BMJ* (2020) 369:m1966. doi: 10.1136/bmj.m1966
3. Docherty AB, Harrison EM, Green CA, Hardwick HE, Pius R, Norman L, et al. ISARIC4C Investigators. Features of 20 133 UK Patients in Hospital With covid-19 Using the ISARIC Who Clinical Characterization Protocol: Prospective Observational Cohort Study. *BMJ* (2020) 369:m1985. doi: 10.1136/bmj.m1985
4. Zhu H, Wang L, Fang C, Peng S, Zhang L, Chang G, et al. Clinical Analysis of 10 Neonates Born to Mothers With 2019-nCoV Pneumonia. *Transl Pediatr* (2020) 9(1):51–60. doi: 10.21037/tp.2020.02.06
5. Zeng H, Xu C, Fan J, Tang Y, Deng Q, Zhang W, et al. Antibodies in Infants Born to Mothers With COVID-19 Pneumonia. *JAMA* (2020) 323(18):1848–9. doi: 10.1001/jama.2020.4861
6. Dong L, Tian J, He S, Zhu C, Wang J, Liu C, et al. Possible Vertical Transmission of SARS-CoV-2 From an Infected Mother to Her Newborn. *JAMA* (2020) 323(18):1846–8. doi: 10.1001/jama.2020.4621
7. Alzamora MC, Paredes T, Caceres D, Webb CM, Valdez LM, La Rosa M. Severe COVID-19 During Pregnancy and Possible Vertical Transmission. *Am J Perinatol* (2020) 37(8):861–5. doi: 10.1055/s-0040-1710050
8. Zeng L, Xia S, Yuan W, Yan K, Xiao F, Shao J, et al. Neonatal Early-Onset Infection With SARS-CoV-2 in 33 Neonates Born to Mothers With COVID-19 in Wuhan, China. *JAMA Pediatr* (2020) 174(7):722–5. doi: 10.1001/jamapediatrics.2020.0878
9. Hecht JL, Quade B, Deshpande V, Mino-Kenudson M, Ting DT, Desai N, et al. SARS-CoV-2 can Infect the Placenta and is Not Associated With Specific Placental Histopathology: A Series of 19 Placentas From COVID-19-positive Mothers. *Mod Pathol* (2020) 33(11):2092–103. doi: 10.1038/s41379-020-0639-4
10. Mulvey JJ, Magro CM, Ma LX, Nuovo GJ, Baergen RN. Analysis of Complement Deposition and Viral RNA in Placentas of COVID-19 Patients. *Ann Diagn Pathol* (2020) 46:151530. doi: 10.1016/j.anndiagpath.2020.151530
11. Smithgall MC, Liu-Jarin X, Hamele-Bena D, Cimic A, Mourad M, Debelenko L, et al. Third-Trimester Placentas of Severe Acute Respiratory Syndrome Coronavirus 2 (SARS-CoV-2)-positive Women: Histomorphology, Including Viral Immunohistochemistry and in-Situ Hybridization. *Histopathology* (2020) 77(6):994–9. doi: 10.1111/his.14215
12. Penfield CA, Brubaker SG, Limaye MA, Lighter J, Ratner AJ, Thomas KM, et al. Detection of Severe Acute Respiratory Syndrome Coronavirus 2 in Placental and Fetal Membrane Samples. *Am J Obstet Gynecol MFM* (2020) 2(3):100133. doi: 10.1016/j.ajogmf.2020.100133
13. Patanè L, Morotti D, Giunta MR, Sigismondi C, Piccoli MG, Frigerio L, et al. Vertical Transmission of Coronavirus Disease 2019: Severe Acute Respiratory Syndrome Coronavirus 2 RNA on the Fetal Side of the Placenta in Pregnancies With Coronavirus Disease 2019-Positive Mothers and Neonates at Birth. *Am J Obstet Gynecol MFM* (2020) 2(3):100145. doi: 10.1016/j.ajogmf.2020.100145
14. Lamouroux A, Attie-Bitach T, Martinovic J, Leruez-Ville M, Ville Y. Evidence for and Against Vertical Transmission for Severe Acute Respiratory Syndrome Coronavirus 2. *Am J Obstet Gynecol* (2020) 223(1):91.e1–4. doi: 10.1016/j.ajog.2020.04.039
15. Joudi N, Henkel A, Lock WS, Lyell D. Preeclampsia Treatment in Severe Acute Respiratory Syndrome Coronavirus 2. *Am J Obstet Gynecol MFM* (2020) 2(3):100146. doi: 10.1016/j.ajogmf.2020.100146
16. Gidlöf S, Savchenko J, Brune T, Josefsson H. COVID-19 in Pregnancy With Comorbidities: More Liberal Testing Strategy is Needed. *Acta Obstet Gynecol Scand* (2020) 99(7):948–9. doi: 10.1111/aogs
17. Lokken EM, Walker CL, Delaney S, Kachikis A, Kretzer NM, Erickson A, et al. Clinical Characteristics of 46 Pregnant Women With a Severe Acute Respiratory Syndrome Coronavirus 2 Infection in Washington State. *Am J Obstet Gynecol* (2020) 223(6):911.e1–911.e14. doi: 10.1016/j.ajog.2020.05.031
18. Pierce-Williams RAM, Burd J, Felder L, Khoury R, Bernstein PS, Avila K, et al. Clinical Course of Severe and Critical Coronavirus Disease 2019 in Hospitalized Pregnancies: A United States Cohort Study. *Am J Obstet Gynecol MFM* (2020) 2(3):100134. doi: 10.1016/j.ajogmf.2020.100134
19. Kirtsman M, Diambomba Y, Poutanen SM, Malinowski A, Vlachodimitropoulou E, Parks W, et al. Probable Congenital SARS-CoV-2 Infection in a Neonate Born to a Woman With Active SARS-CoV-2 Infection. *CMAJ* (2020) 192(24):E647–50. doi: 10.1503/cmaj.200821
20. Vivanti AJ, Vauloup-Fellous C, Prevot S, Zupan V, Suffee C, Do Cao J, et al. Transplacental Transmission of SARS-CoV-2 Infection. *Nat Commun* (2020) 11(1):3572. doi: 10.1038/s41467-020-17436-6
21. Sisman J, Jaleel MA, Moreno W, Rajaram V, Collins RRJ, Savani RC, et al. Intrauterine Transmission of SARS-COV-2 Infection in a Preterm Infant. *Pediatr Infect Dis J* (2020) 39(9):e265–7. doi: 10.1097/INF.0000000000002815
22. Baud D, Greub G, Favre G, Gengler C, Jaton K, Dubruc E, et al. Second-Trimester Miscarriage in a Pregnant Woman With SARS-CoV-2 Infection. *JAMA* (2020) 323(21):2198–200. doi: 10.1001/jama.2020.7233
23. Walker KF, O'Donoghue K, Grace N, Dorling J, Comeau JL, Li W, et al. Maternal Transmission of SARS-COV-2 to the Neonate, and Possible Routes for Such Transmission: A Systematic Review and Critical Analysis. *BJOG* (2020) 127(11):1324–36. doi: 10.1111/1471-0528.16362
24. Schwartz DA, Thomas KM. Characterizing COVID-19 Maternal-Fetal Transmission and Placental Infection Using Comprehensive Molecular Pathology. *EBioMedicine* (2020) 60:102983. doi: 10.1016/j.ebiom.2020.102983
25. Raschetti R, Vivanti AJ, Vauloup-Fellous C, Loi B, Benachi A, De Luca D. Synthesis and Systematic Review of Reported Neonatal SARS-CoV-2 Infections. *Nat Commun* (2020) 11(1):5164. doi: 10.1038/s41467-020-18982-9
26. Benirschke B, Burton GJ, Baergen RN. *Pathology of the Human Placenta. 6th ed.* Berlin, Heidelberg: Springer (2012). doi: 10.1007/978-3-642-23941-0
27. Garcia AG, Fonseca EF, Marques RL, Lobato YY. Placental Morphology in Cytomegalovirus Infection. *Placenta* (1989) 10(1):1–18. doi: 10.1016/0143-4004(89)90002-7

28. de Noronha L, Zanluca C, Burger M, Suzukawa AA, Azevedo M, Rebutini PZ, et al. Zika Virus Infection at Different Pregnancy Stages: Anatomopathological Findings, Target Cells and Viral Persistence in Placental Tissues. *Front Microbiol* (2018) 9:2266. doi: 10.3389/fmicb.2018.02266
29. Ribeiro CF, Silami VG, Brasil P, Nogueira RM. Sickle-Cell Erythrocytes in the Placentas of Dengue-Infected Women. *Int J Infect Dis* (2012) 16(1):e72. doi: 10.1016/j.ijid.2011.09.005
30. Shanes ED, Mithal LB, Otero S, Azad HA, Miller ES, Goldstein JA. Placental Pathology in COVID-19. *Am J Clin Pathol* (2020) 154(1):23–32. doi: 10.1093/ajcp/aqaa089
31. Baergen RN, Heller DS. Placental Pathology in Covid-19 Positive Mothers: Preliminary Findings. *Pediatr Dev Pathol* (2020) 23(3):177–80. doi: 10.1177/1093526620925569
32. Hosier H, Farhadian SF, Morotti RA, Deshmukh U, Lu-Culligan A, Campbell KH, et al. SARS-CoV-2 Infection of the Placenta. *J Clin Invest* (2020) 130 (9):4947–53. doi: 10.1172/JCI139569
33. Gulersen M, Prasannan L, Tam Tam H, Metz CN, Rochelson B, Meirowitz N, et al. Histopathologic Evaluation of Placentas After Diagnosis of Maternal Severe Acute Respiratory Syndrome Coronavirus 2 Infection. *Am J Obstet Gynecol MFM* (2020) 2(4):100211. doi: 10.1016/j.ajogmf.2020.100211
34. Smithgall MC, Liu-Jarin X, Hamele-Bena D, Cimic A, Mourad M, Debelenko L, et al. Third-Trimester Placentas of Severe Acute Respiratory Syndrome Coronavirus 2 (SARS-CoV-2)-positive Women: Histomorphology, Including Viral Immunohistochemistry and in-Situ Hybridization. *Histopathology* (2020) 77(6):994–9. doi: 10.1111/his.14215
35. Khong TY, Mooney EE, Ariel I, Balmus NC, Boyd TK, Brundler MA, et al. Sampling and Definitions of Placental Lesions: Amsterdam Placental Workshop Group Consensus Statement. *Arch Pathol Lab Med* (2016) 140 (7):698–713. doi: 10.5858/arpa.2015-0225-CC
36. Malaquias MAS, Oyama LA, Jericó PC, Costa I, Padilha G, Nagashima S, et al. Effects of Mesenchymal Stromal Cells Play a Role the Oxidant/Antioxidant Balance in a Murine Model of Asthma. *Allergol Immunopathol* (2018) 46 (2):136–43. doi: 10.1016/j.aller.2017.06.003
37. Fajgenbaum DC, June CH. Cytokine Storm. *N Engl J Med* (2020) 383 (23):2255–73. doi: 10.1056/NEJMra2026131
38. Nagashima S, Mendes MC, Martins APC, Borges NH, Godoy TM, Miggiolaro AFRS, et al. Endothelial Dysfunction and Thrombosis in Patients With COVID-19—Brief Report. *Arterioscler Thromb Vasc Biol* (2020) 40:2404–7. doi: 10.1161/atvbaha.120.314860
39. Lippi G, Plebani M. Laboratory Abnormalities in Patients With COVID-2019 Infection. *Clin Chem Lab Med* (2020) 58(7):1131–4. doi: 10.1515/cclm-2020-0198
40. Lippi G, Plebani M, Henry BM. Thrombocytopenia is Associated With Severe Coronavirus Disease 2019 (COVID-19) Infections: A Meta-Analysis. *Clin Chim Acta* (2020) 506:145–8. doi: 10.1016/j.cca.2020.03.022
41. Tang N, Li D, Wang X, Sun Z. Abnormal Coagulation Parameters are Associated With Poor Prognosis in Patients With Novel Coronavirus Pneumonia. *J Thromb Haemost* (2020) 18(4):844–7. doi: 10.1111/jth.14768
42. Benhamou D, Keita H, Ducloy-Bouthors ASCARO Working Group. Coagulation Changes and Thromboembolic Risk in COVID-19 Obstetric Patients. *Anaesth Crit Care Pain Med* (2020) 39(3):351–3. doi: 10.1016/j.accpm.2020.05.003
43. Ribes A, Vardon-Bounes F, Mémier V, Poette M, Au-Duong J, Garcia C, et al. Thromboembolic Events and Covid-19. *Adv Biol Regul* (2020) 77:100735. doi: 10.1016/j.jbior.2020.100735
44. Klok FA, Kruip MJHA, van der Meer NJM, Arbous MS, Gommers D, Kant KM, et al. Confirmation of the High Cumulative Incidence of Thrombotic Complications in Critically Ill ICU Patients With COVID-19. *Thromb Res* (2020) 191:148–50. doi: 10.1016/j.thromres.2020.04.041
45. Zhang Y, Cao W, Xiao M, Li YJ, Yang Y, Zhao J, et al. [Clinical and Coagulation Characteristics of 7 Patients With Critical COVID-2019 Pneumonia and Acro-Ischemia]. *Zhonghua Xue Ye Xue Za Zhi* (2020) 41 (0):E006. doi: 10.3760/cma.j.issn.0253-2727.2020.0006
46. Menter T, Mertz KD, Jiang S, Chen H, Monod C, Tzankov A, et al. Placental Pathology Findings During and After SARS-CoV-2 Infection: Features of Villitis and Malperfusion. *Pathobiology* (2021) 88(1):69–77. doi: 10.1159/000511324
47. Levitan D, London V, McLaren RA, Mann JD, Cheng K, Silver M. Histologic and Immunohistochemical Evaluation of 65 Placentas From Women With Polymerase Chain Reaction-Proven Severe Acute Respiratory Syndrome Coronavirus 2 (SARS-CoV-2) Infection. *Arch Pathol Lab Med* (2021). doi: 10.5858/arpa.2020-0793-SA
48. Schwartz DA, Morotti D. Placental Pathology of COVID-19 With and Without Fetal and Neonatal Infection: Trophoblast Necrosis and Chronic Histiocytic Intervillositis as Risk Factors for Transplacental Transmission of SARS-CoV-2. *Viruses* (2020) 12(11):1308. doi: 10.3390/v12111308
49. Schwartz DA, Baldewijns M, Benachi A, Bugatti M, Collins RRJ, De Luca D, et al. Chronic Histiocytic Intervillositis With Trophoblast Necrosis are Risk Factors Associated With Placental Infection From Coronavirus Disease 2019 (COVID-19) and Intrauterine Maternal-Fetal Severe Acute Respiratory Syndrome Coronavirus 2 (SARS-CoV-2) Transmission in Liveborn and Stillborn Infants. *Arch Pathol Lab Med* (2020) 145(5):517–28. doi: 10.5858/arpa.2020-0771-SA
50. Knight M, Bunch K, Vousden N, Morris E, Simpson N, Gale C, et al. UK Obstetric Surveillance System SARS-CoV-2 Infection in Pregnancy Collaborative Group. Characteristics and Outcomes of Pregnant Women Admitted to Hospital With Confirmed SARS-CoV-2 Infection in UK: National Population-Based Cohort Study. *BMJ* (2020) 369:m2107. doi: 10.1136/bmj.m2107
51. Breslin N, Baptiste C, Gyamfi-Bannerman C, Miller R, Martinez R, Bernstein K, et al. Coronavirus Disease 2019 Infection Among Asymptomatic and Symptomatic Pregnant Women: Two Weeks of Confirmed Presentations to an Affiliated Pair of New York City Hospitals. *Am J Obstet Gynecol MFM* (2020) 2(2):100118. doi: 10.1016/j.ajogmf.2020.100118
52. Blitz MJ, Grünebaum A, Tekbali A, Bornstein E, Rochelson B, Nimaroff M, et al. Intensive Care Unit Admissions for Pregnant and Non-Pregnant Women With Coronavirus Disease 2019. *Am J Obstet Gynecol* (2020) 223 (2):290–1. doi: 10.1016/j.ajog.2020.05.004
53. Kayem G, Lecarpentier E, Deruelle P, Bretelle F, Azria E, Blanc J, et al. A Snapshot of the Covid-19 Pandemic Among Pregnant Women in France. *J Gynecol Obstet Hum Reprod* (2020) 49(7):101826. doi: 10.1016/j.jogoh.2020.101826
54. World Health Organization. *Definition and Categorization of the Timing of Mother-to-Child Transmission of SARS-CoV-2* (2021). Available at: https://www.who.int/publications/i/item/WHO-2019-nCoV-mother-to-child-transmission-2021 (Accessed April 26, 2021).
55. Egloff C, Vauloup-Fellous C, Picone O, Mandelbrot L, Roques P. Evidence and Possible Mechanisms of Rare Maternal-Fetal Transmission of SARS-CoV-2. *J Clin Virol* (2020) 128:104447. doi: 10.1016/j.jcv.2020.104447
56. Schwartz DA, Morotti D, Beigi B, Moshfegh F, Zafaranloo N, Patanè L. Confirming Vertical Fetal Infection With Coronavirus Disease 2019: Neonatal and Pathology Criteria for Early Onset and Transplacental Transmission of Severe Acute Respiratory Syndrome Coronavirus 2 From Infected Pregnant Mothers. *Arch Pathol Lab Med* (2020) 144(12):1451–6. doi: 10.5858/arpa.2020-0442-SA
57. Stonoga ES, de Almeida Lanzoni L, Rebutini P, Permegiani de Oliveira A, Chiste J, Fugaça C, et al. Intrauterine Transmission of SARS-CoV-2. *Emerg Infect Dis* (2021) 27(2):638–41. doi: 10.3201/eid2702.203824
58. Jackson MR, Mayhew TM, Boyd PA. Quantitative Description of the Elaboration and Maturation of Villi From 10 Weeks of Gestation to Term. *Placenta* (1992) 13(4):357–70. doi: 10.1016/0143-4004(92)90060-7
59. Vangrieken P, Vanterpool SF, van Schooten FJ, Al-Nasiry S, Andriessen P, Degreef E, et al. Histological Villous Maturation in Placentas of Complicated Pregnancies. *Histol Histopathol* (2020) 35(8):849–62. doi: 10.14670/HH-18-205
60. Redline RW, Ravishankar S. Fetal Vascular Malperfusion, An Update. *APMIS* (2018) 126(7):561–9. doi: 10.1111/apm.12849
61. Schwartz DA. Viral Infection, Proliferation, and Hyperplasia of Hofbauer Cells and Absence of Inflammation Characterize the Placental Pathology of Fetuses With Congenital Zika Virus Infection. *Arch Gynecol Obstet* (2017) 295 (6):1361–8. doi: 10.1007/s00404-017-4361-5
62. Simoni MK, Jurado KA, Abrahams VM, Fikrig E, Guller S. Zika Virus Infection of Hofbauer Cells. *Am J Reprod Immunol* (2017) 77(2):10.1111/aji.12613. doi: 10.1111/aji.12613

63. Rosenberg AZ, Yu W, Hill DA, Reyes CA, Schwartz DA. Placental Pathology of Zika Virus: Viral Infection of the Placenta Induces Villous Stromal Macrophage (Hofbauer Cell) Proliferation and Hyperplasia. *Arch Pathol Lab Med* (2017) 141(1):43–8. doi: 10.5858/arpa.2016-0401-OA

9

Pregnancy Galectinology: Insights into a Complex Network of Glycan Binding Proteins

Sandra M. Blois[1,2]*, *Gabriela Dveksler*[3], *Gerardo R. Vasta*[4], *Nancy Freitag*[2], *Véronique Blanchard*[5] *and Gabriela Barrientos*[6]

[1] *Reproductive Medicine Research Group, Division of General Internal and Psychosomatic Medicine, Berlin Institute of Health, Charité – Universitätsmedizin Berlin, Corporate Member of Freie Universität Berlin, Humboldt-Universität zu Berlin, Berlin, Germany,* [2] *Experimental and Clinical Research Center, a Cooperation Between the Max Delbrück Center for Molecular Medicine in the Helmholtz Association, and Charité - Universitätsmedizin Berlin, Berlin, Germany,* [3] *Department of Pathology, Uniformed Services University of the Health Sciences, Bethesda, MD, United States,* [4] *Department of Microbiology and Immunology, Institute of Marine and Environmental Technology, University of Maryland School of Medicine, UMB, Baltimore, MD, United States,* [5] *Berlin Institute of Health, Institute of Laboratory Medicine, Clinical Chemistry and Pathobiochemistry, Charité – Universitätsmedizin Berlin, Corporate Member of Freie Universität Berlin, Humboldt-Universität zu Berlin, Berlin, Germany,* [6] *Laboratory of Experimental Medicine, Hospital Alemán, School of Medicine, University of Buenos Aires, CONICET, Buenos Aires, Argentina*

***Correspondence:**
Sandra M. Blois
sandra.blois@charite.de

Galectins are a phylogenetically conserved family of soluble β-galactoside binding proteins, consisting of 15 different types, each with a specific function. Galectins contribute to placentation by regulating trophoblast development, migration, and invasion during early pregnancy. In addition, galectins are critical players regulating maternal immune tolerance to the embedded embryo. Recently, the role of galectins in angiogenesis during decidualization and in placenta formation has gained attention. Altered expression of galectins is associated with abnormal pregnancies and infertility. This review focuses on the role of galectins in pregnancy-associated processes and discusses the relevance of galectin-glycan interactions as potential therapeutic targets in pregnancy disorders.

Keywords: galectins, pregnancy, placentation, glycans, preeclampsia

INTRODUCTION

During pregnancy, a delicately regulated interplay of endocrine, immune and metabolic processes is established in order to sustain offspring development. The coordination of a series of simultaneous events occurring at both sides of the maternal-fetal interface, including multiple signaling pathways driving cell growth and differentiation, vascular development, and immune regulation, is critical for a successful pregnancy outcome. At the maternal site, complex immunoregulatory mechanisms support active tolerance of fetal alloantigens while also remaining competent to elicit an effective response toward pathogenic insults (1). Throughout pregnancy the uterine vascular bed experiences dramatical changes with extensive remodeling of existing vessels and formation of new networks through the process of angiogenesis (2), allowing for the proper delivery of oxygen and nutrients to the developing fetus. In parallel, at the fetal site, the process of placentation relies on a complex interaction between invasive trophoblasts and maternal immune cells involving developmentally regulated periods of branching angiogenesis, non-branching angiogenesis, trophoblast differentiation and syncytium formation. Disruption of this normal pattern of placental development will directly impact placental function, with well-recognized consequences leading to suboptimal pregnancy outcomes (3).

The placenta sustains pregnancy by providing an immunological barrier between the mother and fetus, mediating the transfer of gases, nutrients and water and secreting a variety of hormones, cytokines, and signaling factors. As the active interface mediating maternal-fetal communication, the placenta plays a key role in sensing and modulating perturbations in the maternal environment and transmitting these stimuli to the developing fetus, with potential consequences in long-term offspring health. Indeed, it is now well-recognized than an adverse intrauterine environment during early development can modify disease predisposition in adult life as stated in the so-called "developmental origins of health and disease" or "fetal programming" paradigm. From the time of pioneer studies correlating birth weight and altered fetal growth with predisposition to chronic conditions as cardiovascular disease and diabetes (4), accumulating experimental evidence has contributed to the identification of multiple maternal constitutional and life style factors that can impact long-term individual health as well as the mechanisms involved in the transmission of these programming stimuli across the placenta (5–7).

Among the multiple mediators involved in pregnancy orchestration, the galectin family of β-galactoside binding proteins elicits great interest in the reproductive medicine field due to their unique ability to modulate diverse developmental processes and their potential use as biomarkers for gestational disorders. In this review we discuss the current knowledge on the role of galectins in supporting maternal adaptations to pregnancy and placental development, the impact of their dysregulation for development of disease and the potential application of galectinome profiling studies for diagnostic and therapeutic interventions in adverse pregnancy outcomes.

GENERAL ASPECTS OF GALECTINS

Complex carbohydrates on the cell surface and the extracellular matrix (ECM) encode abundant structural information that when decoded by specific carbohydrate-binding proteins (lectins) modulates interactions between cells, or cells and the ECM (8, 9). Based on their structural folds and canonical sequence motifs in the carbohydrate recognition domain (CRD), lectins have been organized into several families that include galectins (formerly S-type lectins), C-type, F-type, X-type, R-type, P-type, and several other families [Reviewed in (10)]. The taxonomic distribution of selected lectin families and their structural analysis have yielded critical information about their functional aspects and evolutionary history. While F- and C-type lectins—are largely heterogeneous and evolutionary diversified lectin families (11, 12), from a structural standpoint, galectins are relatively conserved (13, 14). Galectins are non-glycosylated soluble proteins characterized by a unique sequence motif in their CRDs and affinity for β-galactosides (13). Most galectins show preference for N-acetylated disaccharides such as N-acetyl-lactosamine (LacNAc; Galβ1,4GlcNAc) and related structures, whereas others have preference for blood group oligosaccharides (13–15).

Galectins are synthesized in the cytoplasm, and can be translocated into the nucleus where they can form part of the spliceosome (16, 17). Galectins can also be secreted to the extracellular space by non-classical mechanisms as they lack a typical signal peptide possibly by direct transport across the plasma membrane (18). Once secreted, galectins bind to carbohydrate ligands in the ECM and the cell surface, namely glycans that display LacNAc and polylactosamine chains [(Galβ1, 4GlcNAc)n] (13) (**Figure 1**). These include laminin and fibronectin, mucins, lysosome-associated membrane proteins, and numerous cell surface glycoproteins (19–22). Among the latter, galectins bind with high affinity to glycosylated cell surface signaling molecules such as α and β integrins (21) and the signaling mucin MUC1 (22). Integrins are the predominant laminin and fibronectin-binding proteins expressed on differentiating cells and represent important ligands for galectins involved in cell adhesion, motility and differentiation (21–24). For some galectins, the immediate binding to ligands in the oxidative extracellular environment is key to the stability of their carbohydrate-binding activity (25). The crystal structure of galectin-1 (Lgals1) revealed six key cysteine residues, some of which are located on the surface of the molecule on the face opposite to the CRD and are potentially susceptible to oxidation (26–28). Under non-reducing conditions, intramolecular disulfide bridges are formed resulting in conformational changes that preclude Lgals1 from forming a dimer (29). A critical interplay takes place between the oxidation state of cysteine sulfhydryl groups and the ligand binding and dimerization equilibrium, suggesting that specific binding to glycan ligands enhances dimerization and reduces sensitivity to oxidative inactivation (25). In addition, extracellular galectins can also recognize exogenous ligands, such as glycans on the surface of viruses, bacterial pathogens and parasites (30–33), a hallmark of other lectin types, such as C-type lectins (11). Furthermore, galectin secretion into the extracellular space upon stress has been proposed to constitute non-infectious "danger signals" that can initiate or exacerbate inflammatory responses (34).

STRUCTURAL ASPECTS OF GALECTINS

Galectins are characterized by their extensive taxonomic distribution and striking evolutionary conservation of primary structures, gene organization, and structural fold (11). The identification of galectin-like proteins in the fungus *Coprinopsis cinerea* (35) and in the sponge *Geodia cydonium* (36) revealed structural conservation of galectins in eukaryotic evolution. Furthermore, proteins sharing the galectin structural fold identified in the protozoan parasite *Toxoplasma gondii* (37, 38) and in rotaviruses (39–41) suggest either early emergence of the galectin fold or horizontal transfer from the vertebrate hosts, respectively. In general, galectin polypeptide subunits exhibit a relatively simple domain organization, housing one, two, or four galectin CRDs (11).

Although galectins have been evolutionarily conserved (42), the galectin repertoire in any given mammalian species is

Galectin	Classification	Glycan specificity	Source of expression	Function	Dysregulation in pregnancy disorders
gal-1	Prototype One CRD, which can dimerize	Asn; α2-3 sialylation; Ser/Thr	Endometrium/ decidua (stromal cells), uNK cells Trophectoderm/ICM Placenta (VT, EVT)	Immune modulation, embryo implantatiion, trophoblast invasion, angiogenesis	Placenta expression: ↑GDM, ↓ early onset PE, ↑ late onset PE, ↑ HELLP, ↓ SA Systemic levels: ↓GDM, ↑late onset PE, ↓SA
gal-3	Chimera One CRD fused with a non-lectin domain	Asn; Ser/Thr	Endometrium/ decidua (epithelium), Placenta (VT, EVT)	Immune modulation, embryo implantation, uNK cell regulation?	Placenta expression: ↓ IUGR, ↑ PE, ↑ HELLP, ↑GTDs Systemic levels: unknown
gal-8	Tandem-repeat Two different CRD	α2-3 sialylation; SO_4; GD1a; GM3; Ser; Ser	Decidua (stromal cells, glands) Placenta (VT, EVT, Syn)	ECM remodeling?, angiogenesis?, immune modulation?	Placenta expression: ↓ IUGR (gender specific) Systemic levels: unknown
gal-9	Tandem-repeat Two different CRD	Asn; GM1; GA1; Ser; Ser	Endothelium/decidua (Epithelium) Placenta (VT)	Immune modulation	Placenta expression: ↓ SA (Lgals9 D5/10), ↑/↓ IUGR (gender specific), ↑ PE Systemic levels: ↓SA
gal-13 (PP13)	Prototype One CRD, which can dimerize	GB-O; BG-A; BG-B	Placenta (Syn, endovascular trophoblasts)	Immune modulation, Arterial remodeling and vasodilation	Placenta expression: ↓PE, ↓GDM Systemic levels: ↑PE (↓ 1st trimester), ↑ HELLP, ↑GDM

FIGURE 1 | Summary of galectins' glycan specificity, functions and sources of expression in mammalian pregnancies. Question marks (?) denote putative functions (not yet experimentally confirmed in the context of pregnancy). BG, blood group; uNK, uterine natural killer; ICM, inner cell mass; VT, villous cytotrophoblast; EVT, extravillous trophoblast; Syn, syncytiotrophoblast; GDM, gestational *diabetes mellitus;* SA, spontaneous abortion; PE, preeclampsia; HELLP, hemolysis elevated liver enzymes and low platelet syndrome; GTD, gestational trophoblastic disease; IUGR, intrauterine growth restriction. ↑ and ↓ denote increased/peak and decreased expression, respectively. ● Mannose ● Galactose ■ N-acetylglucosamine ■ N-acetylgalactosamine ◆ Sialic Acid ▲ Fucose.

constituted by multiple galectin types, subtypes, and isoforms (13). Based on the CRD organization of the polypeptide monomer, mammalian galectins (and by extension, galectins in all vertebrate taxa) have been classified in three major types: "proto," "chimera," and "tandem-repeat" (TR) types (43) (**Figure 1**). Proto-type galectins contain one CRD per subunit and can form concentration-dependent non-covalently linked homodimers. Dimerization of proto-type galectins is key to their function in mediating cell-cell or cell-ECM interactions (44, 45). Two Lgals1 monomers interact via amino acid residues from a hydrophobic core that establish a dimerization equilibrium with a Kd of 7 μM (16). Both proto- and TR-type galectins comprise several distinct subtypes, all numbered in the order of their discovery, while chimera galectins include a single subtype (13). Lgals1,−2,−5,−7,−10,−11,−13,−14, and−15, are included in the proto-type. Chimera-type galectins, represented by Lgals3, have a C-terminal CRD and a proline- and glycine-rich N-terminal "tail." Ligand-driven interactions of Lgals3 subunits via the N-terminal domain mediate their oligomerization into trimers and pentamers (46). TR galectins display two similar—albeit not identical—CRDs connected by a functional linker peptide (47), and comprise the Lgals4, −6, −8, −9, and −12 subtypes. Galectin subtypes may be expressed as multiple isoforms in a single cell type or as tissue-specific variants generated by alternative splicing (13, 48), positive selection, and amino acid replacements in carbohydrate-recognition domains (49). Among the proto, chimera and TR galectin types, several subtypes, that include human Lgals1, Lgals2, Lgals3, Lgals9, and three galectins that cluster in the human chromosome 19 [Lgals13 (pp. 13), −14, and −16], have been recently investigated with regards to their potential roles in fertilization, embryo implantation, placentation, and the various stages of normal and pathological pregnancy (49–52).

The structural fold of Lgals1 and the amino acid residues of the CRD that directly or indirectly—via water molecules—interact with the hydroxyl groups on the carbohydrate ligands have been identified by the resolution of the crystal structure of the Lgals1/LacNAc complex (26, 27, 53). The Lgals1 subunit is a β-sandwich consisting of a 135 amino acid-long polypeptide that folds into two antiparallel β-sheets of five and six strands each (S1–S6 and F1–F5). This globular structure contains one carbohydrate binding cleft formed by three continuous concave strands (S4–S6) that includes all amino acid residues that interact with LacNAc and are responsible for the carbohydrate specificity of Lgals1: histidine 44, asparagine 46, arginine 48, histidine 52, asparagine 61, tryptophan 68, glutamic acid 71, and arginine 73 (27). Tryptophan 68 establishes a hydrophobic stacking interaction with the non-reducing terminal galactose ring. Additional water-mediated interactions between His52, Asp54, and Arg73 in the Lgals1 CRD with the nitrogen of the NAc group rationalize the higher affinity for LacNAc over lactose. The rigorous assessment of the galectins' carbohydrate-binding affinity has been enabled by biophysical approaches, such as microcalorimetry measurements and surface plasmon resonance analysis. For example, the dissociation constants of bovine Lgals1 for Lac, LacNAc, and thiodigalactoside measured by microcalorimetry were in the range of 10^{-5} M, with two binding sites per Lgals1 dimer (54). The overall structure of the Lgals3 CRD is very similar to the Lgals1 CRD although in the former the carbohydrate-binding site is shaped as a cleft open at both ends, exposing the GlcNAc of the LacNAc to the solvent (55). This extended binding site in Lgals3 results in increased affinity for polylactosamines and for ABH blood group oligosaccharides [Fucα1, 2; GalNAcα1,3(Fucα1,2); and Galα1,3(Fucα1,2)] (55). The structures of the individual N- and C-terminal CRDs of TR galectins, such as galectins-4,- 8, and−9, have been resolved by either crystallization or NMR spectroscopy. Results have shown that the two CRDs in the same galectin molecule are structurally similar but exhibit either different affinities for the same ligand such as observed in Lgals4, or different fold and specificities altogether, such as reported for Lgals8 (56–58).

Based on analysis of the galectin primary structure and intron-exon position in various vertebrate species it has been proposed that along the vertebrate lineages leading to mammals, galectins evolved by duplication of a primordial single CRD galectin gene that produced a bi-CRD gene, with the N- and C-terminal CRDs later diverging into two subtypes (F4-CRD and F3-CRD) of distinct exon-intron organization. Single-CRD galectins display the F3- (e.g., Lgals1, −2, −3, −5) or F4- (e.g., Lgals7, −10, −13, −14) subtypes, while TR galectins display both F4 and F3 subtypes (Lgals4, −6, −8, −9, and −12) (13, 42). In invertebrate species, galectins exhibit one, two, or four tandem-arrayed CRDs (59–61). In those invertebrate galectins that carry multiple CRDs, these are structurally similar but not identical, suggesting that they differ in their fine carbohydrate specificity (61). How the multiple CRD galectins from invertebrates relate to the vertebrate TR galectins remains to be fully understood, but a preliminary phylogenetic analysis revealed that individual CRDs of a four-CRD galectin clusters with the mammalian single CRD galectins rather with the TR galectins, suggesting that this gene is the product of two consecutive duplications of a single-CRD galectin gene (61).

FUNCTIONAL ASPECTS OF GALECTINS

As discussed above, TR galectins display two CRDs in a single polypeptide, that can interact with and cross-link multivalent ligands, either soluble glycoproteins or glycolipids, or ECM and complex glycans on the cell surface. Although proto- and chimera-type galectin subunits possess a single CRD, they can organize as oligomeric structures that also bind multivalent ligands with increased avidity (44, 45). The density of the cell surface glycans and their scaffolding (as glycoproteins, glycolipids or polysaccharides) modulates affinity of the CRD-ligand interaction via negative co-operativity (45), and can lead to ligand cross-linking, and formation of lattices that cluster these ligands into lipid raft microdomains (44). These interactions can promote reorganization or association of cell surface components, regulate turnover of endocytic receptors, activate or attenuate signaling pathways, and in turn, modulate cell function (44). Further, because galectin types and subtypes exhibit notable differences in carbohydrate specificity and affinity and bind a broad range of glycans that display the requisite topologies, the galectin repertoire displays considerable diversity in recognition properties that together with their distinct and unique tissue distribution and local concentrations, supports extensive functional diversification (13, 30). Thus, the biological function of a particular galectin may vary among cells, tissues and fluids, depending on their concentration, the availability and multivalent presentation of suitable carbohydrate ligands, and the redox properties of any particular intra- or extracellular microenvironment (30).

EARLY DEVELOPMENT AND TISSUE REGENERATION

The initial description in the early "80s of developmentally-regulated galectins in chicken muscle suggested that their biological roles were related to embryogenesis and early development. Further, the finding that chicken galectins preferentially recognized the abundant polylactosamines present on the myoblast surface and the ECM, suggested that galectins mediate myoblast fusion [reviewed in (14)]. Later studies suggested roles of murine Lgals1 and Lgals3 in notochord development and somitogenesis, and in skeletal muscle and central nervous system development (62, 63). In recent years, the increasing availability of null mice for selected galectins enabled their developmental phenotypic analysis. Although the phenotypes identified have been in some cases rather subtle, which hindered a rigorous assignment of the galectins" biological roles, the use of galectin deficient models and tissue-specific knockouts is one of the most complete available tools for the analysis of the biological role of galectins. In addition, rodents express a complex galectin repertoire; this was attributed to functional redundancy of the multiple galectin types and subtypes. However, as the binding properties and natural ligands of each galectin have been rigorously characterized in recent years, it has become clear that this is not the case, and their unique biological roles are being elucidated in increasing detail. In the past few years, Drosophila, *C. elegans*, and zebrafish (*Danio rerio*) have become useful model systems to address the biological roles of galectins (64–68). For example, antisense knockdown approaches in zebrafish embryos for a Lgals1 isoform (Drgal1-L2) revealed a key role in differentiation and development of the myotome (69). The zebrafish model was also useful to assess the roles of galectins in tissue repair and regeneration (53, 70). Experimentally light-induced retinal injury in adult zebrafish was used in combination with an antisense knockdown approach to demonstrate that photoreceptor cell death upregulates expression and secretion of DrGal1-L2 by stem cells and neuronal progenitors in the Müller glia, and selectively regulates the regeneration of rod photoreceptors (70).

GENOME ORGANIZATION OF GALECTIN FAMILY MEMBERS

While galectins are usually grouped based on their architecture, a potential relationship between gene location and function has been investigated (42, 50). Genes encoding Lgals1 and Lgals2, named *LGALS* in humans and *Lgals* in mice and other chordates, map to syntenic regions of chromosome 22 and chromosome 15, in humans and mice, respectively. Studies of the promoter sequences and expression of murine *Lgals1*, *-2* and *-7* revealed significant differences in the proximal promoter regions for putative transcription factor binding sites in these genes, which is believed to correlate with the ubiquitous gene expression of *Lgals*1 and a more restricted expression of *Lgals*2 and *Lgals*7 (71).

Members of the human galectin gene family are found in different chromosomes, including chromosome 1, 11, 14, 17, 19, and 22. Than et al. proposed that some of the human galectin genes clustered in chromosome 19 and expressed in villous trophoblasts, including *LGALS13, LGALS14, LGALS16*, are developmentally regulated by DNA methylation and induced by transcription factors that drive villous trophoblast differentiation and trophoblast-specific gene expression (49). In addition, dysregulation of these galectin genes with a potential role in immune tolerance to the semi-allogeneic fetus was proposed to be associated with preeclampsia (49).

Interestingly, the *Lgals*3 gene is different from other galectin genes in which gene duplication and inversion within a cluster has been reported. A single member has been identified per species hinting at a conserved function of Lgals3 during evolution (42). In addition, *LGALS3* contains an internal gene, which is much less abundant than *LGALS3* transcripts and is expressed mostly in peripheral blood leukocytes producing an entirely distinct protein from Lgals3 (72).

ROLE OF GALECTINS IN PREGNANCY ASSOCIATED PROCESSES

Expression profiling studies in reproductive tissues have shed important insights on the biological roles played by galectins in pregnancy orchestration, highlighting the importance of a delicate interplay between maternal and fetal sources of galectin expression for healthy outcomes (**Figure 1**). The following section provides a brief overview of the role of individual galectins expressed at the maternal-fetal interface in the establishment and maintenance of pregnancy.

GALECTIN-1 (LGALS1)

The functions of Lgals1 in the context of pregnancy are the best characterized when compared to other members of the galectin family (**Figure 1**), likely due to its high level of expression by decidual stromal cells and trophoblast cell populations which suggested an important function (73). Indeed, Lgals1 has been shown to play a role in a variety of biological processes highly relevant for pregnancy orchestration including angiogenesis, immune response regulation, cell adhesion, invasion, and cell cycle progression through intracellular or extracellular mechanisms (23, 74–76).

Lgals1 expression is observed in 3–5 days human embryos potentially increasing trophoblast attachment to the uterine epithelium (77). After embryo attachment as the trophoblast layer differentiates, Lgals1 localizes to villous cytotrophoblast where it may play a role in promoting syncytium formation, although this function has only been studied *in vitro* using the BeWo trophoblast tumor cell line (78, 79). More recently, Lgals1 has been demonstrated to drive the differentiation of mouse trophoblast stem (TS) cells *in vitro*, by enhancing cell migration and invasiveness associated with a shift in the expression of matrix metalloproteinases, epithelial-mesenchymal transition markers and the TGF-β signaling pathway (80). Circulating levels of Lgals1 increase significantly during pregnancy and several studies indicate the potential use of Lgals1 as a biomarker for miscarriage, recurrent fetal loss and preeclampsia (PE) (77, 81–84). Whether circulating Lgals1 retains carbohydrate binding activity within the oxidative nature of the extracellular environment remains unknown as Lgals1 exhibits exquisite sensitivity to oxidative inactivation (25, 85). In addition, a further question regarding concentration of galectins in serum or plasma is whether high picomolar concentrations are sufficient for galectins to act at a distance similar to circulating hormones (86). In this regard, some galectin-mediated cellular activities (e.g., Lgals3 and Lgals7) (87, 88) might be sufficiently sensitive to be elicited by serum levels of galectins.

Lgals1 is highly expressed in the most invasive trophoblast cells of the placenta and membrane bound Lgals1 has been proposed to regulate migration of primary trophoblasts and of an extravillous trophoblast (EVT) cell line (77, 89–91). Modulation of EVT migration by Lgals1 could be related to its interaction with the β1 integrin chain on the EVT membrane (90, 92–94, 94). Another reported ligand for Lgals1 on the EVT membrane is the mucin MUC1 (95). Expression of *MUC1* is increased during placental development and was found to be elevated in severe pre-eclamptic placentas (96) although the significance of this finding is unclear as MUC1 has been shown to have adhesive and anti-adhesive properties (97). Interestingly, adhesion and invasion of the HTR-8 SV/neo EVT cell line to ECM components is negatively affected by *MUC1* overexpression (98). In endothelial cells, the membrane protein neuropilin-1 was identified as a ligand for Lgals1 and the expression of neuropilin-1 in decidual cells, intermediate trophoblasts, and syncytiotrophoblasts has been recently reported (99, 100). The potential interaction of Lgals1 with neuropilin-1 in these placental cells could potentially have functional consequences for placentation. As stated above, besides interacting with glycoproteins on the cell membrane, Lgals1 interacts with glycoproteins deposited in the ECM and has been shown to have both anti-adhesive as well as pro-adhesive extracellular functions (23). In the placental ECM, Lgals1 ligands include fibronectin, laminin, and osteopontin, which are also integrin ligands (19, 101–104).

The importance of Lgals1 as a contributor to feto-maternal tolerance has been described by many investigators and has been extensively reviewed (51). Several immune cells with essential roles in the establishment and maintenance of pregnancy synthesize and respond to Lgals1, e.g., CD4+ CD25+ regulatory T-cells, which play a very important role in tolerating the immunogenic paternal alloantigens (83, 105–110). In addition, *in vitro* studies showed that Lgals1 regulates the expression of human leucocyte antigen (HLA-G) in EVTs demonstrating that Lgals1 contributes to tolerance via its interaction with immune and trophoblast cells (77).

GALECTIN-2 (LGALS2)

Lgals2 is predominantly expressed in the gastrointestinal tract and has been identified as one of the main gastric mucosal proteins proposed to have a protective role in the stomach by interacting with mucins (111). In addition, immune functions of Lgals2 have been proposed including its ability to induce apoptosis in activated $CD8^+$ T-cells and its effects on monocytes (112, 113). Lgals2 was shown to polarize monocytes and macrophages to a pro-inflammatory, non-arteriogenic M1 phenotype, and reduce monocyte motility. Interestingly, Lgals2 regulation of monocyte/macrophage phenotype were attributed to its interaction with the lipopolysaccharide-binding protein CD14 in a non-carbohydrate dependent manner (112, 113). Lgals2 expression in the placenta was reported in both VT and EVT cells and was shown to be expressed at higher levels in VT and EVT of male compared to female placentas. Interestingly, in cases of intrauterine growth restriction (IUGR), there was no change in expression in female placentas compared to controls; however, expression of Lgals2 in male IUGR placentas was reported to be decreased compared to controls (114). While these studies should be repeated with a larger sample number, they may serve to caution investigators for the need to take the gender of the fetus into account as an important variable when analyzing possible changes in galectin expression when comparing normal to pathologic pregnancies. In addition, *Lgals2* expression was decreased in third-trimester EVT trophoblast cells in cases of PE on the protein and mRNA level (115) and also significantly down-regulated in the VT and EVT trophoblast of spontaneous and recurrent abortion placentas (116).

GALECTIN-3 (LGALS3)

Lgals3 has been implicated in the regulation of innate and adaptive immune responses, where it participates in the activation or differentiation of immune cells and contributes to phagocytic clearance of microorganisms and apoptotic cells by macrophages (117, 118). Lgals3 has been reported to promote but also to inhibit T-cell apoptosis depending on whether it binds to glycoproteins on the cell surface (CD45 and CD71) or to intracellular ligands (Bcl-2) (119, 120). In the placenta, Lgals3 was detected in all trophoblastic lineages including villous cytotrophoblasts (CTB) and EVT with a reduction of Lgals3 expression observed from the VT to the trophoblastic cell columns (121). This pattern of Lgals3 expression correlates with the switch from a proliferative to a migratory trophoblast phenotype and while placental Lgals3 dysregulation has been associated with some obstetric complications including spontaneous or recurrent miscarriages, further studies are needed to understand its contribution to trophoblast biology (81, 122). In addition to trophoblasts, Lgals3 is expressed by maternal decidual cells (73). While showing a different expression pattern, both Lgals1 and Lgals3 have been proposed to play a role in cell-cell and cell-matrix interactions of trophoblast during placentation (121). Studies of the importance of Lgals3 in murine pregnancy by Yang et al. indicate that Lgals3 is expressed in the luminal and glandular epithelium and that an increase in Lgals3 is required for proper embryo implantation (123). In addition, Lgals3 affects chemotaxis and morphology of endothelial cells and stimulates capillary tube formation and angiogenesis *in vivo* (124). Therefore, besides its proposed roles in embryo implantation, immune regulation and trophoblast-matrix interactions, Lgals3 has a potential role in placental angiogenesis. It must be noted, however, that despite considerable research efforts over the past years, the precise physiological relevance of this lectin during pregnancy remains ill-defined. Comprehensive analysis of the placental phenotype, the regulation of vascular development and maternal adaptations in *Lgals3* deficient models could greatly aid our understanding of this lectin's role in pregnancy orchestration.

GALECTIN-7 (LGALS7)

Lgals7 is produced by the premenstrual and menstrual endometrial luminal and glandular epithelium, where it accumulates in menstrual fluid and has been proposed to act as a paracrine factor to facilitate post-menstrual endometrial re-epithelialization (125). While *Lgals7* mRNA was not detected in term placenta by real time-PCR, using immunohistochemistry, expression of Lgals7 was reported in the syncytiotrophoblast (STB), EVT and glandular epithelium in first trimester placenta, decidua and in the STB and endothelial cells of normal term placenta (50, 126). Menkhorst et al. suggested that Lgals7 may facilitate adhesion of the embryo to the endometrium and reported that the serum concentration of Lgals7 was significantly elevated in women (weeks 10–12 and 17–20) who subsequently developed PE compared to women with healthy pregnancies (126, 127). Another study, also explored the potential value of Lgals7 measurement as a biomarker and indicated that maternal serum Lgals7 levels had no value to predict the risk of spontaneous abortion (128). Clearly, further studies are required to confirm the expression of Lgals7 in placental cells and the potential usefulness of Lgals7 measurements in maternal serum as a biomarker for pregnancy pathologies should be evaluated with larger patient cohorts.

GALECTIN-8 (LGALS8)

Lgals8 is ubiquitously expressed and analysis of its expression in normal first trimester placentas indicated that *Lgals8* is expressed by VT and EVT, and is highly expressed in decidual stromal cells (129). Lgals8 has been referred to as an "angiogenesis regulator" in vascular and lymphatic endothelium by binding to podoplanin in lymphatic vessels and CD166 (ALCAM, activated leukocyte cell adhesion molecule) in vascular endothelial cells (130). The role of this galectin in placental angiogenesis has not been explored but an initial report indicates that Lgals8 is not expressed in the endothelium of the placenta (130). The human gene (*LGALS8*) encodes seven different isoforms resulting from alternative splicing but the functional consequences of *Lgals8* splicing are poorly understood (130). Pro-inflammatory and immunosuppressive functions have been both attributed to this galectin in different experimental systems but so far, no studies on its possible role as an immunomodulator during pregnancy have been reported (131–135). Potentially, Lgals8 could play a role in trophoblast cell adhesion and migration as was reported in other cell types, but experimental evidence for the regulation of trophoblast function by this lectin is also lacking (136).

GALECTIN-9 (LGALS9)

The tandem-repeat Lgals9 has been implicated in immune regulation through binding to TIM-3, CD44 and the cell surface protein disulfide isomerase (PDI) (137–139). This galectin is expressed by many cell types including epithelial cells of the endometrium, trophoblasts, stromal cells of the decidua, endothelial cells including those in the placenta, and several types of immune cells (140–143). Splice variants of *Lgals9* have been reported with six of them expressed in human decidua, which may differ in their biological functions (143–145).

Compared to non-pregnant individuals, regulatory T cells show higher level of *Lgals9* expression as pregnancy proceeds and the level of Lgals9 in serum is significantly higher in women with normal pregnancies compared to post-partum and non-pregnant female controls (146). Interestingly, the serum levels of Lgals9 in pregnancy varied with the gender of the fetus as was also reported for some inflammatory cytokines and pro-angiogenic factors; Lgals9 is further increased in the serum of women carrying a male compared to a female fetus (147, 148). Li et al. proposed that Lgals9 contributes to the generation of $CD25^{+}$ $FoxP3^{+}$ T regulatory cells in -circulation and in the spleen and that engagement of Tim-3 by Lgals9 in peripheral NK cells facilitates the immunosuppressive activity of these cells during the first trimester of pregnancy (149). Additionally, they report that the concentration of Lgals9 in the plasma of women with normal pregnancies is significantly higher from that in women suffering from recurrent miscarriages but caution should be taken as the sample size was small and fetal gender was not considered in these studies (149).

Recently, lower levels of Lgals9 expression analyzed by immunohistochemistry were described in trophoblasts of the DBA/2-mated CBA/J mouse model of spontaneous abortion/PE when compared to normal CBA/J × BALB/c matings, further showing that Lgals9 blockade promoted a significant imbalance of Th1/Th2 immunity in this model (150). Additionally, altered placental Lgals9 expression together with dysregulated Tim-3 signaling in distinct NK and T cell subsets have been suggested to mediate the abortifacient effects of mifepristone in mouse pregnancies (151). Furthermore, activation of Tim-3/Lgals9 signaling pathway promotes decidual macrophages polarization to M2 subtype, alleviating the PE-like syndrome induced by LPS in a rat model (152). In conclusion, while a role for Lgals9 in immune tolerance during pregnancy has been reported by a handful of investigators, more studies considering splice variants, fetal gender, and Lgals9 receptors on target cells are required to better understand the potential role for this galectin as a contributor of the systemic and local immune regulation during pregnancy.

GALECTIN-10 (LGALS10)

Prototype Lgals10, also known as eosinophil Charcot-Leyden crystal protein, appears to play an important role in the differentiation of neutrophils and the functional properties of CD25+Treg cells (153, 154). Subsequently, expression of this lectin at the maternal-fetal interface has been described mainly in the STB and to a smaller extent in the decidua during the first trimester, showing decreased levels in spontaneous abortion patients (116, 155). The precise physiological role played by this lectin in pregnancy is still unknown but interestingly, its expression is driven from a chromosome 19 gene cluster comprising also galectins −13, −14, −16, and −17, which emerged during primate evolution as a result of duplication and rearrangement of genes via a birth-and-death process (49, 50). Galectins in the chromosome 19 cluster show primarily placental expression and may be involved in the regulation of unique pregnancy associated processes, including maternal immune tolerance and villous trophoblast differentiation (49, 50, 156).

GALECTIN 13 (LGALS13)

Lgals13 is also known as placental protein 13 (PP13) and was first isolated from human placenta (157). This galectin is predominantly expressed by STB cells of the placenta, in which nuclear staining and strong labeling of the brush border membrane is observed (158, 159). Although originally reported to be absent in serum of pregnant women, Lgals13 is detected in increasing concentration in maternal serum as pregnancy progresses becoming undetectable 2–5 weeks post-partum (158, 160, 161). Besides being found in a soluble form in circulation, Lgals13 is also located inside and on all types of STB-derived extracellular vesicles (162).

Lgals13 has been proposed to have immune regulatory functions, and in studies in rodents it has been shown to reduce blood pressure associated with activation of endothelial prostaglandin and nitric oxide signaling pathways (163–166). The potential for Lgals13 as a useful biomarker for PE has been suggested by Burger and co-workers. They reported that in the 1st trimester, lower than normal Lgals13 levels were found in IUGR and PE, particularly in the early-onset form. In the 2nd and 3rd trimesters, higher than normal concentrations were found in PE, IUGR and in preterm delivery (PTD) (160). On the other hand, lower placental *Lgals13* mRNA and protein expression were found in preterm PE and HELLP syndrome, although the immunoreactivity of the STB microvillous membrane was reported to be stronger in these pregnancies than in age-matched controls suggesting increased membrane shedding (167). The usefulness of Lgals13 as a biomarker for PE has been questioned as late second-trimester Lgals13 alone does not increase the ability to predict PE when compared to second-trimester Doppler pulsatility index and other potential biochemical markers (168), highlighting the need to consider the interactions between different signaling pathways in disease pathogenesis when in search for sensitive, reliable biomarkers. In this regard, recent studies suggest that the kinetics of Lgals13 expression in PE would result from the concerted actions of this protein and antiangiogenic factors as sFlt-1 on the maternal vascular system, with a dual role for Lgals13: first in low levels acting as a priming insult promoting endothelial activation and angiogenic imbalance, and increasing later in the third trimester as a natural rescue response promoting maternal vasodilation to lower blood pressure (169). In the context of gestational diabetes mellitus (GDM), increased Lgals13 serum levels during the early second trimester and lower expression in trophoblast cells of the term placenta have been reported (170, 171). Dysregulation of *Lgals13* was suggested to contribute to an imbalance in inflammatory processes in the placenta during pregnancy and therefore possibly lead to GDM.

Interestingly, while Lgals13 has hemagglutination activity when tested with chicken erythrocytes, a recent report suggested that contrary to what was observed for other galectins, Lgals13 may not bind carbohydrates (172). Prior studies, however, had reported that not only the binding of Lgals13 to erythrocytes or T cells is carbohydrate-dependent (50, 173), but also that N-acetyllactosamine is the preferred disaccharide ligand for Lgals13 (50, 159). This inconsistency in the results from the aforementioned laboratories may reside in that Su et al. (172) had tested lactose as an inhibitor for Lgals13, as well as other carbohydrates, such as xylose and arabinose, that are unrelated to the structures recognized by most galectins. Nevertheless, the identification of natural ligand(s) for Lgals13 at the cell surface and extracellular matrix will be of great importance to better understand its role(s) during pregnancy (165).

GALECTIN-GLYCAN INTERACTIONS AS REGULATORS OF THE FETAL-MATERNAL DIALOGUE

Glycosylation is the most common and structurally diverse type of post-translational modification, affecting proteins, lipids and the extracellular matrix. Glycans play fundamental roles in most biological processes, thus it is not surprising that glycans are profusely expressed in the mammalian uterus (174). During implantation, the uterine epithelium and the outer trophoblast cell layer of the implanting embryo interact in a glyco-specific manner, such that perturbations of the system generally result in failure of implantation or poor placentation and compromised pregnancy outcomes. Glycans are essential functional groups that facilitate and influence the reproduction process. The synthesis of glycans relies on specific modification enzymes (glycosyltransferases and glycosidases) (**Figure 2**), and the glycocode expressed in a particular tissue is highly dependent on the cell type and its developmental, nutritional, and pathological state. The glycans within the glycome can have multiple functions during pregnancy. For example, N-linked glycans (attached to the nitrogen of an asparagine side-chain) play an important role in trophoblast cell invasion in early pregnancy (175, 176) and maternal-fetal tolerance (177, 178). O-Linked glycans (attached to the hydroxyl oxygen of serine, threonine, tyrosine, hydroxylysine or hydroxyproline side-chains) can influence recognition events during fertilization (e.g., sperm-egg interactions) (179). As a detailed discussion about the role of glycosylation—in pregnancy outcome is beyond the scope of this review, we will focus on modifications that affect binding and function of members of the galectin family during gestation.

Extracellularly galectins act by cross-linking *N*- and *O*-glycans on the surface glycoproteins of maternal immune cells, trophoblasts and endothelial cells at the fetal-maternal interface. As glycosylation often represent highly regulated post-translational modifications related to the physiological cellular status, alterations in glycan composition can fundamentally impact galectin activity (180–182). Given the prominent expression of galectins (e.g., Lgals1 and Lgals3) at the fetal-maternal interface, studies designed to examine the relevance of cell surface glycans on maternal/ placental compartments are of key importance. In a physiological context, enhanced expression of N-acetylglucosaminyl transferase V [GnTV, encoded by the *Mgat5* gene (**Figure 2**)] was found in placentas from the first trimester compared with those from full-term pregnancies (175). GnTV generates β1-6-N-acetylglucosamine branches in complex N-glycans which are recognized by Lgals1. LacNAc motives are a glycan signature of EVT (91, 183) as their presence was detected not only on their surface but also on their secretion product HLA-G (91, 184). Since Lgals1 promotes trophoblast invasion and EVT differentiation during early pregnancy (90), it is possible that the increased activity of GnTV results in enhanced Lgals1 signaling (176); particularly, by promoting the interaction of Lgals1 with β1 integrin at the trophoblast cell membrane (94, 176, 185–190) (**Figure 3**). Furthermore, the presence of (β-6) branches and the expression of the glycosyltransferase GnTV involved in the generation of these glycan structures were reduced in villous tissues from early spontaneous miscarriages in comparison with healthy pregnancy villous tissues (191). Thus, differences in the glycan composition of trophoblast related-proteins at the same gestational age could be important disease biomarkers that should be further explored with newly available mass spectroscopy techniques. Indeed, the expression of GnTV was reported to be elevated in PE placentas compared to normal placentas (192). We have shown that *Lgals1* expression is increased in late onset PE and could represent a compensatory mechanism of the trophoblast to overcome the severe inflammation microenvironment that characterizes PE disease (74) (**Figure 3**). This is an interesting link to the metabolic status of trophoblast cells, which is mediated by the intracellular levels of GnTV that affect quality and branching of complex N-glycans and therefore regulate galectin binding.

During pregnancy the STB layer of the placenta releases extracellular vesicles (STBEV) containing a complex cargo of RNAs, proteins, lipids, and also glycans into the maternal

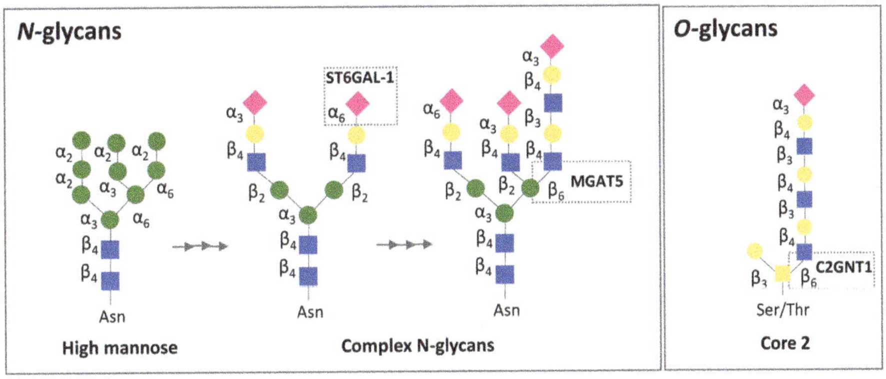

FIGURE 2 | Simplified schematic representation of *N*-and *O*-glycan biosynthesis focusing on galectin-1 binding affinity. N-glycans are attached to asparagine (Asn) residues, whereas O-glycans are attached to either serine (Ser) or threonine (Thr) residues. Gal-1 recognizes galactose on complex *N*-glycans and sialylation on the terminal galactose in the α2,6-linkage, but not in the α2,3-linkage, prevents the binding of gal-I. Regarding *O*-glycans, gal-1 binds to the N-acetyllactosamine (LacNAc) motif in core 2 *O*-glycans. ST6GAL-1, β-galactoside α2,6-sialyltransferase 1; *MGATS*, α1,6-mannosylglycoprotein 6β-N-acetylglucosaminyltransferase; *C2GnT*, core 2 β1,6 N-acetylglucosaminyltransferase.

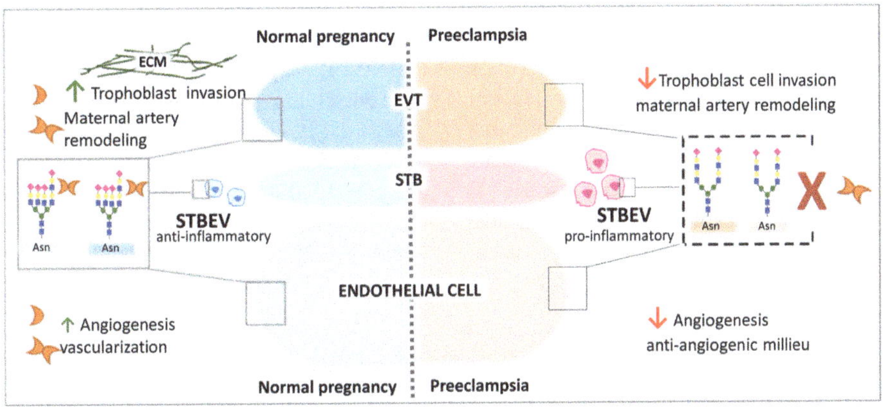

FIGURE 3 | Galectin-1-Giycan axis in the control of pregnancy protective programs. Galectin-1 regulates key process during the course of normal gestation including trophoblast invasion, maternal immune regulation, and angiogenesis. Relevant examples are illustrated. During Preeclampsia an aberrant α2-6 sialylation decorates α5β1integrin on the cell surface of EVT trophoblast, cell surface of STVEV released from the STB trophoblast and on endothelial cells. The high expression of α2-6 sialylated *N*-glycans impairs gal-1-mediated trophoblast ETV cell migration process interfering with the binding to the ECM and subsequently invasion. High α2-6 sialylation on STBEV and impaired gal-I binding might contribute to the pro-inflammatory milieu in maternal circulation and endothelial dysfunction. On vascular endothelial cells, the aberrant α2-6 sialylation may disrupt gal-1-mediated angiogenesis and early vascularization promoting the anti-angiogenesis status typical of the syndrome.

circulation potentially to induce maternal immune adaption. Under pathological conditions such as preeclampsia, however, STBEV exhibit a differential glycan composition compared to uneventful pregnancies. In particular, STBEV derived from PE placentas depict an increased content α2-6-linked sialic acid (193). The presence of α2-6-linked sialic acid on cell surface glycoproteins—is mainly determined—by the activity of the sialyltransferase gene *ST6GAL1* and results in blocking of Lgals1 signaling (194, 195). The selective glycosyltransferase expression (e.g., ST6Gal-1) on trophoblast cells may be an early pathological mechanism of masking Lgals1 activity in modulating the maternal immune response to the developing embryo. Moreover, an increased α2-6 sialylation was observed on the STB layer and also in placenta vessels derived from pregnancies complicated with hypertensive disorders including superimposed PE, PE, and PE + HELLP (196). This is important since high α2-6 sialylation on endothelial cells can reduce Lgals1 mediated angiogenesis (195), which is in line with our *in vivo* experiment showing that blocking Lgals1 mediated angiogenesis with anginex during early gestation in mice induced spontaneously PE development (74) (**Figure 3**). Moreover, the inhibition of Lgals1 binding by sialylation at the position 6 of galactose has been suggested to make Th1 cells resistant to apoptosis (197) and might contribute to uncontrolled maternal inflammation during preeclampsia. Thus, analysis of the glycosylation signature of trophoblast and placental vessels constitute a valuable approach to unravel the importance of galectin signaling through VEGFR2 during gestation.

CONCLUSIONS AND FUTURE DIRECTIONS

There is ample evidence showing that galectins are expressed widely at the feto-maternal interface. Their expression is regulated during pregnancy and galectins are highly specific to certain trophoblast and maternal cell types. Multiple galectin functions have been described in the orchestration of healthy pregnancy, which include maternal immune adaptation, placental development, and angiogenesis. Studies on the association of pregnancy pathologies with dysregulated galectin expression are still at an early stage, with most of our knowledge on the biological role of galectins in pregnancy being inferred from *in vitro* models and clinical correlations. However, sufficient evidence is already available to suggest galectins, especially Lgals1 and Lgals13, are promising candidates for further investigation aimed at understanding the pathogenesis of pregnancy complications including life threatening pregnancy related diseases such as PE. Because galectins are unique proteins with ability to recognize and decode a complex array of glycan motifs, future research could include: (1) a systemic study of the trophoblast cell-type glycome and galectin expression at the maternal-fetal interface in health and disease to determine whether glycomodifications on trophoblast cells that prevent galectin binding are responsible for the development of some pregnancy disorders and what is the galectin distribution in the maternal and placental compartments in health and disease; (2) a comprehensive analysis of the role of galectins in maternal circulation during pregnancy to establish whether galectins act at distance and if the presence of galectins in maternal circulation is a consequence of leakage from placenta tissue; (3) a deep analysis of galectin-glycan interactions either at the maternal or placental compartments with the goal to reveal the critical contribution of the physiological and pathophysiological galectin functions during gestation. In the years ahead, the development of novel *in vivo* strategies to test hypotheses related to the biology of galectin-glycan interactions during pregnancy represents a worthwhile pursuit, which will greatly advance reproductive medicine

AUTHOR CONTRIBUTIONS

All authors listed have made a substantial, direct and intellectual contribution to the work, and approved it for publication.

FUNDING

We acknowledge support from the German Research Foundation (DFG) and the Open Access Publication Fund of Charité—Universitätsmedizin Berlin. Research reviewed herein was supported by the DFG through grants BL1115/2-1, BL1115/3-1, BL1115/4-1 to SMB and the bilateral cooperation project 01DN16022 between Ministerio de Ciencia y Tecnología (MINCYT, Argentina) and Bundesministerium für Bildung und Forschung—Deutschen Zentrum für Luft und Raumfahrt (BMBF-DLR, Germany) to SMB and GB; Grant R01GM070589 from the National Institutes of Health, and Grants IOS-1656720 and IOS-1050518 from the National Science Foundation to GV; Grant R21AI120918 from the National Institutes of Health and Grant 401738 from the Collaborative Health Initiative Research Program at USUHS to GD.

REFERENCES

1. Hyde KJ, Schust DJ. Immunologic challenges of human reproduction: an evolving story. *Fertil Steril.* (2016) 106:499–510. doi: 10.1016/j.fertnstert.2016.07.1073
2. Cross JC, Hemberger M, Lu Y, Nozaki T, Whiteley K, Masutani M, et al. Trophoblast functions, angiogenesis and remodeling of the maternal vasculature in the placenta. *Mol Cell Endocrinol.* (2002) 187:207–12. doi: 10.1016/S0303-7207(01)00703-1
3. Norwitz ER. Defective implantation and placentation: laying the blueprint for pregnancy complications. *Reprod Biomed Online.* (2007) 14:101–9. doi: 10.1016/S1472-6483(10)61464-2
4. Barker DJ. *In utero* programming of chronic disease. *Clin Sci.* (1998) 95:115–28. doi: 10.1042/cs0950115
5. Jansson T, Powell TL. Role of the placenta in fetal programming: underlying mechanisms and potential interventional approaches. *Clin Sci.* (2007) 113:1–13. doi: 10.1042/CS20060339
6. Cheong JN, Wlodek ME, Moritz KM, Cuffe JS. Programming of maternal and offspring disease: impact of growth restriction, fetal sex and transmission across generations. *J Physiol.* (2016) 594:4727–40. doi: 10.1113/JP271745
7. Fajersztajn L, Veras MM. Hypoxia: from placental development to fetal programming. *Birth Defects Res.* (2017) 109:1377–85. doi: 10.1002/bdr2.1142
8. Kasai K, Hirabayashi J. Galectins: a family of animal lectins that decipher glycocodes. *J Biochem.* (1996) 119:1–8. doi: 10.1093/oxfordjournals.jbchem.a021192
9. Andre S, Kaltner H, Manning JC, Murphy PV, Gabius HJ. Lectins: getting familiar with translators of the sugar code. *Molecules.* (2015) 20:1788–823. doi: 10.3390/molecules20021788
10. Vasta GR, Ahmed H. *Animal Lectins: A Functional View.* (2008). Boca Raton, FL: CRC Press.
11. Zelensky AN, Gready JE. The C-type lectin-like domain superfamily. *FEBS J.* (2005) 272:6179–217. doi: 10.1111/j.1742-4658.2005.05031.x
12. Vasta GR, Amzel LM, Bianchet MA, Cammarata M, Feng C, Saito K. F-type lectins: a highly diversified family of fucose-binding proteins with a unique sequence motif and structural fold, involved in self/non-self-recognition. *Front Immunol.* (2017) 8:1648. doi: 10.3389/fimmu.2017.01648
13. Cooper DN. Galectinomics: finding themes in complexity. *Biochim Biophys Acta.* (2002) 1572:209–31. doi: 10.1016/S0304-4165(02)00310-0
14. Cummings RD, Liu FT, Vasta GR. Chapter 36: Galectins. In: A Varki, RD Cummings, JD Esko, P Stanley, GW Hart, M Aebi, AG Darvill, T Kinoshita, NH Packer, JH Prestegard, RL Schnaar, and PH Seeberger, editors. *Essentials of Glycobiology*, 3rd ed. Cold Spring Harbor, NY: Cold Spring Harbor Laboratory Press (2015–2017). p. 469–80.
15. Hirabayashi J, Hashidate T, Arata Y, Nishi N, Nakamura T, Hirashima M, et al. Oligosaccharide specificity of galectins: a search by frontal affinity chromatography. *Biochim Biophys Acta.* (2002) 1572:232–54. doi: 10.1016/S0304-4165(02)00311-2
16. Cho M, Cummings RD. Galectin-1, a beta-galactoside-binding lectin in Chinese hamster ovary cells. II Localization and biosynthesis. *J Biol Chem.* (1995) 270:5207–12. doi: 10.1074/jbc.270.10.5207
17. Tsay YG, Lin NY, Voss PG, Patterson RJ, Wang JL. Export of galectin-3 from nuclei of digitonin-permeabilized mouse 3T3 fibroblasts. *Exp Cell Res.* (1999) 252:250–61. doi: 10.1006/excr.1999.4643
18. Cooper DN, Barondes SH. Evidence for export of a muscle lectin from cytosol to extracellular matrix and for a novel secretory mechanism. *J Cell Biol.* (1990) 110:1681–91. doi: 10.1083/jcb.110.5.1681
19. Ozeki Y, Matsui T, Yamamoto Y, Funahashi M, Hamako J, Titani K. Tissue fibronectin is an endogenous ligand for galectin-1. *Glycobiology.* (1995) 5:255–61. doi: 10.1093/glycob/5.2.255

20. Parsons MJ, Pollard SM, Saude L, Feldman B, Coutinho P, Hirst EM, et al. Zebrafish mutants identify an essential role for laminins in notochord formation. *Development.* (2002) 129:3137–46.
21. Nabi IR, Shankar J, Dennis JW. The galectin lattice at a glance. *J Cell Sci.* (2015) 128:2213–9. doi: 10.1242/jcs.151159
22. Piyush T, Chacko AR, Sindrewicz P, Hilkens J, Rhodes JM, Yu LG. Interaction of galectin-3 with MUC1 on cell surface promotes EGFR dimerization and activation in human epithelial cancer cells. *Cell Death Differ.* (2017) 24:1937–47. doi: 10.1038/cdd.2017.119
23. Elola MT, Wolfenstein-Todel C, Troncoso MF, Vasta GR, Rabinovich GA. Galectins: matricellular glycan-binding proteins linking cell adhesion, migration, and survival. *Cell Mol Life Sci.* (2007) 64:1679–700. doi: 10.1007/s00018-007-7044-8
24. Markowska AI, Cao Z, Panjwani N. Glycobiology of ocular angiogenesis. *Glycobiology.* (2014) 24:1275–82. doi: 10.1093/glycob/cwu078
25. Stowell SR, Cho M, Feasley CL, Arthur CM, Song X, Colucci JK, et al. Ligand reduces galectin-1 sensitivity to oxidative inactivation by enhancing dimer formation. *J Biol Chem.* (2009) 284:4989–99. doi: 10.1074/jbc.M808925200
26. Lobsanov YD, Gitt MA, Leffler H, Barondes SH, Rini JM. X-ray crystal structure of the human dimeric S-Lac lectin, L-14-II, in complex with lactose at 2.9-A resolution. *J Biol Chem.* (1993) 268:27034–8. doi: 10.2210/pdb1hlc/pdb
27. Liao DI, Kapadia G, Ahmed H, Vasta GR, Herzberg O. Structure of S-lectin, a developmentally regulated vertebrate beta-galactoside-binding protein. *Proc Natl Acad Sci USA.* (1994) 91:1428–32. doi: 10.1073/pnas.91.4.1428
28. Di Lella S, Marti MA, Croci DO, Guardia CM, Diaz-Ricci JC, Rabinovich GA, et al. Linking the structure and thermal stability of beta-galactoside-binding protein galectin-1 to ligand binding and dimerization equilibria. *Biochemistry.* (2010) 49:7652–8. doi: 10.1021/bi100356g
29. Lopez-Lucendo MF, Solis D, Andre S, Hirabayashi J, Kasai K, Kaltner H, et al. Growth-regulatory human galectin-1: crystallographic characterization of the structural changes induced by single-site mutations and their impact on the thermodynamics of ligand binding. *J Mol Biol.* (2004) 343:957–70. doi: 10.1016/j.jmb.2004.08.078
30. Vasta GR. Roles of galectins in infection. *Nat Rev Microbiol.* (2009) 7:424–38. doi: 10.1038/nrmicro2146
31. Cerliani JP, Stowell SR, Mascanfroni ID, Arthur CM, Cummings RD, Rabinovich GA. Expanding the universe of cytokines and pattern recognition receptors: galectins and glycans in innate immunity. *J Clin Immunol.* (2011) 31:10–21. doi: 10.1007/s10875-010-9494-2
32. Vasta GR. Galectins as pattern recognition receptors: structure, function, and evolution. *Adv Exp Med Biol.* (2012) 946:21–36. doi: 10.1007/978-1-4614-0106-3_2
33. Thiemann S, Baum LG. Galectins and immune responses-just how do they do those things they do? *Annu Rev Immunol.* (2016) 34:243–64. doi: 10.1146/annurev-immunol-041015-055402
34. Sato S, St-Pierre C, Bhaumik P, Nieminen J. Galectins in innate immunity: dual functions of host soluble beta-galactoside-binding lectins as damage-associated molecular patterns (DAMPs) and as receptors for pathogen-associated molecular patterns (PAMPs). *Immunol Rev.* (2009) 230:172–87. doi: 10.1111/j.1600-065X.2009.00790.x
35. Walser PJ, Kues U, Aebi M, Kunzler M. Ligand interactions of the *Coprinopsis cinerea* galectins. *Fungal Genet Biol.* (2005) 42:293–305. doi: 10.1016/j.fgb.2004.12.004
36. Stalz H, Roth U, Schleuder D, Macht M, Haebel S, Strupat K, et al. The *Geodia cydonium* galectin exhibits prototype and chimera-type characteristics and a unique sequence polymorphism within its carbohydrate recognition domain. *Glycobiology.* (2006) 16:402–14. doi: 10.1093/glycob/cwj086
37. Saouros S, Edwards-Jones B, Reiss M, Sawmynaden K, Cota E, Simpson P, et al. A novel galectin-like domain from *Toxoplasma gondii* micronemal protein 1 assists the folding, assembly, and transport of a cell adhesion complex. *J Biol Chem.* (2005) 280:38583–91. doi: 10.1074/jbc.C500365200
38. Huynh J, Dawson D, Roberts D, Bentley-Lewis R. A systematic review of placental pathology in maternal diabetes mellitus. *Placenta.* (2015) 36:101–14. doi: 10.1016/j.placenta.2014.11.021
39. Dormitzer PR, Sun ZY, Wagner G, Harrison SC. The rhesus rotavirus VP4 sialic acid binding domain has a galectin fold with a novel carbohydrate binding site. *EMBO J.* (2002) 21:885–97. doi: 10.1093/emboj/21.5.885
40. Monnier N, Higo-Moriguchi K, Sun ZY, Prasad BV, Taniguchi K, Dormitzer PR. High-resolution molecular and antigen structure of the VP8* core of a sialic acid-independent human rotavirus strain. *J Virol.* (2006) 80:1513–23. doi: 10.1128/JVI.80.3.1513-1523.2006
41. Sun X, Li D, Peng R, Guo N, Jin M, Zhou Y, et al. Functional and structural characterization of P[19] rotavirus VP8* interaction with histo-blood group antigens. *J Virol.* (2016) 90:9758–65. doi: 10.1128/JVI.01566-16
42. Houzelstein D, Goncalves IR, Fadden AJ, Sidhu SS, Cooper DN, Drickamer K, et al. (2004). Phylogenetic analysis of the vertebrate galectin family. *Mol Biol Evol.* 21:1177–87. doi: 10.1093/molbev/msh082
43. Hirabayashi J, Kasai K. The family of metazoan metal-independent beta-galactoside-binding lectins: structure, function and molecular evolution. *Glycobiology.* (1993) 3:297–304. doi: 10.1093/glycob/3.4.297
44. Rabinovich GA, Toscano MA, Jackson SS, Vasta GR. Functions of cell surface galectin-glycoprotein lattices. *Curr Opin Struct Biol.* (2007) 17:513–20. doi: 10.1016/j.sbi.2007.09.002
45. Dam TK, Brewer CF. Effects of clustered epitopes in multivalent ligand-receptor interactions. *Biochemistry.* (2008) 47:8470–6. doi: 10.1021/bi801208b
46. Hsu DK, Chen HY, Liu FT. Galectin-3 regulates T-cell functions. *Immunol Rev.* (2009) 230:114–27. doi: 10.1111/j.1600-065X.2009.00798.x
47. Hirashima M, Kashio Y, Nishi N, Yamauchi A, Imaizumi TA, Kageshita T, et al. Galectin-9 in physiological and pathological conditions. *Glycoconj J.* (2002) 19:593–600. doi: 10.1023/B:GLYC.0000014090.63206.2f
48. Heusschen R, Schulkens IA, Van Beijnum J, Griffioen AW, Thijssen VL. Endothelial LGALS9 splice variant expression in endothelial cell biology and angiogenesis. *Biochim Biophys Acta.* (2014) 1842:284–92. doi: 10.1016/j.bbadis.2013.12.003
49. Than NG, Romero R, Xu Y, Erez O, Xu Z, Bhatti G, et al. Evolutionary origins of the placental expression of chromosome 19 cluster galectins and their complex dysregulation in preeclampsia. *Placenta.* (2014b) 35:855–65. doi: 10.1016/j.placenta.2014.07.015
50. Than NG, Romero R, Goodman M, Weckle A, Xing J, Dong Z, et al. A primate subfamily of galectins expressed at the maternal-fetal interface that promote immune cell death. *Proc Natl Acad Sci USA.* (2009) 106:9731–6. doi: 10.1073/pnas.0903568106
51. Barrientos G, Freitag N, Tirado-Gonzalez I, Unverdorben L, Jeschke U, Thijssen VL, et al. Involvement of galectin-1 in reproduction: past, present and future. *Hum Reprod Update.* (2014) 20:175–93. doi: 10.1093/humupd/dmt040
52. Blois SM, Barrientos G. Galectin signature in normal pregnancy and preeclampsia. *J Reprod Immunol.* (2014) 101–2:127–34. doi: 10.1016/j.jri.2013.05.005
53. Craig SE, Thummel R, Ahmed H, Vasta GR, Hyde DR, Hitchcock PF. The zebrafish galectin Drgal1-l2 is expressed by proliferating Muller glia and photoreceptor progenitors and regulates the regeneration of rod photoreceptors. *Invest Ophthalmol Vis Sci.* (2010) 51:3244–52. doi: 10.1167/iovs.09-4879
54. Schwarz FP, Ahmed H, Bianchet MA, Amzel LM, Vasta GR. Thermodynamics of bovine spleen galectin-1 binding to disaccharides: correlation with structure and its effect on oligomerization at the denaturation temperature. *Biochemistry.* (1998) 37:5867–77. doi: 10.1021/bi9716478
55. Seetharaman J, Kanigsberg A, Slaaby R, Leffler H, Barondes SH, Rini JM. X-ray crystal structure of the human galectin-3 carbohydrate recognition domain at 2.1-A resolution. *J Biol Chem.* (1998) 273:13047–52. doi: 10.1074/jbc.273.21.13047
56. Ideo H, Seko A, Ishizuka I, Yamashita K. The N-terminal carbohydrate recognition domain of galectin-8 recognizes specific glycosphingolipids with high affinity. *Glycobiology.* (2003) 13:713–23. doi: 10.1093/glycob/cwg094
57. Ideo H, Matsuzaka T, Nonaka T, Seko A, Yamashita K. Galectin-8-N-domain recognition mechanism for sialylated and sulfated glycans. *J Biol Chem.* (2011) 286:11346–55. doi: 10.1074/jbc.M110.195925
58. Krejcirikova V, Pachl P, Fabry M, Maly P, Rezacova P, Brynda J. Structure of the mouse galectin-4 N-terminal carbohydrate-recognition domain reveals

the mechanism of oligosaccharide recognition. *Acta Crystallogr D Biol Crystallogr.* (2011) 67:204–11. doi: 10.1107/S0907444911004082

59. Yoshino TP, Dinguirard N, Kunert J, Hokke CH. Molecular and functional characterization of a tandem-repeat galectin from the freshwater snail *Biomphalaria glabrata*, intermediate host of the human blood fluke *Schistosoma mansoni*. *Gene.* (2008) 411:46–58. doi: 10.1016/j.gene.2008.01.003
60. Shi XZ, Wang L, Xu S, Zhang XW, Zhao XF, Vasta GR, et al. A galectin from the kuruma shrimp (*Marsupenaeus japonicus*) functions as an opsonin and promotes bacterial clearance from hemolymph. *PLoS ONE.* (2014) 9:e91794. doi: 10.1371/journal.pone.0091794
61. Vasta GR, Feng C, Bianchet MA, Bachvaroff TR, Tasumi S. Structural, functional, and evolutionary aspects of galectins in aquatic mollusks: from a sweet tooth to the Trojan horse. *Fish Shellfish Immunol.* (2015) 46:94–106. doi: 10.1016/j.fsi.2015.05.012
62. Colnot C, Sidhu SS, Balmain N, Poirier F. Uncoupling of chondrocyte death and vascular invasion in mouse galectin 3 null mutant bones. *Dev Biol.* (2001) 229:203–14. doi: 10.1006/dbio.2000.9933
63. Georgiadis V, Stewart HJ, Pollard HJ, Tavsanoglu Y, Prasad R, Horwood J, et al. Lack of galectin-1 results in defects in myoblast fusion and muscle regeneration. *Dev Dyn.* (2007) 236:1014–24. doi: 10.1002/dvdy.21123
64. Ahmed H, Bianchet MA, Amzel LM, Hirabayashi J, Kasai K, Giga-Hama Y, et al. Novel carbohydrate specificity of the 16-kDa galectin from *Caenorhabditis elegans*: binding to blood group precursor oligosaccharides (type 1, type 2, Talpha, and Tbeta) and gangliosides. *Glycobiology.* (2002) 12:451–61. doi: 10.1093/glycob/cwf052
65. Pace KE, Lebestky T, Hummel T, Arnoux P, Kwan K, Baum LG. Characterization of a novel *Drosophila melanogaster* galectin. Expression in developing immune, neural, and muscle tissues. *J Biol Chem.* (2002) 277:13091–8. doi: 10.1074/jbc.M112105200
66. Vasta GR, Ahmed H, Du S, Henrikson D. Galectins in teleost fish: Zebrafish (*Danio rerio*) as a model species to address their biological roles in development and innate immunity. *Glycoconj J.* (2004) 21:503–21. doi: 10.1007/s10719-004-5541-7
67. Nemoto-Sasaki Y, Hayama K, Ohya H, Arata Y, Kaneko MK, Saitou N, et al. *Caenorhabditis elegans* galectins LEC-1-LEC-11: structural features and sugar-binding properties. *Biochim Biophys Acta.* (2008) 1780:1131–42. doi: 10.1016/j.bbagen.2008.07.003
68. Feng C, Nita-Lazar M, Gonzalez-Montalban N, Wang J, Mancini J, Ravindran C, et al. Manipulating galectin expression in zebrafish (*Danio rerio*). *Methods Mol Biol.* (2015) 1207:327–41. doi: 10.1007/978-1-4939-1396-1_22
69. Ahmed H, Du SJ, Vasta GR. Knockdown of a galectin-1-like protein in zebrafish (*Danio rerio*) causes defects in skeletal muscle development. *Glycoconj J.* (2009) 26:277–83. doi: 10.1007/s10719-008-9178-9
70. Eastlake K, Heywood WE, Tracey-White D, Aquino E, Bliss E, Vasta GR, et al. Comparison of proteomic profiles in the zebrafish retina during experimental degeneration and regeneration. *Sci Rep.* (2017) 7:44601. doi: 10.1038/srep44601
71. Lohr M, Lensch M, Andre S, Kaltner H, Siebert HC, Smetana K Jr, et al. Murine homodimeric adhesion/growth-regulatory galectins-1,−2 and−7: comparative profiling of gene/ promoter sequences by database mining, of expression by RT-PCR/immunohistochemistry and of contact sites for carbohydrate ligands by computational chemistry. *Folia Biol.* (2007) 53:109–28.
72. Guittaut M, Charpentier S, Normand T, Dubois M, Raimond J, Legrand A. Identification of an internal gene to the human Galectin-3 gene with two different overlapping reading frames that do not encode Galectin-3. *J Biol Chem.* (2001) 276:2652–7. doi: 10.1074/jbc.M002523200
73. Von Wolff M, Wang X, Gabius HJ, Strowitzki T. Galectin fingerprinting in human endometrium and decidua during the menstrual cycle and in early gestation. *Mol Hum Reprod.* (2005) 11:189–94. doi: 10.1093/molehr/gah144
74. Freitag N, Tirado-Gonzalez I, Barrientos G, Herse F, Thijssen VL, Weedon-Fekjaer SM, et al. Interfering with Gal-1-mediated angiogenesis contributes to the pathogenesis of preeclampsia. *Proc Natl Acad Sci USA.* (2013) 110:11451–6. doi: 10.1073/pnas.1303707110
75. Than NG, Romero R, Balogh A, Karpati E, Mastrolia SA, Staretz-Chacham O, et al. Galectins: double-edged swords in the cross-roads of pregnancy complications and female reproductive tract inflammation and neoplasia. *J Pathol Transl Med.* (2015) 49:181–208. doi: 10.4132/jptm.2015.02.25
76. Mendez-Huergo SP, Blidner AG, Rabinovich GA. Galectins: emerging regulatory checkpoints linking tumor immunity and angiogenesis. *Curr Opin Immunol.* (2017) 45:8–15. doi: 10.1016/j.coi.2016.12.003
77. Tirado-Gonzalez I, Freitag N, Barrientos G, Shaikly V, Nagaeva O, Strand M, et al. Galectin-1 influences trophoblast immune evasion and emerges as a predictive factor for the outcome of pregnancy. *Mol Hum Reprod.* (2013) 19:43–53. doi: 10.1093/molehr/gas043
78. Fischer I, Redel S, Hofmann S, Kuhn C, Friese K, Walzel H, et al. Stimulation of syncytium formation *in vitro* in human trophoblast cells by galectin-1. *Placenta.* (2010) 31:825–32. doi: 10.1016/j.placenta.2010.06.016
79. Hutter S, Morales-Prieto DM, Andergassen U, Tschakert L, Kuhn C, Hofmann S, et al. Gal-1 silenced trophoblast tumor cells (BeWo) show decreased syncytium formation and different miRNA production compared to non-target silenced BeWo cells. *Cell Adh Migr.* (2016b) 10:28–38. doi: 10.1080/19336918.2015.1089377
80. You JL, Wang W, Tang MY, Ye YH, Liu AX, Zhu YM. A potential role of galectin-1 in promoting mouse trophoblast stem cell differentiation. *Mol Cell Endocrinol.* (2018) 470:228–39. doi: 10.1016/j.mce.2017.11.003
81. Jeschke U, Mayr D, Schiessl B, Mylonas I, Schulze S, Kuhn C, et al. Expression of galectin-1,−3 (gal-1, gal-3) and the Thomsen-Friedenreich (TF) antigen in normal, IUGR, preeclamptic and HELLP placentas. *Placenta.* (2007) 28:1165–73. doi: 10.1016/j.placenta.2007.06.006
82. Than NG, Erez O, Wildman DE, Tarca AL, Edwin SS, Abbas A, et al. Severe preeclampsia is characterized by increased placental expression of galectin-1. *J Matern Fetal Neonatal Med.* (2008b) 21:429–42. doi: 10.1080/14767050802041961
83. Ramhorst RE, Giribaldi L, Fraccaroli L, Toscano MA, Stupirski JC, Romero MD, et al. Galectin-1 confers immune privilege to human trophoblast: implications in recurrent fetal loss. *Glycobiology.* (2012) 22:1374–86. doi: 10.1093/glycob/cws104
84. Schnabel A, Blois SM, Meint P, Freitag N, Ernst W, Barrientos G, et al. Elevated systemic galectin-1 levels characterize HELLP syndrome. *J Reprod Immunol.* (2016) 114:38–43. doi: 10.1016/j.jri.2016.02.002
85. Guardia CM, Caramelo JJ, Trujillo M, Mendez-Huergo SP, Radi R, Estrin DA, et al. Structural basis of redox-dependent modulation of galectin-1 dynamics and function. *Glycobiology.* (2014) 24:428–41. doi: 10.1093/glycob/cwu008
86. Johannes L, Jacob R, Leffler H. Galectins at a glance. *J Cell Sci.* (2018) 131:jcs208884. doi: 10.1242/jcs.208884
87. Lakshminarayan R, Wunder C, Becken U, Howes MT, Benzing C, Arumugam S, et al. Galectin-3 drives glycosphingolipid-dependent biogenesis of clathrin-independent carriers. *Nat Cell Biol.* (2014) 16:595–606. doi: 10.1038/ncb2970
88. Advedissian T, Proux-Gillardeaux V, Nkosi R, Peyret G, Nguyen T, Poirier F, et al. E-cadherin dynamics is regulated by galectin-7 at epithelial cell surface. *Sci Rep.* (2017) 7:17086. doi: 10.1038/s41598-017-17332-y
89. Vicovac L, Jankovic M, Cuperlovic M. Galectin-1 and−3 in cells of the first trimester placental bed. *Hum Reprod.* (1998) 13:730–5. doi: 10.1093/humrep/13.3.730
90. Kolundzic N, Bojic-Trbojevic Z, Kovacevic T, Stefanoska I, Kadoya T, Vicovac L. Galectin-1 is part of human trophoblast invasion machinery–a functional study *in vitro*. *PLoS ONE.* (2011) 6:e28514. doi: 10.1371/journal.pone.0028514
91. Chen Q, Pang PC, Cohen ME, Longtine MS, Schust DJ, Haslam SM, et al. Evidence for differential glycosylation of trophoblast cell types. *Mol Cell Proteomics.* (2016) 15:1857–66. doi: 10.1074/mcp.M115.055798
92. Fischer C, Sanchez-Ruderisch H, Welzel M, Wiedenmann B, Sakai T, Andre S, et al. Galectin-1 interacts with the α5β1 fibronectin receptor to restrict carcinoma cell growth via induction of p21 and p27. *J Biol Chem.* (2005) 280:37266–77. doi: 10.1074/jbc.M411580200
93. Sanchez-Ruderisch H, Detjen KM, Welzel M, Andre S, Fischer C, Gabius HJ, et al. Galectin-1 sensitizes carcinoma cells to anoikis via the

fibronectin receptor α5β1-integrin. *Cell Death Differ.* (2011) 18:806–16. doi: 10.1038/cdd.2010.148
94. Bojic-Trbojevic Z, Krivokuca MJ, Stefanoska I, Kolundzic N, Vilotic A, Kadoya T, et al. Integrin beta1 is bound to galectin-1 in human trophoblast. *J Biochem.* (2018) 163:39–50. doi: 10.1093/jb/mvx061
95. Bojic-Trbojevic Z, Jovanovic Krivokuca M, Kolundzic N, Petronijevic M, Vrzic-Petronijevic S, Golubovic S, et al. Galectin-1 binds mucin in human trophoblast. *Histochem Cell Biol.* (2014) 142:541–53. doi: 10.1007/s00418-014-1229-7
96. Shyu MK, Chen CW, Lin NY, Liao WC, Chen CH, Lin CJ, et al. MUC1 expression is elevated in severe preeclamptic placentas and suppresses trophoblast cell invasion via beta1-integrin signaling. *J Clin Endocrinol Metab.* (2011) 96:3759–67. doi: 10.1210/jc.2011-1368
97. Swanson BJ, Mcdermott KM, Singh PK, Eggers JP, Crocker PR, Hollingsworth MA. MUC1 is a counter-receptor for myelin-associated glycoprotein (Siglec-4a) and their interaction contributes to adhesion in pancreatic cancer perineural invasion. *Cancer Res.* (2007) 67:10222–9. doi: 10.1158/0008-5472.CAN-06-2483
98. Shyu MK, Lin MC, Liu CH, Fu YR, Shih JC, Lee CN, et al. MUC1 expression is increased during human placental development and suppresses trophoblast like cell invasion *in vitro*. *Biol Reprod.* (2008) 79:233–9. doi: 10.1095/biolreprod.108.067629
99. Hsieh SH, Ying NW, Wu MH, Chiang WF, Hsu CL, Wong TY, et al. Galectin-1, a novel ligand of neuropilin-1, activates VEGFR-2 signaling and modulates the migration of vascular endothelial cells. *Oncogene.* (2008) 27:3746–53. doi: 10.1038/sj.onc.1211029
100. Arad A, Nammouz S, Nov Y, Ohel G, Bejar J, Vadasz Z. The expression of neuropilin-1 in human placentas from normal and preeclamptic pregnancies. *Int J Gynecol Pathol.* (2017) 36:42–9. doi: 10.1097/PGP.0000000000000283
101. Zhou Q, Cummings RD. L-14 lectin recognition of laminin and its promotion of *in vitro* cell adhesion. *Arch Biochem Biophys.* (1993) 300:6–17. doi: 10.1006/abbi.1993.1002
102. Moiseeva EP, Javed Q, Spring EL, De Bono DP. Galectin 1 is involved in vascular smooth muscle cell proliferation. *Cardiovasc Res.* (2000) 45:493–502. doi: 10.1016/S0008-6363(99)00276-X
103. Johnson GA, Burghardt RC, Bazer FW, Spencer TE. Osteopontin: roles in implantation and placentation. *Biol Reprod.* (2003) 69:1458–71. doi: 10.1095/biolreprod.103.020651
104. Kim J, Erikson DW, Burghardt RC, Spencer TE, Wu G, Bayless KJ, et al. Secreted phosphoprotein 1 binds integrins to initiate multiple cell signaling pathways, including FRAP1/mTOR, to support attachment and force-generated migration of trophectoderm cells. *Matrix Biol.* (2010) 29:369–82. doi: 10.1016/j.matbio.2010.04.001
105. Koopman LA, Kopcow HD, Rybalov B, Boyson JE, Orange JS, Schatz F, et al. Human decidual natural killer cells are a unique NK cell subset with immunomodulatory potential. *J Exp Med.* (2003) 198:1201–12. doi: 10.1084/jem.20030305
106. Aluvihare VR, Kallikourdis M, Betz AG. Regulatory T cells mediate maternal tolerance to the fetus. *Nat Immunol.* (2004) 5:266–71. doi: 10.1038/ni1037
107. Blois SM, Ilarregui JM, Tometten M, Garcia M, Orsal AS, Cordo-Russo R, et al. A pivotal role for galectin-1 in fetomaternal tolerance. *Nat Med.* (2007) 13:1450–7. doi: 10.1038/nm1680
108. Garin MI, Chu CC, Golshayan D, Cernuda-Morollon E, Wait R, Lechler RI. Galectin-1: a key effector of regulation mediated by CD4+CD25+ T cells. *Blood.* (2007) 109:2058–65. doi: 10.1182/blood-2006-04-016451
109. Kopcow HD, Rosetti F, Leung Y, Allan DS, Kutok JL, Strominger JL. T cell apoptosis at the maternal-fetal interface in early human pregnancy, involvement of galectin-1. *Proc Natl Acad Sci USA.* (2008) 105:18472–7. doi: 10.1073/pnas.0809233105
110. Than NG, Romero R, Erez O, Weckle A, Tarca AL, Hotra J, et al. Emergence of hormonal and redox regulation of galectin-1 in placental mammals: implication in maternal-fetal immune tolerance. *Proc Natl Acad Sci USA.* (2008c) 105:15819–24. doi: 10.1073/pnas.0807606105
111. Tamura M, Sato D, Nakajima M, Saito M, Sasaki T, Tanaka T, et al. Identification of galectin-2-mucin interaction and possible formation of a high molecular weight lattice. *Biol Pharm Bull.* (2017) 40:1789–95. doi: 10.1248/bpb.b17-00221
112. Loser K, Sturm A, Voskort M, Kupas V, Balkow S, Auriemma M, et al. Galectin-2 suppresses contact allergy by inducing apoptosis in activated CD8+ T cells. *J Immunol.* (2009) 182:5419–29. doi: 10.4049/jimmunol.0802308
113. Yildirim C, Vogel DY, Hollander MR, Baggen JM, Fontijn RD, Nieuwenhuis S, et al. Galectin-2 induces a proinflammatory, anti-arteriogenic phenotype in monocytes and macrophages. *PLoS ONE.* (2015) 10:e0124347. doi: 10.1371/journal.pone.0124347
114. Hutter S, Knabl J, Andergassen U, Hofmann S, Kuhn C, Mahner S, et al. Placental expression patterns of galectin-1, galectin-2, galectin-3 and galectin-13 in cases of intrauterine growth restriction (IUGR). *Int J Mol Sci.* (2016a) 17:523. doi: 10.3390/ijms17040523
115. Hutter S, Martin N, Von Schonfeldt V, Messner J, Kuhn C, Hofmann S, et al. Galectin 2 (gal-2) expression is downregulated on protein and mRNA level in placentas of preeclamptic (PE) patients. *Placenta.* (2015) 36:438–45. doi: 10.1016/j.placenta.2015.01.198
116. Unverdorben L, Haufe T, Santoso L, Hofmann S, Jeschke U, Hutter S. Prototype and chimera-type galectins in placentas with spontaneous and recurrent miscarriages. *Int J Mol Sci.* (2016a) 17:644. doi: 10.3390/ijms17050644
117. Sano H, Hsu DK, Apgar JR, Yu L, Sharma BB, Kuwabara I, et al. Critical role of galectin-3 in phagocytosis by macrophages. *J Clin Invest.* (2003) 112:389–97. doi: 10.1172/JCI200317592
118. Chen HY, Liu FT, Yang RY. Roles of galectin-3 in immune responses. *Arch Immunol Ther Exp (Warsz).* (2005) 53:497–504.
119. Yang RY, Hsu DK, Liu FT. Expression of galectin-3 modulates T-cell growth and apoptosis. *Proc Natl Acad Sci USA.* (1996) 93:6737–42. doi: 10.1073/pnas.93.13.6737
120. Stillman BN, Hsu DK, Pang M, Brewer CF, Johnson P, Liu FT, et al. Galectin-3 and galectin-1 bind distinct cell surface glycoprotein receptors to induce T cell death. *J Immunol.* (2006) 176:778–89. doi: 10.4049/jimmunol.176.2.778
121. Maquoi E, Van Den Brule FA, Castronovo V, Foidart JM. Changes in the distribution pattern of galectin-1 and galectin-3 in human placenta correlates with the differentiation pathways of trophoblasts. *Placenta.* (1997) 18:433–9. doi: 10.1016/S0143-4004(97)80044-6
122. Bozic M, Petronijevic M, Milenkovic S, Atanackovic J, Lazic J, Vicovac L. Galectin-1 and galectin-3 in the trophoblast of the gestational trophoblastic disease. *Placenta.* (2004) 25:797–802. doi: 10.1016/j.placenta.2004.03.006
123. Yang H, Lei C, Zhang W. Expression of galectin-3 in mouse endometrium and its effect during embryo implantation. *Reprod Biomed Online.* (2012) 24:116–22. doi: 10.1016/j.rbmo.2011.09.003
124. Nangia-Makker P, Honjo Y, Sarvis R, Akahani S, Hogan V, Pienta KJ, et al. Galectin-3 induces endothelial cell morphogenesis and angiogenesis. *Am J Pathol.* (2000) 156:899–909. doi: 10.1016/S0002-9440(10)64959-0
125. Evans J, Yap J, Gamage T, Salamonsen L, Dimitriadis E, Menkhorst E. Galectin-7 is important for normal uterine repair following menstruation. *Mol Hum Reprod.* (2014) 20:787–98. doi: 10.1093/molehr/gau032
126. Menkhorst E, Koga K, Van Sinderen M, Dimitriadis E. Galectin-7 serum levels are altered prior to the onset of pre-eclampsia. *Placenta.* (2014a) 35:281–5. doi: 10.1016/j.placenta.2014.01.009
127. Menkhorst EM, Gamage T, Cuman C, Kaitu'u-Lino TJ, Tong S, Dimitriadis E. Galectin-7 acts as an adhesion molecule during implantation and increased expression is associated with miscarriage. *Placenta.* (2014b) 35:195–201. doi: 10.1016/j.placenta.2014.01.004
128. Cagli F, Uysal G, Oz L, Akkaya H, Aksoy H, Ulku Karakilic E, et al. Serum galectin 7 is not useful to predict abortion in the first trimester. *Fetal Pediatr Pathol.* (2018) 37:1–6. doi: 10.1080/15513815.2018.1453001
129. Kolundzic N, Bojic-Trbojevic Z, Radojcic L, Petronijevic M, Vicovac L. Galectin-8 is expressed by villous and extravillous trophoblast of the human placenta. *Placenta.* (2011c) 32:909–11. doi: 10.1016/j.placenta.2011.07.087
130. Troncoso MF, Ferragut F, Bacigalupo ML, Cardenas Delgado VM, Nugnes LG, Gentilini L, et al. Galectin-8: a matricellular lectin with key roles in angiogenesis. *Glycobiology.* (2014) 24:907–14. doi: 10.1093/glycob/cwu054
131. Cattaneo V, Tribulatti MV, Carabelli J, Carestia A, Schattner M, Campetella O. Galectin-8 elicits pro-inflammatory activities in the endothelium. *Glycobiology.* (2014) 24:966–73. doi: 10.1093/glycob/cwu060

132. Sampson JF, Suryawanshi A, Chen WS, Rabinovich GA, Panjwani N. Galectin-8 promotes regulatory T-cell differentiation by modulating IL-2 and TGFbeta signaling. *Immunol Cell Biol.* (2016) 94:213–9. doi: 10.1038/icb.2015.72
133. Carabelli J, Quattrocchi V, D'antuono A, Zamorano P, Tribulatti MV, Campetella O. Galectin-8 activates dendritic cells and stimulates antigen-specific immune response elicitation. *J Leukoc Biol.* (2017) 102:1237–47. doi: 10.1189/jlb.3A0816-357RR
134. Pardo E, Carcamo C, Uribe-San Martin R, Ciampi E, Segovia-Miranda F, Curkovic-Pena C, et al. Galectin-8 as an immunosuppressor in experimental autoimmune encephalomyelitis and a target of human early prognostic antibodies in multiple sclerosis. *PLoS ONE.* (2017) 12:e0177472. doi: 10.1371/journal.pone.0177472
135. Carabelli J, Prato CA, Sanmarco LM, Aoki MP, Campetella O, Tribulatti MV. Interleukin-6 signaling mediates Galectin-8 costimulatory activity of antigen-specific CD4 T cell response. *Immunology.* (2018) 155:379–86. doi: 10.1111/imm.12980
136. Zick Y, Eisenstein M, Goren RA, Hadari YR, Levy Y, Ronen D. Role of galectin-8 as a modulator of cell adhesion and cell growth. *Glycoconj J.* (2002) 19:517–26. doi: 10.1023/B:GLYC.0000014081.55445.af
137. Sanchez-Fueyo A, Tian J, Picarella D, Domenig C, Zheng XX, Sabatos CA, et al. Tim-3 inhibits T helper type 1-mediated auto- and alloimmune responses and promotes immunological tolerance. *Nat Immunol.* (2003) 4:1093–101. doi: 10.1038/ni987
138. Bi S, Hong PW, Lee B, Baum LG. Galectin-9 binding to cell surface protein disulfide isomerase regulates the redox environment to enhance T-cell migration and HIV entry. *Proc Natl Acad Sci USA.* (2011) 108:10650–5. doi: 10.1073/pnas.1017954108
139. Wu C, Thalhamer T, Franca RF, Xiao S, Wang C, Hotta C, et al. Galectin-9-CD44 interaction enhances stability and function of adaptive regulatory T cells. *Immunity.* (2014) 41:270–82. doi: 10.1016/j.immuni.2014.06.011
140. Popovici RM, Krause MS, Germeyer A, Strowitzki T, Von Wolff M. Galectin-9: a new endometrial epithelial marker for the mid- and late-secretory and decidual phases in humans. *J Clin Endocrinol Metab.* (2005) 90:6170–6. doi: 10.1210/jc.2004-2529
141. Shimizu Y, Kabir-Salmani M, Azadbakht M, Sugihara K, Sakai K, Iwashita M. Expression and localization of galectin-9 in the human uterodome. *Endocr J.* (2008) 55:879–87. doi: 10.1507/endocrj.K08E-111
142. Thijssen VL, Hulsmans S, Griffioen AW. The galectin profile of the endothelium: altered expression and localization in activated and tumor endothelial cells. *Am J Pathol.* (2008) 172:545–53. doi: 10.2353/ajpath.2008.070938
143. Heusschen R, Freitag N, Tirado-Gonzalez I, Barrientos G, Moschansky P, Munoz-Fernandez R, et al. Profiling Lgals9 splice variant expression at the fetal-maternal interface: implications in normal and pathological human pregnancy. *Biol Reprod.* (2013) 88:22. doi: 10.1095/biolreprod.112.105460
144. Zhang F, Zheng M, Qu Y, Li J, Ji J, Feng B, et al. Different roles of galectin-9 isoforms in modulating E-selectin expression and adhesion function in LoVo colon carcinoma cells. *Mol Biol Rep.* (2009) 36:823–30. doi: 10.1007/s11033-008-9251-2
145. Li Y, Feng J, Geng S, Geng S, Wei H, Chen G, et al. The N- and C-terminal carbohydrate recognition domains of galectin-9 contribute differently to its multiple functions in innate immunity and adaptive immunity. *Mol Immunol.* (2011) 48:670–7. doi: 10.1016/j.molimm.2010.11.011
146. Meggyes M, Miko E, Polgar B, Bogar B, Farkas B, Illes Z, et al. Peripheral blood TIM-3 positive NK and CD8+ T cells throughout pregnancy: TIM-3/galectin-9 interaction and its possible role during pregnancy. *PLoS ONE.* (2014) 9:e92371. doi: 10.1371/journal.pone.0092371
147. Enninga EA, Nevala WK, Creedon DJ, Markovic SN, Holtan SG. Fetal sex-based differences in maternal hormones, angiogenic factors, and immune mediators during pregnancy and the postpartum period. *Am J Reprod Immunol.* (2015) 73:251–62. doi: 10.1111/aji.12303
148. Enninga EAL, Harrington SM, Creedon DJ, Ruano R, Markovic SN, Dong H, et al. Immune checkpoint molecules soluble program death ligand 1 and galectin-9 are increased in pregnancy. *Am J Reprod Immunol.* (2018) 79:e12795. doi: 10.1111/aji.12795
149. Li Y, Zhang J, Zhang D, Hong X, Tao Y, Wang S, et al. Tim-3 signaling in peripheral NK cells promotes maternal-fetal immune tolerance and alleviates pregnancy loss. *Sci Signal.* (2017) 10:eaah4323. doi: 10.1126/scisignal.aah4323
150. He M, Jiang M, Zhou Y, Li F, Yang M, Fan Y, et al. Impaired Gal-9 dysregulates the PBMC-induced Th1/Th2 imbalance in abortion-prone matings. *J Immunol Res.* (2018) 2018:9517842. doi: 10.1155/2018/9517842
151. Lajko A, Meggyes M, Polgar B, Szereday L. The immunological effect of Galectin-9/TIM-3 pathway after low dose Mifepristone treatment in mice at 14.5 day of pregnancy. *PLoS ONE.* (2018) 13:e0194870. doi: 10.1371/journal.pone.0194870
152. Li ZH, Wang LL, Liu H, Muyayalo KP, Huang XB, Mor G, et al. Galectin-9 alleviates LPS-induced preeclampsia-like impairment in rats via switching decidual macrophage polarization to M2 subtype. *Front Immunol.* (2018) 9:3142. doi: 10.3389/fimmu.2018.03142
153. Abedin MJ, Kashio Y, Seki M, Nakamura K, Hirashima M. Potential roles of galectins in myeloid differentiation into three different lineages. *J Leukoc Biol.* (2003) 73:650–6. doi: 10.1189/jlb.0402163
154. Kubach J, Lutter P, Bopp T, Stoll S, Becker C, Huter E, et al. Human CD4+CD25+ regulatory T cells: proteome analysis identifies galectin-10 as a novel marker essential for their anergy and suppressive function. *Blood.* (2007) 110:1550–8. doi: 10.1182/blood-2007-01-069229
155. Unverdorben L, Jeschke U, Santoso L, Hofmann S, Kuhn C, Arck P, et al. Comparative analyses on expression of galectins1-4, 7-10 and 12 in first trimester placenta, decidua and isolated trophoblast cells *in vitro*. *Histol Histopathol.* (2016b) 31:1095–111. doi: 10.14670/HH-11-739.
156. Than NG, Romero R, Kim CJ, Mcgowen MR, Papp Z, Wildman DE. Galectins: guardians of eutherian pregnancy at the maternal-fetal interface. *Trends Endocrinol Metab.* (2012) 23:23–31. doi: 10.1016/j.tem.2011.09.003
157. Bohn H, Kraus W, Winckler W. Purification and characterization of two new soluble placental tissue proteins (PP13 and PP17). *Oncodev Biol Med.* (1983) 4:343–50.
158. Than NG, Sumegi B, Than GN, Berente Z, Bohn H. Isolation and sequence analysis of a cDNA encoding human placental tissue protein 13 (PP13), a new lysophospholipase, homolog of human eosinophil Charcot-Leyden Crystal protein. *Placenta.* (1999) 20:703–10. doi: 10.1053/plac.1999.0436
159. Than NG, Pick E, Bellyei S, Szigeti A, Burger O, Berente Z, et al. Functional analyses of placental protein 13/galectin-13. *Eur J Biochem.* (2004) 271:1065–78. doi: 10.1111/j.1432-1033.2004.04004.x
160. Burger O, Pick E, Zwickel J, Klayman M, Meiri H, Slotky R, et al. Placental protein 13 (PP-13): effects on cultured trophoblasts, and its detection in human body fluids in normal and pathological pregnancies. *Placenta.* (2004) 25:608–22. doi: 10.1016/j.placenta.2003.12.009
161. Huppertz B, Sammar M, Chefetz I, Neumaier-Wagner P, Bartz C, Meiri H. Longitudinal determination of serum placental protein 13 during development of preeclampsia. *Fetal Diagn Ther.* (2008) 24:230–6. doi: 10.1159/000151344
162. Sammar M, Dragovic R, Meiri H, Vatish M, Sharabi-Nov A, Sargent I, et al. Reduced placental protein 13 (PP13) in placental derived syncytiotrophoblast extracellular vesicles in preeclampsia - a novel tool to study the impaired cargo transmission of the placenta to the maternal organs. *Placenta.* (2018) 66:17–25. doi: 10.1016/j.placenta.2018.04.013
163. Boronkai A, Bellyei S, Szigeti A, Pozsgai E, Bognar Z, Sumegi B, et al. Potentiation of paclitaxel-induced apoptosis by galectin-13 overexpression via activation of Ask-1-p38-MAP kinase and JNK/SAPK pathways and suppression of Akt and ERK1/2 activation in U-937 human macrophage cells. *Eur J Cell Biol.* (2009) 88:753–63. doi: 10.1016/j.ejcb.2009.07.005
164. Gizurarson S, Huppertz B, Osol G, Skarphedinsson JO, Mandala M, Meiri H. Effects of placental protein 13 on the cardiovascular system in gravid and non-gravid rodents. *Fetal Diagn Ther.* (2013) 33:257–64. doi: 10.1159/000345964
165. Than NG, Balogh A, Romero R, Karpati E, Erez O, Szilagyi A, et al. Placental protein 13 (PP13) - a placental immunoregulatory galectin protecting pregnancy. *Front Immunol.* (2014a) 5:348. doi: 10.3389/fimmu.2014.00348
166. Drobnjak T, Gizurarson S, Gokina NI, Meiri H, Mandala M, Huppertz B, et al. Placental protein 13 (PP13)-induced vasodilation of resistance arteries from pregnant and nonpregnant rats occurs via endothelial-signaling pathways. *Hypertens Pregn.* (2017) 36:186–95. doi: 10.1080/10641955.2017.1295052

167. Than NG, Abdul Rahman O, Magenheim R, Nagy B, Fule T, Hargitai B, et al. Placental protein 13 (galectin-13) has decreased placental expression but increased shedding and maternal serum concentrations in patients presenting with preterm pre-eclampsia and HELLP syndrome. *Virchows Arch.* (2008a) 453:387–400. doi: 10.1007/s00428-008-0658-x
168. Spencer K, Cowans NJ, Chefetz I, Tal J, Kuhnreich I, Meiri H. Second-trimester uterine artery Doppler pulsatility index and maternal serum PP13 as markers of pre-eclampsia. *Prenat Diagn.* (2007) 27:258–63. doi: 10.1002/pd.1664
169. Huppertz B. Biology of preeclampsia: combined actions of angiogenic factors, their receptors and placental proteins. *Biochim Biophys Acta Mol Basis Dis.* (2018). S0925-4439(18)30486-1. doi: 10.1016/j.bbadis.2018.11.024 [Epub ahead of print].
170. Unverdorben L, Huttenbrenner R, Knabl J, Jeschke U, Hutter S. Galectin-13/PP-13 expression in term placentas of gestational diabetes mellitus pregnancies. *Placenta.* (2015) 36:191–8. doi: 10.1016/j.placenta.2014.11.019
171. Zhao B, Han X, Meng Q, Luo Q. Early second trimester maternal serum markers in the prediction of gestational diabetes mellitus. *J Diabetes Investig.* (2018) 9:967–74. doi: 10.1111/jdi.12798
172. Su J, Wang Y, Si Y, Gao J, Song C, Cui L, et al. Galectin-13, a different prototype galectin, does not bind beta-galacto-sides and forms dimers via intermolecular disulfide bridges between Cys-136 and Cys-138. *Sci Rep.* (2018) 8:980. doi: 10.1038/s41598-018-19465-0
173. Than NG, Romero R, Meiri H, Erez O, Xu Y, Tarquini F, et al. PP13, maternal ABO blood groups and the risk assessment of pregnancy complications. *PLoS ONE.* (2011) 6:e21564. doi: 10.1371/journal.pone.0021564
174. Dent J, Mcgovern PT, Hancock JL. Immunological implications of ultrastructural studies of goat X sheep hybrid placentae. *Nature.* (1971) 231:116–7. doi: 10.1038/231116a0
175. Tomiie M, Isaka S, Miyoshi E, Taniguchi N, Kimura T, Ogita K, et al. Elevated expression of N-acetylglucosaminyltransferase V in first trimester human placenta. *Biochem Biophys Res Commun.* (2005) 330:999–1004. doi: 10.1016/j.bbrc.2005.02.186
176. Yamamoto E, Ino K, Miyoshi E, Inamori K, Abe A, Sumigama S, et al. N-acetylglucosaminyltransferase V regulates extravillous trophoblast invasion through glycosylation of alpha5beta1 integrin. *Endocrinology.* (2009) 150:990–9. doi: 10.1210/en.2008-1005
177. Ji L, Brkic J, Liu M, Fu G, Peng C, Wang YL. Placental trophoblast cell differentiation: physiological regulation and pathological relevance to preeclampsia. *Mol Aspects Med.* (2013) 34:981–1023. doi: 10.1016/j.mam.2012.12.008
178. Jansen BC, Bondt A, Reiding KR, Lonardi E, De Jong CJ, Falck D, et al. Pregnancy-associated serum N-glycome changes studied by high-throughput MALDI-TOF-MS. *Sci Rep.* (2016) 6:23296. doi: 10.1038/srep23296
179. Varki A. Biological roles of oligosaccharides: all of the theories are correct. *Glycobiology.* (1993) 3:97–130. doi: 10.1093/glycob/3.2.97
180. Acheson A, Sunshine JL, Rutishauser U. NCAM polysialic acid can regulate both cell-cell and cell-substrate interactions. *J Cell Biol.* (1991) 114:143–53. doi: 10.1083/jcb.114.1.143
181. Lauc G, Zoldos V. Protein glycosylation–an evolutionary crossroad between genes and environment. *Mol Biosyst.* (2010) 6:2373–9. doi: 10.1039/c0mb00067a
182. Kaszuba K, Grzybek M, Orlowski A, Danne R, Rog T, Simons K, et al. N-Glycosylation as determinant of epidermal growth factor receptor conformation in membranes. *Proc Natl Acad Sci USA.* (2015) 112:4334–9. doi: 10.1073/pnas.1503262112
183. Jones CJ, Carter AM, Aplin JD, Enders AC. Glycosylation at the fetomaternal interface in hemomonochorial placentae from five widely separated species of mammal: is there evidence for convergent evolution? *Cells Tissues Organs.* (2007) 185:269–84. doi: 10.1159/000102175
184. Mcmaster M, Zhou Y, Shorter S, Kapasi K, Geraghty D, Lim KH, et al. HLA-G isoforms produced by placental cytotrophoblasts and found in amniotic fluid are due to unusual glycosylation. *J Immunol.* (1998) 160:5922–8.
185. Moss L, Prakobphol A, Wiedmann TW, Fisher SJ, Damsky CH. Glycosylation of human trophoblast integrins is stage and cell-type specific. *Glycobiology.* (1994) 4:567–75. doi: 10.1093/glycob/4.5.567
186. Gleeson LM, Chakraborty C, Mckinnon T, Lala PK. Insulin-like growth factor-binding protein 1 stimulates human trophoblast migration by signaling through alpha 5 beta 1 integrin via mitogen-activated protein Kinase pathway. *J Clin Endocrinol Metab.* (2001) 86:2484–93. doi: 10.1210/jc.86.6.2484
187. Jovanovic M, Stefanoska I, Radojcic L, Vicovac L. Interleukin-8 (CXCL8) stimulates trophoblast cell migration and invasion by increasing levels of matrix metalloproteinase (MMP)2 and MMP9 and integrins alpha5 and beta1. *Reproduction.* (2010) 139:789–98. doi: 10.1530/REP-09-0341
188. Li CM, Hou L, Zhang H, Zhang WY. CCL17 induces trophoblast migration and invasion by regulating matrix metalloproteinase and integrin expression in human first-trimester placenta. *Reprod Sci.* (2014) 1933719113519170. doi: 10.1177/1933719113519170 [Epub ahead of print].
189. Liao WC, Liu CH, Chen CH, Hsu WM, Liao YY, Chang HM, et al. beta-1,4-Galactosyltransferase III suppresses extravillous trophoblast invasion through modifying beta1-integrin glycosylation. *Placenta.* (2015) 36:357–64. doi: 10.1016/j.placenta.2015.01.008
190. Furmento VA, Marino J, Blank VC, Cayrol MF, Cremaschi GA, Aguilar RC, et al. Granulocyte colony-stimulating factor (G-CSF) upregulates beta1 integrin and increases migration of human trophoblast Swan 71 cells via PI3K and MAPK activation. *Exp Cell Res.* (2016) 342:125–34. doi: 10.1016/j.yexcr.2016.03.005
191. Zhang M, Wang M, Gao R, Liu X, Chen X, Geng Y, et al. Altered beta1,6-GlcNAc and bisecting GlcNAc-branched N-glycan on integrin beta1 are associated with early spontaneous miscarriage in humans. *Hum Reprod.* (2015) 30:2064–75. doi: 10.1093/humrep/dev153
192. Deng Q, Chen Y, Yin N, Shan N, Luo X, Yuan Y, et al. The role of MGAT5 in human umbilical vein endothelial cells. *Reprod Sci.* (2017) 24:313–23. doi: 10.1177/1933719116655602
193. Tannetta D, Masliukaite I, Vatish M, Redman C, Sargent I. Update of syncytiotrophoblast derived extracellular vesicles in normal pregnancy and preeclampsia. *J Reprod Immunol.* (2017) 119:98–106. doi: 10.1016/j.jri.2016.08.008
194. Toscano MA, Bianco GA, Ilarregui JM, Croci DO, Correale J, Hernandez JD, et al. Differential glycosylation of TH1, TH2 and TH-17 effector cells selectively regulates susceptibility to cell death. *Nat Immunol.* (2007) 8:825–34. doi: 10.1038/ni1482
195. Cerliani JP, Blidner AG, Toscano MA, Croci DO, Rabinovich GA. Translating the 'Sugar Code' into immune and vascular signaling programs. *Trends Biochem Sci.* (2017) 42:255–73. doi: 10.1016/j.tibs.2016.11.003
196. Marini M, Bonaccini L, Thyrion GD, Vichi D, Parretti E, Sgambati E. Distribution of sugar residues in human placentas from pregnancies complicated by hypertensive disorders. *Acta Histochem.* (2011) 113:815–25. doi: 10.1016/j.acthis.2010.12.001
197. Di Lella S, Sundblad V, Cerliani JP, Guardia CM, Estrin DA, Vasta GR, et al. When galectins recognize glycans: from biochemistry to physiology and back again. *Biochemistry.* (2011) 50:7842–57. doi: 10.1021/bi201121m

10

Differential Longevity of Memory CD4 and CD8 T Cells in a Cohort of the Mothers With a History of ZIKV Infection and Their Children

Jessica Badolato-Corrêa[1†], Fabiana Rabe Carvalho[2†], Iury Amancio Paiva[1], Débora Familiar-Macedo[1], Helver Gonçalves Dias[1], Alex Pauvolid-Corrêa[3,4], Caroline Fernandes-Santos[1], Monique da Rocha Queiroz Lima[1], Mariana Gandini[5], Andréa Alice Silva[2], Silvia Maria Baeta Cavalcanti[6], Solange Artimos de Oliveira[7], Renata Artimos de Oliveira Vianna[7], Elzinandes Leal de Azeredo[1], Claudete Aparecida Araújo Cardoso[2,7], Alba Grifoni[8], Alessandro Sette[8,9], Daniela Weiskopf[8] and Luzia Maria de-Oliveira-Pinto[1]*

[1] Laboratory of Viral Immunology, Fundação Oswaldo Cruz, Rio de Janeiro, Brazil, [2] Multiuser Laboratory for Research in Nephrology and Medical Science, School of Medicine, Universidade Federal Fluminense, Niterói, Brazil, [3] Department of Veterinary Integrative Biosciences, Texas A&M University, College Station, TX, United States, [4] Laboratory of Respiratory Viruses and Measles, Fiocruz, Rio de Janeiro, Brazil, [5] Laboratory of Cellular Microbiology, Fundação Oswaldo Cruz, Rio de Janeiro, Brazil, [6] Laboratory of Virological Diagnosis, Biomedical Institute, Universidade Federal Fluminense, Niterói, Brazil, [7] Department of Maternal and Child, School of Medicine, Universidade Federal Fluminense, Niterói, Brazil, [8] Center for Infectious Disease and Vaccine Research, La Jolla Institute for Immunology (LJI), San Diego, CA, United States, [9] Division of Infectious Diseases and Global Public Health, Department of Medicine, University of California, San Diego, San Diego, CA, United States

***Correspondence:**
Luzia Maria de-Oliveira-Pinto
lpinto@ioc.fiocruz.br

Background: Zika virus (ZIKV) infection causes for mild and self-limiting disease in healthy adults. In newborns, it can occasionally lead to a spectrum of malformations, the congenital Zika syndrome (CZS). Thus, little is known if mothers and babies with a history of ZIKV infection were able to develop long-lasting T-cell immunity. To these issues, we measure the prevalence of ZIKV T-cell immunity in a cohort of mothers infected to the ZIKV during pregnancy in the 2016–2017 Zika outbreak, who gave birth to infants affected by neurological complications or asymptomatic ones.

Results: Twenty-one mothers and 18 children were tested for IFN-γ ELISpot and T-cell responses for flow cytometry assays in response to CD4 ZIKV and CD8 ZIKV megapools (CD4 ZIKV MP and CD8 ZIKV MP). IFN-γ ELISpot responses to ZIKV MPs showed an increased CD4 and CD8 T-cell responses in mothers compared to children. The degranulation activity and IFN-γ-producing CD4 T cells were detected in most mothers, and children, while in CD8 T-cells, low responses were detected in these study groups. The total Temra T cell subset is enriched for IFN-γ+ CD4 T cells after stimulation of CD4 ZIKV MP.

Conclusion: Donors with a history of ZIKV infection demonstrated long-term CD4 T cell immunity to ZIKV CD4 MP. However, the same was not observed in CD8 T cells with the ZIKV CD8 MP. One possibility is that the cytotoxic and pro-inflammatory activities of CD8 T cells are markedly demonstrated in the early stages of infection, but less detected in the disease resolution phase, when the virus has already been eliminated. The responses of mothers' T cells to ZIKV MPs do not appear to be related to their children's clinical outcome. There was also no marked difference in the T cell responses to ZIKV MP between children affected or not with CZS. These data still need to be investigated, including the evaluation of the response of CD8 T cells to other ZIKV peptides.

Keywords: Zika, T cells, memory, pregnancy, congenital Zika syndrome (CZS)

INTRODUCTION

The emergence of ZIKV in dengue-endemic regions creates a potentially alarming scenario, as those caused by the ZIKV epidemic spread across countries, especially the Americas, during 2015–2016 (1, 2). At present, half of the world's population is considered at risk of dengue virus (DENV), and cases of ZIKV continue to be reported globally (3, 4).

DENV and ZIKV are members of the family *Flaviviridae* and are among the several medically important viruses (5). Both are spread *via* the bite of infected mosquitoes, *Aedes spp.*, whose ecological niches expand beyond the tropical and subtropical regions (6). Moreover, ZIKV can be transmitted *via* sexual contact (7, 8). It persists for weeks in the reproductive tract (9–11) and undergoes vertical transmission from a mother to fetus (12–15). During Latin America and French Polynesia outbreaks, ZIKV infection typically produces mild symptoms that resolve rapidly. However, when an infection occurs during pregnancy, occasional vertical transmission can lead to a spectrum of devastating neurodevelopmental aberrations, collectively referred to as congenital Zika syndrome (CZS) (16). Conflicting data sets indicate that infants born to mothers infected with ZIKV during pregnancy carry up to 42% risk of developing overt clinical or neuroimaging abnormalities (17–21).

ZIKV is closely related to four serotypes of DENV. They are a positive-sense, single-stranded enveloped RNA virus. The genome encodes a polyprotein, which is processed into three structural proteins [the capsid (C), premembrane (prM), and the envelope (E) protein] and seven non-structural proteins (NS1, NS2A, NS2B, NS3, NS4A, NS4B, and NS5) (22). DENV and ZIKV share 55.1–56.3% amino acid sequence identity (23).

Tonnerre et al. performed a remarkably interesting longitudinal study with samples from 10 non-pregnant women with ZIKV-confirmed acute infection. For the T cell response, the authors confirmed different virus-specific targets for CD4 and CD8 T cells (24). They found that previous DENV infections largely affect the humoral response to ZIKV, with effects on the T cell side limited to increasing the frequency of ZIKV-specific CD8 T cells in some patients (24, 25).

Although viral infections are common during pregnancy, transplacental passage, and fetal infection appear to be the exception rather than the rule. Viral infections during pregnancy have been linked to adverse pregnancy outcomes and birth defects in offspring. Unfortunately, there are limited therapeutic or preventive tools to protect both mother and fetus during pandemics (26).

In the present study, we studied ZIKV memory T cell responses from a cohort of mothers infected with ZIKV during pregnancy in the 2016–2017 Zika outbreak who gave birth to infants affected by neurological complications or asymptomatic ones. These donors with a history of ZIKV infection were evaluated in 2018–2019, 2–3 years after ZIKV infection. This cohort provides a unique opportunity to study ZIKV immunity in an infection occurring during pregnancy and compare it with longitudinal follow-up samples.

MATERIALS AND METHODS

Study Design, Volunteers, and Samples

A cross-sectional study was carried out in pregnant mothers infected with ZIKV and children born to mothers who reported rash during pregnancy overlapping with the ZIKV Public Health Emergency of National Concern in Brazil period (November 2015 and May 2017). These donors' cohort was referred from the Exanthematic Diseases Unit at the Hospital Universitário Antonio Pedro of the Universidade Federal Fluminense (HUAP/UFF) located in Niteroi, Rio de Janeiro (Brazil). Laboratory evidence for ZIKV infection during pregnancy was based on a mother's positive quantitative real-time (qRT)-PCR test result on serum and/or urine samples, done at the flavivirus reference laboratory of Rio de Janeiro State (LACEN, RJ, Brazil) and confirmed by Multiuser Laboratory for Research Support in Nephrology and Medical Science (LAMAP, UFF, Brazil) (27). A qRT-PCR positive test result at any point after maternal rash onset confirmed the ZIKV infection within the first 5 days of rash and/or the urine sample was tested by the 14th day. So, we included 21 pregnant mothers who presented rash, with or without other clinical symptoms suggestive of arbovirus infections, such as arthralgia, myalgia, fever, headache, and conjunctival hyperemia. The exclusion criteria were mothers who were positive with a qRT-PCR for other arboviruses such as chikungunya and dengue. Moreover, mothers who presented positive test results to syphilis, toxoplasmosis, rubella, cytomegalovirus, and HIV infection were excluded. All serology tests were performed by the Service of Clinical Pathology (HUAP, UFF Brazil) (**Figure 1**). Three mothers were infected in the first trimester of pregnancy, 14 in the second trimester, 3 in the third trimester, and 1 before pregnancy (**Table 1**), thus making any laboratory diagnosis of acute Zika infection in babies impossible.

Eighteen children aged 17–38 months with a history of intrauterine exposure to ZIKV were classified as asymptomatic or with CZS if the test was negative for other congenital infections. The asymptomatic ZIKV group (positive maternal qRT-PCR, $n = 9$) consisted of patients with maternal exposure to ZIKV during pregnancy and no clinical evidence of CZS.

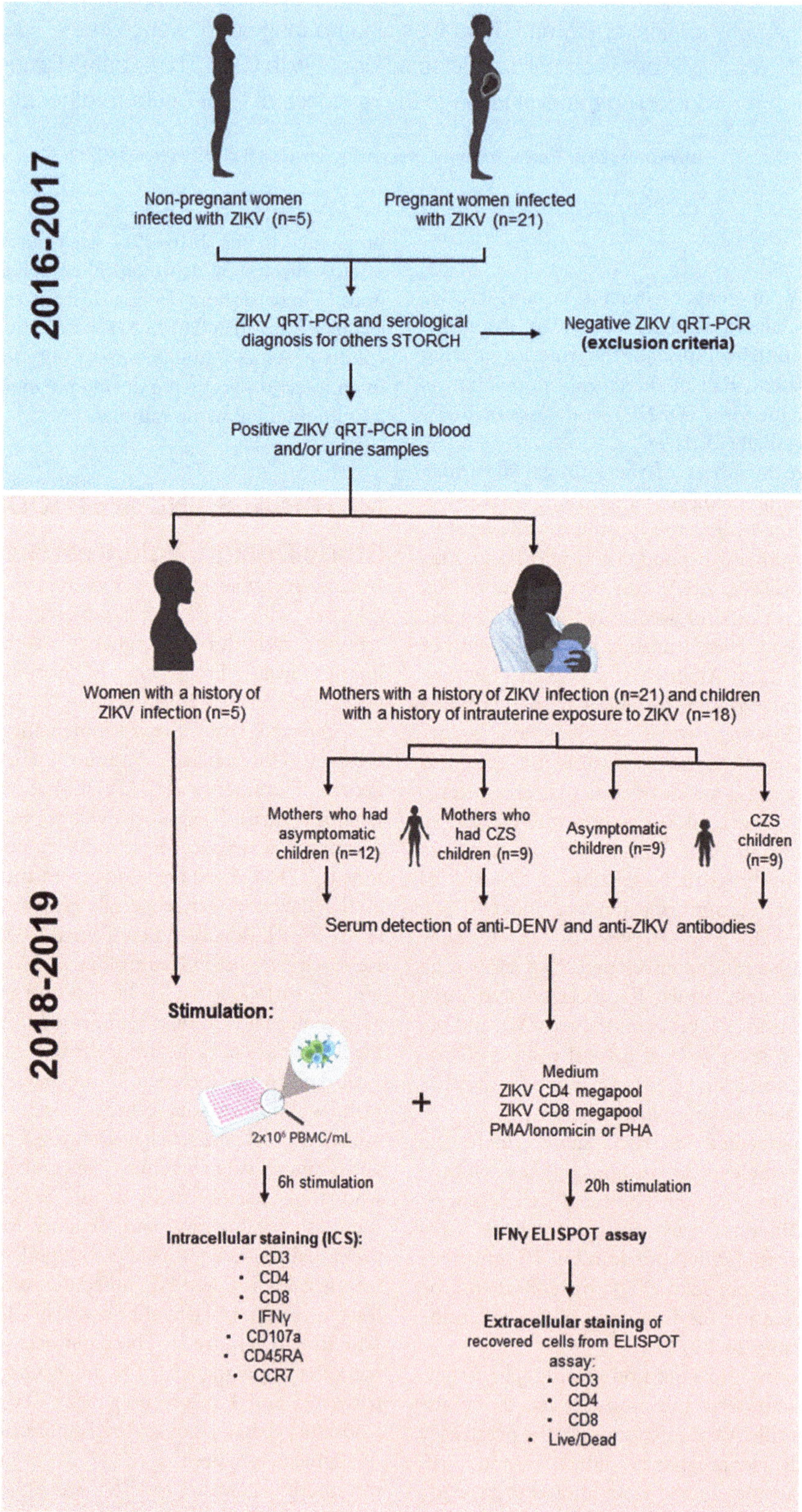

FIGURE 1 | The experimental design used in this study.

TABLE 1 | Characteristics of the recovered mothers infected to Zika virus during pregnancy and their intrauterine exposed children recruited from 2018 to 2019.

Group	Outcome at birth	ID	Age[a,b]	Illness time[b]	Gestational trimester at onset rash	State	RT-aPCR ZIKV	ZIKV anti-IgG	DENV anti-IgG	PRNT 90 ZIKV	PRNT 90 DENV-1	CD4+CD3+ T cells	CD8+CD3+ T cells	CD4/CD8
Women		W1	40	36		RJ	pos	pos	pos	<10	≥10	77.5	13.8	5.6
		W2	40	40		RJ	pos	pos	pos	<10	<10	74.2	18.0	4.1
		W3	23	38		RJ	pos	pos	pos	<10	≥10	60.1	29.4	2.0
		W4	25	42		RJ	pos	pos	pos	<10	≥10	58.9	22.2	2.7
		W5	27	35		RJ	pos	pos	pos	<10	≥10	76.3	20.0	3.8
			27.0 (23–40)[a]	38.0 (35–42)								69.9 (4[illegible].5–76.7)	20.0 (13.8–29.4)	3.8 (2–5.6)
Mothers	Asympt.	M1	22	38	3rd	RJ	pos	pos	neg	160	<10	81.6	9.81	8.3
	Asympt.	M2	36	40	3rd	RJ	pos	pos	pos	>320	≥10	65.2	22.3	2.9
	Asympt.	M3	37	38	2nd	RJ	pos	pos	pos	>320	≥10	62.5	16.5	3.8
	Asympt.	M4	23	24	2nd	RJ	pos	pos	neg	>320	<10	66.6	20.2	3.3
	Asympt.	M5	27	40	2nd	RJ	pos	pos	neg	>320	≥10	71.9	19.5	3.7
	Asympt.	M6	33	38	2nd	RJ	pos	pos	pos	<10	<10	61.0	29.2	2.1
	Asympt.	M7	37	38	2nd	RJ	pos	pos	pos	>320	≥10	73.7	21.1	3.5
	Asympt.	M8	41	x	2nd	RJ	pos	neg	neg	>320	<10	61.6	31.1	2.0
	Asympt.	M9	21	38	2nd	RJ	pos	pos	pos	>320	≥10	72.9	17.1	4.3
	Asympt.	M10	32	40	2nd	RJ	pos	pos	pos	>320	≥10	66.9	20.7	3.2
	Asympt.	M11	30	39	2nd	RJ	pos	pos	pos	>320	≥10	69.5	5.49	12.7
	Asympt.	M12	33	39	2nd	RJ	pos	pos	pos	>320	≥10	66.0	16.7	4.0
			32.5 (21–41)[a]	38.0 (24–40)								66.8 (61–81.6)	19.9 (5.5–31.1)	3.6 (2–12.7)
Mothers	CZS	M13	24	23	1st	RJ	pos	pos	neg	>320	<10	71.6	21.6	3.3
	CZS	M14	42	39	2nd	RJ	pos	pos	pos	>320	<10	67.1	22.5	3.0
	CZS	M15	25	37	3rd	RJ	pos	pos	neg	>320	≥10	66.0	17.4	3.8
	CZS	M16	21	42	1st	RJ	pos	pos	pos	>320	≥10	57.4	24.3	2.4
	CZS	M17	40	40	2nd	RJ	pos	pos	pos	>320	≥10	76.5	17.7	4.3
	CZS	M18	41	36	2nd	RJ	pos	pos	pos	>320	<10	71.3	22.3	3.2
	CZS	M19	28	38	2nd	RJ	pos	pos	pos	>320	≥10	80.5	13.9	5.8
	CZS	M20	21	39	before	RJ	pos	pos	pos	>320	<10	62.7	23.2	2.7
	CZS	M21	28	41	1st	RJ	pos	neg	pos	>320	≥10	78.9	14.9	5.3
			28.0 (21–42)[a]	39.0 (23–42)								71.3 (57.4–80.5)	21.6 (13.9–24.3)	3.3 (2.4–5.8)
Children	Asympt.	C1	35	36		RJ	x	neg	neg	x	x	56.1	29.2	1.9
	Asympt.	C2	29	38		RJ	x	neg	neg	<10	≥10	63.9	25.3	2.5
	Asympt.	C3	31	38		RJ	x	neg	pos	x	x	59.2	17.3	3.4

(Continued)

TABLE 1 | Continued

Group	Outcome at birth	ID	Age[a,b]	Illness time[b]	Gestational trimester at onset rash	State	RT-aPCR ZIKV	ZIKV anti-IgG	DENV anti-IgG	PRNT 90 ZIKV	PRNT 90 DENV-1	CD4+CD3+ T cells	CD8+CD3+ T cells	CD4/CD8
	Asympt.	C4	34	37		RJ	x	pos	pos	>320	≥10	80.0	15.2	5.3
	Asympt.	C5	41	39		RJ	x	neg	neg	<10	≥10	70.9	19.4	3.7
	Asympt.	C6	32	38		RJ	x	neg	neg	<10	<10	54.7	30.7	1.8
	Asympt.	C7	38	37		RJ	x	neg	neg	<10	<10	53.5	35.5	1.5
	Asympt.	C8	24	39		RJ	x	neg	neg	<10	≥10	72.6	15.3	4.7
	Asympt.	C9	x	x		RJ	x	neg	neg	<10	≥10	74.1	8.12	9.1
			33.0 (24–41)[b]	38 (24–39)								67.4 (53.5–80.2)	18.4 (14.2–35.5)	3.5 (1.5–5.4)
Children	CZS	C10	29	46		RJ	x	neg	neg	<10	≥10	41.5	31.3	1.3
	CZS	C11	17	26		RJ	x	neg	pos	<10	≥10	58.8	32.9	1.8
	CZS	C12	22	22		RJ	x	neg	pos	160	≥10	80.3	11.7	6.9
	CZS	C13	30	30		RJ	x	x	x	x	x	74.8	11.7	6.4
	CZS	C14	23	38		RJ	x	neg	neg	<10	≥10	76.9	7.37	10.4
	CZS	C15	24	40		RJ	x	neg	neg	<10	≥10	50.9	35.1	1.5
	CZS	C16	32	35		RJ	x	neg	pos	<10	<10	76.5	11.3	6.8
	CZS	C17	32	43		RJ	x	neg	pos	<10	≥10	64.1	29.8	2.2
	CZS	C18	29	30		RJ	x	pos	pos	<10	<10	69.9	18.6	3.8
			29.0 (17–32)[b]	36.5 (22–46)								69.9 (41.5–80.3)	18.6 (7.4–35.1)	3.8 (1.3–10.4)

Age[a], years.
Age[b], months.
Illness time[b], months.
median (minimum–maximum)[a].

The CZS ZIKV group (positive maternal qRT-PCR, $n = 9$) consisted of patients with exposure to ZIKV during pregnancy and with clinical evidence of CZS. Under both ZIKV conditions, mothers had negative results for other infectious agents (syphilis, toxoplasmosis, rubella, cytomegalovirus, and HIV). All participants were clinically evaluated by a multidisciplinary team and are included in an ongoing clinical follow-up program (28). Neuroimaging, such as skull ultrasound, CT or MRI, was performed to investigate radiological factors compatible with congenital infectious diseases. In symptomatic children, according to the Ministry of Health of Brazil, the presence of CZS is defined by maternal ZIKV infection confirmed through qRT-PCR, with two or more clinical parameters, such as microcephaly or other neurological changes; visual or auditory anomalies; and functional disorders, such as irritability, dysphagia, and spasms (29). However, even if the mother has compatible symptoms and is qRT-PCR ZIKV+, it is not possible to state what exposure children who were born asymptomatic had (**Figure 1**).

From 2018 to 2019, blood donations from these donors with a history of ZIKV infection were collected at HUAP/UFF to be used in our study. Previous exposure to DENV or ZIKV were determined by the presence of detectable DENV-specific immunoglobulin G (IgG) titers (30) or ZIKV-specific IgG titers (31) (**Table 1**).

As a control group, we had 5 non-pregnant women infected with ZIKV in the same timeframe (2015–2017). These controls were invited to participate in this study because they had confirmed the diagnosis of ZIKV by qRT-PCR and had positive anti-ZIKV IgG serology. All participants were similar in age compared to the group of mothers (**Table 1**). DENV and chikungunya RNA were not detected in all tested patients, excluding coinfections.

Detection of Dengue IgG and Zika Antibodies With an in-House ELISA

Serum samples were tested using ELISA IgG specific for ZIKV and DENV. Detection of dengue-specific IgG antibodies (Panbio, Australian) and Zika-specific IgG antibodies (Euroimmun, Germany) was performed according to the manufacturer's protocol. These ELISAs were standardized to be used as recommended after studies by the Brazilian Ministry of Health. However, there are concerns about the genuine potential for serological cross-reactivity as a confounding factor in ELISA screening.

The Plaque Reduction Neutralization Test (PRNT)

The PRNT was performed for the laboratory confirmation of Zika cases. The ZIKV/H.sapiens/Brasil/ES2916/2015 strain identified in the State of Espírito Santo, Brazil was used. The cutoff value for PRNT positivity was defined as 90% ($PRNT_{90}$). Samples with neutralizing antibodies for ZIKV were also submitted to $PRNT_{90}$ for dengue virus serotype 1 (DENV-1 from West Pacific). Reference viruses were provided by Laboratório de Flavivírus (LABFLA) of Fiocruz from their arbovirus stocks. The $PRNT_{90}$ was performed to determine the maximum plasma dilution (1:10–1:320) needed to reduce arbovirus plaque formation by 90% among Vero ATCC CCL-81 cells, following standard protocols (32, 33). All plasma was heat-inactivated (56°C, 30 min) before neutralization testing. Next, a final volume of each inactivated sample and virus mixture was transferred to a well-containing Vero cells and then initially screened at a dilution of 1:10 in 6-well-plates at 37°C for 60 min. Those that neutralized ZIKV by at least 90% were further tested at serial 2-fold dilutions to determine 90% endpoint titers. Plasma samples were considered to have DENV-neutralizing antibodies when a plasma dilution of at least ≥10 reduced no <90% of the formation of DENV viral plaques.

PBMC Isolation

Briefly, peripheral blood mononuclear cells (PBMCs) and plasma were isolated by Ficoll-Paque PLUS density gradient centrifugation (GE Healthcare, United States) and frozen in fetal bovine serum (FBS, Gibco, Invitrogen Co, United States) containing 10% (vol/vol) dimethyl sulfoxide (DMSO) (Sigma-Aldrich, United States). Cells were thawed on the day of the experiment and were used directly for *in vitro* assay.

ZIKV CD4 and CD8 MegaPools Description

ZIKV CD4 and CD8 megapool peptides (MP) have been designed and validated, as previously reported (34, 35). Briefly, a consensus sequence was generated by MAFFT alignment after querying the availability of NCBI polyprotein ZIKV sequences and BLAST to a corresponding ZIKV isolate being able to represent most of the viral sequence analyzed (ID: 64320) (36). Two different strategies have been then applied based on the ZIKV polyprotein sequence to predict CD4 and CD8 epitopes using the TepiTool (37) available in the immune epitope database analysis resource (IEDB-AR) (38). Specifically, to design the ZIKV CD4 MP, the "7-allele-method" (39) was applied with a cutoff of ≤20, while, for the ZIKV CD8 MP, the epitopes were predicted using the panel of 27 most frequent A and B alleles with custom selection to consider both 9-mers and 10-mers for the prediction (40) and consensus percentile rank cutoff ≤1.5. The resulting predicted epitopes have been separately clustered for CD4 and CD8 using an IEDB cluster 2.0 tool, applying the cluster-break method with a 70% cutoff for sequence identity (41). The corresponding peptides derived by the bioinformatic analyses were synthesized as a crude material (A&A, San Diego, CA), resuspended in DMSO, and pooled according to CD4 or CD8 MP composition followed by sequential lyophilization.

Thus, the MP approach was designed by taking into account the 27 most frequent HLA class I allelic variants worldwide, thus making it possible to capture reactivity independently from geographical location, as previously shown in the context of both ZIKV- and DENV-specific CD8+ T cell responses (25, 40, 42, 43). While we cannot rule out the possibility that the specific population considered might express an allelic variant that is infrequent in the worldwide population, the MPs are still designed to provide a worldwide population coverage of 90% or more.

IFN-γ ELISpot Assay

Frozen collected PBMCs were assayed for IFN-γ cell responses, as previously described (44). Briefly, mouse anti-human IFN-γ antibody (clone 1-DK1; Mabtech) was added to 96-well-plates (Multiscreen HTS; Millipore) coated at 2.5 μg/ml, diluted in phosphate buffer saline (PBS), pH 7.2–7.4 (Sigma-Aldrich). PBMCs were then added in triplicate to wells (2×10^5 cells/well) in the presence or not of ZIKV MPs at 1 μg/ml, followed by incubation at 37°C, 5% CO_2 for 18–20 h. After washing with PBS–Tween 20, 1 μg/ml of IgG biotinylated anti-human IFN-γ (clone 7-B6-1; Mabtech) was added and incubated for 2 h at room temperature. After washing, streptavidin–alkaline phosphatase substrate (Mabtech) was prepared and added to the plate, for 1 h at room temperature. Plates were washed, and alkaline phosphatase substrate of 5-bromo-4-chloro-3-indolyl-phosphate/nitro blue tetrazolium chloride (BCIP-NBT) from KPL (Gaithersburg) was added after allowing spots to develop. The reaction was stopped by washing with tap water. Spots were counted using an automated ELISpot reader (ImmunoSpot1S6UV Ultra, Cleveland). The number of IFN-γ-producing cells was expressed as spot-forming cells (SFC) relative to 10^6 PBMCs. Values were calculated by subtracting the number of spots detected in unstimulated control wells. Values were considered positive if they were equal or >20 spots and at least two times above the mean of unstimulated control wells. The stimulation with phytohemagglutinin (PHA, 5 μg/mL) was done for all individuals analyzed as a positive control of *in vitro* stimulation.

We have previously established an approach in which, prior to initiating the ELISpot assay, we recovered stimulated PBMCs for 20 h and stained with Abs listed in **Supplementary Table 1** for extracellular staining used for flow cytometry experiments.

Intracellular Cytokine Staining

Peripheral blood mononuclear cells (2×10^5 cells/well) were cultured for 6 h with 1 μg/ml ZIKV MPs and brefeldin A (44). Subsequently, the stimulated PBMC were stained with the Abs used for flow cytometry experiments listed in **Supplementary Table 1**. The intracellular cytokine staining (ICS) was performed, permeabilized with saponin (0.05%), and stained with anti-IFNγ antibody. The stimulation with phorbol and ionomycin myristate acetate (PMA plus ionomycin) was performed on all individuals analyzed as a positive control of *in vitro* stimulation. The data were collected using BD FACSAria III flow cytometer and analyzed using FlowJo 10.5.2 software (Tree Star1, USA).

Statistical Analysis

Comparisons between different groups were performed using either the non-parametric Mann–Whitney rank sum test or the parametric unpaired *t*-test (two-tailed analyses). When data followed a normal distribution, the paired Wilcoxon's test was used. Outcome variables were compared among the groups of study using the Kruskal–Wallis test followed by the Dunn's multiple comparisons test. Multiple comparison tests were used to compute *post-hoc* comparisons for all pairs of groups. The statistical significance of differences in frequency of "Responders" was performed using the Fisher's exact test. The planned statistical comparisons rely on the accurate classification of outcome and detection of arbovirus infections and CZS in infants. Data in all figure parts in which error bars are shown were presented as the median with interquartile range (25–75%). An analysis was performed with GraphPad PRISM (version 5) (GraphPad Software). The value of $p < 0.05$ was considered statistically significant.

RESULTS

Detection of ZIKV and DENV-Specific IgG Antibodies by Commercial ELISA and of Neutralizing Antibodies to ZIKV and DENV

Zika virus (ZIKV)- and DENV-specific IgG antibody detection was initially determined using the commercial capture ELISA assay. Out of the 21 symptomatic mothers tested, who were qRT-PCR ZIKV+, 14 (66.7%) had both anti-ZIKV IgG and anti-DENV IgG. Similar percentages were observed between mothers who had asymptomatic children (8 out of 12; 66.7%) and those who had children with CZS (6 out of 9; 66.7%). Five out of 21 (23.8%) had anti-ZIKV IgG but not anti-DENV IgG, and similar percentages were also observed between those who had asymptomatic children (3 out of 12; 25%) and those who had children with CZS (2 out of 9; 22.2%). Only one mother who had a child with CZS (1 out of 21; 4.8%) had anti-DENV IgG but not anti-ZIKV IgG. Another mother who had a child with CZS (1 out of 21; 4.8%) had neither anti-DENV IgG nor anti-ZIKV IgG.

Regarding the 18 children with a history of intrauterine exposure to ZIKV, it was not possible to perform the assay on one child with CZS because the sample volume was insufficient. Most of the children, i.e., 10 out of 17 (58.8%), had neither anti-DENV IgG nor anti-ZIKV IgG, among whom seven were asymptomatic (7 out 9; 77.8%) and three had CZS (3 out of 8; 37.5%). Five out of 17 (29.4%) had anti-DENV IgG but not anti-ZIKV IgG, among whom one was asymptomatic (1 out 9; 11.1%) and four had CZS (4 out of 8; 50%). Two out of 17 (11.8%) had both anti-ZIKV IgG and anti-DENV IgG: one was asymptomatic (1 out of 9) and another had CZS (1 out 8). None of them had anti-ZIKV IgG but not anti-ZIKV IgG.

To confirm previous ZIKV and DENV exposure, plasma samples were tested using $PRNT_{90}$ for the detection of ZIKV and DENV-1-neutralizing antibodies. We could not perform PRNT for all four DENV serotypes since the plasma volume was insufficient for this. Thus, we chose to evaluate DENV-1 since this had the highest prevalence in Rio de Janeiro in the period in which the samples were collected (2015–2016) (45). Out of 19 mothers who had anti-ZIKV IgG, 18 (94.7%) presented with ZIKV-neutralizing antibodies with $PRNT_{90}$ titer > 320, thus confirming the exposure to ZIKV. Interestingly, out of 14 mothers who had both anti-ZIKV IgG and anti-DENV IgG that were detectable, 10 had a $PRNT_{90}$ titer for ZIKV and DENV, thus indicating exposure to both viruses, while 3 presented a $PRNT_{90}$ titer for ZIKV and 1 did not have any detectable $PRNT_{90}$ titer. Regarding the children, it was not possible to perform PRNT on three of them because the sample volume was insufficient. Thus, two out of 15 children had both anti-ZIKV IgG and anti-DENV IgG that were detectable, and 1 asymptomatic child presented both ZIKV and DENV-neutralizing antibodies.

The frequency of T cell subpopulations was assessed by flow cytometry assay. Data on the percentage of CD4 and CD8 T cells and the ratio between the two subpopulations showed no statistically significant difference between the two donor cohorts (**Table 1**).

Detection of IFN-γ-Producing Cells in Response to ZIKV Peptides in Women and Mothers With a History of ZIKV Infection, but Not in Children With a History of Intrauterine Exposure to ZIKV

Next, we focused on the analysis of T cell responses in donors with a history of ZIKV infection. *Ex vivo* T cell responses to CD4 and CD8 ZIKV MPs (CD4 ZIKV MP and CD8 ZIKV MP) employing the ELISpot assay were measured to quantify the number of IFN-γ secreting cells. The general characteristics of these donors' cohorts are summarized in **Table 1**.

To ensure the comparable quality of samples, we first compared responses induced by the positive control stimulus PHA. As expected, T cells from women (non-pregnant women infected with ZIKV, see **Figure 1** in Materials and Methods) and mothers (pregnant mothers infected with ZIKV, see **Figure 1** in Materials and Methods) with a history of ZIKV infection responded to PHA with values above 250 SFC per 10^6 PBMC, as well as most of the children with a history of intrauterine exposure to ZIKV (from children born to mothers infected with ZIKV during pregnancy, see **Figure 1** in Materials and Methods). One of the samples collected from children responded to PHA with just over 70 SFC per 10^6 PBMC, which resulted in 15 times greater stimulation with PHA compared to the medium; therefore, we decided to maintain this child from the analysis (**Figure 2A**).

In the ELISpot assay, we were able to successfully detect T cell responses using CD4 ZIKV MP and CD8 ZIKV MP. The T cells of all non-pregnant women responded to ZIKV CD4 MP and four out of the five responded to CD8 MP. The frequency of responders was slightly lower in mothers, so the CD4 T cells of 8 out of 10 mothers responded to ZIKV CD4 MP and 6 out of 10 responded to ZIKV CD8 MP. These data demonstrated an important reactivity of donors exposed to ZIKV, both in frequency and magnitude of CD4 and CD8 T cell responses to ZIKV peptides. However, children's T cell responses to ZIKV MP were uncommon as no child responded to CD4 ZIKV MP and only 2 out of 11 responded to CD8 ZIKV MP (**Figure 2B**).

The T cells of all mothers who had asymptomatic children responded to CD4 ZIKV MP and 4 out of the 5 responded to CD8 ZIKV MP. Among those who had children with CZS, the T cells of 3 out of 5 responded to CD4 ZIKV MP and 2 out of 5 to CD8 ZIKV MP. No significant difference was found between the two groups of mothers regarding the magnitude or frequency of responses to the ZIKV MP (**Figure 2C**).

Regarding children, regardless of the clinical outcome, T cells did not respond to CD4 ZIKV MP, and only 1 out of 5 asymptomatic and 1 out of 6 with CZS responded to the CD8 ZIKV MP (**Figure 2D**).

Higher CD4 T Cell Degranulation Ability Compared to CD8 T Cell Degranulation in Donors With a History of ZIKV Infection

Cytotoxic activity is one of the key components of the virus-specific protective immunity (25). In this study, we measured the degranulation capacity of T cells by staining of the expression of the CD107a molecule (**Figure 3A**). Our results were very surprising since we detected an increase in the magnitude of the CD107a-expressing CD4 T cells after stimulation with CD4 ZIKV MP. This response was more intense in mothers and children and less in women. Thus, regarding the response of CD4 T cells to CD4 ZIKV MP, 10 out of 12 mothers, 5 out of 9 children and 2 out of 5 women were responsive to CD4 ZIKV MP with an increase in the frequency and magnitude of CD107a-expressing CD4 T cells. In contrast, no donor responded to CD8 ZIKV MP by inducing the CD107a-expressing CD8 T cell responses (**Figure 3B**).

Further analysis revealed that the response of CD4 T cells to CD4 ZIKV MP was similar among mothers who had asymptomatic or SCZ children (**Figure 3C**). Among children, this response was also independent of whether they had neurological impairment associated with ZIKV (**Figure 3D**).

Higher IFN-γ Producing ZIKV CD4 T Cell Responses Persist in Donors With a History of ZIKV Infection by ICS Assay

By using a ZIKV MP stimulation and ICS assays (**Figure 4A**), we were able to determine the responding T cell subsets as well as the memory subset. Donors cells with a history of ZIKV infection were stimulated with polyclonal PMA plus ionomycin, confirming the viability of all samples (**Figure 4B**).

In a further series of experiments, CD4 T cells from all donors responded to the CD4 ZIKV MP in terms of frequency and magnitude of responses.

CD4 T cells responded to the CD4 ZIKV MP with IFN-γ production in most donors exposed to ZIKV; 3 out of 5 women, 10 out of 13 mothers, and 8 out of 13 children. Regarding the responses of CD8 T cells after stimulation with CD8 ZIKV MP, we observed a lower frequency of responders in all groups: only one out of 5 women, 3 out of 13 mothers, and only 1 out of 13 children (**Figure 4C**). Thus, all donors showed appreciable reactivity, both in terms of increased frequency and magnitude of IFN-γ-producing CD4 responses but a lower response for CD8 responses.

We went to see if there is a difference between the groups of mothers and children. The CD4 T cells of all mothers who had asymptomatic children responded to CD4 ZIKV MP with IFN-γ production, while 4 out of 7 mothers who had CZS children responded, but this difference was not statistical. Regarding CD8 T cell responses, CD8 ZIKV MP responses were remarkably close (**Figure 4D**). Among children, T cell responses to ZIKV MP were quite similar, therefore, regardless of whether they had any neurological impairment associated with ZIKV (**Figure 4E**).

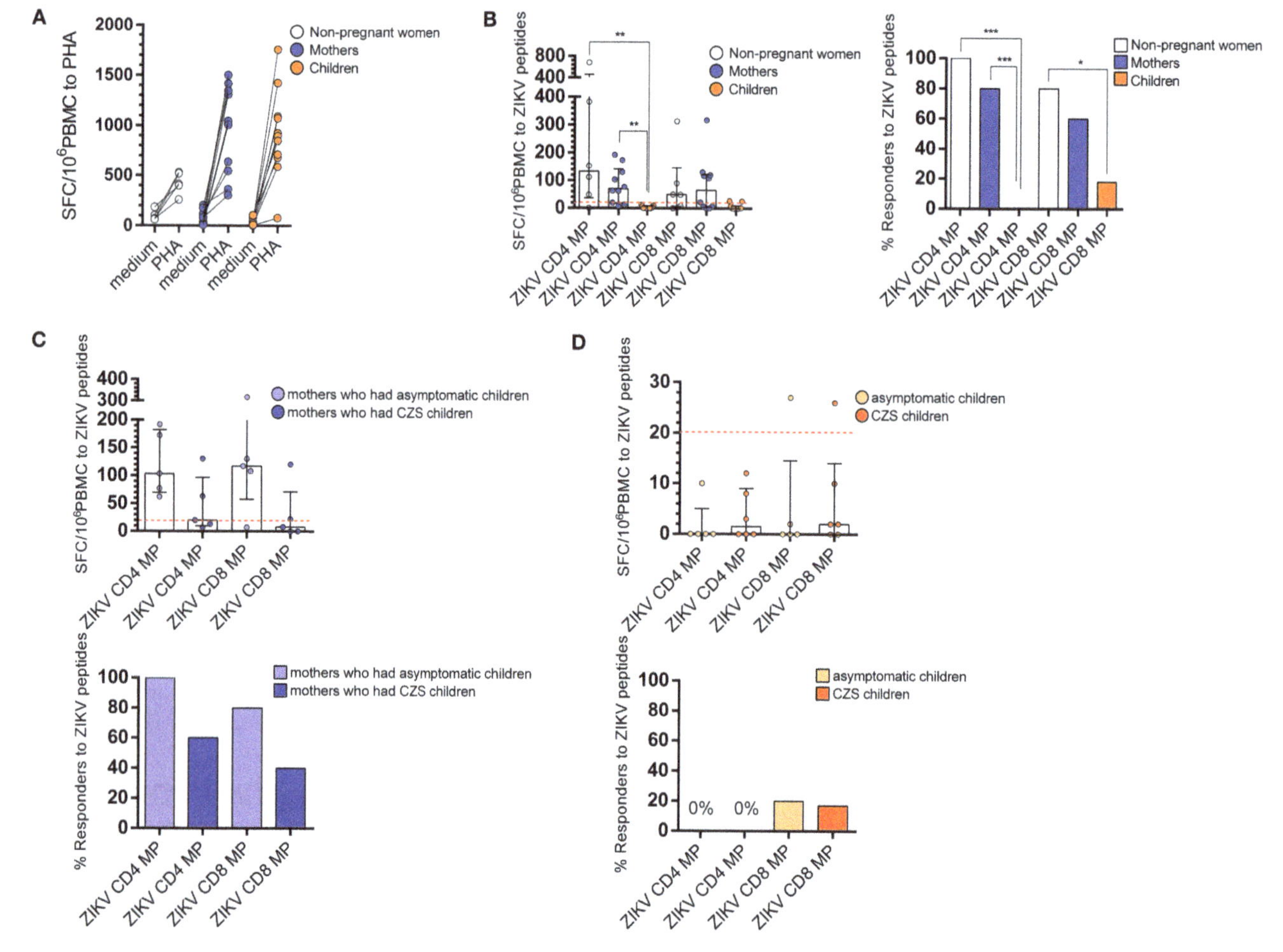

FIGURE 2 | *Ex vivo* reactivity to CD4 and CD8 ZIKV MPs in donors with a history of ZIKV infection. T cell response to by ELISpot *ex vivo* experiments are shown for women (from non-pregnant women infected with ZIKV, white, $n = 5$), mothers (from pregnant mothers infected with ZIKV, blue, $n = 10$), and children (from children born to mothers infected with ZIKV during pregnancy, orange, $n = 11$) with a history of ZIKV infection. In **(A)**, T cell response to PHA stimulation and, in **(B)**, the magnitude of CD4 and CD8 T cell reactivity to ZIKV MPs are expressed as medians and interquartile range (25th and 75th percentiles). Donors were considered "Responders" if the net SFC/106 PBMC after ZIKV MP was ≤20 after 20 h of *in vitro* stimulation. **(C)** CD4 and CD8 T cell reactivity to a ZIKV MP are shown among mothers who had asymptomatic children (light blue) compared with those who had CZS children (dark blue). **(D)** CD4 and CD8 T cell reactivity to ZIKV MPs are shown among children grouped in asymptomatic children (light orange) compared with CZS children (dark orange). Responses were expressed as the number of IFN-g-secreting cells per 106 PBMC. Statistical differences were tested using the one-way analysis of variance (ANOVA) and the Kruskal-Wallis test followed by the Dunn's multiple comparisons test. Bars represent median with interquartile range. Statistical significance for differences in the frequency of "Responders" was performed using Fisher's exact test. $^{*}p < 0.05$, $^{**}p < 0.001$, $^{***}p < 0.001$. ZIKV, Zika virus; MP, megapool peptide; CZS, congenital Zika syndrome; PBMC, peripheral blood mononuclear cell.

Regarding the IFN-γ producing CD4 and CD8 T cells, we observed that there is a greater degree of reactivity of CD4 T cells after CD4 ZIKV MP compared to CD8 T cells after CD8 ZIKV MP in all studied groups (**Figure 4F** and **Supplementary Figure 1**). We performed an analysis of the mother and child pairs to assess whether the responses agreed (pairs tested $n = 7$). Only two of the seven mother and child pairs responded to CD4 ZIKV MP. For the response of CD8 T cells to CD8 ZIKV MP, in 4 pairs, mothers and children did not respond to CD8 ZIKV MP and, in three cases, mothers responded, but children did not (**Figure 4G**).

When the ELISpot and ICS data for all mothers, relating to CD4 ZIKV MP or CD8 ZIKV MP, were combined, we found a significant positive correlation between ELISpot and ICS ($p = 0.002$ for CD4 ZIKV MP and $p = 0.008$ for CD8 ZIKV MP; the Wilcoxon signed-rank test). Thus, in a broad and collective sense, ICS does not fundamentally conflict with ELISpot in the group of mothers. A similar analysis was performed for children, but no significant correlation between ELISpot and ICS was found for either CD4 ZIKV MP or CD8 ZIKV MP (the Wilcoxon signed-rank test). In the ELISpot 20-h cultures, we evaluated susceptibility to death of PBMCs. In particular, the children's PBMCs had a viability ≥100%. We speculate that the kinetics of cytokine production may have more influence on children's PBMCs than on those of their mothers. Other kinetics should therefore be evaluated in future studies.

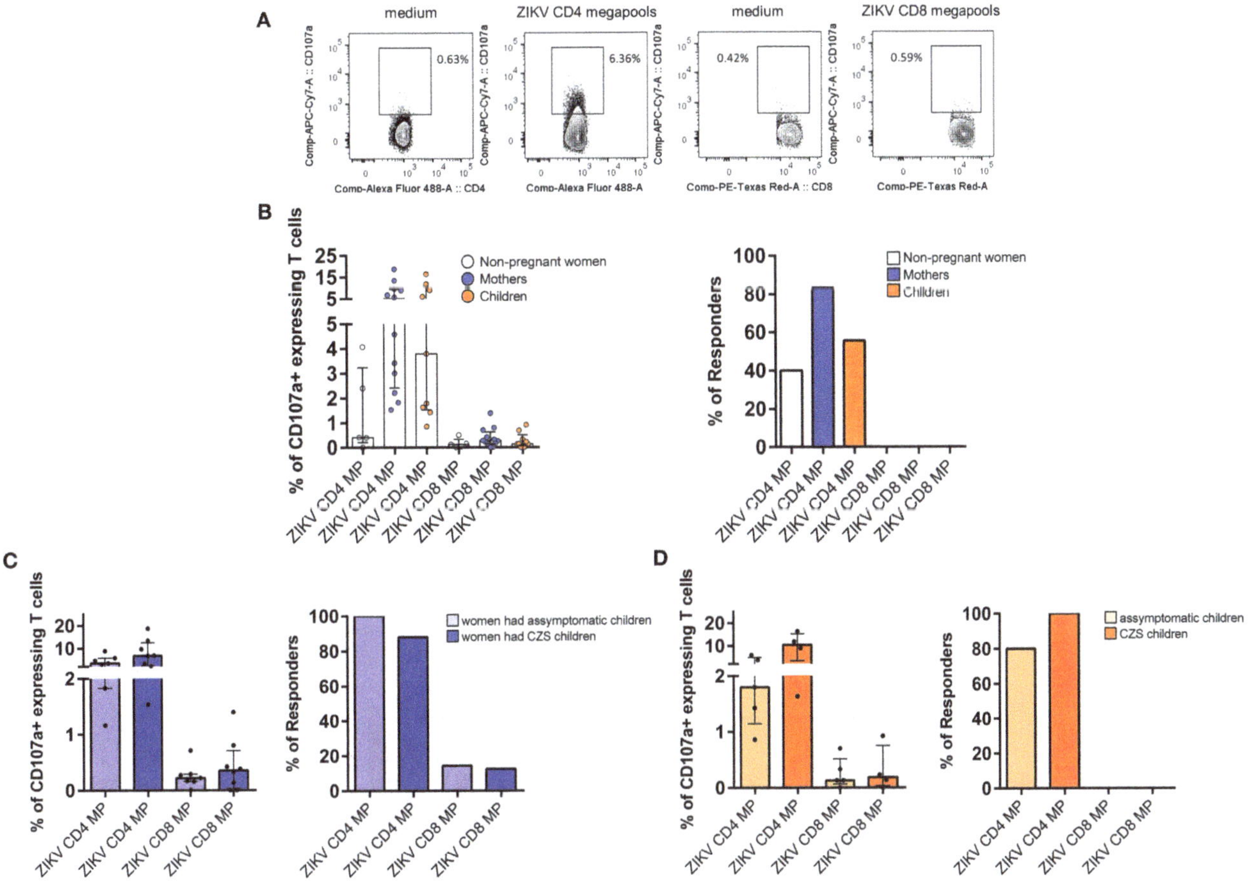

FIGURE 3 | Degranulation activity of T cells from donors with a history of ZIKV infection after ZIKV MP *in vitro* stimulation. **(A)** Gating strategies to the flow cytometry profiles of the degranulation activity of CD4 and CD8 T cells measured by CD107a mobilization after stimulation with ZIKV MPs are shown in a representative of one of the women (from non-pregnant women infected with ZIKV, white, $n = 5$), mothers (from pregnant mothers infected with ZIKV, blue, $n = 12$), and children (from children born to mothers infected with ZIKV during pregnancy, orange, $n = 9$) with a history of ZIKV infection. **(B)** Cumulative data (medians and interquartile range) of the proportion of CD107a+ cells among CD4 and CD8 T cells after ZIKV MP stimulation. Regarding the criteria of positivity of the assay or "Responder," the background in the unstimulated controls was subtracted to ZIKV peptide conditions, and the responder was considered as those who had two times more CD107a-positive cells after subtraction of the background. **(C)** CD4 and CD8 T cell reactivity to ZIKV MPs are shown among mothers who had asymptomatic children (light blue) compared with those who had CZS children (dark blue). **(D)** CD4 and CD8 T cell reactivity to ZIKV MPs are shown among asymptomatic children (light orange) compared with CZS children (dark orange). The magnitude of responses is expressed in medians and interquartile range, and statistical analyses were performed with Mann-Whitney U-test. No statistical difference was found. ZIKV, Zika virus; MP, megapool peptide; CZS, congenital Zika syndrome.

Additionally, we have measured IL-8 levels by ELISA in PBMC supernatants from ZIKV donors recovered from the 20-h cultures for the ELISPOT assay. No statistical difference was found between the groups when comparing the different conditions (data not shown).

The Memory CD4 T Cells Re-Expressing CD45RA (Temra) in Donors With a History of ZIKV Infection Is Enriched for ZIKA-Specific T Cells

We initially analyzed the expression of CD45RA and CCR7 on the total CD4 and CD8 population (**Figure 5A**). In women, the majority of the unspecific CD4 T cells displayed a frequency of naïve (Tn, CD45RA+CCR7+; 50%) phenotype followed by the central memory (Tcm, CD45RA-CCR7+; 37%) phenotype, effector memory (Tem, CD45RA–CCR7–; 15%) phenotype, and finally by effector memory re-expressing CD45RA (Temra, CD45RA+CCR7–; 0.9%) phenotype. In mothers, it was observed that a similar frequency of the unspecific CD4 T cells displayed a Tcm (47%) phenotype and a Tn (41%) phenotype, and then an Tem (11%) phenotype, followed by a Temra (0.5%). As expected, in children, the most CD4 T cells exhibited a Tn (72%) phenotype, followed by a Tcm (23%) phenotype, an Tem (4%) phenotype, and an Temra (0.4%) phenotype (**Figure 5B**).

For the unspecific CD8 T cells, women, mothers, and children had a comparable frequency of all subsets of T cells, exhibiting predominantly a Tn cell (64% in women, 58% in mothers, and 63% in children), followed by a Tem phenotype (23% in women and 16% in both mothers and children donors), a Temra (9, 15, and 11%, respectively), and lastly

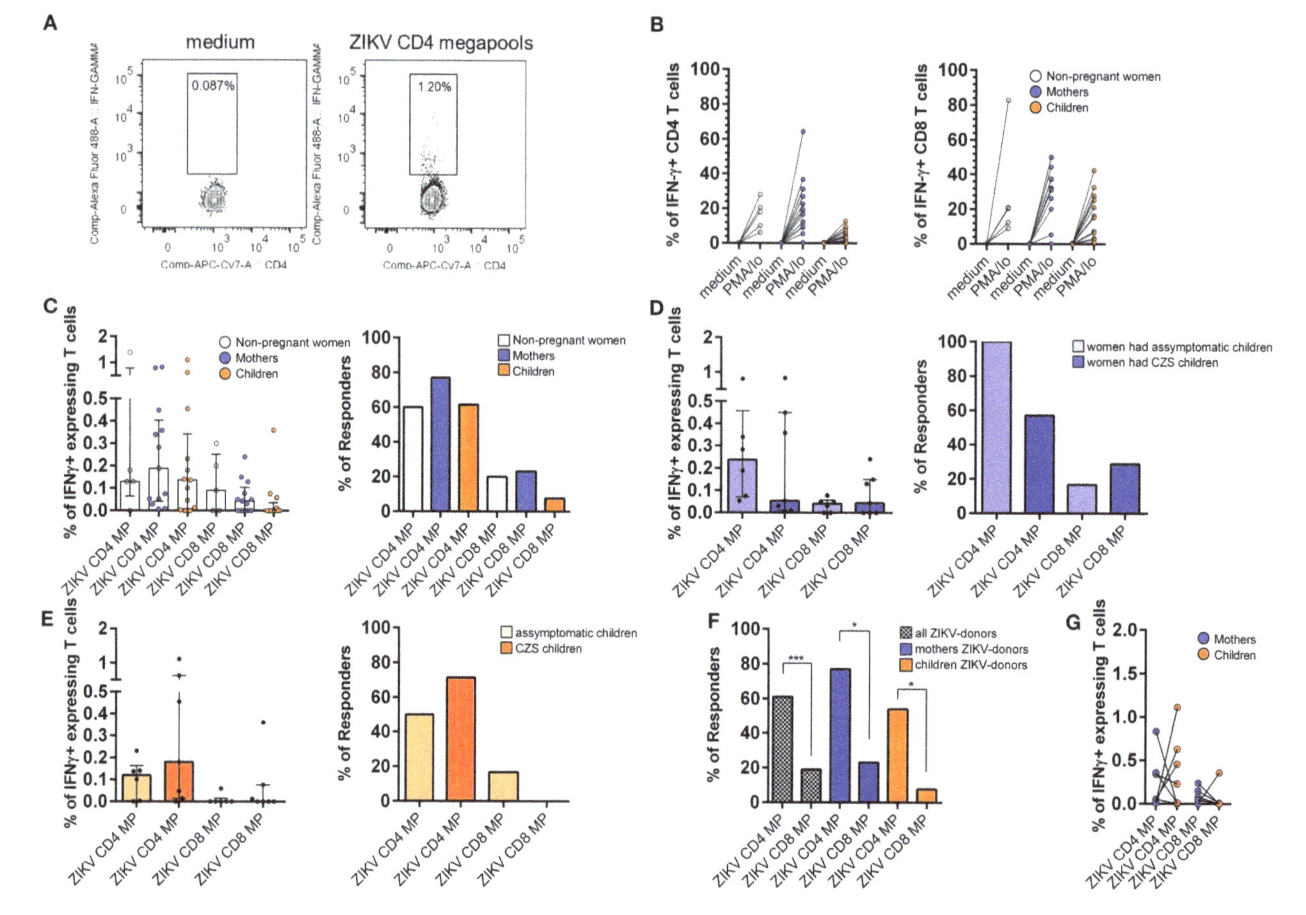

FIGURE 4 | *Ex vivo* reactivity with IFN-γ production of donors with a history with ZIKV infection to CD4 and CD8 ZIKV MPs. CD4 and CD8 ZIKV-restricted responses in women (from non-pregnant women infected with ZIKV, white, $n = 5$), mothers (from pregnant mothers infected with ZIKV, blue, $n = 13$), and children (from children born to mothers infected with ZIKV during pregnancy, orange, $n = 13$) with a history of ZIKV infection after 6-h of *in vitro* stimulation. **(A)** Gating strategy to the flow cytometry plots identifies IFN-g-producing ZIKV-specific T cells. **(B)** Each data point represents the response of a single donor tested with the PMA + io and **(C-E)** two different sets of two protein pools, ZIKV CD4 MP and ZIKV CD8 MP. **(C)** Magnitude of CD4 and CD8 responses and frequency of responders (right) were performed from women, mothers, and children donors to the ZIKV CD4 or CD8 MPs. **(D,E)** Each group is further divided into asymptomatic or CZS. **(D)** Magnitude of CD4 and CD8 responses (left) and frequency of responders (right) were performed from mothers who had asymptomatic children (light blue, $n = 6$) and those who had children with CZS (dark blue, $n = 7$) to the ZIKV CD4 or CD8 peptides. **(E)** Magnitude of CD4 and CD8 responses (left) and frequency of responders (right) were performed from asymptomatic children (light orange, $n = 6$) and CZS children (dark orange, $n = 7$) to the ZIKV CD4 or CD8 MPs. **(F)** Frequency of responders were performed from all (dashed white, $n = 31$), mothers (blue, $n = 13$), and children (orange, $n = 13$) donors to the ZIKV CD4 or CD8 MPs. **(G)** The frequencies of ZIKV-specific IFN-γ-positive CD4 and CD8 cells were compared between the mother-child pairs (tested pairs $n = 7$). The p-values were calculated using the paired t-test. The magnitude of responses is expressed medians and interquartile range, and statistical analyses were performed with the Mann-Whitney U-test. Statistical significance for differences in frequency of responders was performed using a Fisher test. Asterisks indicate significant differences (*$p < 0.05$, ***$p < 0.001$). ZIKV, Zika virus; MP, megapool peptide; CZS, congenital Zika syndrome; INF, interferon.

a Tcm cell (6, 10, and 7%, respectively) (**Figure 5B**). Thus, the majority of unspecific CD4 and CD8 T cells are in the Tn population.

To further determine the memory T cell responses to ZIKV MP, we compared it to responding IFN-γ-secreting Tn out of the total of Tn cells, responding IFN-γ-secreting Tcm out of the total of Tcm cells, responding IFN-γ-secreting Tem out of the total of Tem cells, and finally responding IFN-γ-secreting Temra out of the total of Temra cells (**Figure 5A**).

Further analysis demonstrated that phenotypic analysis of the total of Temra subsets is enriched for responding IFN-γ-secreting CD4 T cells for ZIKV epitopes in women, mothers, and children (**Figure 5C**). In terms of the IFN-γ+-responding CD8 T cells for ZIKV epitopes, no difference was seen in the frequency of Tn or Tcm phenotype in donors with a history of ZIKV infection (**Figure 5C**).

DISCUSSION

In the present study, we aimed to evaluate the T cell response in donors with a history of ZIKV infection during pregnancy. Regarding the few current studies that raise the same questions, our group has progressed when compared to non-pregnant

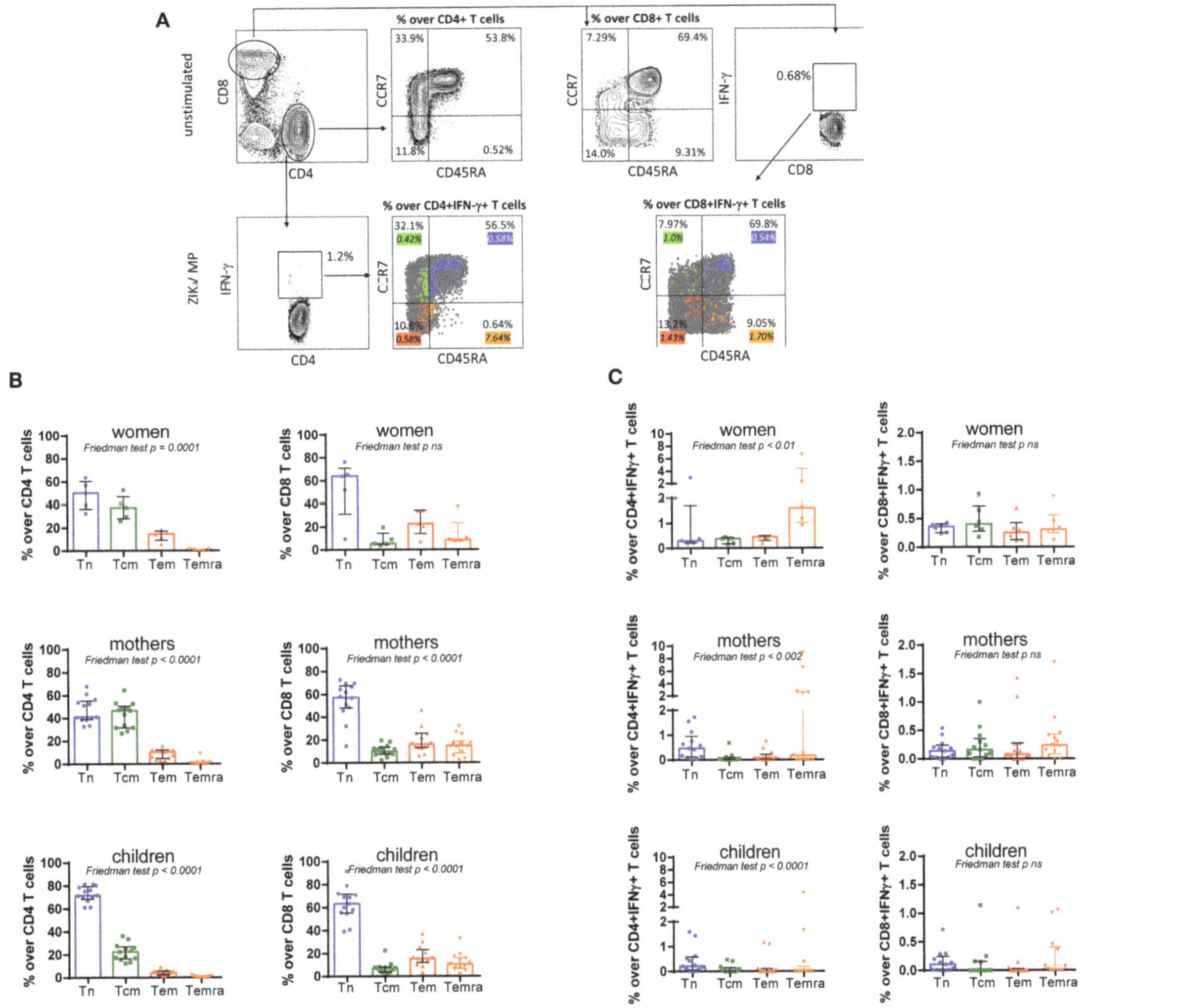

FIGURE 5 | Subpopulations of specific memory from ZIKV donors with a history of ZIKV infection. (A) Gating strategy to identify the CD4 T cell and CD8 T cell subsets, and of the T cell memory subpopulations. Lymphocytes were identified and electronically gated on orthogonal light scatter signals and CD3 immunopositivity. Then, CD3+CD4+T cells and CD3+CD8+T cells were identified. Gating on CD3+CD4+T cells or CD3+CD8+T cells, Tn and Tcm cells were identified as CD45RA negative/positive and CCR7 negative/positive. In unstimulated cells, the percentage of unspecific CD4 and CD8 T cell subsets [Tn: CD45RA+CCR7+; Tcm: CD45RA−CCR7+; effector memory (Tem): CD45RA−CCR7− and effector memory re-expressing CD45RA T cells (Temra): CD45RA+CCR7−] was gated in a representative subject with a history of ZIKV. The percentage values are represented in the graphs. To determine the memory T cell responses to ZIKV MP, the percentage of CD4 and CD8 T cell subsets were demonstrated. The color values represent the frequency of the responding IFN-γ-secreting Tn out of the total of Tn cells, responding IFN-g-secreting Tcm out of the total of Tcm cells, responding IFN-γ-secreting Tem out of the total of Tem cells, and responding IFN-γ-secreting Temra out of the total of Temra cells. The color percentage values are represented in the graphs. **(B)** Percentage of unspecific CD4 and CD8 T cell subsets (Tn, Tcm, Tem, and Temra) gated in unstimulated cells from women (from non-pregnant women infected with ZIKV), mothers (from pregnant mothers infected with ZIKV), and children (from children born to mothers infected with ZIKV during pregnancy) with a history of ZIKV. **(C)** The phenotypic analysis of the responding IFN-γ-secreting T cells for ZIKV epitopes out of a total of Tn or Tcm cell subsets in women, mothers, and children. Data are expressed as median ± the interquartile range for each cohort (n = 5-13 in both panels). Differences between T cell subsets among cohorts were analyzed using the Friedman test. Each data point represents a single donor determination. ZIKV, Zika virus; MP, megapool peptide; CZS, congenital Zika syndrome; INF, interferon; Tn, naïve T cell; Tcm, central memory T cell; Tem, effector memory T cell; Temra, effector memory re-expressing CD45RA T cell.

women, pregnant mothers, and both asymptomatic and CZS children born to mothers infected with ZIKV during pregnancy.

It is essential to understand the repertoires of the ZIKV effector T cell response to the point of extrapolating if the development of a non-protective immunity in mothers is related to the affected children. In addition, in pregnancy and congenital infection scenarios, it is not known if there is a development of long-lasting T cell immunity to ZIKV. To address these issues, the ZIKV T cell immunity in a cohort of mothers infected with ZIKV during pregnancy and children affected (or not) by neurological complications was assessed 2–3 years after the initial infection.

If previous DENV cross-reactive immunity contributes or not to protection against ZIKV infection during pregnancy, it is still unclear. During the Brazilian ZIKV epidemic (2016–2017), 94 pregnant women who gave birth to infants with or without microcephaly were evaluated. Based on previous studies, DENV immunity is not a prerequisite for ZIKV entry into the fetal compartment (46). Halai et al. supported Araújo's findings (47). In contrast, ZIKV-infected human placental tissues showed increased replication in the presence of DENV antibodies, dependent on FcγR engagement (48). In mouse models, the presence of DENV-specific antibodies in ZIKV-infected pregnant mice significantly increased fetal resorption in immune-compromised mice (48) and also displayed CZS, including microcephaly, in immune-competent mice (49, 50).

Thus, conflicting datasets regarding the impact of ADE (antibody-dependent enhancement) on congenital malformations in babies have emerged from different studies, including mouse and non-human primates' models and human donors. Based on Zimmerman's review, additional prospective epidemiologic studies, *ex vivo* studies, and animal model experimentation are needed to fully dissect the complex risk factors and pathways through which ZIKV can seed and infect the fetal compartment (51).

Even so, this can be framed if the mothers' ZIKV T cell effector immune response repertoires are "weak" to the point of not giving protective immunity to the affected children. So far, data addressing this issue is only available in the murine model (52). The authors evaluated adapted mouse models established for ZIKV infection during pregnancy. Interestingly, they observed a reduction in a load of ZIKV in maternal and fetal tissues and an increase in fetal viability and growth in immune mice to DENV compared to non-immune mice. The depletion or genetic deficiency of CD8 T cells nullified this effect, even under ADE conditions (52). A single study on pregnancy and immunity to ZIKV in human patients was recently developed by Reynolds et al. The authors showed that almost all mothers with a history of ZIKV infection have serological evidence of immunity to dengue, suggesting that their children who had microcephaly were born to mothers' immune to DENV. In addition, they showed that different viral products can induce a multifunctional response to E and NS1 antigens and also immunoregulatory responses to NS5 and C ZIKV proteins, which could impact immunopathogenesis (53). From our dataset, it is not yet clear if children who had microcephaly were born of mothers with "an altered" T cell responses. It would be necessary to have acute samples of pregnant mothers to answer this question with greater propriety.

Outside the context of donors infected during pregnancy or by congenital infection, several studies have been evaluating the T cell responses to ZIKV proteins in human donors immune or not to DENV. It is known that ZIKV-reactive T cells in the acute phase of infection are detected earlier and in greater magnitude in DENV-immune patients. Conversely, the pattern of CD4 responses to ZIKV-restricted class II peptides was remarkably similar in acute and convalescent phases, while a lower frequency and magnitude of responses were observed with the CD8 counterpart (44). In another study, Grifoni's data indicated an immunological signature for CD8 T cell responses reproducible and temporally stable after Ag-specific stimulation even 1–2 years after ZIKV infection (25). Moreover, circulating tetramer-positive ZIKV-specific CD8 T cells peaked at early convalescence day post-infection with elevated levels persisting for months from a volunteer woman (54). On the other hand, whereas C-, prM-, E-, and NS5-specific cytokine-expressing CD4 T cells were readily detected in all patients tested, absent or low detection of functional CD8 effector T cells against peptides spanning ZIKV C, prM, E, and NS5 was identified (55). We agree with Lai's study using peptides that span all 10 ZIKV proteins. Our data indicate that after *in vitro* stimulation with the ZIKV MP, CD4 T cells maintain their degranulation and IFN-γ production capacity, which was not observed by CD8 T cells. One possibility is that the cytotoxic and pro-inflammatory activities of CD8 T cells are high at an early stage of ZIKV infection but do not persist in the disease resolution phase when the virus has apparently been eliminated. Our experimental design was based on well-established protocols, with stimulation with ZIKV or DENV MP of cells cultured for 6 h to perform a flow cytometry assay or for 20 h for the ELISpot assay (25, 34, 42, 44, 56). Additionally, studies have already been carried out on *in vitro* expansion of peptide-specific T cells for 14 days (34, 56, 57). Thus, our future proposal is to perform *in vitro* expansion of peptide-specific T cells in the kinetics of up to 14 days, in order to confirm our observations on the role of CD8 T cells.

The protective role of CD8 T cells has been demonstrated in several studies using mouse models. Huang's study demonstrated that an adoptive transfer of ZIKV-immune CD8 T cells can protect against ZIKV infection (58). Indeed, polyfunctional, cytotoxic CD8 T cells are activated (59), reducing ZIKV burden, and, in the same sense, CD8 depletion or genetic absence resulted in greater ZIKV infection and mortality in mice (60). Moreover, ZIKV-specific and ZIKV/DENV cross-reactive CD8 T cells in DENV-immune mice expanded post-ZIKV challenge and reduced infectious ZIKV levels, and CD8 T cell depletion confirmed this protection (61). Nevertheless, within a susceptible mouse model, CD8 T cells appear as an important mediator of ZIKV neuropathogenesis (62, 63). It is currently impossible to determine what the impact of the short duration of ZIKV-specific CD8 T cells will be for donors with a history of ZIKV infection. Unfortunately, only with the emergence of new ZIKV epidemics, this issue can be assessed.

In relation to ZIKV-specific CD4 T cell responses in Zika patients, Koblischke et al. showed a strong impact of structural ZIKV protein on immunodominant CD4 T cell responses (64). Interestingly, most of the CD4 Temra cells are DENV-specific in donors with previous DENV infection (43). Patil et al. revealed in patients with dengue that these CD4 T cells in the Temra subsets are highly enriched with CD4 cytotoxic T lymphocytes expressing several genes linked to cytotoxic and costimulatory function, compared with CD4 T cells in the Tcm and Tem subsets (65). Tian et al. revealed that the CD4 Temra cells can be subdivided into two major subsets between DENV-immune individuals based on the expression of the adhesion G protein-coupled receptor GPR56. While GPR56+ Temra cells display a transcriptional and proteomic program with cytotoxic features, GPR56+ Temra cells have higher levels of clonal expansion and contain the majority of virus-specific Temra cells (66). Overall, like DENV infection, our data indicate that the Temra CD4 T cell subset is enriched for responding IFN-γ-secreting CD4 T cells for ZIKV epitopes in donors with a history of ZIKV infection. Future efforts will be underway in our laboratory to assess whether the heterogeneity of CD4 Temra T cells could provide insights to differentiate the outcome of the child's congenital infection in T cell responses against ZIKV.

Some limitations should be considered when interpreting our findings. First, to understand the evolution of the acquired ZIKV immunity, the best would be a "longitudinal study" in which donors were monitored in the acute and convalescent phases and after complete recovery from the disease. Second, the diagnosis of ZIKV through qRT-PCR was not made in newborns, so we cannot affirm that they were vertically infected, especially in asymptomatic cases. Recently, Ribeiro et al. published data from analyses on the positivity of PRNT and serological tests among a total of 88 children in northeastern Brazil who presented clinical cases of CZS between 2016 and 2018. Six (6.8%) were positive for IgG anti-ZIKV, and 2 (2.3%) of them were ZIKV $PRNT_{90}$-positive (67). Although our initial goal was not to make correlations like those made by Ribeiro et al., our data are very close. In our study, only 2 out of 17 children (11.8%) had anti-ZIKV IgG (but also anti-DENV IgG), and 2 out of 15 (13.3%) were ZIKV and DENV $PRNT_{90}$-positive. This frequency of positivity was much lower than we expected, as were the data of Ribeiro et al. Like in their study, our data cannot be attributed to problems in the execution of $PRNT_{90}$, since the protocol established by Baer and Kehn-Hall (36) was strictly followed. The ZIKV/H.sapiens/Brasil/ES2916/2015 strain was identified in the State of Espírito Santo at the time of the CZS epidemic in Brazil (68). In a case report, it was shown that a child was positive for ZIKV IgG at birth and at the age of 12 months but was negative at 21 and 24 months of age. The child's mother was ZIKV RT-PCR, IgM, IgG, and PRNT-positive during the pregnancy. Three hypotheses were raised by the authors of that study: (a) low and transient ZIKV viremia could lead to the lack of detection of the antigen and absence of a strong immune response in the child; (b) specific and direct tropism of ZIKV to the central nervous system could cause ZIKV to become a silent virus that would escape the host's response; and (c) ZIKV could prevent the triggering of a strong innate immune response because active viral replication might have ceased during intrauterine life or shortly thereafter (69). Moreover, methodologically, the use of the recombinant NS1 antigen as a target in the commercial kit may explain the low anti-ZIKV IgG seropositivity in newborns (70).

Third, it was not possible to carry out many analyzes of paired mothers and children, mainly due to the clinical complications of the children during the study, which made it difficult to define a close association between the immunity of mothers and the clinical outcome of their children. Fourth, a caveat to this study is that the T cell responses detected after ZIKV MP restimulations may actually cover specific ZIKV responses and responses from cross-reactions due to previous flavivirus infections, particularly DENV.

Given the similarity between DENV and ZIKV and their common regions of endemicity, questions have arisen about whether immunity to one virus can provide cross-protection against another. Grifoni et al. published data that demonstrated that the degree of MP sequence homology for different flaviviruses directly influenced cross-reactivity in terms of CD4 and CD8 T cell responses. It is important to note that the CD8 MP of ZIKV used in our study was provided by Dr. Sette's team and, therefore, is the same as used by Grifoni et al. According to them, 33% of the DENV and ZIKV CD8 MP have homology ≥70% of sequence similarity with the consensus sequence, which in fact means that one-third of the peptides present in the MPs that we tested can cross-react with DENV (34). Here, our data showed that more than 70% of mothers who had both anti-ZIKV IgG and anti-DENV IgG had a $PRNT_{90}$ test positive for ZIKV and DENV. Among the children, 50% of those who had both anti-ZIKV IgG and anti-DENV IgG presented ZIKV and DENV-neutralizing antibodies. Several human studies have investigated cross-reactivity in T cell responses, targeting a variety of viral proteins (71). Grifoni et al. found that prior DENV exposure did not have any impact on the CD4 T cell response to ZIKV infection: patients in the acute phase of ZIKV infection had more IFN-γ+ CD8 T cells after restimulation with ZIKV-derived peptides (44). However, prior DENV immunity did not have any impact on either the transcriptional profile of the CD8 T cells or the capacity of CD4 or CD8 T cells to produce IFN-γ at later stages of infection (25). Therefore, we have no way of knowing with certainty whether the T cell response that we are evaluating is directed only to primary ZIKV infection and not to DENV. We believe that the most important thing is that, despite the high degree of cross-reactivity between T cell responses to DENV and ZIKV, no indication has yet been provided that this may have a negative impact on disease outcomes.

Our data did not show any notable differences between children with CZS and asymptomatic children or between mothers who gave birth to children with CZS and those who gave birth to asymptomatic children, 2–3 years after primary infection. Recently, Macedo-da-Silva et al. used the same cohort of children as in our study, also in the recovery phase. They demonstrated that asymptomatic children presented changes in proteins that participated in processes relating to neuronal death and cerebrovascular abnormalities, low regulation of proteins relating to vision, and increased activity of metalloproteinases, namely MMP-2 and MMP-9, associated with neuronal death. Interestingly, these changes are not common among control children, but they are also characteristic of children with CZS (72). Together with Macedo-da-Silva et al. we think that, perhaps, marked differences between the groups occurred in the acute phase of Zika but were not so evident in the recovery phase.

In summary, we studied donors with a history of ZIKV infection that occurred in the 2016–2017 outbreak in Brazil, including non-pregnant women, mothers infected with ZIKV during pregnancy, and children with a history of intrauterine exposure. In general, donors demonstrated long-term immunity from CD4 T cells to ZIKV CD4 MP, but the same was not observed in CD8 T cells with ZIKV CD8 MP. It is possible that the cytotoxic and pro-inflammatory activities of CD8 T cells are markedly exhibited in the early stages of the disease but less detected in the resolution phase. The responses of mothers'

T cells and children's T cells to ZIKV MPs do not appear to be related to the clinical outcome. These data still need to be investigated, including the evaluation of CD8 T cell response to other ZIKV peptides.

STUDY APPROVAL

These patients were recruited from the Exanthematic Diseases Unit at the Hospital Universitário Antonio Pedro of the Universidade Federal Fluminense, Niteroi city, RJ, Brazil. All activities were performed after obtaining the informed consent of mothers and parents of children. This approved study is titled "Clinical follow-up of pregnant women with rash and their children: prospective study cohort" with approval number 56913416.9.0000.5243.

ETHICS STATEMENT

The studies involving human participants were reviewed and approved by these patients were recruited from the Exanthematic Diseases Unit at the HUAP/UFF, Niteroi city, RJ, Brazil. All activities were performed after obtaining the informed consent of mothers and parents of children. This approved study is titled Clinical follow-up of pregnant women with rash and their children: prospective study cohort with approval number 56913416.9.0000.5243. Written informed consent to participate in this study was provided by the participants' legal guardian/next of kin.

AUTHOR CONTRIBUTIONS

JB-C, IAP and, DF-M developed and performed experiments, analyzed, and interpreted data. HGD, AP-C, and CF-S clinically characterized patients for the study including the PRNT90 trials for ZIKV and DENV-1 and additional cytokines ELISA. MG made the sample acquisitions on the flow cytometer. FRC, AAS, RAOV, and CAAC recruited the clinical cohort for the study. FRC, MRQL, AAS, SMBC, and CAAC clinically characterized patients for the study including DENV IgG and ZIKV IgG ELISA. SAO, ELA, and CAAC helped prepare the manuscript. AG, AS, and DW designed and validated the ZIKV megapools. LMO-P and JB-C conceived and designed the study, interpreted the data, and wrote the manuscript. CAAC and LMO-P supervised the research. All the authors discussed the results and commented on the manuscript.

ACKNOWLEDGMENTS

JB-C, FRC, IAP, DF-M, HGD, and CF-S are recipient of doctoral fellowship from Brazilian research institutions CNPq, CAPES and IOC/Fiocruz. This work was funded by the National Institutes of Health contract Nr. 75N9301900065 (AS and DW). This study was financed in part by the Coordination for the Improvement of Higher Education Personnel (Coordenação de Aperfeiçoamento de Pessoal de Nível Superior - CAPES) - Finance Code 001. We thank children and their families that participated in the study, the Multi-function Laboratory to support research in Nephrology and Medical Sciences/LAMAP, the Clinical Research Unit/UPC, Zika Collaborative Group, and Dr. Remberto Mauricio de la Cruz Vargas Vilte for his valuable and stimulating scientific discussions. We also thank the Laboratório de Flavivírus (LabFLA) of Fiocruz, which provided reference viruses from their arbovirus stocks.

REFERENCES

1. Perkins TA, Siraj AS, Ruktanonchai CW, Kraemer MU, Tatem AJ. Model-based projections of Zika virus infections in childbearing women in the Americas. *Nat Microbiol.* (2016) 1:16126. doi: 10.1038/nmicrobiol.2016.126
2. Fauci AS, Morens DM. Zika virus in the Americas-yet another arbovirus threat. *N Engl J Med.* (2016) 374:601-4. doi: 10.1056/NEJMp16 00297
3. Brady OJ, Gething PW, Bhatt S, Messina JP, Brownstein JS, Hoen AG, et al. Refining the global spatial limits of dengue virus transmission by evidence-based consensus. *PLoS Negl Trop Dis.* (2012) 6:e1760. doi: 10.1371/journal.pntd.0001760
4. Brady OJ, Hay SI. The first local cases of Zika virus in Europe. *Lancet.* (2019) 394:1991–2. doi: 10.1016/S0140-6736(19)32790-4
5. Bhatt S, Gething PW, Brady OJ, Messina JP, Farlow AW, Moyes CL, et al. The global distribution and burden of dengue. *Nature.* (2013) 496:504–7. doi: 10.1038/nature12060
6. Messina JP, Kraemer MU, Brady OJ, Pigott DM, Shearer FM, Weiss DJ, et al. Mapping global environmental suitability for Zika virus. *Elife.* (2016) 19:e15272. doi: 10.7554/eLife.15272.017
7. D'Ortenzio E, Matheron S, Yazdanpanah Y, de Lamballerie X, Hubert B, Piorkowski G, et al. Evidence of sexual transmission of Zika virus. *N Engl J Med.* (2016) 374:2195–8. doi: 10.1056/NEJMc16 04449
8. Fréour T, Mirallié S, Hubert B, Splingart C, Barrière P, Maquart M, et al. Sexual transmission of Zika virus in an entirely asymptomatic couple returning from a Zika epidemic area, France, April 2016. *Euro Surveill.* (2016) 21:23. doi: 10.2807/1560-7917
9. Govero J, Esakky P, Scheaffer SM, Fernandez E, Drury A, Platt DJ, et al. Zika virus infection damages the testes in mice. *Nature.* (2016) 540:438–42. doi: 10.1038/nature20556
10. Ma W, Li S, Ma S, Jia L, Zhang F, Zhang Y, et al. Zika virus causes testis damage and leads to male infertility in mice. *Cell.* (2017) 168:542. doi: 10.1016/j.cell.2017.01.009
11. Tang WW, Young MP, Mamidi A, Regla-Nava JA, Kim K, Shresta S. A mouse model of Zika virus sexual transmission and vaginal viral replication. *Cell Rep.* (2016) 17:3091–8. doi: 10.1016/j.celrep.2016.11.070
12. Cugola FR, Fernandes IR, Russo FB, Freitas BC, Dias JL, Guimarães KP, et al. The Brazilian Zika virus strain causes birth defects in experimental models. *Nature.* (2016) 534:267–71. doi: 10.1038/nature18296

13. Miner JJ, Cao B, Govero J, Smith AM, Fernandez E, Cabrera OH, et al. Zika virus infection during pregnancy in mice causes placental damage and fetal demise. *Cell.* (2016) 165:1081–91. doi: 10.1016/j.cell.2016.05.008
14. Venturi G, Zammarchi L, Fortuna C, Remoli ME, Benedetti E, Fiorentini C, et al. An autochthonous case of Zika due to possible sexual transmission, Florence, Italy, (2014). *Euro Surveill.* (2016) 21:30148. doi: 10.2807/1560-7917.ES.2016.21.8.30148
15. Yockey LJ, Varela L, Rakib T, Khoury-Hanold W, Fink SL, et al. Vaginal exposure to Zika virus during pregnancy leads to fetal brain infection. *Cell.* (2016) 166:1247–56. doi: 10.1016/j.cell.2016.08.004
16. Lima GP, Rozenbaum D, Pimentel C, Frota ACC, Vivacqua D, Machado ES, et al. Factors associated with the development of congenital Zika syndrome: a case-control study. *BMC Infect Dis.* (2019) 19:277. doi: 10.1186/s12879-019-3908-4
17. Brasil P, Pereira JP Jr, Moreira ME, Ribeiro Nogueira RM, Damasceno L, Wakimoto M, et al. Zika virus infection in pregnant women in Rio de Janeiro. *N Engl J Med.* (2016) 375:2321–34. doi: 10.1056/NEJMoa16 02412
18. Costa F, Sarno M, Khouri R, de Paula Freitas B, Siqueira I, Ribeiro GS, et al. Emergence of congenital Zika syndrome: viewpoint from the front lines. *Ann Intern Med.* (2016) 164:689–91. doi: 10.7326/M16-0332
19. França GV, Schuler-Faccini L, Oliveira WK, Henriques CM, Carmo EH, Pedi VD, et al. Congenital Zika virus syndrome in Brazil: a case series of the first 1501 livebirths with complete investigation. *Lancet.* (2016) 388:891–7. doi: 10.1016/S0140-6736(16)30902-3
20. Kleber de Oliveira W, Cortez-Escalante J, De Oliveira WT, do Carmo GM, Henriques CM, Coelho GE, et al. Increase in reported prevalence of microcephaly in infants born to women living in areas with confirmed Zika virus transmission during the first trimester of pregnancy - Brazil, 2015. *MMWR Morb Mortal Wkly Rep.* (2016) 65:242–7. doi: 10.15585/mmwr.mm6509e2
21. Mlakar J, Korva M, Tul N, Popović M, Poljšak-Prijatelj M, Mraz J, et al. Zika virus associated with microcephaly. *N Engl J Med.* (2016) 374:951–8. doi: 10.1056/NEJMoa1600651
22. Hamel R, Dejarnac O, Wichit S, Ekchariyawat P, Neyret A, Luplertlop N, et al. Biology of Zika virus infection in human skin cells. *J Virol.* (2015) 89:8880–96. doi: 10.1128/JVI.00354-15
23. Ngono AE, Shresta S. Immune response to dengue and Zika. *Annu Rev Immunol.* (2018) 36:279–308. doi: 10.1146/annurev-immunol-042617-053142
24. Tonnerre P, Melgaço JG, Torres-Cornejo A, Pinto MA, Yue C, Blümel J, et al. Evolution of the innate and adaptive immune response in women with acute Zika virus infection. *Nat Microbiol.* (2020) 5:76–83. doi: 10.1038/s41564-019-0618-z
25. Grifoni A, Costa-Ramos P, Pham J, Tian Y, Rosales SL, Seumois G, et al. Cutting edge: transcriptional profiling reveals multifunctional and cytotoxic antiviral responses of Zika virus-specific CD8+ T cells. *J Immunol.* (2018) 201:3487–91. doi: 10.4049/jimmunol.1801090
26. Racicot K, Mor G. Risks associated with viral infections during pregnancy. *J Clin Invest.* (2017) 127:1591–9. doi: 10.1172/JCI87490
27. Lanciotti RS, Kosoy OL, Laven JJ, Velez JO, Lambert AJ, Johnson AJ, et al. Genetic and serologic properties of Zika virus associated with an epidemic, yap state, Micronesia, 2007. *Emerg Infect Dis.* (2008) 14:1232–9. doi: 10.3201/eid1408.080287
28. Vianna RAO, Lovero KL, Oliveira SA, Fernandes AR, Santos TCSD, Lima LCSS, et al. Children born to mothers with rash during Zika virus epidemic in Brazil: first 18 months of life. *J Trop Pediatr.* (2019) 65:592–602. doi: 10.1093/tropej/fmz019
29. Brazil. Ministry of Health of Brazil. *Health Surveillance Department. Zika Virus in Brazil : the SUS response (electronic resource)/Ministry of Health of Brazil, Health Surveillance Department.* Brasilia: Ministry of Health of Brazil (2017).
30. Miagostovich MP, Nogueira RM, dos Santos FB, Schatzmayr HG, Araújo ES, Vorndam V. Evaluation of an IgG enzyme-linked immunosorbent assay for dengue diagnosis. *J Clin Virol.* (1999) 14:183–9. doi: 10.1016/S1386-6532(99)00059-1
31. Steinhagen K, Probst C, Radzimski C, Schmidt-Chanasit J, Emmerich P, van Esbroeck M, et al. Serodiagnosis of Zika virus (ZIKV) infections by a novel NS1-based ELISA devoid of cross-reactivity with dengue virus antibodies: a multicohort study of assay performance, 2015 to 2016. *Euro Surveill.* (2016) 21:30426. doi: 10.2807/1560-7917.ES.2016.21.50.30426
32. Russell PK, Nisalak A, Sukhavachana P, Vivona S. A plaque reduction test for dengue virus neutralizing antibodies. *J Immunol.* (1967) 99:285–90.
33. Roehrig JT, Hombach J, Barrett AD. Guidelines for plaque-reduction neutralization testing of human antibodies to dengue viruses. *Viral Immunol.* (2008) 21:123–32. doi: 10.1089/vim.2008.0007
34. Grifoni A, Voic H, Dhanda SK, Kidd CK, Brien JD, Buus S, et al. T cell responses induced by attenuated flavivirus vaccination are specific and show limited cross-reactivity with other flavivirus species. *J Virol.* (2020) 94:e00089-20. doi: 10.1128/JVI.00089-20
35. Grifoni A, Tian Y, Sette A, Weiskopf D. Transcriptomic immune profiles of human flavivirus-specific T-cell responses. *Immunology.* (2020) 160:3–9. doi: 10.1111/imm.13161
36. Xu X, Vaughan K, Weiskopf D, Grifoni A, Diamond MS, Sette A, et al. Identifying candidate targets of immune responses in Zika virus based on homology to epitopes in other flavivirus species. *PLoS Curr.* (2016) 8. doi: 10.1371/currents.outbreaks.9aa2e1fb61b0f632f58a098773008c4b
37. Paul S, Sidney J, Sette A, Peters B. TepiTool: a pipeline for computational prediction of T cell epitope candidates. *Curr Protoc Immunol.* (2016) 114:18.19.1–24. doi: 10.1002/cpim.12
38. Dhanda SK, Mahajan S, Paul S, Yan Z, Kim H, Jespersen MC et al. IEDB-AR: immune epitope database-analysis resource in 2019. *Nucleic Acids Res.* (2019) 47:W502–6. doi: 10.1093/nar/gkz452
39. Paul S, Lindestam Arlehamn CS, Scriba TJ, Dillon MB, Oseroff C, Hinz D et al. Development and validation of a broad scheme for prediction of HLA class II restricted T cell epitopes. *J Immunol Methods.* (2015) 422:28–34. doi: 10.1016/j.jim.2015.03.022
40. Paul S, Weiskopf D, Angelo MA, Sidney J, Peters B, Sette A. HLA class I alleles are associated with peptide-binding repertoires of different size, affinity, and immunogenicity. *J Immunol.* (2013) 191:5831–9. doi: 10.4049/jimmunol.1302101
41. Dhanda SK, Vaughan K, Schulten V, Grifoni A, Weiskopf D, Sidney J, et al. Development of a novel clustering tool for linear peptide sequences. *Immunology.* (2018) 155:331–45. doi: 10.1111/imm.12984
42. Weiskopf D, Angelo MA, de Azeredo EL, Sidney J, Greenbaum JA, Fernando AN, et al. Comprehensive analysis of dengue virus-specific responses supports an HLA-linked protective role for CD8+ T cells. *Proc Natl Acad Sci USA.* (2013) 110:E2046–53. doi: 10.1073/pnas.1305227110
43. Weiskopf D, Bangs DJ, Sidney J, Kolla RV, De Silva AD, de Silva AM, et al. Dengue virus infection elicits highly polarized CX3CR1+ cytotoxic CD4+ T cells associated with protective immunity. *Proc Natl Acad Sci USA.* (2015) 112:E4256–63. doi: 10.1073/pnas.1505956112
44. Grifoni A, Pham J, Sidney J, O'Rourke PH, Paul S, Peters B, et al. Prior dengue virus exposure shapes T cell immunity to Zika virus in humans. *J Virol.* (2017) 91:e01469-17. doi: 10.1128/JVI.01469-17
45. Secretaria Estadual de Saúde do Rio de Janeiro. *Boletim Epidemiológico 005/2016.* Rio de Janeiro: Secretaria Estadual de Saúde do Rio de Janeiro (2016).
46. de Araújo TVB, Rodrigues LC, de Alencar Ximenes RA, de Barros Miranda-Filho D, Montarroyos UR, de Melo APL, et al. Association between Zika virus infection and microcephaly in Brazil, January to May, 2016: preliminary report of a case-control study. *Lancet Infect Dis.* (2016) 16:1356–3. doi: 10.1016/S1473-3099(16)30318-8
47. Halai UA, Nielsen-Saines K, Moreira ML, de Sequeira PC, Junior JPP, de Araujo Zin A, et al. Maternal Zika virus disease severity, virus load, prior dengue antibodies, and their relationship to birth outcomes. *Clin Infect Dis.* (2017) 65:877–83. doi: 10.1093/cid/cix472
48. Brown JA, Singh G, Acklin JA, Lee S, Duehr JE, Chokola AN, et al. Dengue virus immunity increases Zika virus-induced damage during pregnancy. *Immunity.* (2019) 50:751–62. doi: 10.1016/j.immuni.2019.01.005
49. Camargos VN, Foureaux G, Medeiros DC, da Silveira VT, Queiroz-Junior CM, Matosinhos ALB, et al. In-depth characterization of congenital Zika syndrome in immunocompetent mice: antibody-dependent enhancement and an antiviral peptide therapy. *EBioMedicine.* (2019) 44:516–29. doi: 10.1016/j.ebiom.2019.05.014

50. Rathore APS, Saron WAA, Lim T, Jahan N, St John AL. Maternal immunity and antibodies to dengue virus promote infection and Zika virus-induced microcephaly in fetuses. *Sci Adv.* (2019) 5:eaav3208. doi: 10.1126/sciadv.aav3208
51. Zimmerman MG, Wrammert J, Suthar MS. Cross-reactive antibodies during Zika virus infection: protection, pathogenesis, and placental seeding. *Cell Host Microbe.* (2020) 27:14–24. doi: 10.1016/j.chom.2019.12.003
52. Regla-Nava JA, Elong Ngono A, Viramontes KM, Huynh AT, Wang YT, Nguyen AT, et al. Cross-reactive dengue virus-specific CD8+ T cells protect against Zika virus during pregnancy. *Nat Commun.* (2018) 9:3042. doi: 10.1038/s41467-018-05458-0
53. Reynolds CJ, Suleyman OM, Ortega-Prieto AM, Skelton JK, Bonnesoeur P, Blohm A, et al. T cell immunity to Zika virus targets immunodominant epitopes that show cross-reactivity with other Flaviviruses. *Sci Rep.* (2018) 8:672. doi: 10.1038/s41598-017-18781-1
54. Ricciardi MJ, Magnani DM, Grifoni A, Kwon YC, Gutman MJ, Grubaugh ND, et al. Ontogeny of the B- and T-cell response in a primary Zika virus infection of a dengue-naïve individual during the 2016 outbreak in Miami, FL. *PLoS Negl Trop Dis.* (2017) 11:e0006000. doi: 10.1371/journal.pntd.0006000
55. Lai L, Rouphael N, Xu Y, Natrajan MS, Beck A, Hart M, et al. Innate, T-, and B-cell responses in acute human Zika patients. *Clin Infect Dis.* (2018) 66:1–10. doi: 10.1093/cid/cix732
56. Angelo MA, Grifoni A, O'Rourke PH, Sidney J, Paul S, Peters B, et al. Human CD4+ T cell responses to an attenuated tetravalent dengue vaccine parallel those induced by natural infection in magnitude, HLA restriction, and antigen specificity. *J Virol.* (2017) 91:e02147–16. doi: 10.1128/JVI.02147-16
57. Grifoni A, Moore E, Voic H, Sidney J, Phillips E, Jadi R, et al. Characterization of magnitude and antigen specificity of HLA-DP, DQ, and DRB3/4/5 restricted DENV-specific CD4+ T cell responses. *Front Immunol.* (2019) 10:1568. doi: 10.3389/fimmu.2019.01568
58. Huang H, Li S, Zhang Y, Han X, Jia B, Liu H, et al. CD8+ T cell immune response in immunocompetent mice during Zika virus infection. *J Virol.* (2017) 91:e00900–17. doi: 10.1128/JVI.00900-17
59. Pardy RD, Rajah MM, Condotta SA, Taylor NG, Sagan SM, Richer MJ. Analysis of the T cell response to Zika virus and identification of a novel CD8+ T cell epitope in immunocompetent mice. *PLoS Pathog.* (2017) 13:e1006184. doi: 10.1371/journal.ppat.1006184
60. Elong Ngono A, Vizcarra EA, Tang WW, Sheets N, Joo Y, Kim K, et al. Mapping and role of the CD8+ T cell response during primary Zika virus infection in mice. *Cell Host Microbe.* (2017) 21:35–46. doi: 10.1016/j.chom.2016.12.010
61. Wen J, Tang WW, Sheets N, Ellison J, Sette A, Kim K, et al. Identification of Zika virus epitopes reveals immunodominant and protective roles for dengue virus cross-reactive CD8+ T cells. *Nat Microbiol.* (2017) 2:17036. doi: 10.1038/nmicrobiol.2017.36
62. Manangeeswaran M, Ireland DD, Verthelyi D. Zika (PRVABC59) infection is associated with T cell infiltration and neurodegeneration in CNS of immunocompetent neonatal C57Bl/6 mice. *PLoS Pathog.* (2016) 12:e1006004. doi: 10.1371/journal.ppat.1006004
63. Jurado KA, Yockey LJ, Wong PW, Lee S, Huttner AJ, Iwasaki A. Antiviral CD8 T cells induce Zika-virus-associated paralysis in mice. *Nat Microbiol.* (2018) 3:141–7. doi: 10.1038/s41564-017-0060-z
64. Koblischke M, Stiasny K, Aberle SW, Malafa S, Tsouchnikas G, Schwaiger J, et al. Structural influence on the dominance of virus-specific CD4 T cell epitopes in Zika virus infection. *Front Immunol.* (2018) 9:1196. doi: 10.3389/fimmu.2018.02083
65. Patil VS, Madrigal A, Schmiedel BJ, Clarke J, O'Rourke P, de Silva AD, et al. Precursors of human CD4+ cytotoxic T lymphocytes identified by single-cell transcriptome analysis. *Sci Immunol.* (2018) 3:eaan8664. doi: 10.1126/sciimmunol.aan8664
66. Tian Y, Babor M, Lane J, Schulten V, Patil VS, Seumois G, et al. Unique phenotypes and clonal expansions of human CD4 effector memory T cells re-expressing CD45RA. *Nat Commun.* (2017) 8:1473. doi: 10.1038/s41467-017-01728-5
67. Ribeiro MRC, Khouri R, Sousa PS, Branco MRFC, Batista RFL, Costa EPF, et al. Plaque reduction neutralization test (PRNT) in the congenital Zika syndrome: positivity and associations with laboratory, clinical, and imaging characteristics. *Viruses.* (2020) 12:1244. doi: 10.3390/v12111244
68. Pauvolid-Corrêa A, Gonçalves Dias H, Marina Siqueira Maia L, Porfírio G, Oliveira Morgado T, Sabino-Santos G, et al. Zika virus surveillance at the human-animal interface in west-central Brazil, 2017-2018. *Viruses.* (2019) 11:1164. doi: 10.3390/v11121164
69. Sulleiro E, Frick MA, Rodó C, Espasa M, Thome C, Espiau M, et al. The challenge of the laboratory diagnosis in a confirmed congenital Zika virus syndrome in utero: a case report. *Medicine.* (2019) 98:1–6. doi: 10.1097/MD.0000000000015532
70. Robbiani DF, Olsen PC, Costa F, Wang Q, Oliveira TY, Nery N Jr, et al. Risk of Zika microcephaly correlates with features of maternal antibodies. *J Exp Med.* (2019) 216:2302–15. doi: 10.1084/jem.20191061
71. Pardy RD, Richer MJ. Protective to a T: the role of T cells during Zika virus infection. *Cells.* (2019) 8:820. doi: 10.3390/cells8080820
72. Macedo-da-Silva J, Rosa-Fernandes L, Barbosa RH, Angeli CB, Carvalho FR, de Oliveira Vianna RA, et al. Serum proteomics reveals alterations in protease activity, axon guidance, and visual phototransduction pathways in infants with in utero exposure to Zika virus without congenital Zika syndrome. *Front Cell Infect Microbiol.* (2020) 10:577819. doi: 10.3389/fcimb.2020.577819

11

Placental Galectins are Key Players in Regulating the Maternal Adaptive Immune Response

Andrea Balogh[1,2], Eszter Toth[1], Roberto Romero[3,4,5,6], Katalin Parej[1,7], Diana Csala[1], Nikolett L. Szenasi[1], Istvan Hajdu[7], Kata Juhasz[1], Arpad F. Kovacs[8], Hamutal Meiri[9], Petronella Hupuczi[10], Adi L. Tarca[3,11,12], Sonia S. Hassan[3,11,13], Offer Erez[14], Peter Zavodszky[7], Janos Matko[2], Zoltan Papp[10,15], Simona W. Rossi[16], Sinuhe Hahn[16], Eva Pallinger[8] and Nandor Gabor Than[1,10,17]*

[1] Systems Biology of Reproduction Momentum Research Group, Institute of Enzymology, Research Centre for Natural Sciences, Hungarian Academy of Sciences, Budapest, Hungary, [2] Department of Immunology, Eotvos Lorand University, Budapest, Hungary, [3] Perinatology Research Branch, Eunice Kennedy Shriver National Institute of Child Health and Human Development, National Institutes of Health, U.S. Department of Health and Human Services, Bethesda, MD and Detroit, MI, United States, [4] Department of Obstetrics and Gynecology, University of Michigan, Ann Arbor, MI, United States, [5] Department of Epidemiology and Biostatistics, Michigan State University, East Lansing, MI, United States, [6] Center for Molecular Medicine and Genetics, Wayne State University, Detroit, MI, United States, [7] Structural Biophysics Research Group, Institute of Enzymology, Research Centre for Natural Sciences, Hungarian Academy of Sciences, Budapest, Hungary, [8] Department of Genetics, Cell and Immunobiology, Semmelweis University, Budapest, Hungary, [9] TeleMarpe Ltd, Tel Aviv, Israel, [10] Maternity Private Clinic of Obstetrics and Gynecology, Budapest, Hungary, [11] Department of Obstetrics and Gynecology, Wayne State University School of Medicine, Detroit, MI, United States, [12] Department of Computer Science, Wayne State University College of Engineering, Detroit, MI, United States, [13] Department of Physiology, Wayne State University School of Medicine, Detroit, MI, United States, [14] Division of Obstetrics and Gynecology, Maternity Department "D", Faculty of Health Sciences, Soroka University Medical Center, School of Medicine, Ben Gurion University of the Negev, Beer-Sheva, Israel, [15] Department of Obstetrics and Gynecology, Semmelweis University, Budapest, Hungary, [16] Department of Biomedicine, University and University Hospital Basel, Basel, Switzerland, [17] First Department of Pathology and Experimental Cancer Research, Semmelweis University, Budapest, Hungary

***Correspondence:**
Nandor Gabor Than
than.gabor@ttk.mta.hu

Galectins are potent immunomodulators that regulate maternal immune responses in pregnancy and prevent the rejection of the semi-allogeneic fetus that also occurs in miscarriages. We previously identified a gene cluster on Chromosome 19 that expresses a subfamily of galectins, including galectin-13 (Gal-13) and galectin-14 (Gal-14), which emerged in anthropoid primates. These galectins are expressed only by the placenta and induce the apoptosis of activated T lymphocytes, possibly contributing to a shifted maternal immune balance in pregnancy. The placental expression of Gal-13 and Gal-14 is decreased in preeclampsia, a life-threatening obstetrical syndrome partly attributed to maternal anti-fetal rejection. This study is aimed at revealing the effects of Gal-13 and Gal-14 on T cell functions and comparing the expression of these galectins in placentas from healthy pregnancies and miscarriages. First-trimester placentas were collected from miscarriages and elective termination of pregnancies, tissue microarrays were constructed, and then the expression of Gal-13 and Gal-14 was analyzed by immunohistochemistry and immunoscoring. Recombinant Gal-13 and Gal-14 were expressed and purified, and their effects were investigated on primary peripheral blood T cells. The binding of Gal-13 and Gal-14 to T cells and the effects of these galectins on apoptosis, activation marker (CD25, CD71, CD95, HLA-DR) expression and cytokine (IL-1β, IL-6, IL-8, IL-10, IFNγ) production of T cells were examined by flow cytometry.

Gal-13 and Gal-14 are primarily expressed by the syncytiotrophoblast at the maternal-fetal interface in the first trimester, and their placental expression is decreased in miscarriages compared to first-trimester controls. Recombinant Gal-13 and Gal-14 bind to T cells in a population- and activation-dependent manner. Gal-13 and Gal-14 induce apoptosis of Th and Tc cell populations, regardless of their activation status. Out of the investigated activation markers, Gal-14 decreases the cell surface expression of CD71, Gal-13 increases the expression of CD25, and both galectins increase the expression of CD95 on T cells. Non-activated T cells produce larger amounts of IL-8 in the presence of Gal-13 or Gal-14. In conclusion, these results show that Gal-13 and Gal-14 already provide an immunoprivileged environment at the maternal-fetal interface during early pregnancy, and their reduced expression is related to miscarriages.

Keywords: angiogenesis, glycomics, immune privilege, PP13, trophoblast differentiation, trophoblast invasion

INTRODUCTION

The mechanisms sustaining maternal immune tolerance to the semi-allogeneic fetus while shielding against microbial infections during pregnancy as well as the changes and interplay of maternal, fetal, and placental immune responses during pregnancy are of major interest in reproductive research (1–41). These immune tolerance mechanisms are complex and dynamic given that implantation involves decidual inflammation; the second trimester of pregnancy is characterized by a predominantly anti-inflammatory milieu in the womb, while at the end of the third trimester, the initiation of parturition requires a transition toward physiologic pro-inflammatory responses (42–44). Recent evolutionary evidence has shown that the pro-inflammatory implantation reaction in humans, as in all eutherian mammals, is derived from an inflammatory attachment reaction in the uterus of the ancestral therian mammals that directly leads to parturition, and that a key innovation in eutherian mammals was the shift from this inflammatory attachment reaction to the non-inflammatory mid-pregnancy period, which allowed an extended period of intimate placentation (45, 46). Although the molecular changes of this evolutionary shift in uterine immune responses are not yet explored in detail, these may include the placental expression of molecules that down-regulate maternal immune responses (47–67). This is substantiated by the fact that the dysregulated expression of immunoregulatory molecules at the maternal-fetal interface and the consequent disturbances in maternal-fetal immune regulation and pro-inflammatory processes are associated with the development of the great obstetrical syndromes, including miscarriage (68–71), preterm labor (72–80), or preeclampsia (81–87).

Regulation of the immune system is mediated by a complex network of cellular and molecular interactions, including glycan recognition by endogenous lectins (61, 88–90). Galectins, a subfamily of lectins specifically bind β-galactoside-containing glycoconjugates, also on immune cell surfaces where they modify immune responses by cross-linking receptors (61, 89, 91–93). Galectins have pleiotropic functions given their binding to a diverse set of cell surface ligands on immune and other cells including trophoblasts (94, 95). In mammals, 19 galectins have been identified, of which 13 are expressed in human tissues (56, 61, 92, 93). Studies of past decades began the exploration of the diverse functions of human galectins, primarily galectins-1, -3, and -9, in innate and adaptive immune responses including the regulation of leukocyte homing, adhesion, apoptosis, pathogen sensing, and immune signaling, also observed in reproductive processes (52, 96–102). Of major interest, several human galectins have an abundant expression at the maternal-fetal interface (31, 52, 53, 56, 58, 97, 103–109), and galectins-13, -14, and -16 are solely expressed by the human placenta (53, 56, 58, 61). These three galectins are expressed from a gene cluster on Chromosome 19 that had emerged in anthropoid primates (53, 56, 61, 110).

We recently started to explore the biological functions of Chromosome 19 galectins in pregnancy (53). Galectin-13 and galectin-14 (Gal-13 and Gal-14), originally described as placental protein 13 (PP13) (111) and placental protein 13-like (PPL13) (112), respectively, are strongly expressed in the syncytiotrophoblast at the lining of the maternal-fetal interface (53, 106, 110, 113, 114). The expression of these galectins is dependent on trophoblast differentiation, and this developmentally regulated process in the trophoblast emerged during primate evolution (110). Of importance, Gal-13 is secreted from the syncytiotrophoblast into the maternal circulation, and low Gal-13 concentration in the maternal circulation in the first trimester was found in women who subsequently developed preterm preeclampsia (115–122), a severe obstetrical syndrome with a strong systemic immune dysregulation (51, 82, 86, 123–128) that already exists in the first trimester (129). Our studies have also shown that the placental expression of Gal-13 and Gal-14 is down-regulated in preterm preeclampsia (81, 110, 113, 129), where the placental pathology and the pro-inflammatory changes are similar to that of miscarriage (130–135).

Since we and our collaborators have shown that Gal-13 and Gal-14 induce the apoptosis of pre-activated T lymphocytes (53) and that Gal-13 increased IL-1α and IL-6 secretion from peripheral blood mononuclear cells (PBMCs) in pregnant women (114), an unanswered question remained: are Gal-13

TABLE 1 | Demographic and clinical data of the first-trimester placental study groups.

Groups	Control	Miscarriage
Number of cases[a]	30	10
Maternal age (years)[b]	30 (19–41)	36 (27–42)*
Gestational age at surgery (weeks)[b]	8.7 (5.0–11.9)	9.4 (7.0–13.0)
Gravidity[b,d]	2 (1–6)	2 (1–7)
Parity[b,d]	0 (0–4)	0 (0–1)
Habitual abortion[c,d]	3	30**

All women were Caucasian
[a]*Values are presented as numbers.*
[b]*Values are presented as medians (interquartile (IQR) range).*
[c]*Values are presented as a percentages.*
[d]*Data were available for 29 cases in the control group.*
**$p < 0.05$ compared to gestational age-matched controls.*
***$p < 0.01$ compared to gestational age-matched controls.*

and Gal-14 critical regulators of immune processes at the early maternal-fetal interface that can be considerably dysregulated in miscarriage? Therefore, we investigated the placental expression of Gal-13 and Gal-14 in miscarriage and also the effects of Gal-13 and Gal-14 on human T lymphocyte functions, which may play a critical role in immune tolerance and rejection. Indeed, we show herein that these placenta-specific galectins moderate adaptive immune responses and are down-regulated in miscarriages, suggesting that their reduced expression is related to the immunopathology of miscarriage.

MATERIALS AND METHODS

Study Groups, Clinical Definitions, and Sample Collection

Placental tissue samples, collected from Caucasian women, were processed immediately after sample collection as previously described (81, 136), fixed in 10% neutral-buffered formalin, and were then embedded in paraffin (FFPE). First- ($n = 40$) and third- ($n = 2$) trimester placentas were collected prospectively at the Maternity Private Department, Semmelweis University (Budapest, Hungary). Pregnancies were dated according to ultrasound scans collected between 5 and 13 weeks of gestation. Patients with a twin gestation were excluded. Women were enrolled in two groups: those who underwent elective termination of pregnancy (control, $n = 30$) and those who miscarried their pregnancy (cases, $n = 10$) (**Table 1**). Miscarriage was defined according to the American College of Obstetricians and Gynecologists Practice Bulletin, as a non-viable, intrauterine pregnancy with a gestational sac containing an embryo or fetus without fetal heart activity within the first 12 6/7 weeks of gestation (137).

Clinical samples and data collection were approved by the Health Science Board of Hungary (ETT-TUKEB 4834-0/2011-1018EKU). Written informed consent was obtained from women prior to sample collection and the experiments conformed to the principles set out in the World Medical Association Declaration of Helsinki. Specimens and data were stored anonymously.

Histopathologic Evaluation of the Placentas

Five-micrometers-thick sections were cut from FFPE tissue blocks and stained with hematoxylin and eosin for histopathological evaluation at the 1st Department of Pathology and Experimental Cancer Research, Semmelweis University. The sections were examined using light microscopy by a perinatal pathologist blinded to the clinical information. Histopathologic changes were defined according to published criteria (136, 138, 139).

Tissue Microarray Construction, and Galectin-13 and Galectin-14 Immunostainings

As previously described (140–143), representative areas were selected for the construction of tissue microarrays (TMAs), which contained 2 mm cores in diameter. To investigate protein expressions, two TMAs were created, using an automated tissue arrayer (TMA Master II, 3DHISTECH Ltd.), to contain one block of each first-trimester ($n = 40$) placenta as well as a positive control (third-trimester healthy placenta) and a negative control (liver) in triplicate.

Five-micrometers-thick sections were cut from TMAs and placed on silanized slides. After deparaffinization and rehydration, antigen retrieval was performed using citrate buffer (10 mM Sodium citrate, 0.05% Tween 20, pH = 6) for 5 min at 100°C in a pressure cooker. Endogen peroxidase blocking was performed using 10% H_2O_2 for 20 min. Immunostaining was carried out using the Novolink Polymer Detection System (Novocastra Laboratories), according to the manufacturer's protocol, as detailed in **Supplementary Table 1**. Slides were blocked for 10 min with Protein Block. To evaluate Gal-13 expression, slides were incubated with anti-galectin-13 mouse monoclonal antibody (clone 215-28-3) in 1% BSA-TBS for 60 min at 37°C. To evaluate Gal-14 expression, slides were incubated with anti-galectin-14 recombinant human antibody in 1% BSA-TBS for 60 min at room temperature. In the case of Gal-14 staining, after three washes with Tris buffer saline with 0.05% Tween 20 (TBST), slides were incubated with anti-His_6 mouse monoclonal antibody for 30 min at room temperature. In both circumstances, subsequent steps were the same. Briefly, after three washes with TBST and Post Primary treatment (30 min, at room temperature), Novolink Polymer was used as the secondary antibody for 30 min at room temperature. This was followed by three washes with TBST, and then the sections were developed using 3,3′-diaminobenzidine (DAB, Novolink) in 1:20 dilution. Finally, sections were counterstained with hematoxylin, and these were mounted with DPX Mountant (Sigma-Aldrich) after dehydration.

Evaluation of Immunostainings

Gal-13 or Gal-14 immunostained placental TMAs were digitally scanned by a high-resolution bright field slide scanner (Pannoramic Scan, 3DHISTECH Ltd.), and cytoplasmic staining in the syncytiotrophoblast was evaluated on virtual slides using Pannoramic Viewer 1.15.4 (3DHISTECH Ltd.) by two examiners blinded to the clinical information. All villi were scored semi-quantitatively. The intensity of immunostaining was graded from 0 to 3. The average intensity was determined for each core as the representative data for that core. By averaging immunoscores of the cores, the overall intensity score was assigned to each placenta and then to each patient group.

Expression and Purification of Recombinant Galectin-13 and Galectin-14

Recombinant Gal-13/Gal-14 was expressed as previously described (53) with modifications. Expression plasmids used earlier (53) were modified by the N-terminal insertion of maltose-binding protein (MBP) tag on these galectins. These modified plasmids, containing either full-length Gal-13 or Gal-14 as well as N-terminal maltose-binding protein (MBP)- and C-terminal His_6-tags, were transformed into ClearColi BL21 (DE3) (Lucigen). For protein expression, cells were grown in LB-Miller broth to $OD_{600} = 0.6$ at 37°C, induced with 0.4 mM isopropyl β-D-1-thiogalactopyranoside (IPTG), and further grown for 4 h at 30°C. The following purification steps were applied: affinity purification on MBPTrap HP column (GE Healthcare Life Sciences); size exclusion chromatography (Superdex 200 Increase SEC column, GE Healthcare Life Sciences) for elimination of aggregates (only for Gal-14); MBP cleavage by Tobacco Etch virus (TEV) protease [expressed and purified according to Kapust et al. (144)]; affinity chromatography on HisTrap HP columns (GE Healthcare Life Sciences); desalting and buffer exchange on Bio-Gel P-6 Desalting Cartridge (Bio-Scale Mini, Bio-Rad). All steps were carried out in the presence of 1 mM dithiothreitol (DTT). Finally, Gal-13 and Gal-14 in PBS, supplemented with 1 mM DTT, were aliquoted and stored at −80°C.

Checking the Purity and Carbohydrate Binding Properties of Recombinant Gal-13 and Gal-14

The purity of the recombinant galectins was verified by heating the samples in Laemmli buffer for 10 min at 70°C, followed by 15% SDS polyacrylamide gel electrophoresis (SDS-PAGE) (Bio-Rad). After gel electrophoresis, recombinant galectins were either subjected to Coomassie blue staining (**Supplementary Figure 1A**) or transferred to nitrocellulose membranes. Membranes were blocked with 5% non-fat dry milk in TBST for 1 h, and then these were incubated overnight at 4°C with primary antibodies to Gal-13 (clone 27-3-2) or Gal-14 in TBST with 5% BSA. After repeated washing with TBST, blots were incubated for 1 h with HRP-goat anti-mouse IgG antibody (ThermoFisher Scientific) for Gal-13 or with HRP-goat anti-human IgG F(ab')2 antibody (Bio-Rad) for Gal-14 (**Supplementary Table 2**). After repeated washing with TBST, protein bands were visualized by enhanced chemiluminescence (ECL; Amersham International) (**Supplementary Figure 1B**).

To determine their functional activity, the binding of purified galectins to asialofetuin (ASF), a naturally occurring multivalent glycoprotein serving as a ligand for several galectins, was assayed by ELISA (145, 146). Briefly, ASF (50 μL of 10 μg/mL bovine ASF in sodium carbonate buffer pH = 9.6) was immobilized in microtiter plates overnight. After blocking residual binding sites with BSA (5% in PBS-Tween, PBST) for 2 h, different amounts of Gal-13 or Gal-14 were incubated for 1 h in PBST with 0.5% BSA. Washing with PBS was done three times between the incubation steps. Bound galectins were detected by incubation with anti-His_6-HRP antibody in PBST with 0.5% BSA (Biolegend, 1:1,000) and by the subsequent conversion of 3,3′5,5′-tetramethylbenzidine (TMB; Sigma-Aldrich) with a readout at 450 nm (reference filter: 620 nm). The reaction was stopped by 4N H_2SO_4 (**Supplementary Figure 1C**). Additionally, 50 μg/mL recombinant galectins were pre-incubated with gentle rotation on lactose-agarose beads (Sigma-Aldrich) for 1 h at room temperature prior to performing ELISA to also check for lactose inhibition. The inhibition was moderate for Gal-13 and weak for Gal-14, as we found differential binding of Gal-13 and Gal-14 to lactose and other carbohydrates in a previous study (53).

Isolation of Primary Immune Cells

Blood samples were obtained from a donor pool of non-pregnant, healthy, human females ($n = 18$ in total, $n = 4$–8 per assay, median age: 29.5) who were in the pre-ovulatory phase. PBMCs were isolated by Ficoll-Hypaque (Sigma-Aldrich) density-gradient centrifugation and washed in RPMI 1640 medium (ThermoFisher Scientific) before experimentations. T cells were isolated from PBMCs with the Dynabeads untouched human T cell kit (ThermoFisher Scientific) according to the manufacturer's protocol. PBMCs or T lymphocytes were kept in RPMI 1640 medium supplemented with 10% FBS and gentamycin or were activated for 48/72 h with the Dynabeads human T-Activator CD3/CD28 (ThermoFisher Scientific), according to the manufacturer's instructions, before treatment with Gal-13 or Gal-14 for 24 h.

Binding of Gal-13 and Gal-14 to Peripheral Blood T Cells

Fresh PBMCs from three donors, or PBMCs activated or not with human T-Activator for 72 h, were used for the Gal-13/Gal-14 binding study. To measure the binding of recombinant Gal-13 or Gal-14 to the surface of T cells, 2×10^5 PBMCs were initially washed in PBS containing 1% BSA. Recombinant Gal-13 or Gal-14 (4 μM), which we conjugated with CF488 fluorophore using the Mix-n-Stain CF488 kit (Sigma-Aldrich) according to the technical bulletin, was added to the cells, and samples were incubated for 45 min on ice. After washing, Fc receptors were blocked with human FcR blocking reagent (Miltenyi Biotec) for 5 min on ice. Anti-CD3-APC, anti-CD4-PerCP, and anti-CD8-APC/Fire750 antibodies (Biolegend) were applied to discriminate between T lymphocyte populations. All antibodies and reagents are listed in **Supplementary Table 3**. Flow cytofluorimetric measurements were carried out on a CytoFLEX device (Beckman Coulter) by collecting data from 50,000 cells. Data were analyzed using FlowJo v10 software (FlowJo, LLC).

Apoptosis Assay

PBMCs (5×10^5), previously activated or not with human T-Activator for 48 h, were incubated for 24 h on tissue culture plates with 0.25 or 4 μM recombinant Gal-13 or Gal-14 in RPMI 1640 medium supplemented with 10% FBS. The 10^5 cells were stained with anti-CD3-APC and anti-CD8-FITC antibodies, as described above. Cells were then incubated in 100 μL of annexin-binding buffer containing phycoerythrin-conjugated Annexin V (Annexin V-PE) and 7-amino-actinomycin D (7-AAD) (Annexin-V Apoptosis Detection Kit, ThermoFisher Scientific; **Supplementary Table 3**) for 15 min at room temperature in the dark. After incubation, 400 μL annexin binding buffer was added, and samples were measured immediately on a FACSCalibur cytofluorimeter using Cell Quest software (BD Biosciences). The Annexin V-PE$^-$/7-AAD$^-$ population was regarded as normal, while the Annexin V-PE$^+$/7-AAD$^-$ and Annexin V-PE$^+$/7-AAD$^+$ populations were taken as measurements of early and late apoptotic cells, respectively. Data were analyzed using FlowJo v10 software.

Flow Cytometry Measurement of Activation Markers

The PBMCs (5×10^5), previously activated or not with human T-Activator for 72 h, were incubated for 24 h on tissue culture plates with 4 μM recombinant Gal-13 or Gal-14 in RPMI 1640 medium supplemented with 10% FBS. To examine cell surface markers, 2×10^5 PBMCs were initially washed in PBS containing 1% FBS. Fc receptors were blocked with human FcR blocking reagent for 5 min on ice; then, specific antibodies to mid-late and late activation markers CD25 (Interleukin-2 Receptor alpha, IL-2Rα), CD71 (Transferrin Receptor, TfR), CD95 (Fas Cell Surface Death Receptor, Fas), and HLA-DR (Human Leukocyte Antigen, DR isotype; member of MHC-II) were added to the cells. Anti-CD3-APC and anti-CD8-FITC antibodies were added simultaneously and samples were incubated for 20 min on ice. All antibodies are listed in **Supplementary Table 3**. After washing, cells were measured in a CytoFLEX flow cytofluorimeter. A total of 20,000 cells were collected and data were analyzed using FlowJo v10 software.

Measurement of Cytokine Production by Bead Array

The T lymphocytes were isolated as described above. The 5×10^5 cells, previously activated or not with human T-Activator for 72 h, were incubated for 24 h on tissue culture plates with 4 μM recombinant Gal-13 or Gal-14 in RPMI 1640 medium supplemented with 10% FBS. Supernatants were collected in all cases, centrifuged at 400 g for 10 min, aliquoted and stored at −80°C until use. LEGENDplex bead-based immunoassays (Biolegend) were applied to measure the concentration of IL-8, IL-10, IFNγ, IL-1β, and IL-6 cytokines in cell culture supernatants of T cells, according to the manufacturer's instruction. Beads were measured in a FACSCalibur flow cytofluorimeter and data were analyzed using FlowJo v10 software.

Statistical Analysis

Statistical analysis was performed using GraphPad Prism 5.0 (GraphPad Software). An unpaired *t*-test with or without Welch's correction was used to analyze demographic data. An unpaired *t*-test was also used to analyze Gal-13 and Gal-14 immunostainings when comparing first-trimester control and miscarriage groups. The Fisher's exact test was performed to test the distribution of Gal-13 or Gal-14 immunoscores between the control and miscarriage groups. Repeated ANOVA tests with Tukey's *post-hoc* test were used for the analysis of galectin binding and CD4:CD8 ratio upon different treatments. One sample *t*-test was used to compare apoptosis of the Gal-13- and Gal-14-treated groups to the PBS-DTT-treated group, and to analyze the binding of Gal-13 and Gal-14 to ASF with or without lactose pre-treatment. Repeated ANOVA tests with Dunnett's *post-hoc* test were used to compare the non-treated group with Gal-13/Gal-14-treated groups in activation marker expression and cytokine production studies. Results were considered statistically significant at $^*p < 0.05$, $^{**}p < 0.01$, and $^{***}p < 0.001$.

RESULTS

Gal-13 and Gal-14 Are Expressed in First-Trimester Placentas and Their Expression Is Decreased in Miscarriage

Immunostainings of TMAs revealed that Gal-13 (**Figures 1A,B**) and Gal-14 (**Figures 1E,F**) are predominantly expressed in the cytoplasm of the syncytiotrophoblast of chorionic villi in the first trimester, and there were no stainings in the cytotrophoblasts and villous stroma, similar to later stages of pregnancy (53, 81, 106, 110, 113). Moreover, chorionic villi exhibited more intense syncytiotrophoblast cytoplasmic staining in the first trimester than in the third trimester (**Supplementary Figure 2**). The specificity of the galectin antibodies was confirmed by previous studies and by the lack of Gal-13 and Gal-14 immunostaining of human livers on our TMAs.

Next, we examined whether the expression of Gal-13 and Gal-14 is dysregulated in first-trimester placentas obtained from women who miscarried, as a potential sign of fetal rejection. There was no significant change in Gal-13 or Gal-14 immunoscores with gestational age in control placentas ($R^2 = 0.0078$ for Gal-14; $R^2 = 10^{-5}$ for Gal-13). However, the average immunoscore of syncytiotrophoblast decreased by 11.5% for Gal-13 ($p = 0.027$, **Figures 1A–D**) and by 20% ($p = 0.001$) for Gal-14 (**Figures 1E–H**) in miscarriages compared to gestational age-matched controls. Also, there was a significant difference in the distribution of Gal-13 and Gal-14 immunoscores ($p = 0.002$ and $p < 0.001$, respectively) between the disease and control groups (**Figures 1D,H**).

Gal-13 and Gal-14 Bind to Peripheral Blood T Cells

As Gal-13 and Gal-14 are released from the placenta into the maternal circulation, where they may regulate maternal T lymphocytes (53), we further characterized their effects on T cell populations. First, we examined the binding of fluorescent

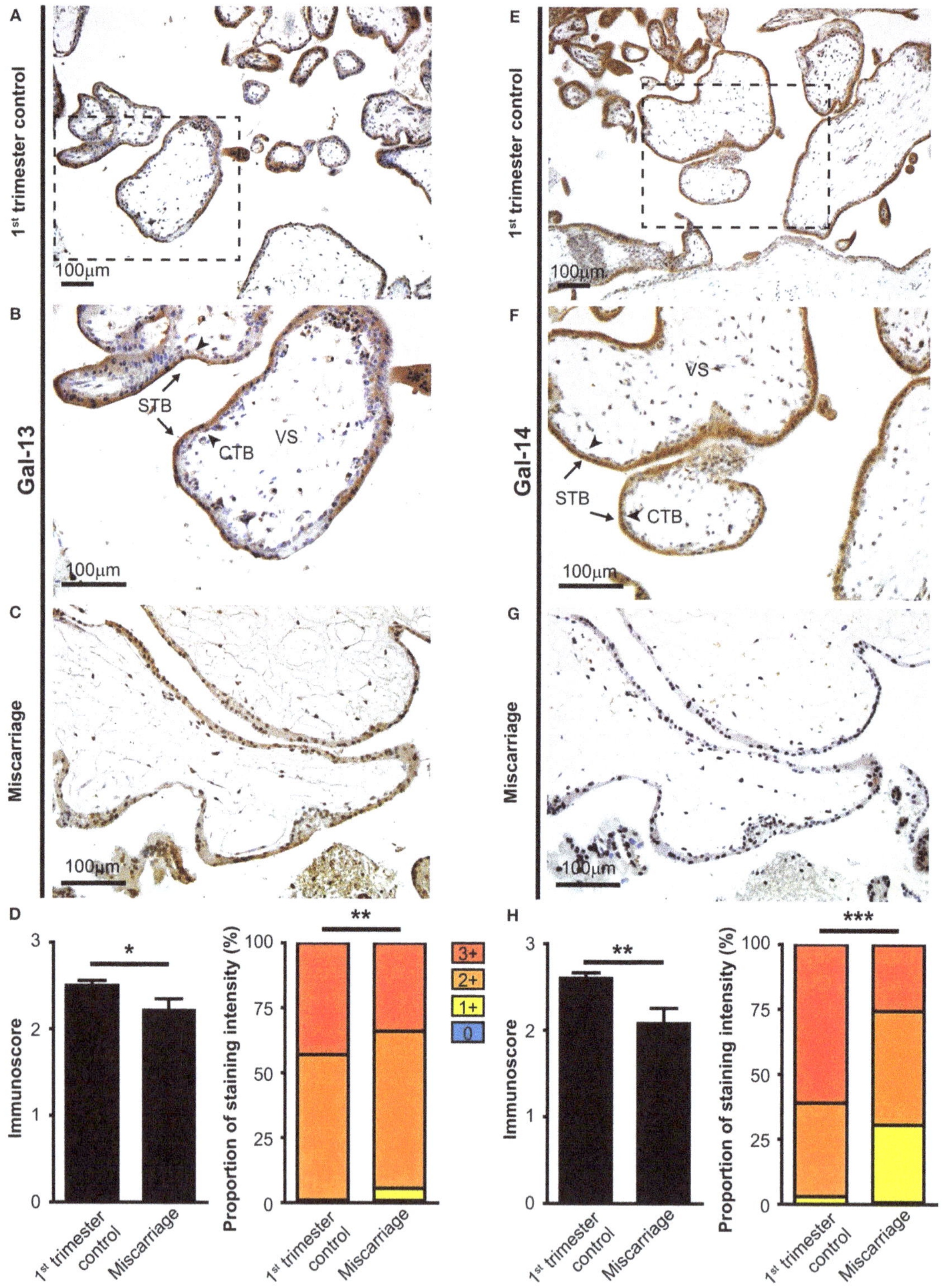

FIGURE 1 | The syncytiotrophoblast expresses galectin-13 and galectin-14 in the first-trimester placenta, which is decreased in miscarriage. Five-micrometers-thick first-trimester placental sections from normal pregnancy **(A,B,E,F)** or from miscarriage **(C,G)** were stained for Gal-13 **(A–C)** or Gal-14 **(E–G)** by specific monoclonal antibodies. Chorionic villi exhibited intense syncytiotrophoblast cytoplasmic staining (arrows, STB), while the villus stroma (VS) and cytotrophoblasts were negative (arrowheads, CTB). Representative images, hematoxylin counterstain, 100x **(A,E)** and 200x **(B,C,F,G)** magnifications. Gal-13 **(D)** and Gal-14 **(H)** immunoscores (mean ± SEM) and proportion of staining intensities in control placentas ($n = 30$) and placentas with miscarriage ($n = 10$) are displayed on left and right graphs, respectively (Gal-13: $n_{total\ villus} = 775$ and $n_{total\ villus} = 106$, respectively; Gal-14: $n_{total\ villus} = 797$ and $n_{total\ villus} = 121$, respectively). Unpaired *t*-test was used for the comparison of the mean immunoscores of the two groups. Fisher's exact test was performed to test the frequency difference of Gal-13 or Gal-14 immunostaining between control and miscarriage groups (*$p < 0.05$, **$p < 0.01$, ***$p < 0.001$).

Gal-13 or Gal-14 to primary T cells. We found that Gal-13 and Gal-14 bound to freshly isolated T lymphocytes, either to helper (Th: 3.4 ± 0.9% and 5.1 ± 1%, respectively) or cytotoxic T (Tc: 3.9 ± 0.8% and 7.7 ± 2.2%, respectively) cells (**Figures 2A,B, Supplementary Figure 3**). Upon activation, binding of Gal-13 to Th and Tc cells was increased by 21% ($p < 0.001$) and 42% ($p < 0.001$), respectively (**Figure 2B, Supplementary Figure 3B**). Binding of Gal-14 was increased by 20% ($p < 0.01$) and by 30% ($p < 0.001$) to activated Th and Tc cells, respectively, compared to non-activated ones (**Figure 2B, Supplementary Figure 3B**). Of note, both galectins tended to bind more to Tc over Th lymphocytes, a difference that reached statistical significance in the case of activated cells ($p < 0.001$ for Gal-13 and $p < 0.05$ for Gal-14).

Gal-13 and Gal-14 Increase Apoptosis of Non-activated and Activated T Cells

Since certain galectins can induce the apoptosis of T cells depending on T cell subsets and their activation status (147–149), we investigated the effects of Gal-13 and Gal-14 on various T cell populations, either in an activated or a non-activated state. Flow cytometry results, overall, show that 4 μM, but not 0.25 μM, of Gal-13 or Gal-14 increased apoptosis of T lymphocytes either pre-activated or not (**Figures 3A,B, Supplementary Figure 4A**). Gal-13 increased apoptosis of both non-activated and pre-activated T cells by 5.3% ($p = 0.010$) and 9%, ($p = 0.011$), respectively. Gal-14 increased apoptosis of pre-activated T cells by 8.9% ($p = 0.040$) compared to PBS-DTT treated cells. We further analyzed Th and Tc lymphocytes separately, based on CD3 and CD8 expression. Tc cell apoptosis was increased for both galectins regardless of the activation state (Gal-13, non-activated: 3.9%, $p = 0.002$; Gal-13, pre-activated: 8.2%, $p = 0.022$; Gal-14, non-activated: 11%, $p = 0.001$; Gal-14, pre-activated: 11.2%, $p = 0.032$), while Gal-13 increased apoptosis rate (8.3%, $p = 0.031$) of non-activated Th cells (**Figures 3A,B**). The proportion of early apoptotic (Annexin V^+ 7-AAD^-) T lymphocytes, Th cells, and Tc cells as well did not change upon Gal-13 or Gal-14 treatment (**Supplementary Figure 4B**).

Gal-13 and Gal-14 Treatment Alters Cell Surface Expression of T Cell Activation Markers

Next, we investigated the impact of Gal-13 and Gal-14 on the expression of well-known activation markers—CD25 (IL-2Rα), CD71 (TfR), CD95 (Fas), and HLA-DR (MHC-II)—of T lymphocytes. Interestingly, Gal-13 treatment increased both the percentage of CD95 positive cells and the cell surface expression of CD95 on Th (% control: 11.3 ± 5.2%, Gal-13: 19.6 ± 7%, $p < 0.05$; RMFI control: 1.7 ± 0.2, Gal-13: 2.2 ± 0.2, $p < 0.01$) and Tc (% control: 6.1 ± 1.7%, Gal-13: 13.7 ± 3.7%, $p < 0.05$; RMFI control: 1.4 ± 0.1, Gal-13: 1.7 ± 0.2, $p < 0.01$) lymphocytes. Gal-14 treatment increased the percentage of CD95 positive cells (18.7 ± 8.5%, $p < 0.05$) and the cell surface expression of CD95 on Th (2.1 ± 0.3, $p < 0.05$) but not on Tc lymphocytes (**Figure 4A, Supplementary Figure 5B**).

The percentage of cells expressing CD71 and the cell surface expression of CD71 decreased upon Gal-14, but not Gal-13 treatment on both Th (% control: 96.9 ± 0.8%, Gal-14: 91 ± 1.3%, $p < 0.05$; RMFI control: 175.1 ± 17, Gal-14: 129 ± 6.1, $p < 0.05$) and Tc (% control: 97 ± 0.5%, Gal-14: 95 ± 1.1%, $p < 0.05$; RMFI control: 191.4 ± 26, Gal-14: 129.3 ± 33.2, $p < 0.01$) lymphocytes (**Figure 4B, Supplementary Figure 5B**).

Neither the percentage of CD25 nor of HLA-DR positive cells changed upon galectin treatment (**Figures 4C,D, Supplementary Figure 5B**). However, cell surface expression of CD25 increased upon Gal-13 treatment (Th RMFI control: 59.1 ± 8.1, Gal-13: 161 ± 30, $p < 0.05$; Tc RMFI control: 42.7 ± 9.6, Gal-13: 103.5 ± 24, $p < 0.05$), and tended to increase upon Gal-14 (RMFI Th: 110.6 ± 23.7; Tc: 64.4 ± 9.1) treatment in both T cell populations (**Figure 4C**). Of note, treatment of non-activated cells with Gal-13 or Gal-14 did not change the expression of these activation markers (**Supplementary Figure 5A**).

Gal-13 and Gal-14 Induce Il-8 Secretion of T Cells

Next, we sought to explore whether T lymphocytes contribute to the altered cytokine production, previously measured in PBMCs (114). IL-1β and IL-6 concentrations were below the detection limit in cell culture supernatants (data not shown). Surprisingly, IL-8 production was increased upon treatment with either Gal-13 (260.7 ± 78 pg/mL, $p < 0.01$) or Gal-14 (237.4 ± 73.5 pg/mL, $p < 0.05$) compared to the control (10.6 ± 9.2 pg/mL), when T cells were not activated. In the case of activation through CD3 and CD28, galectins could not further increase IL-8 production (**Figure 5**). Neither IL-10 nor IFNγ production changed upon galectin treatment (**Figure 5**).

DISCUSSION

Principal Findings of the Study

(1) Gal-13 and Gal-14 are mainly expressed by the syncytiotrophoblast at the maternal-fetal interface in the first trimester, stronger than in the third trimester of pregnancy; (2) the syncytiotrophoblastic expression of both Gal-13 and Gal-14 is down-regulated in miscarriages compared to first trimester control placentas; (3) recombinant Gal-13 and Gal-14 differentially bind to peripheral blood T cell populations, predominantly to Tc over Th cells; (4) Gal-13 and Gal-14 induce the apoptosis of both T cell populations regardless of their activation status; (5) Gal-14 decreases the cell surface expression of CD71, Gal-13 and Gal-14 increase the cell surface expression of CD95 and Gal-13 increases the cell surface expression of CD25 on T cells; and (6) non-activated T cells produce larger amounts of IL-8 in the presence of Gal-13 or Gal-14.

Placental Galectin-13 and Galectin-14 Expression Is Decreased in Miscarriage

This is the first study to characterize the simultaneous expression of Gal-13 and Gal-14 in first-trimester placentas in healthy

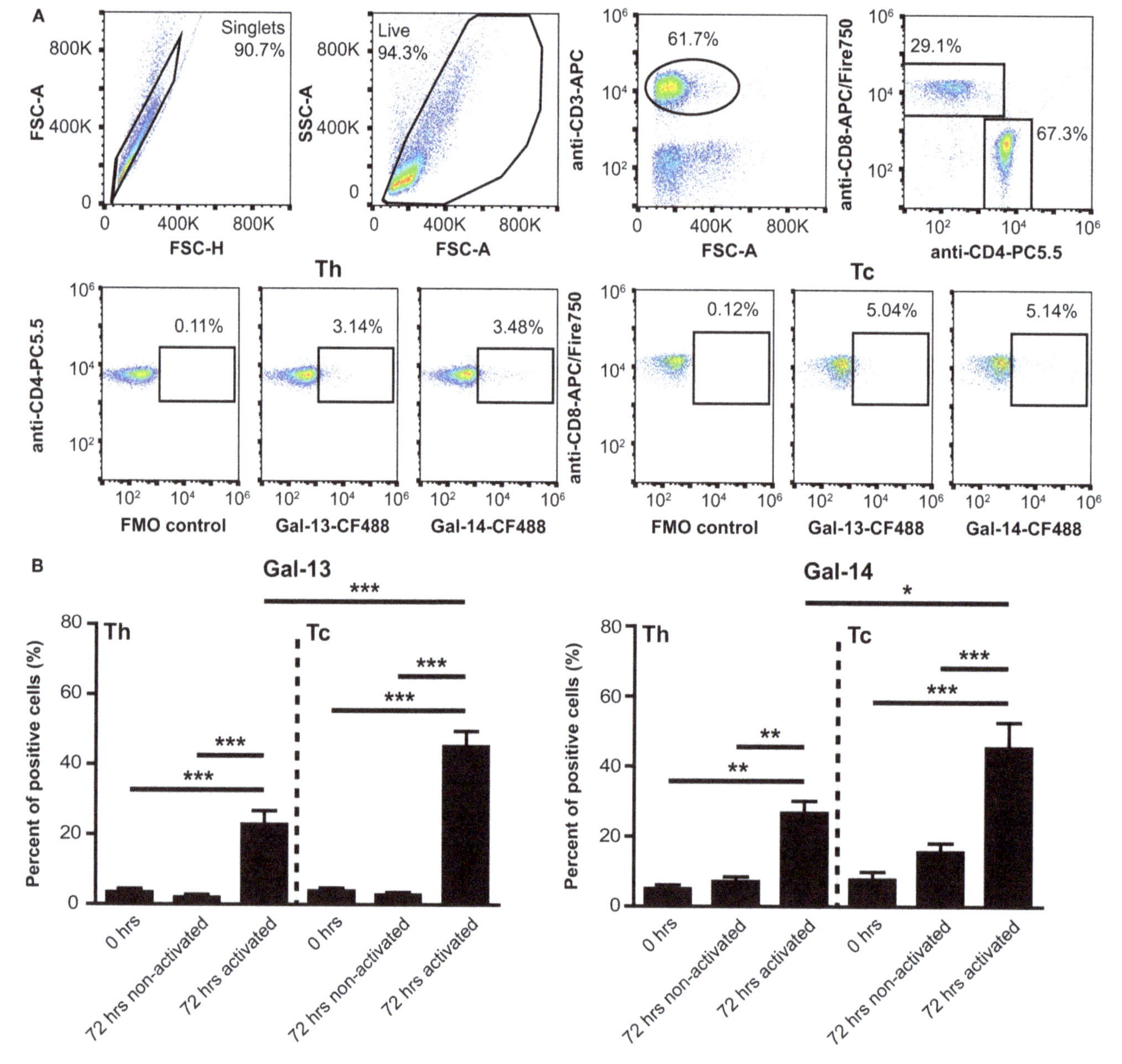

FIGURE 2 | Binding of galectin-13 and galectin-14 to T lymphocytes is population- and activation-dependent. **(A)** Detection of Gal-13 or Gal-14 binding to human T lymphocytes was achieved by flow cytometry with the following cells: freshly isolated PBMCs (0 h) or PBMCs, kept in culture for 72 h in the presence (72 h activated) or absence (72 h non-activated) of anti-CD3/CD28 microbeads. Cells were incubated with 4 μM Gal-13-CF488 or Gal-14-CF488 for 45 min on ice. PBMCs were also stained for CD3 (anti-CD3-APC), CD4 (anti-CD4-PC5.5), and CD8 (anti-CD8-APC/Fire750), in order to distinguish between helper (Th) and cytotoxic (Tc) T lymphocytes. The gating strategy is shown in **(A)**. **(B)** Graphs show the percentage of cells, to which Gal-13 (left) or Gal-14 (right) were bound, as mean ± SEM. Repeated ANOVA with Tukey's *post-hoc* test was used for the comparison of groups ($^{*}p < 0.05$, $^{**}p < 0.01$, $^{***}p < 0.001$). Four non-pregnant female donors were included in each group. FMO, Fluorescence minus one; PBMCs, peripheral blood mononuclear cells.

and complicated pregnancies. We found that these placenta-specific galectins are mainly expressed by the syncytiotrophoblast at the lining of the maternal-fetal interface, similar to these galectins that are expressed in the placenta in the third trimester (53, 106, 110, 113). The expression of these galectins in the syncytiotrophoblast is developmentally regulated during trophoblast differentiation by transcription factors binding to non-coding elements upfront of these galectin genes on Chromosome 19, a process that emerged in anthropoid primates (110). This is particularly interesting from an immunological point of view given that these anthropoids had a long gestation, which necessitated additional immune tolerance mechanisms at their maternal-fetal interface to prevent fetal rejection (53). In this latter evolutionary and immune functional study, we proposed that the emergence of these galectins in anthropoid primates provided additional immune tolerance

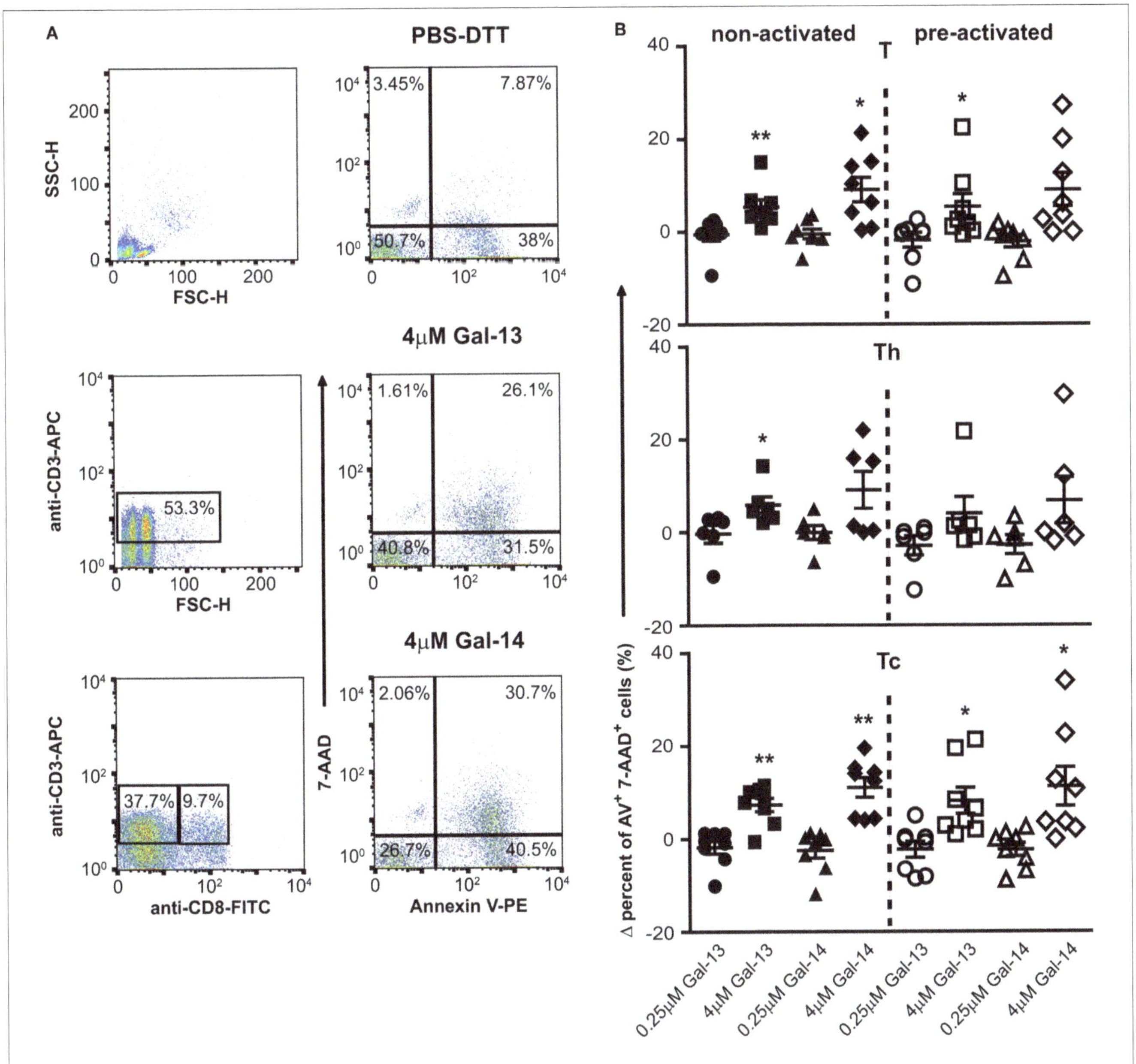

FIGURE 3 | Galectin-13 and galectin-14 increase apoptosis of T lymphocytes. **(A)** PBMCs were kept in culture for 48 h in the presence (activated) or absence (non-activated) of anti-CD3/CD28 microbeads, then treated with Gal-13 or Gal-14 for 24 h. To detect apoptosis of T lymphocytes by flow cytometry, cells were stained with Annexin V-PE and 7-AAD and were also stained for CD3 (anti-CD3-APC), and CD8 (anti-CD8-FITC), in order to distinguish between helper (Th) and cytotoxic (Tc) T cells, respectively. **(A)** The gating strategy (left: $CD3^+$ T gate, $CD3^+CD8^+$ Tc gate, $CD3^+CD8^-$ Th gate) and representative Annexin V and 7-AAD dot plots of vehicle- (PBS-DTT), Gal-13- or Gal-14-treated T cells ($CD3^+$) are displayed. **(B)** Graphs show the Δ percentage of double positive (Annexin $V\text{-}PE^+$ $7\text{-}AAD^+$) cells as mean ± SEM. One sample t-test was used for the comparison of galectin-treated groups with the PBS-DTT-treated group of non-activated or pre-activated cells (**p* < 0.05, ***p* < 0.01). Six-eight non-pregnant female donors were included in each group. PBMCs, Peripheral blood mononuclear cells.

toward the fetus. Previous studies on placentas delivered by women with preeclampsia, a severe obstetrical syndrome with an immune rejection component, revealed the down-regulation of Gal-13 and Gal-14 placental expression, suggesting that this phenomenon may be linked to altered immune tolerance (81, 110, 113, 129).

Herein, we report for the first time that the placental expression of Gal-13 and Gal-14 is also decreased in first-trimester miscarriages. As most of these cases have a normal karyotype, our finding suggests that altered maternal-fetal immune tolerance is not closely associated with chromosomal abnormalities but can be a separate underlying mechanism for miscarriages. Indeed, recent publications presented that miscarriages are associated with immune etiologies (150), where the development of the fetus and placenta is affected by either auto- or alloimmune rejection-type activity (151).

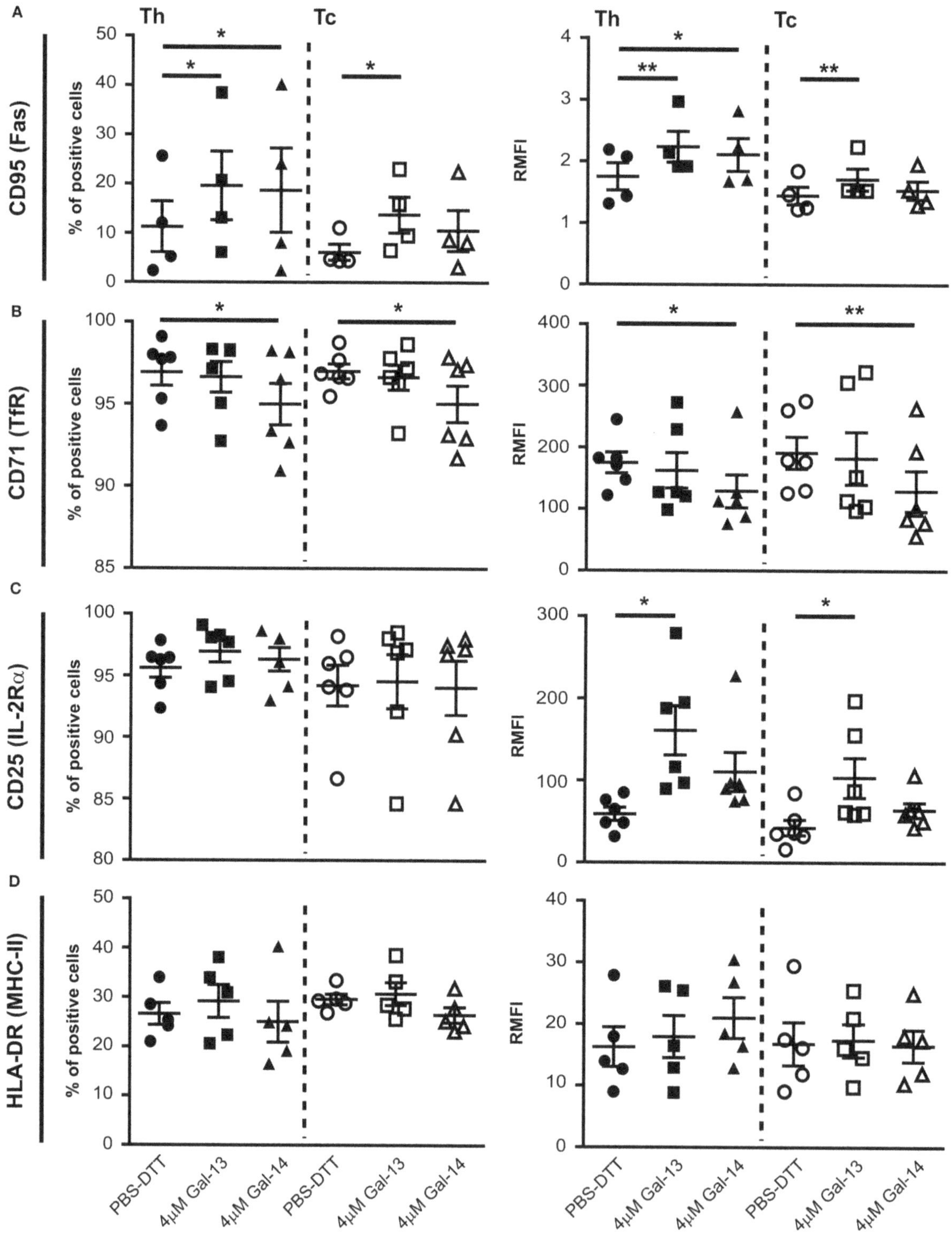

FIGURE 4 | Galectin-13 and galectin-14 affect cell surface expression of activation markers on T lymphocytes. PBMCs were kept in culture for 72 h in the presence of anti-CD3/CD28 microbeads, then treated with Gal-13 or Gal-14 for 24 h. To detect cell surface expression of CD95 **(A)**, CD71 **(B)**, CD25 **(C)**, HLA-DR **(D)** activation markers on T lymphocytes by flow cytometry, cells were stained with anti-CD25-PE and anti-CD71-PerCP/5.5, or anti-CD95-PE and anti-HLA-DR-PerCP/5.5. Cells were also stained for CD3 (anti-CD3-APC), and CD8 (anti-CD8-FITC) in order to distinguish between helper (Th) and cytotoxic (Tc) T cells. Left graphs show the percentage of positive cells and right graphs show relative median fluorescence intensity (RMFI) values (mean ± SEM). RMFI was calculated by dividing specific median fluorescence intensity with the median fluorescence intensity of the isotype control. Repeated ANOVA with Dunnett's *post-hoc* test was used for comparison of the non-treated group with Gal-13/Gal-14-treated groups (*$p < 0.05$, **$p < 0.01$). Four-six non-pregnant female donors were included in each group. HLA-DR, Human leukocyte antigen DR isotype; PBMCs, peripheral blood mononuclear cells.

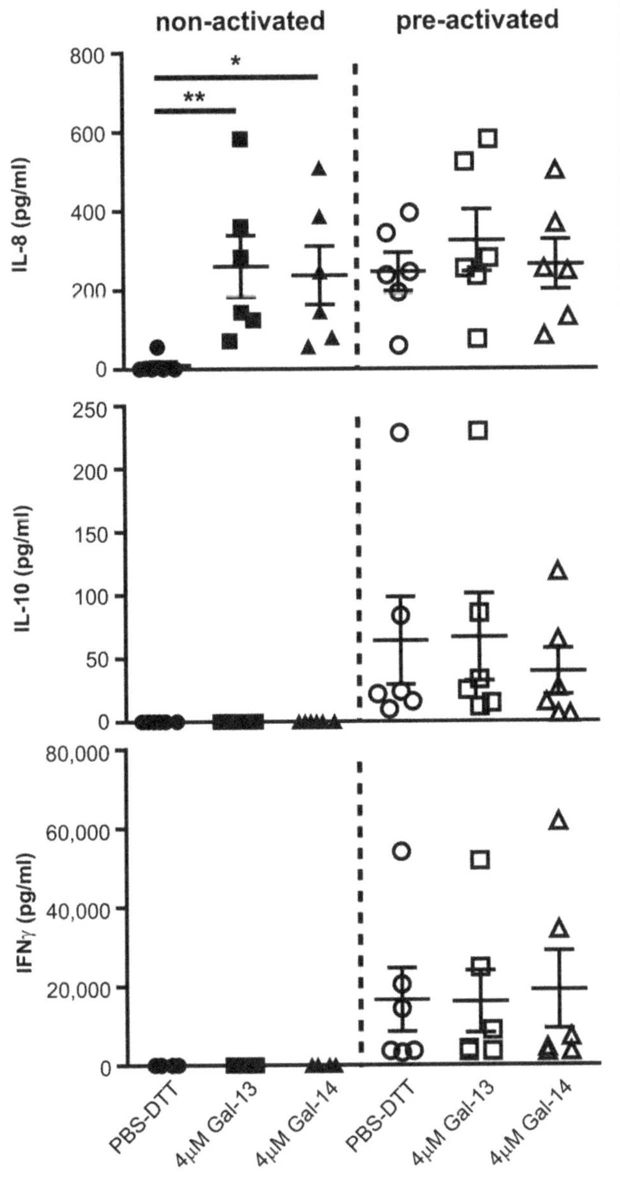

FIGURE 5 | Galectin-13 and galectin-14 induce IL-8 production in resting T lymphocytes. T lymphocytes after negative selection were kept in culture for 72 h in the presence (pre-activated) or absence (non-activated) of anti-CD3/CD28 microbeads, then treated with 4 μM Gal-13 or Gal-14 for 24 h. Supernatants were collected and IL-8, IL-10, and IFNγ cytokines were measured by flow cytometry using LEGENDplex assays. Graphs show calculated cytokine concentrations as mean ± SEM. Repeated ANOVA with Dunnett's *post-hoc* test was used for the comparison of the non-treated group with Gal-13/Gal-14-treated groups (*$p < 0.05$, **$p < 0.01$). Six non-pregnant female donors were included in each group.

Of interest, the expression of other galectins, although in modest extent, is also decreased at the maternal-fetal interface in spontaneous and recurrent miscarriages, including Gal-1, Gal-2, Gal-7, Gal-9, and Gal-10 (152–154). Furthermore, in good accordance, serum concentrations of Gal-1 and Gal-9 were also found to be decreased in miscarriage (99, 154, 155). An elegant study revealed that Gal-1 has pivotal functions supporting maternal-fetal immune tolerance and its decreased expression leads to fetal loss in a mouse model. Gal-1 prevents fetal loss and restores tolerance through multiple mechanisms, including the induction of tolerogenic dendritic cells, which, in turn, promotes the expansion of IL-10-secreting regulatory T cells *in vivo* (107). On the other hand, Gal-9 was found to exert its functions in non-pregnant and pregnant states on NK cells, T cells, and B cells (101, 102, 147, 156–159). In addition, Gal-9 promotes trophoblast invasion in a Tim-3 dependent manner (154). Consistently, a higher proportion of decidual T cells that express activation markers (CD25, and CD69) was found in spontaneous abortion than in elective termination of pregnancy, and decidual lymphocytes from spontaneous abortion increased the apoptosis of trophoblast cells (160). Since Gal-13 and Gal-14 are only expressed in anthropoid primates, it is not possible to investigate the role of these proteins in knock-out mammalian models *in vivo*. Nevertheless, we can conclude that several galectins, including Gal-13 and Gal-14, potentially act in concert and play a role in maintaining pregnancy and that their lower expression at the maternal-fetal interface in early pregnancy may lead to an immune imbalance that interferes with implantation, trophoblast invasion, and placentation, leading to fetal rejection and miscarriages.

Galectin-13 and Galectin-14 Promote Apoptosis of T Cells

The majority of the galectin family regulates adaptive immune responses through the induction of T cell apoptosis, which then leads to a shift in the innate/adaptive, Th1/Th2, and Th17/Treg immune balances (161–163). Similarly, we reported that exogenously added Gal-13 and Gal-14 are able to induce the apoptosis of activated T cells to a similar extent as Gal-1 (53). In accord with these findings, the interesting study from Kliman et al. (114) showed that Gal-13 is secreted from the syncytiotrophoblast and forms perivenous aggregates in the decidual extracellular matrix in the first trimester. These Gal-13 aggregates, found around decidual veins, were associated with T cell-, neutrophil-, and macrophage-containing "decidual zones of necrosis" (ZONEs), in which apoptotic T cells were also found. Based on these findings in normal pregnancies, and also based on cases in which fewer ZONEs and apoptotic T cells were found in association with very low serum Gal-13 levels, the authors hypothesized that Gal-13 is a key placental protein that downregulates maternal immune responses in the first-trimester decidua to avoid rejection of invasive trophoblasts at the maternal-fetal interface, and that low Gal-13 expression leads to heightened immune responses and impaired trophoblast invasion. It is possible that in cases where this mechanism is very defective (e.g., due to the concerted downregulation of Gal-13, Gal-14, Gal-1, and other immunoregulatory molecules in the placenta or decidua), pregnancies will be miscarried.

To better elucidate the role of Gal-13/Gal-14 in the regulation of T cells, we further characterized the pro-apoptotic effect of these galectins on T lymphocytes. We found that both Gal-13 and Gal-14 increased the rate of late-apoptotic T lymphocytes with ~5–10%, which was not affected by the activation status of the cells, while other galectins promote the apoptosis of only activated leukocytes (164, 165). Our result suggests that Gal-13 and Gal-14 have a basic pro-apoptotic activity on T cells. Of note, Tc cells bound more galectins than Th cells and Tc cells were more susceptible to Gal-13/Gal-14 induced apoptosis than Th cells, which may be related to the differential glycosylation pattern on these two T cell populations. This phenomenon has not been deeply explored in other galectins, which, however, were studied for their effects on different Th subsets. For example, Gal-1 selectively induced the apoptosis of pro-inflammatory Th1 and Th17 cell subsets, but not of naïve, Th2, or Treg cells (166). Moreover, Gal-9 induced the apoptosis of Th1 cells (147) in a Tim-3 dependent manner. Our results warrant further characterization of the pro-apoptotic effects of Gal-13 and Gal-14 on different Th subsets and determination of glycophenotype on T cell populations.

Apoptotic cell death in activated T cells is mediated by signaling through the activation marker CD95 (Fas), following binding to its ligand CD95L/FasL (167). In addition, another T cell activation marker CD25 (Il-2Rα), important for T cell proliferation, is also involved in this process by increasing the expression of CD95 (168). Herein, we found that the cell surface expression of CD95 and CD25 are increased upon Gal-14 and/or Gal-13 treatment. This is important since activated T cells are more prone to apoptosis (169); thus, Gal-13 and Gal-14 may increase the sensitivity of activated T cells to die by the activation-induced cell death. This is concordant with an earlier study in which Gal-1 increased the percentage of Th1 cells expressing CD95, although the Gal-1-mediated apoptosis of these cells was independent of CD95 (149). Interestingly, we found decreased expression of another activation marker (CD71) on T cells treated with Gal-14. This is seemingly contradictory, however, CD71 transiently associates with the TCR in response to TCR engagement (170) and is an essential factor for proliferating T cells (171, 172). Thus, galectins may inhibit T cell proliferation, which still needs to be tested in later studies.

Galectin-13 and Galectin-14 Regulate Cytokine Production of T Cells

Several galectins have been shown to alter cytokine production of immune cells. For example, Gal-1 induces IL-10 production in Treg cells (107, 173) and Gal-9 promotes IL-2 and IFNγ production in T cells (164). Herein, we found in the applied experimental settings that Gal-13 and Gal-14 did not alter most pro-inflammatory (IFNγ, IL-1β, and IL-6) or anti-inflammatory (IL-10) cytokine production of T cells; however, both of these galectins induced IL-8 production in non-activated T cells. This is particularly interesting since IL-8 exerts a pro-angiogenic effect on endothelial cells by decreasing the apoptosis of endothelial cells and increasing their proliferation and capillary formation (174). In addition, a novel neutrophil population was identified by recent studies in second-trimester human deciduas, which promoted *in vitro* angiogenesis in an IL-8-dependent manner (175, 176). Furthermore, decidual NK cell subsets release significant amounts of pro-angiogenic factors, such as VEGF and IL-8, necessary for spiral artery formation during decidualization (177–179). Of note, the pro-angiogenic effects of other galectins during gestation have been discovered, as reviewed recently (180). Therefore, it is tempting to speculate that Gal-13 and Gal-14 may induce angiogenesis at the maternal-fetal interface through increasing IL-8 production of T cells. This finding is related to the *in vivo* vasodilator effect of Gal-13 (181–184). In this context, reduced Gal-13 and Gal-14 expression may play a role in the disturbed vascular changes in preterm preeclampsia (58, 185–194). All our data discussed above support the idea that Gal-13 and Gal-14 also have immunoregulatory and vascular effects, as found for galectin-1 or galectin-3 (195, 196). Since the immunomodulatory effects of Gal-13 and Gal-14 could be observed on a broad scale, changing the habit of adaptive immune cells may affect innate immune cells, as well. More experiments are warranted in this direction to comprehensively elucidate the effects of these galectins at the maternal-fetal interface.

Strengths and Limitations of the Study

The strengths of the study are as follows: (1) strict clinical definitions and homogenous patient groups; (2) standardized, quick placental sample collection during pregnancy terminations; (3) standardized histopathological examination of the placentas based on international criteria; (4) protein expression profiling on placentas with tissue microarray and immunostaining followed by semiquantitative immunoscorings and statistical analysis; (5) expression and purification of large amounts of recombinant galectins with standardized methods; and (6) an array of functional experiments with primary cells and recombinant proteins.

Limitations of the study are as follows: (1) the relatively modest number of cases in each patient group due to the strict clinical and histopathological inclusion criteria used for patient enrollment. On the other hand, this was one of the most important strengths of our study; (2) for *in vitro* experiments, only non-pregnant donors were included in the study given the conditions in our patient recruitment. However, this was also a value of our study, since we used a "naïve" population of immune cells to test the effects of Gal-13 and Gal-14, while experiments with PBMCs isolated from the peripheral circulation or decidua of pregnant women pre-exposed to placental Gal-13/Gal-14 might not have revealed the true effects of these molecules. Nevertheless, our results warrant further characterization of the effects of Gal-13 and Gal-14 on peripheral blood and decidual leukocytes isolated from pregnant women, as pregnancy hormones, especially estrogen and progesterone, may impact glycosylation pattern and galectin-biding capacity of these cells; (3) Gal-13 and Gal-14 concentrations applied in our *in vitro* experiments were supraphysiologic, similar to experimental settings in previous studies on the functional effects of galectins (7, 165). The use of higher galectin concentrations is due to the fact that blood concentrations of galectins do not reflect their effective local/cell surface concentrations. In fact, these studies usually applied recombinant galectins between 10 and 100 μg/mL, representing a reasonable range of the local galectin concentration expected in the tissues (197). Another technical reason to use higher galectin concentrations is to prevent their subunit dissociation in the solvent that contains DTT (198); and (4) the evaluation of blood concentrations of Gal-13/Gal-14, which may change in parallel with their placental dysregulation in miscarriages, as also seen in the case of Gal-1 (99, 153, 155, 184), was beyond the scope of this study, but our results warrant further investigation.

CONCLUDING REMARKS

The causes and consequences of the down-regulation of placental Gal-13 and Gal-14 expression in miscarriages still have to be uncovered by later functional studies. This work suggests that Gal-13 and Gal-14 down-regulate adaptive immune responses at the maternal-fetal interface through T cell apoptosis, and that their impaired expression leads to fetal rejection in miscarriages. Another process in which these galectins may function is angiogenesis, which is altered in both miscarriage and preeclampsia, in which Gal-13 and Gal-14 expression is decreased. Since galectins have pleiotropic functions on various immune and non-immune cells given their promiscuous binding to various cell surface receptors via glycan binding, we envision that both actions may be functional in human pregnancy. In conclusion, our results suggest that Gal-13 and Gal-14 provide an immunoprivileged environment at the maternal-fetal interface, already in early pregnancy, either through down-regulating maternal immune responses or via the support of placental development, and their reduced expression is related to the immune pathology of miscarriages.

ETHICS STATEMENT

Clinical sample and data collection were approved by the Health Science Board of Hungary (ETT-TUKEB 4834-0/2011-1018EKU). Written informed consent was obtained from women prior to sample collection and the experiments conformed to the principles set out in the World Medical Association Declaration of Helsinki. Specimens and data were stored anonymously.

AUTHOR CONTRIBUTIONS

AB, IH, SH, JM, SR, EP, and NT conceptualized study and designed research. AB, DC, KJ, AK, EP, KP, NS, and ET performed research. SH, PH, HM, EP, ZP, RR, NT, and PZ contributed new reagents, analytic tools, and clinical specimens. AB, DC, OE, JM, EP, SR, AT, and NT analyzed and interpreted data. All authors contributed to the writing of the paper.

FUNDING

This research was supported by the Perinatology Research Branch, Division of Obstetrics and Maternal-Fetal Medicine, Division of Intramural Research, *Eunice Kennedy Shriver* National Institute of Child Health and Human Development, National Institutes of Health, US Department of Health and Human Services (NICHD/NIH/DHHS); Federal funds from NICHD/NIH/DHHS under Contract No. HHSN275201300006C; grants from the Hungarian National Science Fund (OTKA-PD 104398 to AB and OTKA-K 124862 to NT), from the Hungarian Academy of Sciences (Momentum LP2014-7/2014 to NT), and from the Hungarian National Research, Development and Innovation Fund (ÚNKP-18-3-IV-SE-14 to AK and FIEK_16-1-2016-0005 to NT).

ACKNOWLEDGMENTS

We thank for Judit Baunoch and Dr. Anna Sarai (Hungarian Academy of Sciences), Dorottya Csernus-Horvath, Nora Fekete, Katalin Karaszi, Prof. Ilona Kovalszky, Dr. Tibor Krenacs, Eva Matraine Balogh, and Zsofia Zsibai (Semmelweis University), Jolan Csapai, Laszlo Daru, Hajnalka Nyiro, and Erzsebet Szilagyi (Maternity Private Clinic) for their assistance and Maureen McGerty (Wayne State University) for her critical reading of the manuscript.

REFERENCES

1. Szekeres-Bartho J, Wegmann TG. A progesterone-dependent immunomodulatory protein alters the Th1/Th2 balance. *J Reprod Immunol.* (1996) 31:81–95. doi: 10.1016/0165-0378(96)00964-3
2. Moffett-King A. Natural killer cells and pregnancy. *Nat Rev Immunol.* (2002) 2:656–63. doi: 10.1038/nri886
3. Abrahams VM, Kim YM, Straszewski SL, Romero R, Mor G. Macrophages and apoptotic cell clearance during pregnancy. *Am J Reprod Immunol.* (2004) 51:275–82. doi: 10.1111/j.1600-0897.2004.00156.x
4. Mor G, Romero R, Aldo PB, Abrahams VM. Is the trophoblast an immune regulator? The role of Toll-like receptors during pregnancy. *Crit Rev Immunol.* (2005) 25:375–88. doi: 10.1615/CritRevImmunol.v25.i5.30
5. Richani K, Soto E, Romero R, Espinoza J, Chaiworapongsa T, Nien JK, et al. Normal pregnancy is characterized by systemic activation of the complement system. *J Matern Fetal Neonatal Med.* (2005) 17:239–45. doi: 10.1080/14767050500072722
6. Aluvihare VR, Betz AG. The role of regulatory T cells in alloantigen tolerance. *Immunol Rev.* (2006) 212:330–43. doi: 10.1111/j.0105-2896.2006.00408.x

7. Blois SM, Kammerer U, Alba Soto C, Tometten MC, Shaikly V, Barrientos G, et al. Dendritic cells: key to fetal tolerance? *Biol Reprod.* (2007) 77:590–8. doi: 10.1095/biolreprod.107.060632
8. Holzgreve W, Hahn S, Zhong XY, Lapaire O, Hosli I, Tercanli S, et al. Genetic communication between fetus and mother: short- and long-term consequences. *Am J Obstet Gynecol.* (2007) 196:372–81. doi: 10.1016/j.ajog.2006.12.013
9. Saito S, Shiozaki A, Sasaki Y, Nakashima A, Shima T, Ito M. Regulatory T cells and regulatory natural killer (NK) cells play important roles in feto-maternal tolerance. *Semin Immunopathol.* (2007) 29:115–22. doi: 10.1007/s00281-007-0067-2
10. Zenclussen AC, Schumacher A, Zenclussen ML, Wafula P, Volk HD. Immunology of pregnancy: cellular mechanisms allowing fetal survival within the maternal uterus. *Expert Rev Mol Med.* (2007) 9:1–14. doi: 10.1017/S1462399407000294
11. Kalkunte S, Chichester CO, Gotsch F, Sentman CL, Romero R, Sharma S. Evolution of non-cytotoxic uterine natural killer cells. *Am J Reprod Immunol.* (2008) 59:425–32. doi: 10.1111/j.1600-0897.2008.00595.x
12. Mor G. Inflammation and pregnancy: the role of toll-like receptors in trophoblast-immune interaction. *Ann N Y Acad Sci.* (2008) 1127:121–8. doi: 10.1196/annals.1434.006
13. Robertson SA, Guerin LR, Moldenhauer LM, Hayball JD. Activating T regulatory cells for tolerance in early pregnancy - the contribution of seminal fluid. *J Reprod Immunol.* (2009) 83:109–16. doi: 10.1016/j.jri.2009.08.003
14. Erlebacher A. Immune surveillance of the maternal/fetal interface: controversies and implications. *Trends Endocrinol Metab.* (2010) 21:428–34. doi: 10.1016/j.tem.2010.02.003
15. Robertson SA. Immune regulation of conception and embryo implantation-all about quality control? *J Reprod Immunol.* (2010) 85:51–7. doi: 10.1016/j.jri.2010.01.008
16. Munoz-Suano A, Hamilton AB, Betz AG. Gimme shelter: the immune system during pregnancy. *Immunol Rev.* (2011) 241:20–38. doi: 10.1111/j.1600-065X.2011.01002.x
17. Arck PC, Hecher K. Fetomaternal immune cross-talk and its consequences for maternal and offspring's health. *Nat Med.* (2013) 19:548–56. doi: 10.1038/nm.3160
18. Erlebacher A. Mechanisms of T cell tolerance towards the allogeneic fetus. *Nat Rev Immunol.* (2013) 13:23–33. doi: 10.1038/nri3361
19. Gomez-Lopez N, Vega-Sanchez R, Castillo-Castrejon M, Romero R, Cubeiro-Arreola K, Vadillo-Ortega F. Evidence for a role for the adaptive immune response in human term parturition. *Am J Reprod Immunol.* (2013) 69:212–30. doi: 10.1111/aji.12074
20. Hahn S, Giaglis S, Chowdhury CS, Hosli I, Hasler P. Modulation of neutrophil NETosis: interplay between infectious agents and underlying host physiology. *Semin Immunopathol.* (2013) 35:439–53. doi: 10.1007/s00281-013-0380-x
21. Hemberger M. Immune balance at the foeto-maternal interface as the fulcrum of reproductive success. *J Reprod Immunol.* (2013) 97:36–42. doi: 10.1016/j.jri.2012.10.006
22. Shynlova O, Lee YH, Srikhajon K, Lye SJ. Physiologic uterine inflammation and labor onset: integration of endocrine and mechanical signals. *Reprod Sci.* (2013) 20:154–67. doi: 10.1177/1933719112446084
23. Tilburgs T, Strominger JL. CD8+ effector T cells at the fetal-maternal interface, balancing fetal tolerance and antiviral immunity. *Am J Reprod Immunol.* (2013) 69:395–407. doi: 10.1111/aji.12094
24. Gomez-Lopez N, StLouis D, Lehr MA, Sanchez-Rodriguez EN, Arenas-Hernandez M. Immune cells in term and preterm labor. *Cell Mol Immunol.* (2014) 11:571–81. doi: 10.1038/cmi.2014.46
25. Kwan M, Hazan A, Zhang J, Jones RL, Harris LK, Whittle W, et al. Dynamic changes in maternal decidual leukocyte populations from first to second trimester gestation. *Placenta.* (2014) 35:1027–34. doi: 10.1016/j.placenta.2014.09.018
26. Lima PD, Zhang J, Dunk C, Lye SJ, Croy BA. Leukocyte driven-decidual angiogenesis in early pregnancy. *Cell Mol Immunol.* (2014) 11:522–37. doi: 10.1038/cmi.2014.63
27. Lash GE. Molecular cross-talk at the feto-maternal interface. *Cold Spring Harb Perspect Med.* (2015) 5:a023010. doi: 10.1101/cshperspect.a023010
28. Mor G, Kwon JY. Trophoblast-microbiome interaction: a new paradigm on immune regulation. *Am J Obstet Gynecol.* (2015) 213:S131–7. doi: 10.1016/j.ajog.2015.06.039
29. Schumacher A, Zenclussen AC. The paternal contribution to fetal tolerance. *Adv Exp Med Biol.* (2015) 868:211–25. doi: 10.1007/978-3-319-18881-2_10
30. Giaglis S, Stoikou M, Sur Chowdhury C, Schaefer G, Grimolizzi F, Rossi SW, et al. Multimodal regulation of NET formation in pregnancy: progesterone antagonizes the pro-NETotic effect of estrogen and G-CSF. *Front Immunol.* (2016) 7:565. doi: 10.3389/fimmu.2016.00565
31. El-Azzamy H, Balogh A, Romero R, Xu Y, LaJeunesse C, Plazyo O, et al. Characteristic changes in decidual gene expression signature in spontaneous term parturition. *J Pathol Transl Med.* (2017) 51:264–83. doi: 10.4132/jptm.2016.12.20
32. Kinder JM, Stelzer IA, Arck PC, Way SS. Immunological implications of pregnancy-induced microchimerism. *Nat Rev Immunol.* (2017) 17:483–94. doi: 10.1038/nri.2017.38
33. Liu S, Diao L, Huang C, Li Y, Zeng Y, Kwak-Kim JYH. The role of decidual immune cells on human pregnancy. *J Reprod Immunol.* (2017) 124:44–53. doi: 10.1016/j.jri.2017.10.045
34. Shah NM, Herasimtschuk AA, Boasso A, Benlahrech A, Fuchs D, Imami N, et al. Changes in T cell and dendritic cell phenotype from mid to late pregnancy are indicative of a shift from immune tolerance to immune activation. *Front Immunol.* (2017) 8:1138. doi: 10.3389/fimmu.2017.01138
35. Zhang J, Dunk C, Croy AB, Lye SJ. To serve and to protect: the role of decidual innate immune cells on human pregnancy. *Cell Tissue Res.* (2016) 363:249–65. doi: 10.1007/s00441-015-2315-4
36. Cheng SB, Davis S, Sharma S. Maternal-fetal cross talk through cell-free fetal DNA, telomere shortening, microchimerism, and inflammation. *Am J Reprod Immunol.* (2018) 79:e12851. doi: 10.1111/aji.12851
37. Schumacher A, Sharkey DJ, Robertson SA, Zenclussen AC. Immune cells at the fetomaternal interface: how the microenvironment modulates immune cells to foster fetal development. *J Immunol.* (2018) 201:325–34. doi: 10.4049/jimmunol.1800058
38. Szekeres-Bartho J, Sucurovic S, Mulac-Jericevic B. The role of extracellular vesicles and PIBF in embryo-maternal immune-interactions. *Front Immunol.* (2018) 9:2890. doi: 10.3389/fimmu.2018.02890
39. Vacca P, Vitale C, Munari E, Cassatella MA, Mingari MC, Moretta L. Human innate lymphoid cells: their functional and cellular interactions in decidua. *Front Immunol.* (2018) 9:1897. doi: 10.3389/fimmu.2018.01897
40. Ander SE, Diamond MS, Coyne CB. Immune responses at the maternal-fetal interface. *Sci Immunol.* (2019) 4:eaat6114. doi: 10.1126/sciimmunol.aat6114
41. Yang X, Zhang C, Chen G, Sun C, Li J. Antibodies: the major participants in maternal-fetal interaction. *J Obstet Gynaecol Res.* (2019) 45:39–46. doi: 10.1111/jog.13839
42. Mor G, Cardenas I, Abrahams V, Guller S. Inflammation and pregnancy: the role of the immune system at the implantation site. *Ann N Y Acad Sci.* (2011) 1221:80–7. doi: 10.1111/j.1749-6632.2010.05938.x
43. Racicot K, Kwon JY, Aldo P, Silasi M, Mor G. Understanding the complexity of the immune system during pregnancy. *Am J Reprod Immunol.* (2014) 72:107–16. doi: 10.1111/aji.12289
44. Aghaeepour N, Ganio EA, McIlwain D, Tsai AS, Tingle M, Van Gassen S, et al. An immune clock of human pregnancy. *Sci Immunol.* (2017) 2:eaan2946. doi: 10.1126/sciimmunol.aan2946
45. Chavan AR, Griffith OW, Wagner GP. The inflammation paradox in the evolution of mammalian pregnancy: turning a foe into a friend. *Curr Opin Genet Dev.* (2017) 47:24–32. doi: 10.1016/j.gde.2017.08.004
46. Griffith OW, Chavan AR, Protopapas S, Maziarz J, Romero R, Wagner GP. Embryo implantation evolved from an ancestral inflammatory attachment reaction. *Proc Natl Acad Sci USA.* (2017) 114:E6566–75. doi: 10.1073/pnas.1701129114
47. Uckan D, Steele A, Cherry, Wang BY, Chamizo W, Koutsonikolis A, et al. Trophoblasts express Fas ligand: a proposed mechanism for immune privilege in placenta and maternal invasion. *Mol Hum Reprod.* (1997) 3:655–62. doi: 10.1093/molehr/3.8.655
48. Hunt JS, Petroff MG, McIntire RH, Ober C. HLA-G and immune tolerance in pregnancy. *FASEB J.* (2005) 19:681–93. doi: 10.1096/fj.04-2078rev

49. Mincheva-Nilsson L, Nagaeva O, Chen T, Stendahl U, Antsiferova J, Mogren I, et al. Placenta-derived soluble MHC class I chain-related molecules down-regulate NKG2D receptor on peripheral blood mononuclear cells during human pregnancy: a possible novel immune escape mechanism for fetal survival. *J Immunol.* (2006) 176:3585–92. doi: 10.4049/jimmunol.176.6.3585
50. Trowsdale J, Betz AG. Mother's little helpers: mechanisms of maternal-fetal tolerance. *Nat Immunol.* (2006) 7:241–6. doi: 10.1038/ni1317
51. Rusterholz C, Hahn S, Holzgreve W. Role of placentally produced inflammatory and regulatory cytokines in pregnancy and the etiology of preeclampsia. *Semin Immunopathol.* (2007) 29:151–62. doi: 10.1007/s00281-007-0071-6
52. Than NG, Romero R, Erez O, Weckle A, Tarca AL, Hotra J, et al. Emergence of hormonal and redox regulation of galectin-1 in placental mammals: implication in maternal-fetal immune tolerance. *Proc Natl Acad Sci USA.* (2008) 105:15819–24. doi: 10.1073/pnas.0807606105
53. Than NG, Romero R, Goodman M, Weckle A, Xing J, Dong Z, et al. A primate subfamily of galectins expressed at the maternal-fetal interface that promote immune cell death. *Proc Natl Acad Sci USA.* (2009) 106:9731–6. doi: 10.1073/pnas.0903568106
54. Hunt JS, Pace JL, Gill RM. Immunoregulatory molecules in human placentas: potential for diverse roles in pregnancy. *Int J Dev Biol.* (2010) 54:457–67. doi: 10.1387/ijdb.082831jh
55. Petroff MG, Perchellet A. B7 family molecules as regulators of the maternal immune system in pregnancy. *Am J Reprod Immunol.* (2010) 63:506–19. doi: 10.1111/j.1600-0897.2010.00841.x
56. Than NG, Romero R, Kim CJ, McGowen MR, Papp Z, Wildman DE. Galectins: guardians of eutherian pregnancy at the maternal-fetal interface. *Trends Endocrinol Metab.* (2012) 23:23–31. doi: 10.1016/j.tem.2011.09.003
57. Schumacher A, Costa SD, Zenclussen AC. Endocrine factors modulating immune responses in pregnancy. *Front Immunol.* (2014) 5:196. doi: 10.3389/fimmu.2014.00196
58. Than NG, Balogh A, Romero R, Karpati E, Erez O, Szilagyi A, et al. Placental protein 13 (PP13) - a placental immunoregulatory galectin protecting pregnancy. *Front Immunol.* (2014) 5:348. doi: 10.3389/fimmu.2014.00348
59. Cheng SB, Sharma S. Interleukin-10: a pleiotropic regulator in pregnancy. *Am J Reprod Immunol.* (2015) 73:487–500. doi: 10.1111/aji.12329
60. Kinder JM, Jiang TT, Ertelt JM, Xin L, Strong BS, Shaaban AF, et al. Tolerance to noninherited maternal antigens, reproductive microchimerism and regulatory T cell memory: 60 years after 'Evidence for actively acquired tolerance to Rh antigens'. *Chimerism.* (2015) 6:8–20. doi: 10.1080/19381956.2015.1107253
61. Than NG, Romero R, Balogh A, Karpati E, Mastrolia SA, Staretz-Chacham O, et al. Galectins: double-edged swords in the cross-roads of pregnancy complications and female reproductive tract inflammation and neoplasia. *J Pathol Transl Med.* (2015) 49:181–208. doi: 10.4132/jptm.2015.02.25
62. Zhang YH, Tian M, Tang MX, Liu ZZ, Liao AH. Recent insight into the role of the PD-1/PD-L1 pathway in feto-maternal tolerance and pregnancy. *Am J Reprod Immunol.* (2015) 74:201–8. doi: 10.1111/aji.12365
63. Ferreira LMR, Meissner TB, Tilburgs T, Strominger JL. HLA-G: at the interface of maternal-fetal tolerance. *Trends Immunol.* (2017) 38:272–86. doi: 10.1016/j.it.2017.01.009
64. Le Bouteiller P, Bensussan A. Up-and-down immunity of pregnancy in humans. *F1000Res.* (2017) 6:1216. doi: 10.12688/f1000research.11690.1
65. Schumacher A. Human chorionic gonadotropin as a pivotal endocrine immune regulator initiating and preserving fetal tolerance. *Int J Mol Sci.* (2017) 18:E2166. doi: 10.3390/ijms18102166
66. Chang RQ, Li DJ, Li MQ. The role of indoleamine-2,3-dioxygenase in normal and pathological pregnancies. *Am J Reprod Immunol.* (2018) 79:e12786. doi: 10.1111/aji.12786
67. Robertson SA, Care AS, Moldenhauer LM. Regulatory T cells in embryo implantation and the immune response to pregnancy. *J Clin Invest.* (2018) 128:4224–35. doi: 10.1172/JCI122182
68. Raghupathy R, Al-Mutawa E, Al-Azemi M, Makhseed M, Azizieh F, Szekeres-Bartho J. Progesterone-induced blocking factor (PIBF) modulates cytokine production by lymphocytes from women with recurrent miscarriage or preterm delivery. *J Reprod Immunol.* (2009) 80:91–9. doi: 10.1016/j.jri.2009.01.004
69. Prins JR, Gomez-Lopez N, Robertson SA. Interleukin-6 in pregnancy and gestational disorders. *J Reprod Immunol.* (2012) 95:1–14. doi: 10.1016/j.jri.2012.05.004
70. Whitten AE, Romero R, Korzeniewski SJ, Tarca AL, Schwartz AG, Yeo L, et al. Evidence of an imbalance of angiogenic/antiangiogenic factors in massive perivillous fibrin deposition (maternal floor infarction): a placental lesion associated with recurrent miscarriage and fetal death. *Am J Obstet Gynecol.* (2013) 208:310 e1–310 e11. doi: 10.1016/j.ajog.2013.01.017
71. Shemesh A, Tirosh D, Sheiner E, Tirosh NB, Brusilovsky M, Segev R, et al. First trimester pregnancy loss and the expression of alternatively spliced NKp30 isoforms in maternal blood and placental tissue. *Front Immunol.* (2015) 6:189. doi: 10.3389/fimmu.2015.00189
72. Romero R, Mazor M, Brandt F, Sepulveda W, Avila C, Cotton DB, et al. Interleukin-1 alpha and interleukin-1 beta in preterm and term human parturition. *Am J Reprod Immunol.* (1992) 27:117–23. doi: 10.1111/j.1600-0897.1992.tb00737.x
73. Romero R, Mazor M, Sepulveda W, Avila C, Copeland D, Williams J. Tumor necrosis factor in preterm and term labor. *Am J Obstet Gynecol.* (1992) 166:1576–87. doi: 10.1016/0002-9378(92)91636-O
74. Cherouny PH, Pankuch GA, Romero R, Botti JJ, Kuhn DC, Demers LM, et al. Neutrophil attractant/activating peptide-1/interleukin-8: association with histologic chorioamnionitis, preterm delivery, and bioactive amniotic fluid leukoattractants. *Am J Obstet Gynecol.* (1993) 169:1299–303. doi: 10.1016/0002-9378(93)90297-V
75. Gotsch F, Romero R, Kusanovic JP, Erez O, Espinoza J, Kim CJ, et al. The anti-inflammatory limb of the immune response in preterm labor, intra-amniotic infection/inflammation, and spontaneous parturition at term: a role for interleukin-10. *J Matern Fetal Neonatal Med.* (2008) 21:529–47. doi: 10.1080/14767050802127349
76. Gomez-Lopez N, Laresgoiti-Servitje E, Olson DM, Estrada-Gutierrez G, Vadillo-Ortega F. The role of chemokines in term and premature rupture of the fetal membranes: a review. *Biol Reprod.* (2010) 82:809–14. doi: 10.1095/biolreprod.109.080432
77. Romero R, Dey SK, Fisher SJ. Preterm labor: one syndrome, many causes. *Science.* (2014) 345:760–5. doi: 10.1126/science.1251816
78. Romero R, Grivel JC, Tarca AL, Chaemsaithong P, Xu Z, Fitzgerald W, et al. Evidence of perturbations of the cytokine network in preterm labor. *Am J Obstet Gynecol.* (2015) 213:836 e831–836 e818. doi: 10.1016/j.ajog.2015.07.037
79. Vora B, Wang A, Kosti I, Huang H, Paranjpe I, Woodruff TJ, et al. Meta-analysis of maternal and fetal transcriptomic data elucidates the role of adaptive and innate immunity in preterm birth. *Front Immunol.* (2018) 9:993. doi: 10.3389/fimmu.2018.00993
80. Xu Y, Romero R, Miller D, Silva P, Panaitescu B, Theis KR, et al. Innate lymphoid cells at the human maternal-fetal interface in spontaneous preterm labor. *Am J Reprod Immunol.* (2018) 79:e12820. doi: 10.1111/aji.12820
81. Than NG, Abdul Rahman O, Magenheim R, Nagy B, Fule T, Hargitai B, et al. Placental protein 13 (galectin-13) has decreased placental expression but increased shedding and maternal serum concentrations in patients presenting with preterm pre-eclampsia and HELLP syndrome. *Virchows Arch.* (2008) 453:387–400. doi: 10.1007/s00428-008-0658-x
82. Than NG, Erez O, Wildman DE, Tarca AL, Edwin SS, Abbas A, et al. Severe preeclampsia is characterized by increased placental expression of galectin-1. *J Matern Fetal Neonatal Med.* (2008) 21:429–42. doi: 10.1080/14767050802041961
83. Than NG, Romero R, Meiri H, Erez O, Xu Y, Tarquini F, et al. PP13, maternal ABO blood groups and the risk assessment of pregnancy complications. *PLoS ONE.* (2011) 6:e21564. doi: 10.1371/journal.pone.0021564
84. Hsu P, Nanan RK. Innate and adaptive immune interactions at the fetal-maternal interface in healthy human pregnancy and pre-eclampsia. *Front Immunol.* (2014) 5:125. doi: 10.3389/fimmu.2014.00125
85. Stoikou M, Grimolizzi F, Giaglis S, Schafer G, van Breda SV, Hoesli IM, et al. Gestational diabetes mellitus Is associated with altered neutrophil activity. *Front Immunol.* (2017) 8:702. doi: 10.3389/fimmu.2017.00702

86. Geldenhuys J, Rossouw TM, Lombaard HA, Ehlers MM, Kock MM. Disruption in the regulation of immune responses in the placental subtype of preeclampsia. *Front Immunol.* (2018) 9:1659. doi: 10.3389/fimmu.2018.01659
87. Tsuda S, Zhang X, Hamana H, Shima T, Ushijima A, Tsuda K, et al. Clonally expanded decidual effector regulatory T cells increase in late gestation of normal pregnancy, but not in preeclampsia, in humans. *Front Immunol.* (2018) 9:1934. doi: 10.3389/fimmu.2018.01934
88. Dam TK, Brewer CF. Lectins as pattern recognition molecules: the effects of epitope density in innate immunity. *Glycobiology.* (2010) 20:270–9. doi: 10.1093/glycob/cwp186
89. Vasta GR, Ahmed H, Nita-Lazar M, Banerjee A, Pasek M, Shridhar S, et al. Galectins as self/non-self recognition receptors in innate and adaptive immunity: an unresolved paradox. *Front Immunol.* (2012) 3:199. doi: 10.3389/fimmu.2012.00199
90. Schnaar RL. Glycobiology simplified: diverse roles of glycan recognition in inflammation. *J Leukoc Biol.* (2016) 99:825–38. doi: 10.1189/jlb.3RI0116-021R
91. Gitt MA, Barondes SH. Evidence that a human soluble beta-galactoside-binding lectin is encoded by a family of genes. *Proc Natl Acad Sci USA.* (1986) 83:7603–7. doi: 10.1073/pnas.83.20.7603
92. Cooper DN. Galectinomics: finding themes in complexity. *Biochim Biophys Acta.* (2002) 1572:209–31. doi: 10.1016/S0304-4165(02)00310-0
93. Rabinovich GA, Toscano MA. Turning 'sweet' on immunity: galectin-glycan interactions in immune tolerance and inflammation. *Nat Rev Immunol.* (2009) 9:338–52. doi: 10.1038/nri2536
94. Blois SM, Barrientos G. Galectin signature in normal pregnancy and preeclampsia. *J Reprod Immunol.* (2014) 101–2:127–34. doi: 10.1016/j.jri.2013.05.005
95. Arthur CM, Baruffi MD, Cummings RD, Stowell SR. Evolving mechanistic insights into galectin functions. *Methods Mol Biol.* (2015) 1207:1–35. doi: 10.1007/978-1-4939-1396-1_1
96. Terness P, Kallikourdis M, Betz AG, Rabinovich GA, Saito S, Clark DA. Tolerance signaling molecules and pregnancy: IDO, galectins, and the renaissance of regulatory T cells. *Am J Reprod Immunol.* (2007) 58:238–54. doi: 10.1111/j.1600-0897.2007.00510.x
97. Kopcow HD, Rosetti F, Leung Y, Allan DS, Kutok JL, Strominger JL. T cell apoptosis at the maternal-fetal interface in early human pregnancy, involvement of galectin-1. *Proc Natl Acad Sci USA.* (2008) 105:18472–7. doi: 10.1073/pnas.0809233105
98. Molvarec A, Blois SM, Stenczer B, Toldi G, Tirado-Gonzalez I, Ito M, et al. Peripheral blood galectin-1-expressing T and natural killer cells in normal pregnancy and preeclampsia. *Clin Immunol.* (2011) 139:48–56. doi: 10.1016/j.clim.2010.12.018
99. Ramhorst RE, Giribaldi L, Fraccaroli L, Toscano MA, Stupirski JC, Romero MD, et al. Galectin-1 confers immune privilege to human trophoblast: implications in recurrent fetal loss. *Glycobiology.* (2012) 22:1374–86. doi: 10.1093/glycob/cws104
100. Meggyes M, Miko E, Polgar B, Bogar B, Farkas B, Illes Z, et al. Peripheral blood TIM-3 positive NK and CD8+ T cells throughout pregnancy: TIM-3/galectin-9 interaction and its possible role during pregnancy. *PLoS ONE.* (2014) 9:e92371. doi: 10.1371/journal.pone.0092371
101. Hu XH, Tang MX, Mor G, Liao AH. Tim-3: expression on immune cells and roles at the maternal-fetal interface. *J Reprod Immunol.* (2016) 118:92–9. doi: 10.1016/j.jri.2016.10.113
102. Sun J, Yang M, Ban Y, Gao W, Song B, Wang Y, et al. Tim-3 is upregulated in NK cells during early pregnancy and inhibits NK cytotoxicity toward trophoblast in galectin-9 dependent pathway. *PLoS ONE.* (2016) 11:e0147186. doi: 10.1371/journal.pone.0147186
103. Maquoi E, van den Brule FA, Castronovo V, Foidart JM. Changes in the distribution pattern of galectin-1 and galectin-3 in human placenta correlates with the differentiation pathways of trophoblasts. *Placenta.* (1997) 18:433–9. doi: 10.1016/S0143-4004(97)80044-6
104. Van den Brule FA, Fernandez PL, Buicu C, Liu FT, Jackers P, Lambotte R, et al. Differential expression of galectin-1 and galectin-3 during first trimester human embryogenesis. *Dev Dyn.* (1997) 209:399–405. doi: 10.1002/(SICI)1097-0177(199708)209:4<399::AID-AJA7>3.0.CO;2-D
105. Vicovac L, Jankovic M, Cuperlovic M. Galectin-1 and−3 in cells of the first trimester placental bed. *Hum Reprod.* (1998) 13:730–5. doi: 10.1093/humrep/13.3.730
106. Than NG, Pick E, Bellyei S, Szigeti A, Burger O, Berente Z, et al. Functional analyses of placental protein 13/galectin-13. *Eur J Biochem.* (2004) 271:1065–78. doi: 10.1111/j.1432-1033.2004.04004.x
107. Blois SM, Ilarregui JM, Tometten M, Garcia M, Orsal AS, Cordo-Russo R, et al. A pivotal role for galectin-1 in fetomaternal tolerance. *Nat Med.* (2007) 13:1450–7. doi: 10.1038/nm1680
108. Jeschke U, Mayr D, Schiessl B, Mylonas I, Schulze S, Kuhn C, et al. Expression of galectin-1,−3 (gal-1, gal-3) and the Thomsen-Friedenreich (TF) antigen in normal, IUGR, preeclamptic and HELLP placentas. *Placenta.* (2007) 28:1165–73. doi: 10.1016/j.placenta.2007.06.006
109. Miko E, Meggyes M, Doba K, Barakonyi A, Szereday L. Immune checkpoint molecules in reproductive immunology. *Front Immunol.* (2019) 10:846. doi: 10.3389/fimmu.2019.00846
110. Than NG, Romero R, Xu Y, Erez O, Xu Z, Bhatti G, et al. Evolutionary origins of the placental expression of chromosome 19 cluster galectins and their complex dysregulation in preeclampsia. *Placenta.* (2014) 35:855–65. doi: 10.1016/j.placenta.2014.07.015
111. Bohn H, Kraus W, Winckler W. Purification and characterization of two new soluble placental tissue proteins (PP13 and PP17). *Oncodev Biol Med.* (1983) 4:343–50.
112. Yang QS, Ying K, Yuan HL, Chen JZ, Meng XF, Wang Z, et al. Cloning and expression of a novel human galectin cDNA, predominantly expressed in placenta(1). *Biochim Biophys Acta.* (2002) 1574:407–11. doi: 10.1016/S0167-4781(01)00319-0
113. Balogh A, Pozsgay J, Matko J, Dong Z, Kim CJ, Varkonyi T, et al. Placental protein 13 (PP13/galectin-13) undergoes lipid raft-associated subcellular redistribution in the syncytiotrophoblast in preterm preeclampsia and HELLP syndrome. *Am J Obstet Gynecol.* (2011) 205:156 e151–114. doi: 10.1016/j.ajog.2011.03.023
114. Kliman HJ, Sammar M, Grimpel YI, Lynch SK, Milano KM, Pick E, et al. Placental protein 13 and decidual zones of necrosis: an immunologic diversion that may be linked to preeclampsia. *Reprod Sci.* (2012) 19:16–30. doi: 10.1177/1933719111424445
115. Chafetz I, Kuhnreich I, Sammar M, Tal Y, Gibor Y, Meiri H, et al. First-trimester placental protein 13 screening for preeclampsia and intrauterine growth restriction. *Am J Obstet Gynecol.* (2007) 197:35 e31–7. doi: 10.1016/j.ajog.2007.02.025
116. Romero R, Kusanovic JP, Than NG, Erez O, Gotsch F, Espinoza J, et al. First-trimester maternal serum PP13 in the risk assessment for preeclampsia. *Am J Obstet Gynecol.* (2008) 199:122 e121–122 e111. doi: 10.1016/j.ajog.2008.01.013
117. Grill S, Rusterholz C, Zanetti-Dallenbach R, Tercanli S, Holzgreve W, Hahn S, et al. Potential markers of preeclampsia–a review. *Reprod Biol Endocrinol.* (2009) 7:70. doi: 10.1186/1477-7827-7-70
118. Wortelboer EJ, Koster MP, Cuckle HS, Stoutenbeek PH, Schielen PC, Visser GH. First-trimester placental protein 13 and placental growth factor: markers for identification of women destined to develop early-onset pre-eclampsia. *BJOG.* (2010) 117:1384–9. doi: 10.1111/j.1471-0528.2010.02690.x
119. Huppertz B, Kawaguchi R. First trimester serum markers to predict preeclampsia. *Wien Med Wochenschr.* (2012) 162:191–5. doi: 10.1007/s10354-012-0072-5
120. Allen RE, Rogozinska E, Cleverly K, Aquilina J, Thangaratinam S. Abnormal blood biomarkers in early pregnancy are associated with preeclampsia: a meta-analysis. *Eur J Obstet Gynecol Reprod Biol.* (2014) 182:194–201. doi: 10.1016/j.ejogrb.2014.09.027
121. Meiri H, Sammar M, Herzog A, Grimpel YI, Fihaman G, Cohen A, et al. Prediction of preeclampsia by placental protein 13 and background risk factors and its prevention by aspirin. *J Perinat Med.* (2014) 42:591–601. doi: 10.1515/jpm-2013-0298
122. Madar-Shapiro L, Karady I, Trahtenherts A, Syngelaki A, Akolekar R, Poon L, et al. Predicting the risk to develop preeclampsia in the first trimester combining promoter variant−98A/C of LGALS13 (Placental Protein 13),

black ethnicity, previous preeclampsia, obesity, and maternal age. *Fetal Diagn Ther.* (2018) 43:250–65. doi: 10.1159/000477933

123. Chaiworapongsa T, Gervasi MT, Refuerzo J, Espinoza J, Yoshimatsu J, Berman S, et al. Maternal lymphocyte subpopulations (CD45RA+ and CD45RO+) in preeclampsia. *Am J Obstet Gynecol.* (2002) 187:889–93. doi: 10.1067/mob.2002.127309
124. Saito S, Shiozaki A, Nakashima A, Sakai M, Sasaki Y. The role of the immune system in preeclampsia. *Mol Aspects Med.* (2007) 28:192–209. doi: 10.1016/j.mam.2007.02.006
125. Zhou Y, Bianco K, Huang L, Nien JK, McMaster M, Romero R, et al. Comparative analysis of maternal-fetal interface in preeclampsia and preterm labor. *Cell Tissue Res.* (2007) 329:559–69. doi: 10.1007/s00441-007-0428-0
126. Laresgoiti-Servitje E. A leading role for the immune system in the pathophysiology of preeclampsia. *J Leukoc Biol.* (2013) 94:247–57. doi: 10.1189/jlb.1112603
127. Djurisic S, Hviid TV. HLA Class Ib molecules and immune cells in pregnancy and preeclampsia. *Front Immunol.* (2014) 5:652. doi: 10.3389/fimmu.2014.00652
128. Perez-Sepulveda A, Torres MJ, Khoury M, Illanes SE. Innate immune system and preeclampsia. *Front Immunol.* (2014) 5:244. doi: 10.3389/fimmu.2014.00244
129. Than NG, Romero R, Tarca AL, Kekesi KA, Xu Y, Xu Z, et al. Integrated systems biology approach identifies novel maternal and placental pathways of preeclampsia. *Front Immunol.* (2018) 9:1661. doi: 10.3389/fimmu.2018.01661
130. Burton GJ, Jauniaux E. Placental oxidative stress: from miscarriage to preeclampsia. *J Soc Gynecol Investig.* (2004) 11:342–52. doi: 10.1016/j.jsgi.2004.03.003
131. Gupta AK, Hasler P, Holzgreve W, Hahn S. Neutrophil NETs: a novel contributor to preeclampsia-associated placental hypoxia? *Semin Immunopathol.* (2007) 29:163–7. doi: 10.1007/s00281-007-0073-4
132. Gupta AK, Joshi MB, Philippova M, Erne P, Hasler P, Hahn S, et al. Activated endothelial cells induce neutrophil extracellular traps and are susceptible to NETosis-mediated cell death. *FEBS Lett.* (2010) 584:3193–7. doi: 10.1016/j.febslet.2010.06.006
133. Lynch AM, Salmon JE. Dysregulated complement activation as a common pathway of injury in preeclampsia and other pregnancy complications. *Placenta.* (2010) 31:561–7. doi: 10.1016/j.placenta.2010.03.010
134. Calleja-Agius J, Muttukrishna S, Pizzey AR, Jauniaux E. Pro- and antiinflammatory cytokines in threatened miscarriages. *Am J Obstet Gynecol.* (2011) 205:83 e88–16. doi: 10.1016/j.ajog.2011.02.051
135. Hahn S, Giaglis S, Hoesli I, Hasler P. Neutrophil NETs in reproduction: from infertility to preeclampsia and the possibility of fetal loss. *Front Immunol.* (2012) 3:362. doi: 10.3389/fimmu.2012.00362
136. Hargitai B, Marton T, Cox PM. Best practice no 178. Examination of the human placenta. *J Clin Pathol.* (2004) 57:785–92. doi: 10.1136/jcp.2003.014217
137. Committee on Practice Bulletins-Gynecology. The American College of Obstetricians and Gynecologists Practice Bulletin no. 150. Early pregnancy loss. *Obstet Gynecol.* (2015) 125:1258–67. doi: 10.1097/01.AOG.0000465191.27155.25
138. Redline RW. Placental pathology: a systematic approach with clinical correlations. *Placenta.* (2008) 29(Suppl. A):S86–91. doi: 10.1016/j.placenta.2007.09.003
139. Khong TY, Mooney EE, Ariel I, Balmus NC, Boyd TK, Brundler MA, et al. Sampling and definitions of placental lesions: Amsterdam Placental Workshop Group Consensus Statement. *Arch Pathol Lab Med.* (2016) 140:698–713. doi: 10.5858/arpa.2015-0225-CC
140. Varkonyi T, Nagy B, Fule T, Tarca AL, Karaszi K, Schonleber J, et al. Microarray profiling reveals that placental transcriptomes of early-onset HELLP syndrome and preeclampsia are similar. *Placenta.* (2011) 32(Suppl.):S21–29. doi: 10.1016/j.placenta.2010.04.014
141. Szabo S, Xu Y, Romero R, Fule T, Karaszi K, Bhatti G, et al. Changes of placental syndecan-1 expression in preeclampsia and HELLP syndrome. *Virchows Arch.* (2013) 463:445–58. doi: 10.1007/s00428-013-1426-0
142. Szabo S, Mody M, Romero R, Xu Y, Karaszi K, Mihalik N, et al. Activation of villous trophoblastic p38 and ERK1/2 signaling pathways in preterm preeclampsia and HELLP syndrome. *Pathol Oncol Res.* (2015) 21:659–68. doi: 10.1007/s12253-014-9872-9
143. Karaszi K, Szabo S, Juhasz K, Kiraly P, Kocsis-Deak B, Hargitai B, et al. Increased placental expression of placental protein 5 (PP5) / tissue factor pathway inhibitor-2 (TFPI-2) in women with preeclampsia and HELLP syndrome: relevance to impaired trophoblast invasion? *Placenta.* (2019) 76:30–9. doi: 10.1016/j.placenta.2019.01.011
144. Kapust RB, Tozser J, Fox JD, Anderson DE, Cherry S, Copeland TD, et al. Tobacco etch virus protease: mechanism of autolysis and rational design of stable mutants with wild-type catalytic proficiency. *Protein Eng.* (2001) 14:993–1000. doi: 10.1093/protein/14.12.993
145. Dam TK, Gabius HJ, Andre S, Kaltner H, Lensch M, Brewer CF. Galectins bind to the multivalent glycoprotein asialofetuin with enhanced affinities and a gradient of decreasing binding constants. *Biochemistry.* (2005) 44:12564–71. doi: 10.1021/bi051144z
146. Bocker S, Elling L. Binding characteristics of galectin-3 fusion proteins. *Glycobiology.* (2017) 27:457–68. doi: 10.1093/glycob/cwx007
147. Zhu C, Anderson AC, Schubart A, Xiong H, Imitola J, Khoury SJ, et al. The Tim-3 ligand galectin-9 negatively regulates T helper type 1 immunity. *Nat Immunol.* (2005) 6:1245–52. doi: 10.1038/ni1271
148. Stillman BN, Hsu DK, Pang M, Brewer CF, Johnson P, Liu FT, et al. Galectin-3 and galectin-1 bind distinct cell surface glycoprotein receptors to induce T cell death. *J Immunol.* (2006) 176:778–89. doi: 10.4049/jimmunol.176.2.778
149. Motran CC, Molinder KM, Liu SD, Poirier F, Miceli MC. Galectin-1 functions as a Th2 cytokine that selectively induces Th1 apoptosis and promotes Th2 function. *Eur J Immunol.* (2008) 38:3015–27. doi: 10.1002/eji.200838295
150. Zarnani AH. Recurrent pregnancy loss through the lens of immunology. *J Reprod Infertil.* (2015) 16:59–60.
151. Varla-Leftherioti M, Immunology in reproduction. In: Carp, HJA, Carp H, editors. *Recurrent Pregnancy Loss Causes, Controversies and Treatment*, 2nd ed. Boca Raton: CRC Press (2015). p 233–48.
152. Liu AX, Jin F, Zhang WW, Zhou TH, Zhou CY, Yao WM, et al. Proteomic analysis on the alteration of protein expression in the placental villous tissue of early pregnancy loss. *Biol Reprod.* (2006) 75:414–20. doi: 10.1095/biolreprod.105.049379
153. Unverdorben L, Haufe T, Santoso L, Hofmann S, Jeschke U, Hutter S. Prototype and chimera-type galectins in placentas with spontaneous and recurrent miscarriages. *Int J Mol Sci.* (2016) 17:644. doi: 10.3390/ijms17050644
154. Sun FR, Chen CQ, Yu M, Wang SC, Li DJ, Du MR. Galectin-9 promotes human trophoblast cell invasion through matrix metalloproteinase-2 and p38 signaling pathway. *Reprod Dev Med.* (2018) 2:1–7. doi: 10.4103/2096-2924.232880
155. Tirado-Gonzalez I, Freitag N, Barrientos G, Shaikly V, Nagaeva O, Strand M, et al. Galectin-1 influences trophoblast immune evasion and emerges as a predictive factor for the outcome of pregnancy. *Mol Hum Reprod.* (2013) 19:43–53. doi: 10.1093/molehr/gas043
156. Cao A, Alluqmani N, Buhari FHM, Wasim L, Smith LK, Quaile AT, et al. Galectin-9 binds IgM-BCR to regulate B cell signaling. *Nat Commun.* (2018) 9:3288. doi: 10.1038/s41467-018-05771-8
157. Giovannone N, Liang J, Antonopoulos A, Geddes Sweeney J, King SL, Pochebit SM, et al. Galectin-9 suppresses B cell receptor signaling and is regulated by I-branching of N-glycans. *Nat Commun.* (2018) 9:3287. doi: 10.1038/s41467-018-05770-9
158. He M, Jiang M, Zhou Y, Li F, Yang M, Fan Y, et al. Impaired Gal-9 dysregulates the PBMC-induced Th1/Th2 imbalance in abortion-prone matings. *J Immunol Res.* (2018) 2018:9517842. doi: 10.1155/2018/9517842
159. Lajko A, Meggyes M, Fulop BD, Gede N, Reglodi D, Szereday L. Comparative analysis of decidual and peripheral immune cells and

immune-checkpoint molecules during pregnancy in wild-type and PACAP-deficient mice. *Am J Reprod Immunol.* (2018) 80:e13035. doi: 10.1111/aji.13035
160. Olivares EG, Munoz R, Tejerizo G, Montes MJ, Gomez-Molina F, Abadia-Molina AC. Decidual lymphocytes of human spontaneous abortions induce apoptosis but not necrosis in JEG-3 extravillous trophoblast cells. *Biol Reprod.* (2002) 67:1211–7. doi: 10.1095/biolreprod67.4.1211
161. Sacks G, Sargent I, Redman C. An innate view of human pregnancy. *Immunol Today.* (1999) 20:114–8. doi: 10.1016/S0167-5699(98)01393-0
162. Saito S, Nakashima A, Shima T, Ito M. Th1/Th2/Th17 and regulatory T-cell paradigm in pregnancy. *Am J Reprod Immunol.* (2010) 63:601–10. doi: 10.1111/j.1600-0897.2010.00852.x
163. Figueiredo AS, Schumacher A. The T helper type 17/regulatory T cell paradigm in pregnancy. *Immunology.* (2016) 148:13–21. doi: 10.1111/imm.12595
164. Lhuillier C, Barjon C, Niki T, Gelin A, Praz F, Morales O, et al. Impact of exogenous galectin-9 on human T cells: contribution of the T cell receptor complex to antigen-independent activation but not to apoptosis induction. *J Biol Chem.* (2015) 290:16797–811. doi: 10.1074/jbc.M115.661272
165. Perillo NL, Pace KE, Seilhamer JJ, Baum LG. Apoptosis of T cells mediated by galectin-1. *Nature.* (1995) 378:736–9. doi: 10.1038/378736a0
166. Toscano MA, Bianco GA, Ilarregui JM, Croci DO, Correale J, Hernandez JD, et al. Differential glycosylation of TH1, TH2 and TH-17 effector cells selectively regulates susceptibility to cell death. *Nat Immunol.* (2007) 8:825–34. doi: 10.1038/ni1482
167. Alderson MR, Tough TW, Davis-Smith T, Braddy S, Falk B, Schooley KA, et al. Fas ligand mediates activation-induced cell death in human T lymphocytes. *J Exp Med.* (1995) 181:71–7. doi: 10.1084/jem.181.1.71
168. Richter GH, Mollweide A, Hanewinkel K, Zobywalski C, Burdach S. CD25 blockade protects T cells from activation-induced cell death (AICD) via maintenance of TOSO expression. *Scand J Immunol.* (2009) 70:206–15. doi: 10.1111/j.1365-3083.2009.02281.x
169. Zhan Y, Carrington EM, Zhang Y, Heinzel S, Lew AM. Life and death of activated T cells: how are they different from naive T cells? *Front Immunol.* (2017) 8:1809. doi: 10.3389/fimmu.2017.01809
170. Batista A, Millan J, Mittelbrunn M, Sanchez-Madrid F, Alonso MA. Recruitment of transferrin receptor to immunological synapse in response to TCR engagement. *J Immunol.* (2004) 172:6709–14. doi: 10.4049/jimmunol.172.11.6709
171. Trowbridge IS, Omary MB. Human cell surface glycoprotein related to cell proliferation is the receptor for transferrin. *Proc Natl Acad Sci USA.* (1981) 78:3039–43. doi: 10.1073/pnas.78.5.3039
172. Taetle R, Castagnola J, Mendelsohn J. Mechanisms of growth inhibition by anti-transferrin receptor monoclonal antibodies. *Cancer Res.* (1986) 46:1759–63.
173. van der Leij J, van den Berg A, Blokzijl T, Harms G, van Goor H, Zwiers P, et al. Dimeric galectin-1 induces IL-10 production in T-lymphocytes: an important tool in the regulation of the immune response. *J Pathol.* (2004) 204:511–8. doi: 10.1002/path.1671
174. Li A, Dubey S, Varney ML, Dave BJ, Singh RK. IL-8 directly enhanced endothelial cell survival, proliferation, and matrix metalloproteinases production and regulated angiogenesis. *J Immunol.* (2003) 170:3369–76. doi: 10.4049/jimmunol.170.6.3369
175. Amsalem H, Kwan M, Hazan A, Zhang J, Jones RL, Whittle W, et al. Identification of a novel neutrophil population: proangiogenic granulocytes in second-trimester human decidua. *J Immunol.* (2014) 193:3070–9. doi: 10.4049/jimmunol.1303117
176. Lash GE, Ernerudh J. Decidual cytokines and pregnancy complications: focus on spontaneous miscarriage. *J Reprod Immunol.* (2015) 108:83–9. doi: 10.1016/j.jri.2015.02.003
177. Santoni A, Zingoni A, Cerboni C, Gismondi A. Natural killer (NK) cells from killers to regulators: distinct features between peripheral blood and decidual NK cells. *Am J Reprod Immunol.* (2007) 58:280–8. doi: 10.1111/j.1600-0897.2007.00513.x
178. Bruno A, Pagani A, Pulze L, Albini A, Dallaglio K, Noonan DM, et al. Orchestration of angiogenesis by immune cells. *Front Oncol.* (2014) 4:131. doi: 10.3389/fonc.2014.00131
179. Gamliel M, Goldman-Wohl D, Isaacson B, Gur C, Stein N, Yamin R, et al. Trained memory of human uterine NK cells enhances their function in subsequent pregnancies. *Immunity.* (2018) 48:951–62 e955. doi: 10.1016/j.immuni.2018.03.030
180. Blois SM, Conrad ML, Freitag N, Barrientos G. Galectins in angiogenesis: consequences for gestation. *J Reprod Immunol.* (2015) 108:33–41. doi: 10.1016/j.jri.2014.12.001
181. Gizurarson S, Huppertz B, Osol G, Skarphedinsson JO, Mandala M, Meiri H. Effects of placental protein 13 on the cardiovascular system in gravid and non-gravid rodents. *Fetal Diagn Ther.* (2013) 33:257–64. doi: 10.1159/000345964
182. Gizurarson S, Sigurdardottir ER, Meiri H, Huppertz B, Sammar M, Sharabi-Nov A, et al. Placental protein 13 administration to pregnant rats lowers blood pressure and augments fetal growth and venous remodeling. *Fetal Diagn Ther.* (2016) 39:56–63. doi: 10.1159/000381914
183. Drobnjak T, Gizurarson S, Gokina NI, Meiri H, Mandala M, Huppertz B, et al. Placental protein 13 (PP13)-induced vasodilation of resistance arteries from pregnant and nonpregnant rats occurs via endothelial-signaling pathways. *Hypertens Pregnancy.* (2017) 36:186–95. doi: 10.1080/10641955.2017.1295052
184. Drobnjak T, Jonsdottir AM, Helgadottir H, Runolfsdottir MS, Meiri H, Sammar M, et al. Placental protein 13 (PP13) stimulates rat uterine vessels after slow subcutaneous administration. *Int J Womens Health.* (2019) 11:213–22. doi: 10.2147/IJWH.S188303
185. Levine RJ, Maynard SE, Qian C, Lim KH, England LJ, Yu KF, et al. Circulating angiogenic factors and the risk of preeclampsia. *N Engl J Med.* (2004) 350:672–83. doi: 10.1056/NEJMoa031884
186. Gotsch F, Romero R, Friel L, Kusanovic JP, Espinoza J, Erez O, et al. CXCL10/IP-10: a missing link between inflammation and anti-angiogenesis in preeclampsia? *J Matern Fetal Neonatal Med.* (2007) 20:777–92. doi: 10.1080/14767050701483298
187. Erez O, Romero R, Espinoza J, Fu W, Todem D, Kusanovic JP, et al. The change in concentrations of angiogenic and anti-angiogenic factors in maternal plasma between the first and second trimesters in risk assessment for the subsequent development of preeclampsia and small-for-gestational age. *J Matern Fetal Neonatal Med.* (2008) 21:279–87. doi: 10.1080/14767050802034545
188. Gotsch F, Romero R, Kusanovic JP, Chaiworapongsa T, Dombrowski M, Erez O, et al. Preeclampsia and small-for-gestational age are associated with decreased concentrations of a factor involved in angiogenesis: soluble Tie-2. *J Matern Fetal Neonatal Med.* (2008) 21:389–402. doi: 10.1080/14767050802046069
189. Maynard S, Epstein FH, Karumanchi SA. Preeclampsia and angiogenic imbalance. *Annu Rev Med.* (2008) 59:61–78. doi: 10.1146/annurev.med.59.110106.214058
190. Romero R, Nien JK, Espinoza J, Todem D, Fu W, Chung H, et al. A longitudinal study of angiogenic (placental growth factor) and anti-angiogenic (soluble endoglin and soluble vascular endothelial growth factor receptor-1) factors in normal pregnancy and patients destined to develop preeclampsia and deliver a small for gestational age neonate. *J Matern Fetal Neonatal Med.* (2008) 21:9–23. doi: 10.1080/14767050701830480
191. Chaiworapongsa T, Romero R, Korzeniewski SJ, Kusanovic JP, Soto E, Lam J, et al. Maternal plasma concentrations of angiogenic/antiangiogenic factors in the third trimester of pregnancy to identify the patient at risk for stillbirth at or near term and severe late preeclampsia. *Am J Obstet Gynecol.* (2013) 208:287 e281–287 e215. doi: 10.1016/j.ajog.2013.01.016
192. Giaglis S, Stoikou M, Grimolizzi F, Subramanian BY, van Breda SV, Hoesli I, et al. Neutrophil migration into the placenta: Good, bad or deadly? *Cell Adh Migr.* (2016) 10:208–25. doi: 10.1080/19336918.2016.1148866

193. Tomimatsu T, Mimura K, Endo M, Kumasawa K, Kimura T. Pathophysiology of preeclampsia: an angiogenic imbalance and long-lasting systemic vascular dysfunction. *Hypertens Res.* (2017) 40:305–10. doi: 10.1038/hr.2016.152
194. Sahay AS, Jadhav AT, Sundrani DP, Wagh GN, Mehendale SS, Chavan-Gautam P, et al. VEGF and VEGFR1 levels in different regions of the normal and preeclampsia placentae. *Mol Cell Biochem.* (2018) 438:141–52. doi: 10.1007/s11010-017-3121-y
195. D'Haene N, Sauvage S, Maris C, Adanja I, Le Mercier M, Decaestecker C, et al. VEGFR1 and VEGFR2 involvement in extracellular galectin-1- and galectin-3-induced angiogenesis. *PLoS ONE.* (2013) 8:e67029. doi: 10.1371/journal.pone.0067029
196. Freitag N, Tirado-Gonzalez I, Barrientos G, Herse F, Thijssen VL, Weedon-Fekjaer SM, et al. Interfering with Gal-1-mediated angiogenesis contributes to the pathogenesis of preeclampsia. *Proc Natl Acad Sci USA.* (2013) 110:11451–6. doi: 10.1073/pnas.1303707110
197. Crocker PR. *Mammalian Carbohydrate Recognition Systems.* Berlin; New York, NY: Springer (2001). doi: 10.1007/978-3-540-46410-5
198. Cedeno-Laurent F, Dimitroff CJ. Galectin-1 research in T cell immunity: past, present and future. *Clin Immunol.* (2012) 142:107–16. doi: 10.1016/j.clim.2011.09.011

12

Hormonal Regulation of Physiology, Innate Immunity and Antibody Response to H1N1 Influenza Virus Infection During Pregnancy

Elizabeth Q. Littauer[1,2] *and Ioanna Skountzou*[1,2*]

[1] *Emory Vaccine Center, Emory University School of Medicine, Atlanta, GA, United States,* [2] *Department of Microbiology and Immunology, Emory University School of Medicine, Atlanta, GA, United States*

***Correspondence:**
Ioanna Skountzou
iskount@emory.edu

In 2009, the H1N1 swine flu pandemic highlighted the vulnerability of pregnant women to influenza viral infection. Pregnant women infected with influenza A virus were at increased risk of hospitalization and severe acute respiratory distress syndrome (ARDS), which is associated with high mortality, while their newborns had an increased risk of pre-term birth or low birth weight. Pregnant women have a unique immunological profile modulated by the sex hormones required to maintain pregnancy, namely progesterone and estrogens. The role of these hormones in coordinating maternal immunotolerance in uterine tissue and cellular subsets has been well researched; however, these hormones have wide-ranging effects outside the uterus in modulating the immune response to disease. In this review, we compile research findings in the clinic and in animal models that elaborate on the unique features of H1N1 influenza A viral pathogenesis during pregnancy, the crosstalk between innate immune signaling and hormonal regulation during pregnancy, and the role of pregnancy hormones in modulating cellular responses to influenza A viral infection at mid-gestation. We highlight the ways in which lung architecture and function is stressed by pregnancy, increasing baseline inflammation prior to infection. We demonstrate that infection disrupts progesterone production and upregulates inflammatory mediators, such as cyclooxygenase-2 (COX-2) and prostaglandins, resulting in pre-term labor and spontaneous abortions. Lastly, we profile the ways in which pregnancy alters innate and adaptive cellular immune responses to H1N1 influenza viral infection, and the ways in which these protect fetal development at the expense of effective long-term immune memory. Thus, we highlight advancements in the field of reproductive immunology in response to viral infection and illustrate how that knowledge might be used to develop more effective post-infection therapies and vaccination strategies.

Keywords: pregnancy, H1N1 influenza virus infection, animal models, sex hormones, maternal immune response

INTRODUCTION

Influenza viruses are segmented, negative-stranded enveloped RNA viruses that cause respiratory infections, fever, malaise, coughing, and mucus production. Influenza viruses are divided into A, B, C, and D types; while all A, B, and C can be infectious in humans with influenza A viruses (IAVs) causing the most widespread disease, influenza D virus is not known to infection humans (1, 2).

Influenza A viruses are further classified by the antigenicity of their surface proteins hemagglutinin (HA) and neuraminidase (NA), which are encoded on individual segments of viral RNA, and define the host range of each virus (1, 3). Through a process unique to influenza and other segmented genome viruses, co-infection of different viral subtypes in human, swine, avian or other animal hosts can result in reassortment leading to antigenically unique novel viruses that may take advantage of an immunologically naïve host species (4). This process of reassortment resulted in the emergence of the four major influenza virus strains causing pandemics; the 1918 H1N1 Spanish influenza, the 1957 H2N2 Asian influenza, the 1968 H3N2 Hong Kong influenza, and the 2009 H1N1/09 swine influenza, that infected up to 50% of the global population and caused a significant increase in mortality (2, 3). While infection can occur year-round, the epidemiology of influenza virus infection is seasonal, causing peak illness in November through March in the Northern Hemisphere and approximately 200,000 hospitalizations and 36,000 deaths annually in the United States (3). Currently, the most common circulating influenza A subtypes are H1N1 and H3N2, which are included in quadrivalent vaccines together with the type B influenza lineages Yamagata and Victoria (5). Due to the wide variety of circulating viruses and the frequency of genetic reassortment between subtypes, vaccination is required annually to provide immune protection during each influenza season although it may not be complete if there is mismatch between predicted strains included in the vaccine and the resultant circulating strains in the following season.

Seasonal influenza infections during the second and third trimester of gestation increase the morbidity of pregnant women with higher hospitalization rates than the general population and mortality (6). Pregnant women have been particularly vulnerable to pandemic influenza viruses showing up to 45% increased morbidity and mortality, and they were at an increased risk of higher cardiopulmonary complications and gestational abnormalities during the four major influenza pandemics in the past 100 years (7–9). While pregnant women typically represent 1% of the American population, during the 2009 H1N1 pandemic they comprised 6.4% of all hospitalizations and 4.3% of all deaths (10, 11). Over half of those women hospitalized for H1N1 influenza virus infection had another pre-existing condition, such as asthma, high blood pressure, and diabetes; women with asthma represented 43.5% of deaths from influenza virus infection during pregnancy, which is part of a larger phenomenon of enhanced viral pathogenesis and severe outcomes among asthmatic adults (11, 12).

Influenza infection-related complications in fetuses and neonates have been associated with increased risk of miscarriage, pre-term birth, stillbirth, neonatal death, and low birth weight (6, 9, 13, 14). Clinical reports of influenza-like illness (ILI) during pregnancy have been correlated with a five-fold increase in perinatal morbidity and mortality (15). The incidence of pre-term birth increased from 7 per 1,000 births to 39 per 1,000 births and the incidence of stillbirth from 6 to 27 stillbirths per 1,000 births in the 2009 pandemic (9, 10, 16). Specifically, pregnant women who tested positive for the 2009 swine-origin H1N1 virus were more likely to deliver low birthweight infants than pregnant women who delivered following ILI that was not caused by the pandemic strain (17). There is historical evidence that the 1918 and 1957 pandemics produced similar clinical outcomes for pregnant women; however, modern diagnostic procedures employed during the 2009 H1N1 pandemic allow for more direct linkage between influenza viral infection of pregnant mothers and poor outcomes for maternal and neonatal health (9).

The mortality rates reported for both women and their newborns led to initiatives by the Centers for Disease Control and Prevention (CDC) and the World Health Organization (WHO) to increase influenza vaccination coverage in pregnant women (5, 18). Maternal vaccination during the second or third trimester of pregnancy with seasonal trivalent influenza vaccine substantially reduced the incidence of ILI in both mothers and their newborns (19–21) and has not been associated with pre-term delivery or an increase of adverse outcomes for mothers or their infants. In a review of 7 clinical studies, Bratton et al concluded that maternal vaccination reduced the likelihood of stillbirth compared to unvaccinated pregnant mothers (22–24). However, while the conventional intramuscular vaccination has been determined to be reasonably safe for routine use during pregnancy, promoting the transplacental transfer of anti-influenza virus antibodies from mother to fetus, clinical data is inconclusive regarding the efficiency of immune responses to the vaccine when compared to those induced in non-pregnant women (18, 19, 25–27).

Vaccination is widely recommended during pregnancy for the benefit of mother and child; however, vaccination coverage among pregnant women in the United States remains around 50% (6). Research into the specific mechanisms by which H1N1 influenza virus infection causes pregnancy complications and how pregnancy hormones modulate the immune response to infection and vaccination may reveal improved routes of therapy for women infected with influenza A virus during pregnancy. This review will discuss how H1N1 influenza virus infection disrupts maternal lung and placental function as well as the role of pregnancy hormones in shaping the innate and cellular immune responses to H1N1 influenza virus infection.

The Physiology of Influenza A Virus Infection and Immune Responses

Human influenza A virus is typically transmitted through respiratory droplets and inhaled into the nasopharynx. Initial virus infection occurs when hemagglutinin (HA), a surface protein on influenza virions, binds to α2,6-linked sialic acids that are widely expressed on the surface of ciliated airway epithelial cells throughout the upper respiratory tract (28, 29). Viruses are then endocytosed primarily via a clathrin-mediated pathway; upon acidification of the vesicle containing influenza virions, the HA protein is triggered to fuse viral and cellular membranes, releasing the viral genome into the cell (30–32). The eight negative-stranded RNA segments of the viral genome are then translocated to the nucleus, where they replicate using the associated viral RNA-dependent RNA polymerase through a complementary RNA (cRNA) replication intermediate (33). In parallel, viral transcripts are generated using stretches of capped cellular RNA molecules as primers ("cap-snatching"). After translation of the viral transcripts in the cytoplasm, the eight genome segments are packaged into virions which are released from the apical cellular membranes to infect nearby cells and thus result in viral amplification (32, 34). Viruses shed from the nasopharynx may be inhaled further into the lower respiratory tract causing severe pulmonary infections or transmitted through respiratory droplets from the upper respiratory compartment to the next person. People infected with 2009 H1N1 influenza A virus were contagious as early as 12 hours post-inoculation and typically began experiencing symptoms approximately 2 days following infection (35).

The release of viral RNA within the cell activates innate immune signaling pathways, especially toll-like receptors (TLRs) and retinoic-acid-inducible gene 1 (RIG1), which induce the expression of the pro-inflammatory cytokines interferon-α (IFN-α) and interferon-β (IFN-β) (36, 37). The secretion of these cytokines activates the surrounding epithelial cells to express antiviral genes that hamper viral entry and replication and recruit innate immune cells to the site of infection (37–39). Natural killer (NK) cells and neutrophils kill infected cells, and additional cytokines expressed by activated airway epithelium and innate immune cells induce fever and mucus production, which in turn results in coughing and rhinorrhea to shed the virus and cellular debris from the lungs and the nasopharynx (38, 40). These infection-induced responses are the hallmark of influenza illness symptomatology, and in clinically vulnerable populations, chest congestion due to viral infection and the ensuing immune response can lead to bronchitis, pneumonia, and secondary bacterial infections (41–43). Viral clearance finally occurs around 8 to 10 days after the onset of symptoms when the adaptive immune response mounts virus-specific clearing of infected tissue (38, 44). Viral antigen is taken up and processed by dendritic cells which migrate upon activation to draining mediastinal lymph nodes and prime naïve resident T cells to respond to the infection (45). Humoral memory is developed when naïve B cells are primed by soluble antigen and costimulated by CD4+ T follicular helper (TFH) cells to mature into plasmablasts that will then traffic to the site of the infection and secrete virus-specific neutralizing antibodies (46). Ultimately, following costimulatory help from CD4+ T cells, CD8+ cytotoxic T lymphocytes will traffic to the lungs and eradicate virus-infected cells (38, 46, 47). Upon resolution of disease, alveolar macrophages clear cellular debris, and basal stem cells regenerate airway epithelium to restore healthy tissue (48, 49). In animal models for influenza viral pathogenesis, it was demonstrated that virus-specific CD103$^+$ CD8$^+$ tissue resident memory (TRM) T cells in the lungs could provide rapid response upon the next infection and memory B cells persisted in the mediastinal lymph nodes to secrete virus-neutralizing antibody into circulation upon restimulation (50–52).

Research into the specific mechanisms of H1N1 influenza A virus binding, entry, RNA replication, transmission, and induction of the host immune system has been extensive since the 1918 Spanish influenza pandemic; however, investigations into how these mechanisms manifest in disease in immunologically unique populations, such as infants, the elderly, HIV$^+$ or asthmatic patients, and pregnant women have been limited.

Hormonal Regulation of Pregnancy and Immune Signaling Are Delicately Balanced to Protect Fetal Development

Female reproduction is regulated predominately via estrogen, progesterone, luteinizing hormone (LH), and follicular stimulating hormone (FSH). Estrogen receptors (ERs) and progesterone receptors (PGRs) are typically expressed within the cytosol and translocated to the nucleus upon ligand binding to induce a suite of genes encoding immunomodulators, regulators for tissue remodeling, mammary gland development, metabolism, lung physiology and function (53–55). LH and FSH are synthesized in the anterior pituitary gland and coordinate the decidualization of the uterine endometrium as well as the release of oocytes from mature ovarian follicles into the uterus for fertilization (56). A fertilized oocyte develops into a blastocyst, and then the outer layer of the blastocyst forms a polarized structure called the trophectoderm (57). The trophoctoderm layer implants in the uterine wall to become syncytiotrophoblasts that secrete human chorionic gonadotropin (hCG) and develop into fetal placental chorionic villi (57). Placental hCG expression signals the maternal corpus luteum to produce progesterone, which maintains the appropriate thickness and vascularization of the endometrium to support embryonic growth (56).

Insufficient progesterone production has been associated with infertility and recurrent spontaneous abortions, indicating that variations in progesterone levels as a result of infectious disease are not well tolerated by maternal physiology and may result in miscarriage or pre-term birth (58–60). Sex hormones play a crucial role in organizing endometrial granulated lymphocytes (EGLs) in the innermost layer of epithelial tissue in the uterus and populations of uterine natural killer (NK) cells, dendritic cells, macrophages, and memory and regulatory T cells are tightly controlled throughout the first, second, and third trimesters of pregnancy (56, 61, 62). Estrogens are expressed in several major forms, mainly estradiol (E2) and estriol (E3); each can have biphasic effects in stimulating pro-inflammatory signaling via mitogen-associated protein kinases (MAPKs) and NK activation at low concentrations or enhancing the expression of PD-L1 on T cells and the synthesis of TGF- β and IL-10 at high concentrations (62). Progesterone receptors are expressed broadly on most immune cell subsets and are produced in higher levels in females (62–64). In the uterus, progesterone induces the transition of naïve Th0 cells into IL-4, IL-5, and IL-6 secreting Th2 memory cells upon antigen recognition; these Th2 cells are critical for coordinating immune tolerant cytokine crosstalk between the maternal and fetal sides of the placenta and preventing intrauterine NK cell activation against fetal trophoblasts (61). The expression of IL-4 and IL-6 then promotes hCG secretion from the corpus luteum, which in turn releases more progesterone, creating a positive feedback loop for the amplification of hormone-mediated Th2 polarization (61). This phenomenon has been shown to be important for maintaining immune tolerance, and recurrent miscarriage is associated with a predominance of Th1 memory cells in the endometrium (65). Estrogens have also been implicated in inducing $CD4^+$ $CD25^+$ T regulatory cells (Tregs) and are critical for maintaining tolerance within the maternal-fetal interface (66). Progesterone also upregulates the activity of uterine Tregs, which act as suppressors of inflammatory immune subsets, particularly NK cells and macrophages resident to the endometrium (62, 64). In this way, estrogens and progesterone coordinate an environment in which both uterine epithelial cells and innate immune cells resident to uterine tissue will tolerate the implantation of a fertilized oocyte and the development of a placenta and fetus.

The structure and cellular composition of placenta is critical to maintaining fetal growth and development as well as protection from inflammation. Fetal placenta develops from the cells in the implanted blastocyst as it transitions into the trophoblast which differentiates into cytotrophoblasts and synciotrophoblasts. Both cell types contribute to the development of chorionic villi that form an interface with the uterine decidua (57). Here, maternal blood makes direct contact with fetal cells, allowing for gas, nutrient, and waste exchange but also providing a potential door for entry of bacteria, viruses, and parasites to a fetus with an undeveloped immune system (67). Few pathogens can cross the placental barrier from the mother to the fetus. TORCH pathogens [*Toxoplasma gondii*; other pathogens including, human immunodeficiency virus (HIV), varicella zoster virus (VZV), malaria-causing *Plasmodium* species, *Listeria monocytogenes*, *Treponema pallidum*, parvoviruses B19, enteroviruses, and recently, Zika virus; *r*ubella virus; *c*ytomegalovirus (CMV); and *h*erpes simplex virus 1 and 2 (HSV)] are associated with fetal and neonatal morbidity and mortality from CNS abnormalities, microcephaly, blindness, deafness, premature birth or low birth weight (67, 68). However, there is limited evidence that influenza A virus crosses the maternal-fetal barrier. Despite the demonstrated ability of the 2009 pandemic strain to infect fetal trophoblasts, the development of chorionic villitis and the widespread reports of increased risk of maternal and fetal mortality, there were few conclusive cases of vertical transmission via the placenta (69, 70). Thus, poor fetal outcomes during pregnancy are likely due to indirect exposure to maternal inflammatory cytokine expression and dysregulation of pregnancy-supportive hormones.

In addition to preventing pathogen entry into the fetal bloodstream, it is also critical that cytokines that make it across the placental syncytiotrophoblast layer into the fetal circulatory system do not cause inflammation or immune cell activation that interrupts fetal growth and development (71, 72). Clinical reports of maternal inflammation and infection during pregnancy have been associated, although inconclusively, with the development of autism, bipolar disorders, and schizophrenia in children born to mothers infected with influenza A virus during pregnancy (73–75). Peripheral blood mononuclear cells (PBMCs) isolated from healthy pregnant women and co-cultured with 2009 pandemic influenza A virus subtype H1N1 or circulating rhinovirus strains (HRV43 and HRV1B) had significantly reduced IFN-α and IFN-γ responses, indicating increased susceptibility to severe outcomes of viral infection during pregnancy (76, 77) A shift away from inflammatory Th1 cytokines (TNF-α, IFN-γ, IL-2) can limit potential cytotoxic damage to the fetus and placenta (61, 62). Sex hormones coordinate this shift by activating transcriptional factors via transmembrane and intracellular receptors which activate a suite of anti-abortive, pro-pregnancy genes (63). For example, progesterone activates progesterone-induced binding factor (PIBF) in lymphocytes, which in turn promotes the synthesis of IL-3, IL-4, and IL-10, while reducing the expression of IL-12 (78, 79). PIBF also inhibits NK cell degranulation, and decreased PIBF expression is linked to recurrent spontaneous abortions (79, 80). Thus, hormone-mediated suppression of inflammatory cytokine production and cellular activation is critical to successful pregnancy in the short-term by protecting the placenta from inflammation that could trigger pre-term birth or neurodevelopment damage; however, proper inflammatory signals must still be activated to recruit innate immune cells and $CD8^+$ T cells in order to clear virus-infected tissue.

While pre-term birth and low birth weight neonates have been well-documented outcomes of the 2009 H1N1 influenza virus infection in pregnant women, a mechanism for this phenotype is unclear, though placental transmission of inflammatory cytokines, dysregulated hormone signaling, and oxygen deprivation due to maternal respiratory distress have all been implicated (62, 81, 82). The effect of the hormonal millieu during pregnancy on innate immune responses is complicated, and *ex vivo* modeling of a single subset of cells may not depict the entire story of hormonal, cytokine and immune cell signaling between lung, fetus, and placenta in an infected pregnant woman. Clinical samples from pregnant women are limited to blood, post-partum placenta, and post-mortem tissues, leaving research questions about maternal lung function and immune responses to non-fatal influenza viral infection unanswered.

Rodent models, particularly mice, are a commonly accepted experimental tool for preclinical research studies due to their hemochorial placental structures, recapitulation of influenza viral pathogenesis seen in humans, and their cost effectiveness over multiple time points (29). One approach for the elucidation of these mechanisms is to expose healthy non-pregnant female mice to low doses of sex hormones comparable to birth control or high doses comparable to those of pregnancy. Pazos et al. implanted female C57BL/6 mice with degradable 17β-estradiol (E2 in mice) pellets to yield serum E2 levels of third trimester pregnancy and infected them with H1N1 PR8 virus; mice implanted with E2 exhibited reduced type I IFN signaling and impaired $CD8^+$ T cell function compared to infected non-implanted female mice (83). Robinson et al proposed that 17β-estradiol has protective effect during pregnancy; ovariectomized and E2-implanted female C57BL/6 mice infected with H1N1 PR8 influenza virus exhibited enhanced recruitment of neutrophils and virus-specific T cells, which promote viral clearance (84). In contrast, studies involving pregnant mice demonstrated that while individual expression of estrogen or progesterone may limit inflammation, the condition of pregnancy resulted in elevated inflammatory responses to influenza virus infection compared to the immune responses of infected non-pregnant female mice (85–87). Pregnant mice infected with a mouse-adapted, 2009 H1N1 influenza virus expressed elevated levels of IL-1α, IL-6, granulocyte-colony stimulating factor (G-CSF), monocyte chemotactic protein (MCP-1), CXCL1, and RANTES and experienced more severe pathology and mortality when compared to non-pregnant mice (88). These cytokines were highly expressed in humans who died as a result of 2009 H1N1 influenza A virus (87, 89). These differences in immune responses between hormone-treated mice and pregnant mice infected with influenza virus highlights how immune and endocrine crosstalk between mother, fetus, and placenta has far-reaching consequences beyond classical reproductive tissues and complicates our understanding of typical H1N1 viral pathogenesis.

The genetic background of mouse strain is also significant in the selection of a pregnant mouse model. C57BL/6 mice classically tend toward Th1-type immune responses while mice with BALB/c genetic backgrounds tend toward Th2-type immune responses (90, 91). Differences in genetic background have been shown to cause variability in viral pathogenesis, inflammatory cytokine response, pulmonary microRNA expression, alveolar macrophage viability following intranasal infection with 2009 H1N1 pandemic influenza virus strains (92–94). Strain differences also affect the physiological response to influenza viral infection during pregnancy. Recent findings in C57BL/6 mice have highlighted that pregnancy significantly enhances lung function by increasing respiratory compliance and total lung capacity and that influenza virus infection does not alter lung tidal volume, minute ventilation, diffusing capacity, and compliance as shown in non-pregnant infected mice. The authors observed less inflammation in the lungs of infected pregnant mice and suggested that this is a protective mechanism against maternal respiratory damage during pregnancy (95). However, we and others have shown in the BALB/c mouse model that pregnancy increases lung inflammation and expression of stress-induced prostaglandins (PGs) and cyclooxygenase-2 (COX-2) prior to infection and that IAV infection enhances immunopathology in the lungs of pregnant mice relative to non-pregnant mice (86–88). Oxidative stress interferes with lipid raft clustering and has been shown to inhibit the ability of PIBF to bind its transmembrane receptor and IL-4R to induce the STAT6 signaling pathway; this interference reduces the sensitivity of cells to PIBF (96, 97). Thus, influenza viral infection and subsequent oxidative stress may interfere with the unique lung and mucosal physiology tightly regulated by sex hormones toward successful pregnancy and fetal development.

Humoral Immune Responses Following Infection and Vaccination During Pregnancy

The natural outcome of infection is the development of immunological memory to prevent re-infection and future cellular damage. As discussed previously, soluble viral antigen released from infected cells in the lungs primes naive B cells in the proximal draining lymph nodes by binding to the B cell receptor (BCR), crosslinking several BCRs in the process and amplifying an activation signal (46, 98–100). Additional costimulation by $CD4^+$ helper T cells responding to processed viral antigen in MHC class II proteins on the B cell's surface is required to fully activate B cells and provides a second activation signal, resulting in clonal proliferation and amplification of antibodies specific for influenza viral antigens (46). Selection for B cells with BCRs with highest affinity for the viral antigen occurs in the germinal centers found in secondary lymphoid tissues such as the spleen. In the latter, cells undergo somatic hypermutation, a process by which DNA encoding hypervariable Ig regions is broken by activation-induced deaminase (AID) and uracil-DNA glycosylase (UNG) and repaired by MSH2/6 and REV1. The accumulating mutations may result in the generation of antibodies with an increased affinity to viral antigens (101, 102). Immunoglobulin class switching increases the range of functions by recombining antibody variable regions encoding specificity for influenza viral proteins with constant regions encoding receptors for various innate immune cells and intercellular trafficking (102). Ultimately, most antibody-secreting cells (ASCs) will undergo apoptosis following viral clearance. Only a small percentage of these high-specificity B cell clones will become plasma cells that secrete low levels of antibody into the serum for months, or memory cells that reside in the bone marrow, and can be reactivated to provide antibody responses to a subsequent infection (46, 103).

This system-wide coordination of B cell activation and survival in response to foreign antigen delicately balances the pregnant mother's serum antibody levels to both provide the benefits of transplacental immunity to the fetus and avoid the development of fetal-reactive antibodies. The competing priorities of fetal antigen tolerance and the production of antibodies that can be transplacentally conferred to the fetus to promote neonatal immunity are tightly regulated by pregnancy hormones. Clinical evidence has long documented that the symptoms of autoimmune diseases arising from the generation of antibodies against self-antigen tend to recede during pregnancy and resurge after parturition and breastfeeding, indicating that pregnancy hormones play a role in coordinating immune tolerance at the local uterine and systemic level (62, 64). The development of autoimmune disorders such as multiple sclerosis, rheumatoid arthritis, and systemic lupus erythematosus (SLE), which are more prevalent in women, have been linked to the effects of estrogen on B cell activation and function (104). Estradiol (E2) has been shown to upregulate Bcl-2, inducing survival of autoreactive B cells and changing signaling thresholds required to induce apoptosis (105, 106). In contrast, progesterone has been established as negative regulator of B cell lymphopoiesis (107–109). Reduced expansion of B cells within a pregnant mother may help establish allotolerance to the fetus by preventing antibody recognition of fetal antigen, which might result in inflammation, lymphocyte cytotoxicity, and complement activation (63). Healthy pregnancy has been shown to suppress B cell lymphopoiesis in BALB/c mice, which could be reversed by the exogenous addition of IL-7 (107, 110, 111). These data suggest that pregnancy may reduce or redirect activated B cells during their migration to the lungs or bone marrow. Differential recruitment of IgA^+ plasmablasts to the murine mammary glands after parturition and during nursing has been demonstrated, but specific homing receptors have not been identified, suggesting a role of local chemoattractants such as E-selectin (112, 113). In this way, maintaining immunological tolerance to fetal antigen that reaches the maternal circulatory system may require that B cell activation be altered in order to prevent the proliferation of anti-fetal antibodies.

Understanding how pregnancy impacts the development of immune memory is of clinical significance. Immunization has been reported to reduce hospitalization and ILI of pregnant women and their newborns during the flu season with no record of increased adverse events due to vaccination between this group and the unvaccinated population (21, 23, 114, 115). Clinical trials of seasonal trivalent inactivated influenza vaccination (TIV) in Bangladesh showed improved transplacental transfer of influenza-specific antibodies from mother to child (116). However, there are mixed results in how pregnancy affects humoral immunity following vaccination. Schlaudecker et al. reported that pregnant women seroconverted at the same rate as non-pregnant women following TIV but generated lower geometric mean titers (GMTs) against H1N1 (A/California) and H3N2 (A/Perth) viruses (26). Serological analysis from a cohort of influenza A virus (IAV) vaccinated healthy pregnant and non-pregnant women in California showed similar seroconversion rates and numbers of plasmablasts (18). Thus, while influenza vaccination during pregnancy has been demonstrated to be safe and to reduce the incidence of influenza-induced hospitalization and pre-term birth, further research into antibody functionality and expression is still needed.

Pregnancy hormones may coordinate the down-regulation of class-switching or post-translational modifications (i.e., glycosylation, fucosylation, sialylation, etc.) of the antigen-binding (Fab) or receptor binding (Fc) regions of antibodies in order to attenuate potentially inflammatory or anti-fetal immune responses. There have been reports that pregnant women infected with H1N1 pandemic virus in Shenyang, China in 2009 produced an imbalanced proportion of anti-H1N1 IgG1, IgG2, IgG3, and IgG4 antibody subtypes compared with infected non-pregnant women in the same hospital (117). Interestingly, IgG1 is preferentially transported from maternal circulation across the placenta compared to other IgG classes, especially IgG2, although this phenomenon has not been directly linked to influenza infection and vaccination (118–120). While preferential transport from mother to fetus is linked to neonatal Fc receptor (FcRn) expression on placental syncytiotrophoblasts, how pregnancy shifts expression from virus-specific IgG2 to IgG1 requires further investigation.

Antibody isotype classes and generation of specificity are governed by the class-switching of Ig genes and somatic hypermutation of their variable chain-encoding regions (102, 121). Variability is induced primarily by activation-induced cytidine deaminase (AID) and uracil-DNA glycosylase (UNG) that selectively damage DNA and repair it randomly (102, 121, 122). B cells that have complementarity-determining regions (CDRs) that bind best to antigen are selected for by T follicular helper cells (Tfhs) and clonally amplified to flood the circulatory system with virus neutralizing antibodies (123, 124). Estrogen and progesterone seem to work in opposition to each other on the regulation of AID: estrogen receptors bind the *HoxC4* promoter to induce AID activation, while progesterone receptors can bind directly to the AID promoter to inhibit activation (125–127). Glucocorticoids have also been described as negative regulators of AID activation (128). These phenomena are typically described in the context of autoimmune disease regulation and have not been described in the multi-hormonal environment of pregnancy.

Asymmetric glycosylation, or the single glycosylation of one side rather than both sides of the Fab or Fc antibody chains, can result in fine-tuned interactions with antigen and Fc receptors, and these binding affinities are important for antibody-dependent cellular cytotoxicity (ADCC) (129, 130). Pregnancy has been shown to increase the serum and placental concentrations of asymmetrically glycosylated IgG and may provide an explanation for the reduced avidity and virus-binding capability following viral infection during pregnancy (131, 132). Human and murine placental expression of IL-6 has been shown to induce asymmetrical glycosylation of IgG from hybridomas (133, 134). Trophoblast-produced asymmetric antibodies have been documented throughout the placenta (132, 135). However, whether these signaling effects can extend outside the uterus has yet to be determined and would be a major finding in maternal immunity. By reducing binding specificity for antibody effector cells via asymmetric glycosylation, the maternal immune system may be able to mitigate the negative effects of any anti-fetal antibodies that may have developed while still maintaining a population of semi-functional or selectively-functional antibodies that can neutralize pathogens and non-self-entities (131).

CONCLUSIONS

Influenza viral illness causes significant socioeconomic and clinical burden each year (136). While most research focused on the consequences of influenza A (H1N1) virus infection during pregnancy, there is evidence that influenza B virus can also cause significant maternal and fetal complications following mid-gestation infection (137, 138). It remains unclear if seasonal type A (H3N2) virus infection during pregnancy causes similar poor clinical outcomes compared to the severity of complications following type A (H1N1) or type B virus infection during pregnancy (138–141). Lastly, the recently identified highly neurotropic avian H7N9 and H5N1 influenza A reassortants, which could potentially cause pandemics, have been shown to cause severe disease during pregnancy (142–147). The knowledge gained through research of the 2009 pandemic swine-derived influenza A (H1N1) virus may provide the clinical and research community with an improved capacity for the early detection of a novel pandemic virus entering a naïve pregnant population. These studies we have reviewed demonstrate the vulnerability of pregnant women to infectious diseases and the fact that neonatal health is directly dependent on maternal health, doubles the significance of research that results in improved therapies and treatment strategies.

Respiratory infection during pregnancy is of broad interest. While influenza A virus has generated some of the highest morbidity rates following maternal infection, coronavirus outbreaks have also been associated with similar outcomes in mothers and neonates following mid-gestation infection. Infection with severe acute respiratory syndrome (SARS) coronavirus and Middle Eastern respiratory syndrome (MERS) coronavirus have been associated with spontaneous abortion, fetal growth retardation, and maternal and neonatal mortality (148–150). Mid-gestation infection with respiratory syncytial virus (RSV) has been described in rare severe adult cases and has also been associated with pre-term birth and low birth weight in a cohort in Nepal (151, 152). High rates of mortality among infants and toddlers infected with RSV highlights the need for improved understanding of maternal immunity to RSV infection and vaccination during pregnancy, and there is hope that vaccination of mothers during pregnancy can provide passive immunity that will protect the fetus for months after birth (153). None of the previously mentioned viruses were transmitted transplacentally to fetuses, and yet respiratory infection during pregnancy induced significant maternal illness, pre-term labor, low birth weight, or spontaneous abortion.

Early antiviral therapy following H1N1 influenza A virus infection during pregnancy has been shown to significantly reduce pre-term birth, hospitalization in intensive care units (ICUs), and maternal death (11, 154). Seasonal H1N1 influenza A virus induced increased levels of cyclooxygenase-2 (COX-2) and prostaglandin-F2α in the lungs and placenta, providing a mechanism for lung immunopathology and pre-term labor in pregnant mice (88). The anti-inflammatory potential of COX-2 inhibitor therapy has already been proposed for decreasing disease severity caused by the highly pathogenic avian influenza strains H5N1 and H7N9 (155, 156). In addition, COX inhibitor treatment has demonstrated to attenuate the lung expression of granulocyte colony-stimulating factor (G-CSF) and keratinocyte-derived (KC) cytokines elevated in pregnant mice infected by H1N1 A/Brisbane/59/2007 and H1N1 A/California/07/2009 (157, 158). However, while non-steroidal anti-inflammatory drugs (NSAIDs) have been shown to be safe during pregnancy, COX-2 specific inhibitors may induce pre-term labor and musculoskeletal defects (159–161). Viral load was negatively associated with progesterone concentration, and reduced progesterone expression was correlated with pre-term labor in influenza virus-infected pregnant mice (88). Administration of progesterone to female mice following influenza A(H1N1) virus infection reduced immunopathological changes and improved lung epithelial cell regeneration, although it did not reduce viral load (162, 163). Hence, limiting viral replication should be one of many aims for anti-influenza therapy during pregnancy, including the limiting of immunopathology caused by cytokine dysregulation and promoting the healing of damaged airway epithelium following viral clearance.

The connections between viral pathogenesis and reproductive endocrinology makes the field of infectious disease in pregnant women complicated, exciting, and clinically significant. Investigations into the immunological components of infertility, recurrent miscarriage, and preeclampsia have yielded a wealth of information regarding the requirements of immune tolerance and rejection, and this information can provide a platform for understanding healthy pregnancy and how inflammation and hormonal dysregulation will impact maternal health and fetal development. Development of accurate animal pregnancy models across a range of species in coordination with broader clinical sampling from influenza-infected or -vaccinated pregnant women will provide an effective platform for validation of experimental studies and improved therapeutics and treatment for pregnant women and their offspring.

AUTHOR CONTRIBUTIONS

All authors listed have made a substantial, direct and intellectual contribution to the work, and approved it for publication.

FUNDING

Funding for this research was provided through Centers of Excellence for Influenza Research and Surveillance (HHSN272201400004C).

REFERENCES

1. Webster RG, Bean WJ, Gorman OT, Chambers TM, Kawaoka Y. Evolution and ecology of influenza A viruses. *Microbiol Rev.* (1992) 56:152–79.
2. Kidd M. Influenza viruses: update on epidemiology, clinical features, treatment and vaccination. *Curr Opin Pulm Med.* (2014) 20:242–6. doi: 10.1097/MCP.0000000000000049
3. Taubenberger JK, Kash JC. Influenza virus evolution, host adaptation, and pandemic formation. *Cell Host Microbe* (2010) 7:440–51. doi: 10.1016/j.chom.2010.05.009
4. Tao H, Steel J, Lowen AC. Intrahost dynamics of influenza virus reassortment. *J Virol.* (2014) 88:7485–92. doi: 10.1128/JVI.00715-14
5. Hannoun C. The evolving history of influenza viruses and influenza vaccines. *Expert Rev Vacc.* (2013) 12:1085–94. doi: 10.1586/14760584.2013.824709
6. Cantu J, Tita AT. Management of influenza in pregnancy. *Am J Perinatol.* (2013) 30:99–103. doi: 10.1055/s-0032-1331033
7. Longman RE, Johnson TR. Viral respiratory disease in pregnancy. *Curr Opin Obstet Gynecol.* (2007) 19:120–5. doi: 10.1097/GCO.0b013e328028fdc7
8. Jamieson DJ, Honein MA, Rasmussen SA, Williams JL, Swerdlow DL, Biggerstaff MS, et al. H1N1 2009 influenza virus infection during pregnancy in the USA. *Lancet* (2009) 374:451–8. doi: 10.1016/S0140-6736(09)61304-0
9. Rasmussen SA, Jamieson DJ, Uyeki TM. Effects of influenza on pregnant women and infants. *Am J Obstet Gynecol.* (2012) 207:S3–8. doi: 10.1016/j.ajog.2012.06.068
10. Creanga AA, Johnson TF, Graitcer SB, Hartman LK, Al-Samarrai T, Schwarz AG, et al. Severity of 2009 pandemic influenza A (H1N1) virus infection in pregnant women. *Obstet Gynecol.* (2010) 115:717–26. doi: 10.1097/AOG.0b013e3181d57947
11. Siston AM, Rasmussen SA, Honein MA, Fry AM, Seib K, Callaghan WM, et al. Pandemic 2009 influenza A(H1N1) virus illness among pregnant women in the United States. *JAMA* (2010) 303:1517–25. doi: 10.1001/jama.2010.479
12. Mortensen E, Louie J, Pertowski C, Cadwell BL, Weiss E, Acosta M, et al. Epidemiology and outcomes of adults with asthma who were hospitalized

or died with 2009 pandemic influenza A (H1N1)-California, 2009. *Influenza Other Respir Viruses* (2013) 7:1343–9. doi: 10.1111/irv.12120

13. Jamieson AM, Yu S, Annicelli CH, Medzhitov R. Influenza virus-induced glucocorticoids compromise innate host defense against a secondary bacterial infection. *Cell Host Microbe.* (2010) 7:103–14. doi: 10.1016/j.chom.2010.01.010
14. Vrekoussis T, Kalantaridou SN, Mastorakos G, Zoumakis E, Makrigiannakis A, Syrrou M, et al. The role of stress in female reproduction and pregnancy: an update. *Ann N Y Acad Sci.* (2010) 1205:69–75. doi: 10.1111/j.1749-6632.2010.05686.x
15. Memoli MJ, Harvey H, Morens DM, Taubenberger JK. Influenza in pregnancy. *Influenza Other Respir Viruses* (2013) 7:1033–9. doi: 10.1111/irv.12055
16. Pierce M, Kurinczuk JJ, Spark P, Brocklehurst P, Knight M. Ukoss Perinatal outcomes after maternal 2009/H1N1 infection: national cohort study. *BMJ* (2011) 342:d3214. doi: 10.1136/bmj.d3214
17. Mendez-Figueroa H, Raker C, Anderson BL. Neonatal characteristics and outcomes of pregnancies complicated by influenza infection during the 2009 pandemic. *Am J Obstet Gynecol.* (2011) 204:S58–63. doi: 10.1016/j.ajog.2011.02.058
18. Kay AW, Blish CA. Immunogenicity and clinical efficacy of influenza vaccination in pregnancy. *Front Immunol.* (2015) 6:289. doi: 10.3389/fimmu.2015.00289
19. Omer SB, Bednarczyk R, Madhi SA, Klugman KP. Benefits to mother and child of influenza vaccination during pregnancy. *Hum Vaccin Immunother.* (2012) 8:130–7. doi: 10.4161/hv.8.1.18601
20. Dabrera G, Zhao H, Andrews N, Begum F, Green H, Ellis J, et al. Effectiveness of seasonal influenza vaccination during pregnancy in preventing influenza infection in infants, England, 2013/14. *Euro Surveill.* (2014) 19:20959. doi: 10.2807/1560-7917.ES2014.19.45.20959
21. Takeda S, Hisano M, Komano J, Yamamoto H, Sago H, Yamaguchi K. Influenza vaccination during pregnancy and its usefulness to mothers and their young infants. *J Infect Chemother.* (2015) 21:238–46. doi: 10.1016/j.jiac.2015.01.015
22. Bednarczyk RA, Adjaye-Gbewonyo D, Omer SB. Safety of influenza immunization during pregnancy for the fetus and the neonate. *Am J Obstet Gynecol.* (2012) 207:S38–46. doi: 10.1016/j.ajog.2012.07.002
23. Ahrens KA, Louik C, Kerr S, Mitchell AA, Werler MM. Seasonal influenza vaccination during pregnancy and the risks of preterm delivery and small for gestational age birth. *Paediatr Perinat Epidemiol.* (2014) 28:498–509. doi: 10.1111/ppe.12152
24. Bratton KN, Wardle MT, Orenstein WA, Omer SB. Maternal influenza immunization and birth outcomes of stillbirth and spontaneous abortion: a systematic review and meta-analysis. *Clin Infect Dis.* (2015) 60:e11–19. doi: 10.1093/cid/ciu915
25. Adegbola R, Nesin M, Wairagkar N. Immunogenicity and efficacy of influenza immunization during pregnancy: recent and ongoing studies. *Am J Obstet Gynecol.* (2012) 207:S28–32. doi: 10.1016/j.ajog.2012.07.001
26. Schlaudecker EP, Mcneal MM, Dodd CN, Ranz JB, Steinhoff MC. Pregnancy modifies the antibody response to trivalent influenza immunization. *J Infect Dis.* (2012) 206:1670–3. doi: 10.1093/infdis/jis592
27. Kay AW, Bayless NL, Fukuyama J, Aziz N, Dekker CL, Mackey S, et al. Pregnancy does not attenuate the antibody or plasmablast response to inactivated influenza vaccine. *J Infect Dis.* (2015) 212:861–70. doi: 10.1093/infdis/jiv138
28. Salomon R, Webster RG. The influenza virus enigma. *Cell* (2009) 136:402–10. doi: 10.1016/j.cell.2009.01.029
29. Van Riel D, Den Bakker MA, Leijten LM, Chutinimitkul S, Munster VJ, De Wit E, et al. Seasonal and pandemic human influenza viruses attach better to human upper respiratory tract epithelium than avian influenza viruses. *Am J Pathol.* (2010) 176:1614–8. doi: 10.2353/ajpath.2010.090949
30. Lakadamyali M, Rust MJ, Zhuang X. Endocytosis of influenza viruses. *Microbes Infect.* (2004) 6:929–36. doi: 10.1016/j.micinf.2004.05.002
31. Leung HS, Li OT, Chan RW, Chan MC, Nicholls JM, Poon LL. Entry of influenza A Virus with a alpha2,6-linked sialic acid binding preference requires host fibronectin. *J Virol.* (2012) 86:10704–13. doi: 10.1128/JVI.01166-12
32. Luo M. Influenza virus entry. *Adv Exp Med Biol.* (2012) 726:201–21. doi: 10.1007/978-1-4614-0980-9_9
33. Gu W, Gallagher GR, Dai W, Liu P, Li R, Trombly MI, et al. Influenza A virus preferentially snatches noncoding *RNA* caps. *RNA* (2015b) 21:2067–75. doi: 10.1261/rna.054221.115
34. Watanabe T, Watanabe S, Kawaoka Y. Cellular networks involved in the influenza virus life cycle. *Cell Host Microbe.* (2010) 7:427–39. doi: 10.1016/j.chom.2010.05.008
35. Canini L, Carrat F. Population modeling of influenza A/H1N1 virus kinetics and symptom dynamics. *J Virol.* (2011) 85:2764–70. doi: 10.1128/JVI.01318-10
36. Hsu AC, Parsons K, Barr I, Lowther S, Middleton D, Hansbro PM, et al. Critical role of constitutive type I interferon response in bronchial epithelial cell to influenza infection. *PLoS ONE* (2012) 7:e32947. doi: 10.1371/journal.pone.0032947
37. Kuiken T, Riteau B, Fouchier RA, Rimmelzwaan GF. Pathogenesis of influenza virus infections: the good, the bad and the ugly. *Curr Opin Virol.* (2012) 2:276–86. doi: 10.1016/j.coviro.2012.02.013
38. Fukuyama S, Kawaoka Y. The pathogenesis of influenza virus infections: the contributions of virus and host factors. *Curr Opin Immunol.* (2011) 23:481–6. doi: 10.1016/j.coi.2011.07.016
39. Yamaya M, Nadine LK, Ota C, Kubo H, Makiguchi T, Nagatomi R, et al. Magnitude of influenza virus replication and cell damage is associated with interleukin-6 production in primary cultures of human tracheal epithelium. *Respir Physiol Neurobiol.* (2014) 202:16–23. doi: 10.1016/j.resp.2014.07.010
40. Schultz-Cherry S. Role of NK cells in influenza infection. *Curr Top Microbiol Immunol.* (2015) 386:109–20. doi: 10.1007/82_2014_403
41. Taubenberger JK, Morens DM. The pathology of influenza virus infections. *Annu Rev Pathol.* (2008) 3:499–522. doi: 10.1146/annurev.pathmechdis.3.121806.154316
42. Liderot K, Ahl M, Ozenci V. Secondary bacterial infections in patients with seasonal influenza A and pandemic H1N1. *Biomed Res Int.* (2013) 2013:376219. doi: 10.1155/2013/376219
43. Mccullers JA. The co-pathogenesis of influenza viruses with bacteria in the lung. *Nat Rev Microbiol.* (2014) 12:252–62. doi: 10.1038/nrmicro3231
44. De Serres G, Rouleau I, Hamelin ME, Quach C, Skowronski D, Flamand L, et al. Contagious period for pandemic (H1N1) 2009. *Emerg Infect Dis.* (2010) 16:783–8. doi: 10.3201/eid1605.091894
45. La Gruta NL, Turner SJ. T cell mediated immunity to influenza: mechanisms of viral control. *Trends Immunol.* (2014) 35:396–402. doi: 10.1016/j.it.2014.06.004
46. Chiu C, Ellebedy AH, Wrammert J, Ahmed R. B cell responses to influenza infection and vaccination. *Curr Top Microbiol Immunol.* (2015) 386:381–98. doi: 10.1007/82_2014_425
47. Bot A, Reichlin A, Isobe H, Bot S, Schulman J, Yokoyama WM, et al. Cellular mechanisms involved in protection and recovery from influenza virus infection in immunodeficient mice. *J Virol.* (1996) 70:5668–72.
48. Hogan BL, Barkauskas CE, Chapman HA, Epstein JA, Jain R, Hsia CC, et al. Repair and regeneration of the respiratory system: complexity, plasticity, and mechanisms of lung stem cell function. *Cell Stem Cell* (2014) 15:123–38. doi: 10.1016/j.stem.2014.07.012
49. Grabiec AM, Hussell T. The role of airway macrophages in apoptotic cell clearance following acute and chronic lung inflammation. *Semin Immunopathol.* (2016) 38:409–23. doi: 10.1007/s00281-016-0555-3
50. Boyden AW, Frickman AM, Legge KL, Waldschmidt TJ. Primary and long-term B-cell responses in the upper airway and lung after influenza A virus infection. *Immunol Res.* (2014) 59:73–80. doi: 10.1007/s12026-014-8541-0
51. Laidlaw BJ, Zhang N, Marshall HD, Staron MM, Guan T, Hu Y, et al. CD4+ T cell help guides formation of CD103+ lung-resident memory CD8+ T cells during influenza viral infection. *Immunity* (2014) 41:633–45. doi: 10.1016/j.immuni.2014.09.007
52. Pichyangkul S, Yongvanitchit K, Limsalakpetch A, Kum-Arb U, Im-Erbsin R, Boonnak K, et al. Tissue distribution of memory T and B cells in rhesus monkeys following influenza a infection. *J Immunol.* (2015) 195:4378–86. doi: 10.4049/jimmunol.1501702

53. Mulac-Jericevic B, Conneely OM. Reproductive tissue selective actions of progesterone receptors. *Reproduction* (2004) 128:139–46. doi: 10.1530/rep.1.00189
54. Wetendorf M, Demayo FJ. Progesterone receptor signaling in the initiation of pregnancy and preservation of a healthy uterus. *Int J Dev Biol.* (2014) 58:95–106. doi: 10.1387/ijdb.140069mw
55. Sathish V, Martin YN, Prakash YS. Sex steroid signaling: implications for lung diseases. *Pharmacol Ther.* (2015) 150:94–108. doi: 10.1016/j.pharmthera.2015.01.007
56. Wira CR, Rodriguez-Garcia M, Patel MV. The role of sex hormones in immune protection of the female reproductive tract. *Nat Rev Immunol.* (2015) 15:217–30. doi: 10.1038/nri3819
57. James JL, Carter AM, Chamley LW. Human placentation from nidation to 5 weeks of gestation. Part I: What do we know about formative placental development following implantation? *Placenta* (2012) 33:327–34. doi: 10.1016/j.placenta.2012.01.020
58. Balogh A, Ditroi F, Lampe G. Serum progesterone levels in early imminent abortion. *Acta Physiol Hung.* (1985) 65:275–9.
59. Darland NW. Infertility associated with luteal phase defect. *J Obstet Gynecol Neonatal Nurs.* (1985) 14:212–7. doi: 10.1111/j.1552-6909.1985.tb02229.x
60. Young SL, Lessey BA. Progesterone function in human endometrium: clinical perspectives. *Semin Reprod Med.* (2010) 28:5–16. doi: 10.1055/s-0029-1242988
61. Saito S. Cytokine network at the feto-maternal interface. *J Reprod Immunol.* (2000) 47:87–103. doi: 10.1016/S0165-0378(00)00060-7
62. Robinson DP, Klein SL. Pregnancy and pregnancy-associated hormones alter immune responses and disease pathogenesis. *Horm Behav.* (2012) 62:263–71. doi: 10.1016/j.yhbeh.2012.02.023
63. Druckmann R, Druckmann MA. Progesterone and the immunology of pregnancy. *J Steroid Biochem Mol Biol.* (2005) 97:389–96. doi: 10.1016/j.jsbmb.2005.08.010
64. Tan IJ, Peeva E, Zandman-Goddard G. Hormonal modulation of the immune system - A spotlight on the role of progestogens. *Autoimmun Rev.* (2015) 14:536–42. doi: 10.1016/j.autrev.2015.02.004
65. Szekeres-Bartho J, Polgar B. PIBF: the double edged sword. *Pregnancy and tumor Am J Reprod Immunol.* (2010) 64:77–86. doi: 10.1111/j.1600-0897.2010.00833.x
66. Tai P, Wang J, Jin H, Song X, Yan J, Kang Y, et al. Induction of regulatory T cells by physiological level estrogen. *J Cell Physiol.* (2008) 214:456–64. doi: 10.1002/jcp.21221
67. Coyne CB, Lazear HM. Zika virus - reigniting the TORCH. *Nat Rev Microbiol.* (2016) 14:707–15. doi: 10.1038/nrmicro.2016.125
68. Adams Waldorf KM, Mcadams RM. Influence of infection during pregnancy on fetal development. *Reproduction* (2013) 146:R151–162. doi: 10.1530/REP-13-0232
69. Komine-Aizawa S, Suzaki A, Trinh QD, Izumi Y, Shibata T, Kuroda K, et al. H1N1/09 influenza A virus infection of immortalized first trimester human trophoblast cell lines. *Am J Reprod Immunol.* (2012) 68:226–32. doi: 10.1111/j.1600-0897.2012.01172.x
70. Meijer WJ, Wensing AM, Bruinse HW, Nikkels PG. High rate of chronic villitis in placentas of pregnancies complicated by influenza A/H1N1 infection. *Infect Dis Obstet Gynecol.* (2014) 2014:768380. doi: 10.1155/2014/768380
71. Bastek JA, Weber AL, Mcshea MA, Ryan ME, and Elovitz MA. Prenatal inflammation is associated with adverse neonatal outcomes. *Am J Obstet Gynecol.* (2014) 210:450 e451–10. doi: 10.1016/j.ajog.2013.12.024
72. Goeden N, Velasquez J, Arnold KA, Chan Y, Lund BT, Anderson GM, et al. Maternal inflammation disrupts fetal neurodevelopment via increased placental output of serotonin to the fetal brain. *J Neurosci.* (2016) 36:6041–9. doi: 10.1523/JNEUROSCI.2534-15.2016
73. Brown AS, Derkits EJ. Prenatal infection and schizophrenia: a review of epidemiologic and translational studies. *Am J Psychiatry* (2010) 167:261–80. doi: 10.1176/appi.ajp.2009.09030361
74. Parboosing R, Bao Y, Shen L, Schaefer CA, Brown AS. Gestational influenza and bipolar disorder in adult offspring. *JAMA Psychiatry* (2013) 70:677–85. doi: 10.1001/jamapsychiatry.2013.896
75. Zerbo O, Qian Y, Yoshida C, Fireman BH, Klein NP, Croen LA. Association between influenza infection and vaccination during pregnancy and risk of autism spectrum disorder. *JAMA Pediatr.* (2017) 171:e163609. doi: 10.1001/jamapediatrics.2016.3609
76. Forbes RL, Gibson PG, Murphy VE, Wark PA. Impaired type I and III interferon response to rhinovirus infection during pregnancy and asthma. *Thorax* (2012a) 67:209–14. doi: 10.1136/thoraxjnl-2011-200708
77. Forbes RL, Wark PA, Murphy VE, Gibson PG. Pregnant women have attenuated innate interferon responses to 2009 pandemic influenza A virus subtype H1N1. *J Infect Dis.* (2012b) 206:646–53. doi: 10.1093/infdis/jis377
78. Szekeres-Bartho J, Faust Z, Varga P, Szereday L, Kelemen K. The immunological pregnancy protective effect of progesterone is manifested via controlling cytokine production. *Am J Reprod Immunol.* (1996) 35:348–51. doi: 10.1111/j.1600-0897.1996.tb00492.x
79. Raghupathy R, Al-Mutawa E, Al-Azemi M, Makhseed M, Azizieh F, Szekeres-Bartho J. Progesterone-induced blocking factor (PIBF) modulates cytokine production by lymphocytes from women with recurrent miscarriage or preterm delivery. *J Reprod Immunol.* (2009) 80:91–9. doi: 10.1016/j.jri.2009.01.004
80. Faust Z, Laskarin G, Rukavina D, Szekeres-Bartho J. Progesterone-induced blocking factor inhibits degranulation of natural killer cells. *Am J Reprod Immunol.* (1999) 42:71–5.
81. Raj RS, Bonney EA, Phillippe M. Influenza, immune system, and pregnancy. *Reprod Sci.* (2014) 21:1434–51. doi: 10.1177/1933719114537720
82. Meijer WJ, Van Noortwijk AG, Bruinse HW, Wensing AM. Influenza virus infection in pregnancy: a review. *Acta Obstet Gynecol Scand.* (2015) 94:797–819. doi: 10.1111/aogs.12680
83. Pazos MA, Kraus TA, Munoz-Fontela C, Moran TM. Estrogen mediates innate and adaptive immune alterations to influenza infection in pregnant mice. *PLoS ONE* (2012b) 7:e40502. doi: 10.1371/journal.pone.0040502
84. Robinson DP, Hall OJ, Nilles TL, Bream JH, Klein SL. 17beta-estradiol protects females against influenza by recruiting neutrophils and increasing virus-specific CD8 T cell responses in the lungs. *J Virol.* (2014) 88:4711–20. doi: 10.1128/JVI.02081-13
85. Chan KH, Zhang AJ, To KK, Chan CC, Poon VK, Guo K, et al. Wild type and mutant 2009 pandemic influenza A (H1N1) viruses cause more severe disease and higher mortality in pregnant BALB/c mice. *PLoS ONE* (2010) 5:e13757. doi: 10.1371/journal.pone.0013757
86. Marcelin G, Aldridge JR, Duan S, Ghoneim HE, Rehg J, Marjuki H, et al. Fatal outcome of pandemic H1N1 2009 influenza virus infection is associated with immunopathology and impaired lung repair, not enhanced viral burden, in pregnant mice. *J Virol.* (2011) 85:11208–19. doi: 10.1128/JVI.00654-11
87. Kim HM, Kang YM, Song BM, Kim HS, Seo SH. The 2009 pandemic H1N1 influenza virus is more pathogenic in pregnant mice than seasonal H1N1 influenza virus. *Viral Immunol.* (2012) 25:402–10. doi: 10.1089/vim.2012.0007
88. Littauer EQ, Esser ES, Antao OQ, Vassilieva EV, Compans RW, Skountzou I. H1N1 influenza virus infection results in adverse pregnancy outcomes by disrupting tissue-specific hormonal regulation. *PLoS Pathog.* (2017) 13:e1006757. doi: 10.1371/journal.ppat.1006757
89. Gao R, Bhatnagar J, Blau DM, Greer P, Rollin DC, Denison AM, et al. Cytokine and chemokine profiles in lung tissues from fatal cases of 2009 pandemic influenza A (H1N1): role of the host immune response in pathogenesis. *Am J Pathol.* (2013) 183:1258–68. doi: 10.1016/j.ajpath.2013.06.023
90. Watanabe H, Numata K, Ito T, Takagi K, Matsukawa A. Innate immune response in Th1- and Th2-dominant mouse strains. *Shock* (2004) 22:460–6. doi: 10.1097/01.shk.0000142249.08135.e9
91. Sellers RS, Clifford CB, Treuting PM, Brayton C. Immunological variation between inbred laboratory mouse strains: points to consider in phenotyping genetically immunomodified mice. *Vet Pathol.* (2012) 49:32–43. doi: 10.1177/0300985811429314
92. Otte A, Gabriel G. 2009 pandemic H1N1 influenza A virus strains display differential pathogenicity in C57BL/6J but not BALB/c mice. *Virulence* (2011) 2:563–6. doi: 10.4161/viru.2.6.18148
93. Preusse M, Schughart K, Pessler F. Host genetic background strongly affects pulmonary microrna expression before and during influenza a virus infection. *Front Immunol.* (2017) 8:246. doi: 10.3389/fimmu.2017.00246

94. Califano D, Furuya Y, Metzger DW. Effects of influenza on alveolar macrophage viability are dependent on mouse genetic strain. *J Immunol.* (2018) 201:134–44. doi: 10.4049/jimmunol.1701406
95. Vermillion MS, Nelson A, Vom Steeg LG, Loube JM, Mitzner W, Klein SL. Pregnancy preserves pulmonary function following influenza virus infection in C57BL/6 mice. *Am J Physiol Lung Cell Mol Physiol.* (2018) 315:L517–25. doi: 10.1152/ajplung.00066.2018
96. De La Haba C, Palacio JR, Palkovics T, Szekeres-Bartho J, Morros A, Martinez P. Oxidative stress effect on progesterone-induced blocking factor (PIBF) binding to PIBF-receptor in lymphocytes. *Biochim Biophys Acta* (2014) 1838:148–57. doi: 10.1016/j.bbamem.2013.08.006
97. Liu M, Chen F, Liu T, Chen F, Liu S, Yang J. The role of oxidative stress in influenza virus infection. *Microbes Infect.* (2017) 19:580–6. doi: 10.1016/j.micinf.2017.08.008
98. Niiro H, Clark EA. Regulation of B-cell fate by antigen-receptor signals. *Nat Rev Immunol.* (2002) 2:945–56. doi: 10.1038/nri955
99. Batista FD, Harwood NE. The who, how and where of antigen presentation to B cells. *Nat Rev Immunol.* (2009) 9:15–27. doi: 10.1038/nri2454
100. Harwood NE, Batista FD. Early events in B cell activation. *Annu Rev Immunol.* (2010) 28:185–210. doi: 10.1146/annurev-immunol-030409-101216
101. Shulman Z, Gitlin AD, Targ S, Jankovic M, Pasqual G, Nussenzweig MC, et al. T follicular helper cell dynamics in germinal centers. *Science* (2013) 341:673–7. doi: 10.1126/science.1241680
102. Matthews AJ, Zheng S, Dimenna LJ, Chaudhuri J. Regulation of immunoglobulin class-switch recombination: choreography of noncoding transcription, targeted DNA deamination, and long-range DNA repair. *Adv Immunol.* (2014) 122:1–57. doi: 10.1016/B978-0-12-800267-4.00001-8
103. Chu VT, Berek C. The establishment of the plasma cell survival niche in the bone marrow. *Immunol Rev.* (2013) 251:177–88. doi: 10.1111/imr.12011
104. Assad S, Khan HH, Ghazanfar H, Khan ZH, Mansoor S, Rahman MA, et al. Role of sex hormone levels and psychological stress in the pathogenesis of autoimmune diseases. *Cureus* (2017) 9:e1315. doi: 10.7759/cureus.1315
105. Bynoe MS, Grimaldi CM, Diamond B. Estrogen up-regulates Bcl-2 and blocks tolerance induction of naive B cells. *Proc Natl Acad Sci USA.* (2000) 97:2703–8. doi: 10.1073/pnas.040577497
106. Grimaldi CM, Cleary J, Dagtas AS, Moussai D, Diamond B. Estrogen alters thresholds for B cell apoptosis and activation. *J Clin Invest.* (2002) 109:1625–33. doi: 10.1172/JCI0214873
107. Medina KL, Smithson G, Kincade PW. Suppression of B lymphopoiesis during normal pregnancy. *J Exp Med.* (1993) 178:1507–15. doi: 10.1084/jem.178.5.1507
108. Pazos M, Sperling RS, Moran TM, Kraus TA. The influence of pregnancy on systemic immunity. *Immunol Res.* (2012a) 54:254–61. doi: 10.1007/s12026-012-8303-9
109. Zhang LCK, Li MQ, Li DJ, Yao XY. Mouse endometrial stromal cells and progesterone inhibit the activation and regulate the differentiation and antibody secretion of mouse B cells. *Int J Clin Exp Pathol.* (2014) 7:123–33.
110. Bosco N, Ceredig R, Rolink A. Transient decrease in interleukin-7 availability arrests B lymphopoiesis during pregnancy. *Eur J Immunol.* (2008) 38:381–90. doi: 10.1002/eji.200737665
111. Clark MR, Mandal M, Ochiai K, Singh H. Orchestrating B cell lymphopoiesis through interplay of IL-7 receptor and pre-B cell receptor signalling. *Nat Rev Immunol.* (2014) 14:69–80. doi: 10.1038/nri3570
112. Kruse AMM, Hallmann R, Butcher EC. Evidence of specialized leukocyte-vascular homing interactions at the maternal/fetal interface. *Eur J Immunol.* (1999) 29, 1116–26. doi: 10.1002/(SICI)1521-4141(199904)29:04<1116::AID-IMMU1116>3.0.CO;2-4
113. Tanneau Gm HSOL, Chevaleyre CC, Salmon HP. Differential recruitment of T- and IgA B-lymphocytes in the developing mammary gland in relation to homing receptors and vascular addressins. *J Histochem Cytochem.* (1999) 47:1581–92. doi: 10.1177/002215549904701210
114. Omer SB, Goodman D, Steinhoff MC, Rochat R, Klugman KP, Stoll BJ, et al. Maternal influenza immunization and reduced likelihood of prematurity and small for gestational age births: a retrospective cohort study. *PLoS Med.* (2011) 8:e1000441. doi: 10.1371/journal.pmed.1000441
115. Ludvigsson JF, Zugna D, Cnattingius S, Richiardi L, Ekbom A, Ortqvist A, et al. Influenza H1N1 vaccination and adverse pregnancy outcome. *Eur J Epidemiol.* (2013) 28:579–88. doi: 10.1007/s10654-013-9813-z
116. Steinhoff MC, Omer SB, Roy E, Arifeen SE, Raqib R, Altaye M, et al. Influenza immunization in pregnancy–antibody responses in mothers and infants. *N Engl J Med.* (2010) 362:1644–6. doi: 10.1056/NEJMc0912599
117. Zheng R, Qin X, Li Y, Yu X, Wang J, Tan M, et al. Imbalanced anti-H1N1 immunoglobulin subclasses and dysregulated cytokines in hospitalized pregnant women with 2009 H1N1 influenza and pneumonia in Shenyang, China. *Hum Immunol.* (2012) 73:906–11. doi: 10.1016/j.humimm.2012.06.005
118. Malek A, Sager R, Zakher A, Schneider H. Transport of immunoglobulin G and its subclasses across the *in vitro*-perfused human placenta. *Am J Obstet Gynecol.* (1995) 173:760–7. doi: 10.1016/0002-9378(95)90336-4
119. Malek A. *Ex vivo* human placenta models: transport of immunoglobulin G and its subclasses. *Vaccine* (2003) 21:3362–4. doi: 10.1016/S0264-410X(03)00333-5
120. Malek A. Role of IgG antibodies in association with placental function and immunologic diseases in human pregnancy. *Expert Rev Clin Immunol.* (2013) 9:235–49. doi: 10.1586/eci.12.99
121. Hwang JK, Alt FW, Yeap LS. Related mechanisms of antibody somatic hypermutation and class switch recombination. *Microbiol Spectr* (2015) 3:MDNA3-0037-2014. doi: 10.1128/microbiolspec.MDNA3-0037-2014
122. Muramatsu M, Kinoshita K, Fagarasan S, Yamada S, Shinkai Y, Honjo T. Class switch recombination and hypermutation require activation-induced cytidine deaminase (AID), a potential RNA editing enzyme. *Cell* (2000) 102:553–63. doi: 10.1016/S0092-8674(00)00078-7
123. Gitlin AD, Shulman Z, Nussenzweig MC. Clonal selection in the germinal centre by regulated proliferation and hypermutation. *Nature* (2014) 509:637–40. doi: 10.1038/nature13300
124. Shulman Z, Gitlin AD, Weinstein JS, Lainez B, Esplugues E, Flavell RA, et al. Dynamic signaling by T follicular helper cells during germinal center B cell selection. *Science* (2014) 345:1058–62. doi: 10.1126/science.1257861
125. Pauklin S, Petersen-Mahrt SK. Progesterone inhibits activation-induced deaminase by binding to the promoter. *J Immunol.* (2009) 183:1238–44. doi: 10.4049/jimmunol.0803915
126. Pauklin S, Sernandez IV, Bachmann G, Ramiro AR, Petersen-Mahrt SK. Estrogen directly activates AID transcription and function. *J Exp Med.* (2009) 206:99–111. doi: 10.1084/jem.20080521
127. Mai T, Zan H, Zhang J, Hawkins JS, Xu Z, Casali P. Estrogen receptors bind to and activate the HOXC4/HoxC4 promoter to potentiate HoxC4-mediated activation-induced cytosine deaminase induction, immunoglobulin class switch DNA recombination, and somatic hypermutation. *J Biol Chem.* (2010) 285:37797–810. doi: 10.1074/jbc.M110.169086
128. Benko AL, Olsen NJ, Kovacs WJ. Glucocorticoid inhibition of activation-induced cytidine deaminase expression in human B lymphocytes. *Mol Cell Endocrinol.* (2014) 382:881–7. doi: 10.1016/j.mce.2013.11.001
129. Shatz W, Chung S, Li B, Marshall B, Tejada M, Phung W, et al. Knobs-into-holes antibody production in mammalian cell lines reveals that asymmetric afucosylation is sufficient for full antibody-dependent cellular cytotoxicity. *MAbs* (2013) 5:872–81. doi: 10.4161/mabs.26307
130. Caaveiro JM, Kiyoshi M, Tsumoto K. Structural analysis of Fc/FcgammaR complexes: a blueprint for antibody design. *Immunol Rev.* (2015) 268:201–21. doi: 10.1111/imr.12365
131. Gutierrez G, Gentile T, Miranda S, Margni RA. Asymmetric antibodies: a protective arm in pregnancy. *Chem Immunol Allergy* (2005) 89:158–68. doi: 10.1159/000087964
132. Gu J, Lei Y, Huang Y, Zhao Y, Li J, Huang T, et al. Fab fragment glycosylated IgG may play a central role in placental immune evasion. *Hum Reprod.* (2015a) 30:380–91. doi: 10.1093/humrep/deu323
133. Gutierrez G, Malan Borel I, Margni RA. The placental regulatory factor involved in the asymmetric IgG antibody synthesis responds to IL-6 features. *J Reprod Immunol.* (2001) 49:21–32. doi: 10.1016/S0165-0378(00)00074-7
134. Miranda S, Gentile T, Margni R. Enhancement of *in vitro* hsp72 expression by placental IL-6. *Am J Reprod Immunol.* (2001) 46:358–65. doi: 10.1034/j.1600-0897.2001.d01-24.x
135. Li J, Korteweg C, Qiu Y, Luo J, Chen Z, Huang G, et al. Two ultrastructural distribution patterns of immunoglobulin G in human

placenta and functional implications. *Biol Reprod.* (2014b) 91:128. doi: 10.1095/biolreprod.114.122614
136. Gasparini R, Amicizia D, Lai PL, Panatto D. Clinical and socioeconomic impact of seasonal and pandemic influenza in adults and the elderly. *Hum Vaccin Immunother.* (2012) 8:21–8. doi: 10.4161/hv.8.1.17622
137. Kim JC, Kim HM, Kang YM, Ku KB, Park EH, Yum J, et al. Severe pathogenesis of influenza B virus in pregnant mice. *Virology* (2014) 448:74–81. doi: 10.1016/j.virol.2013.10.001
138. Regan AK, Moore HC, Sullivan SG, NDEK, Effler PV. Epidemiology of seasonal influenza infection in pregnant women and its impact on birth outcomes. *Epidemiol Infect.* (2017) 145:2930–9. doi: 10.1017/S0950268817001972
139. Mackenzie JS, Williams K, Papadimitriou J. Influenza A virus and its influence on the outcome of pregnancy in the mouse. *Dev Biol Stand.* (1977) 39:489–96.
140. Stanwell-Smith R, Parker AM, Chakraverty P, Soltanpoor N, Simpson CN. Possible association of influenza A with fetal loss: investigation of a cluster of spontaneous abortions and stillbirths. *Commun Dis Rep CDR Rev.* (1994) 4:R28–32.
141. Puig-Barbera J, Natividad-Sancho A, Trushakova S, Sominina A, Pisareva M, Ciblak MA, et al. Epidemiology of hospital admissions with influenza during the 2013/2014 Northern hemisphere influenza season: results from the global influenza hospital surveillance network. *PLoS ONE* (2016) 11:e0154970. doi: 10.1371/journal.pone.0154970
142. Xu L, Bao L, Deng W, Qin C. Highly pathogenic avian influenza H5N1 virus could partly be evacuated by pregnant BALB/c mouse during abortion or preterm delivery. *Virol J.* (2011) 8:342. doi: 10.1186/1743-422X-8-342
143. Jang H, Boltz D, Mcclaren J, Pani AK, Smeyne M, Korff A, et al. Inflammatory effects of highly pathogenic H5N1 influenza virus infection in the CNS of mice. *J Neurosci.* (2012) 32:1545–59. doi: 10.1523/JNEUROSCI.5123-11.2012
144. Guo Q, Zhao D, Dong F, Liu S, Chen Y, Jin J, et al. Delivery of fetus death with misoprostol in a pregnant woman with H7N9 avian influenza A virus pneumonia and ARDS. *Crit Care* (2014) 18:589. doi: 10.1186/s13054-014-0589-7
145. Qi X, Cui L, Xu K, Wu B, Tang F, Bao C, et al. Avian influenza A(H7N9) virus infection in pregnant woman, China, 2013. *Emerg Infect Dis.* (2014) 20:333–4. doi: 10.3201/eid2002.131109
146. Siegers JY, Short KR, Leijten LM, De Graaf M, Spronken MI, Schrauwen EJ, et al. Novel avian-origin influenza A (H7N9) virus attachment to the respiratory tract of five animal models. *J Virol.* (2014) 88:4595–9. doi: 10.1128/JVI.03190-13
147. Liu S, Sha J, Yu Z, Hu Y, Chan TC, Wang X, et al. Avian influenza virus in pregnancy. *Rev Med Virol.* (2016) 26:268–84. doi: 10.1002/rmv.1884
148. Wong SF, Chow KM, Leung TN, Ng WF, Ng TK, Shek CC, et al. Pregnancy and perinatal outcomes of women with severe acute respiratory syndrome. *Am J Obstet Gynecol.* (2004) 191:292–7. doi: 10.1016/j.ajog.2003.11.019
149. Alserehi H, Wali G, Alshukairi A, Alraddadi B. Impact of middle east respiratory syndrome coronavirus (MERS-CoV) on pregnancy and perinatal outcome. *BMC Infect Dis.* (2016) 16:105. doi: 10.1186/s12879-016-1437-y
150. Malik A, El Masry KM, Ravi M, Sayed F. Middle east respiratory syndrome coronavirus during pregnancy, Abu Dhabi, United Arab Emirates, 2013. *Emerg Infect Dis.* (2016) 22:515–7. doi: 10.3201/eid2203.151049
151. Wheeler SM, Dotters-Katz S, Heine RP, Grotegut CA, Swamy GK. Maternal effects of respiratory syncytial virus infection during pregnancy. *Emerg Infect Dis.* (2015) 21:1951–5. doi: 10.3201/eid2111.150497
152. Chu HY, Katz J, Tielsch J, Khatry SK, Shrestha L, Leclerq SC, et al. Clinical presentation and birth outcomes associated with respiratory syncytial virus infection in pregnancy. *PLoS ONE* (2016) 11:e0152015. doi: 10.1371/journal.pone.0152015
153. Munoz FM. Respiratory syncytial virus in infants: is maternal vaccination a realistic strategy? *Curr Opin Infect Dis.* (2015) 28:221–4. doi: 10.1097/QCO.0000000000000161
154. Yates L, Pierce M, Stephens S, Mill AC, Spark P, Kurinczuk JJ, et al. Influenza A/H1N1v in pregnancy: an investigation of the characteristics and management of affected women and the relationship to pregnancy outcomes for mother and infant. *Health Technol Assess.* (2010) 14:109–82. doi: 10.3310/hta14340-02
155. Lee SM, Gai WW, Cheung TK, Peiris JS. Antiviral effect of a selective COX-2 inhibitor on H5N1 infection *in vitro*. *Antiviral Res.* (2011) 91:330–4. doi: 10.1016/j.antiviral.2011.07.011
156. Li C, Li C, Zhang AJ, To KK, Lee AC, Zhu H, et al. Avian influenza A H7N9 virus induces severe pneumonia in mice without prior adaptation and responds to a combination of zanamivir and COX-2 inhibitor. *PLoS ONE* (2014a) 9:e107966. doi: 10.1371/journal.pone.0107966
157. Carey MA, Bradbury JA, Seubert JM, Langenbach R, Zeldin DC, Germolec DR. Contrasting effects of cyclooxygenase-1 (COX-1) and COX-2 deficiency on the host response to influenza A viral infection. *J Immunol.* (2005) 175:6878–84. doi: 10.4049/jimmunol.175.10.6878
158. Carey MA, Bradbury JA, Rebolloso YD, Graves JP, Zeldin DC, Germolec DR. Pharmacologic inhibition of COX-1 and COX-2 in influenza A viral infection in mice. *PLoS ONE* (2010) 5:e11610. doi: 10.1371/journal.pone.0011610
159. Chan VS. A mechanistic perspective on the specificity and extent of COX-2 inhibition in pregnancy. *Drug Saf.* (2004) 27:421–6. doi: 10.2165/00002018-200427070-00001
160. Daniel S, Matok I, Gorodischer R, Koren G, Uziel E, Wiznitzer A, et al. Major malformations following exposure to nonsteroidal antiinflammatory drugs during the first trimester of pregnancy. *J Rheumatol.* (2012) 39:2163–9. doi: 10.3899/jrheum.120453
161. Berard A, Sheehy O, Girard S, Zhao JP, Bernatsky S. Risk of preterm birth following late pregnancy exposure to NSAIDs or COX-2 inhibitors. *Pain* (2018) 159:948–55. doi: 10.1097/j.pain.0000000000001163
162. Hall OJ, Limjunyawong N, Vermillion MS, Robinson DP, Wohlgemuth N, Pekosz A, et al. Progesterone-based therapy protects against influenza by promoting lung repair and recovery in females. *PLoS Pathog.* (2016) 12:e1005840. doi: 10.1371/journal.ppat.1005840
163. Hall OJ, Nachbagauer R, Vermillion MS, Fink AL, Phuong V, Krammer F, et al. Progesterone-based contraceptives reduce adaptive immune responses and protection against sequential influenza a virus infections. *J Virol.* (2017) 91:e02160-16. doi: 10.1128/JVI.02160-16

13

Regulation of Placental Extravillous Trophoblasts by the Maternal Uterine Environment

*Jürgen Pollheimer[1], Sigrid Vondra[1], Jennet Baltayeva[2,3], Alexander Guillermo Beristain[2,3] and Martin Knöfler[1]**

[1] Department of Obstetrics and Gynaecology, Medical University of Vienna, Vienna, Austria, [2] British Columbia's Children's Hospital Research Institute, Vancouver, BC, Canada, [3] Department of Obstetrics and Gynecology, University of British Columbia, Vancouver, BC, Canada

***Correspondence:**
Martin Knöfler
martin.knoefler@meduniwien.ac.at

During placentation invasive extravillous trophoblasts (EVTs) migrate into the maternal uterus and modify its vessels. In particular, remodeling of the spiral arteries by EVTs is critical for adapting blood flow and nutrient transport to the developing fetus. Failures in this process have been noticed in different pregnancy complications such as preeclampsia, intrauterine growth restriction, stillbirth, or recurrent abortion. Upon invasion into the decidua, the endometrium of pregnancy, EVTs encounter different maternal cell types such as decidual macrophages, uterine NK (uNK) cells and stromal cells expressing a plethora of growth factors and cytokines. Here, we will summarize development of the EVT lineage, a process occurring independently of the uterine environment, and formation of its different subtypes. Further, we will discuss interactions of EVTs with arteries, veins and lymphatics and illustrate how the decidua and its different immune cells regulate EVT differentiation, invasion and survival. The present literature suggests that the decidual environment and its soluble factors critically modulate EVT function and reproductive success.

Keywords: placental development, extravillous trophoblast, decidual immune cells, trophoblast invasion, uterine natural killer cells, decidual macrophages

INTRODUCTION

Development of the human placenta, its distinct epithelial trophoblast subtypes and their interplay with maternal cells and growth factors of the pregnant uterus are crucial for a successful pregnancy. After implantation the trophectoderm, the outermost cell layer of the blastocyst, gives rise to mononuclear cytotrophoblasts (CTBs) forming placental villi through branching morphogenesis. During the first weeks of gestation primary villi, consisting of proliferative CTBs, transform into secondary mesenchymal villi and mature tertiary villi, the latter undergoing vasculogenesis and angiogenesis (1–3). At term these tree-like structures of the human placenta display a surface area of $\sim$15 m^2, completely covered with multinuclear syncytiotrophoblasts (STBs). STBs are generated by cell fusion of villous CTBs (vCTBs) and fulfill a vast range of functions such as production of pregnancy hormones, transport of oxygen and nutrients from the maternal blood stream to the growing fetus and clearance of fetal waste products (4, 5). However, early placental development and fetal growth occurs in the absence of maternal blood and oxygen and are likely supported by growth factors and proteins secreted from endometrial glands (6). As soon as the utero-placental circulation is established between 10th and 12th week of pregnancy placental villi are bathed in maternal blood, and hence are termed floating villi.

Whereas, STBs of floating villi represent the transport units of the human placenta, anchoring villi of the placental basal plate form another differentiated trophoblast type, the so called invasive extravillous trophoblast (EVT). Upon attachment of villi to the maternal decidua, the endometrium of the pregnant uterus, proliferative proximal cell column trophoblasts (pCCTs) develop which further differentiate into distal CCTs (dCCTs) ceasing their mitotic activity (**Figure 1**). EVTs are formed upon detachment from the distal cell column. These cells deeply migrate into the maternal decidua and the first third of the underlying myometrium (7). Already 2 weeks after fertilization two types of EVTs can be discerned within the maternal uterine compartment, interstitial CTBs (iCTBs), colonizing the decidual stroma, and endovascular CTBs (eCTBs), penetrating the maternal spiral arteries (8). Stepwise modification of these vessels is regarded as a critical step in placentation. In the first weeks of pregnancy, EVTs plug the spiral arteries, likely to prevent precocious onset of blood flow to the developing placenta, hence protecting against early placental damage through oxidative stress and fetal loss (6, 9). However, as the embryo switches from histiotrophic to haemotrophic nutrition after the 10th week gestation, plugs dissolve and the endothelial layer of the spiral arteries is replaced by eCTBs (8, 10). The latter are thought to arise by luminal migration into the myometrial segments of spiral arteries (11). Moreover, iCTBs accumulate in the muscular vessel wall promoting its elastolysis and degradation, where decidual macrophages and uterine natural killer cells (uNKs) also contribute to this process (12). Notably, uNK cells, increasing in numbers during the secretory phase of the menstrual cycle and early pregnancy (13), initiate remodeling by inducing apoptosis of vascular smooth muscle cells, whereas iCTBs are thought to complete this process (14). These modifications transform the spiral arteries into highly dilated vessels ensuring low-pressure blood flow to the placenta and the developing fetus. Both iCTBs and eCTBs upregulate adhesion molecules mimicking an endothelial phenotype which could be instrumental during invasion and for the replacement of maternal endothelial cells (15). Defects in vessel remodeling, in particular in the myometrial part of the spiral arteries, have been reported in various pregnancy complications, such as preeclampsia, fetal growth restriction, preterm labor, abortions, and stillbirth (9, 10, 16–19). Failures in immunological acceptance of the placenta, decidual function and/or abnormal trophoblast invasion and differentiation could be underlying causes (20–23). During the first weeks of gestation EVTs, originating from the trophoblastic shell (24), also migrate into decidual lymphatics and veins, already before arterial remodeling occurs (25–27). Number of EVTs in lymphatic and venous vessels is lower in recurrent abortions suggesting that, along with defects in spiral artery remodeling, failed interactions of EVTs with other types of uterine vessels could contribute to pregnancy complications (26). Similarly, EVTs also invade into the decidual glands which could promote early histiotrophic nutrition (28).

In the decidua basalis, iCTBs communicate with diverse cell types of the fetal-maternal interface, such as decidual stromal cells (DSCs) and different immune cells (**Figure 1**). Amongst those, uNK cells and macrophages have been delineated as the most abundant cell types (29). The role of uNK cells has been extensively investigated throughout the years. Besides their role in the immunological tolerance of the semi-allogenic fetus, uNK cells are thought to affect decidual angiogenesis and EVT function (22, 30). Expression of human leukocyte antigen C (HLA-C) on EVTs, interacting with killer cell immunoglobulin-like (KIR) receptors on uNK cells, could play a role in pregnancy outcome as certain combinations of fetal HLA-C and maternal KIR alleles might increase the risk of developing preeclampsia and recurrent miscarriage (31, 32). It is anticipated that unfavorable HLA-C/KIR interactions impair trophoblast invasion and as a consequence spiral artery remodeling. The role of KIRs and their effects in allorecognition of EVTs has been subject of numerous reviews (22, 33–36) and will be only briefly discussed herein. Instead, we review how uNK cells influence EVTs in a paracrine manner. Further, we will also focus on the other maternal cell types of the decidua and summarize how they might affect cell column growth of anchoring villi, EVT formation and motility. Factors secreted by EVTs, controlling trophoblast migration and invasion in an autocrine manner, have been extensively discussed elsewhere (37, 38), and will not be presented herein. Likewise, the paracrine effects of EVT-secreted factors on decidual immune cell function will not be a topic of this review.

DEVELOPMENT OF THE EVT LINEAGE AND ITS DIFFERENT SUBTYPES

EVTs originate from distal cell columns of anchoring villi at distinct contact sites with the maternal decidua. Numbers of the latter are a consequence of the frequency of villous branching (5). Different to growth of vCTBs, that form a double-rowed epithelium after lateral cell division and fuse into STBs, pCCTs break through the overlying STB layer and form multiple layers of proliferative trophoblasts (**Figure 1**). Similar to early phases of tumor formation, pCCTs detach from the basal membrane and lose their polarity. However, in contrast to cancer cells, growth and invasion of trophoblasts is highly organized and precisely controlled in a spatiotemporal manner. At distal sites of anchoring villi, pCCTs differentiate into non-proliferative dCCTs. Similar to iCTBs which have deeply migrated into the decidua, dCCTs express numerous EVT markers such as HLA-G (39), T-cell factor 4 (TCF-4) (40), integrin $\alpha5$ (ITGA5) and $\beta1$ (41), Notch2 (42), proteoglycan 2 (26). and ErbB2 (43). Hence, formation of dCCTs represents the first step of EVT differentiation. In comparison to dCCTs, iCTBs undergo further differentiation by inducing/upregulating specific proteins, for example ITGA1 (41), matrix metalloproteinase (MMP) 12 (44, 45) or diamine oxidase (DAO) (46). The latter is predominantly expressed in EVTs surrounding decidual vessels and was shown to be decreased in serum samples of early-onset preeclamptic women (46). *In vivo*, DAO is only detected in ~20 and 45% of iCTBs and perivascular CTBs, respectively, providing some evidence for the existence of different iCTB subtypes. Similarly, different EVT populations, identified by single-cell RNA-Seq, have recently been suggested (47). However,

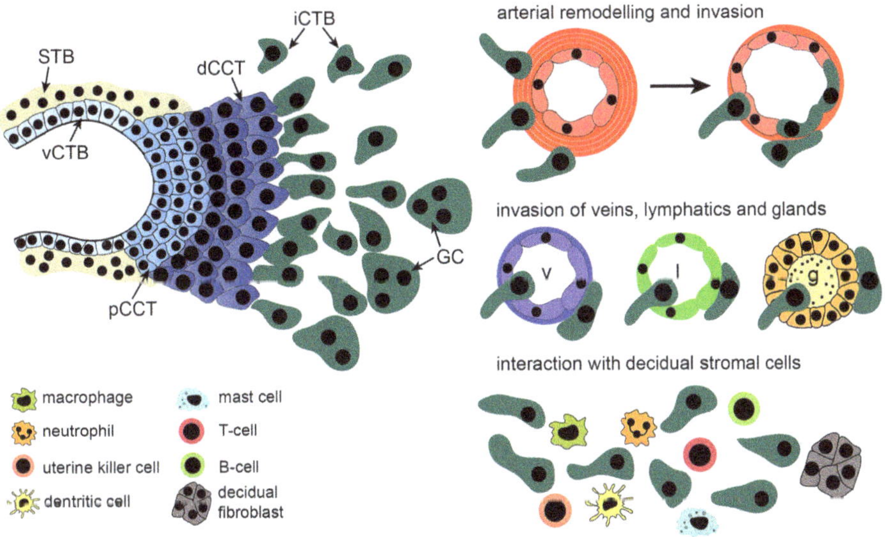

FIGURE 1 | Structure of a placental anchoring villus and its different trophoblast subtypes. Precursors, residing in the villous cytotrophoblast (vCTB) layer either differentiate into multinuclear syncytiotrophoblasts (STBs), surrounded by maternal blood, or give rise to proliferative proximal cell column trophoblasts (pCCTs) upon attachment of villi to the maternal decidua. After differentiation into distal cell column trophoblasts (dCCTs) extravillous trophoblasts (EVTs) develop, breaking through the overlying STB layer. EVTs detach from distal cell columns, migrate into the decidual stroma and the maternal spiral arteries replacing maternal endothelial cells. In the decidual stroma interstitial CTBs (iCTBs) interact with macrophages, B- and T-cells, mast cells, dendritic cells, neutrophils, decidual stromal cells, and uterine natural killer (uNK) cells. Moreover, iCTBs approach the vessel walls of spiral arteries and promote remodeling from outside. Also, veins (v), lymphatics (l) and glands (g) are invaded by these cells forming multinucleated trophoblast giant cells (GC) as an end-stage of differentiation.

it remains largely unknown if variations between iCTBs are specified by the intrinsic genetic program of the placental anchoring villus or determined by the diverse decidual structures. Likewise, the exact route of eCTB migration and the mechanisms specifying these cells have not been unraveled (11). The different phenotypes of EVTs could eventually be influenced by the decidual environment. For example, it was shown that abnormal gene expression of preeclamptic CTBs was reverted back to normal physiological levels when cultured *in vitro* (21). On the other hand, EVT development *per se* occurs independently of the decidual environment and its growth factors. Purified CTBs and villous explant cultures, seeded on extracellular matrix, undergo spontaneous EVT differentiation upregulating dCCT, and iCTB markers in a kinetic manner (48–50). In preeclampsia this endogenous EVT differentiation program could be disturbed (51). Anchoring villi and detaching EVTs of tubal pregnancies show the same pattern in integrin switching as EVTs invading the decidua basalis (52). Similarly, EVTs migrating from implanted villous explants and invading the kidney capsule of SCID mice, were shown to induce HLA-G expression (53).

Although the genome-wide expression profiles of non-migratory CTBs and invasive EVTs have been unraveled (54, 55), mechanisms promoting cell column formation and CTB commitment toward the EVT lineage have been poorly elucidated. Recently, Notch1 has been detected in a subset of proliferative pCCTs, indicating that this particular receptor could mark EVT progenitors (56). Indeed, the active Notch1 intracellular domain promoted pCCT survival and marker expression, but suppressed stemness markers of vCTBs suggesting that Notch1 could convert CTB precursors into EVT progenitors (57). Low oxygen levels, occurring during early phases of placental development (58), were shown to trigger Notch1 expression in primary CTBs (57). Hence, low oxygen could promote expansion of EVT progenitors and promote early stages of EVT differentiation and invasion (59). However, the current literature about the specific role of oxygen in trophoblast biology is controversial, has been extensively discussed (60–63), and will not be subject of the present review. Moreover, changes of the self-renewing conditions of long-term expanding 3-dimensional cytotrophoblast organoid cultures promoted outgrowth of Notch1-positive progenitors and EVT formation (64), further supporting the view that development of different trophoblast subtypes is largely determined by the intrinsic differentiation program of the placenta.

THE IMPACT OF THE DECIDUA ON EXTRAVILLOUS TROPHOBLASTS: GENERAL ASPECTS

In a few species, spontaneous uterine transformation commences during the second half of the menstrual cycle. This process, preceding implantation, is exclusively observed in mammals with menstruation and deep, haemochorial placentation, such as humans and higher primates (65, 66). Shortly after implantation the pregnant uterus undergoes dramatic morphological changes including extracellular matrix remodeling, vascularization, increase in uNK cell numbers and secretory activity of glands as well as transformation of stromal fibroblasts into polygonal decidual cells (67). Decidual glands secrete glycoproteins, such as glycodelin A, carbohydrates and other metabolites nourishing the embryo during the first weeks of pregnancy (68–70). During this phase of histiotrophic nutrition glandular cells also produce various growth factors likely promoting early placental development such as leukemia-inhibitory factors (LIF), epidermal growth factor (EGF), vascular endothelial growth factor (VEGF) and endocrine gland-derived vascular endothelial growth factor (EG-VEGF) (69, 71–74). Indeed, EGF (see below) and EG-VEGF were shown to augment proliferation of vCTBs/CCTs in villous explant cultures (75). Similarly, VEGF was shown to stimulate growth of trophoblast cell lines and primary cultures (76). In contrast, LIF may be mainly involved in the regulation of implantation and trophoblast invasion (77–79).

Differentiation of uterine fibroblasts, commonly referred to as decidualization, initiates during the luteal phase of the menstrual cycle and requires the combined action of cAMP and progesterone on the estrogen-primed endometrium (80). Besides secretion of growth- and- invasion-controlling factors (see below) numerous other functions have been assigned to decidual fibroblasts (DFs). For example, DFs secrete enzymes clearing reactive oxygen species (67, 81) and thereby might protect the decidua and/or EVTs from adverse stress response when local oxygen levels rise between 10th and 12th week of gestation. Trophoblast-derived human chorionic gonadotrophin (hCG) could further increase resistance of DFs against oxidative tissue damage (82). DFs also express various extracellular matrix proteins, such as fibronectin, emilin-1, decorin, fibulins, collagens and laminins (83–86), potentially controlling EVT motility by binding to trophoblast-expressed adhesion molecules and receptors (87).

In women with placenta accreta, EVTs excessively invade the maternal uterus, mostly as a consequence of implantation onto or close to a scar after preceding cesarean section. It is anticipated that the local absence of decidua facilitates trophoblast invasion into the underlying myometrium (88, 89). From this pathology, one might conclude that the decidua restricts migration of trophoblasts thereby controlling depth of invasion in a temporal manner and preventing aberrant, tumor-like expansion of the placenta. Indeed, former concepts suggested that trophoblast-derived MMPs, known to promote invasiveness, are counter-balanced by tissue-inhibitors of metalloproteinases (TIMPs) present in the decidua (90, 91). Similarly, decidual plasminogen activator inhibitors (PAI) 1 and 2 could control timing and depth of trophoblast invasion by inhibiting the plasminogen activator (PA) system expressed by migratory EVTs. However, physiology of trophoblast invasion is more complex since both EVTs and DFs express MMPs, TIMPs, PAs, PAIs as well as urokinase plasminogen activator receptor (uPAR) (90, 92–98). Hence, the decreasing rate of EVT invasion during pregnancy cannot be merely explained by the reciprocal expression of MMPs/uPA and TIMPs/PAI in EVTs and the decidua, respectively. Moreover, potential changes of inhibitor expression throughout gestation or in superficial vs. deeper regions of the decidua have not been measured. Diminished EVT migration at later stages of pregnancy might also be a consequence of the decreasing growth rates of cell columns. As follows, defects in invasion/remodeling, as observed in IUGR, could at least partly be the result of reduced trophoblast growth in this condition (99).

Other data do not support the concept that the decidua restricts trophoblast invasion. In contrast to anchoring villi of normal uterine pregnancies, distal cell columns of ectopic placental villi, isolated from tubal pregnancies, were extended in size. This suggests that the decidua could facilitate EVT detachment from anchoring villi during physiological development of the placental basal plate (52). Indeed, decidualized endometrial stromal cells express a tissue-specific variant of fibronectin favoring trophoblast invasion (100). Whereas, EVTs, generated by first trimester villous explant culture, migrated superficially on dermal fibroblasts, their co-culture with DFs resulted in promotion of interstitial invasion (100). Therefore, the specific features of the decidua may adapt to different stages of pregnancy and precisely control invasion of EVTs by expressing pro- and anti-migratory matrix proteins and factors (37, 38). In return, DFs have a high migratory capacity and could promote implantation by actively moving toward the blastocyst and provoking encapsulation of the conceptus (101). Indeed, EVT supernatants contain chemotactic signals that promote endometrial stromal cell migration (102). Genome-wide expression analyses revealed that trophoblast-conditioned medium of cultivated CTB preparations, containing a mixture of different CTB subtypes, could induce mRNAs encoding chemokines and angiogenic factors in decidualized endometrial fibroblasts (103). However, compared to EVTs, mixed CTB isolates may elicit different responses. In a recent study EVTs increased numbers of resting FoxP3-positive regulatory T cells (Tregs) upon co-cultivation with $CD4^+$ T cells, whereas vCTBs were ineffective (104).

CAVEATS OF *IN VITRO* STUDIES WITH EXTRAVILLOUS TROPHOBLASTS

Decidua-derived growth factors and their role in trophoblast motility have been investigated in numerous publications. However, many of these studies have drawbacks limiting their scientific value. Access to primary trophoblasts of early pregnancy is generally restricted, hence different trophoblast-like cell lines were utilized in invasion and migration assays. Yet, the specific origin of these cell lines is uncertain and their genome-wide gene expression profiles and HLA status differ considerably from purified CTBs (105, 106). Cell lines proliferate in culture whereas EVTs are non-mitotic cells. Hence, discordant results were obtained between cell lines and primary cells, for example in migration assays under hypoxic conditions (107, 108). Similarly, transforming growth factor β (TGFB), expressed by DFs, uNK cells and uterine glands (109, 110), was shown to either promote or inhibit trophoblast proliferation or invasion (111–115). Besides divergence between cell lines and first trimester CTBs, contaminations with highly migratory placental fibroblasts and variations between different cell isolations and primary model systems might account for multiple discrepancies and the high variances observed in trophoblast-related studies. Invasion assays are often performed with pooled fractions of trypsinized primary CTBs representing a mixture of CCTs, EVTs and vCTBs. The latter also invade through 8 μm transwells *in vitro*, whilst undergoing cell fusion *in vivo*. Moreover, nuclear size is a limiting factor in invasion/migration assays (116). Indeed, EVTs become polyploid during differentiation displaying increased nuclear diameter (117, 118). Therefore, EVTs hardly pass membranes with 8 μm pores (50), a fact which has not been considered by the majority of trophoblast invasion/migration studies. Moreover, the high complexity of decidual cell types cannot be mimicked *in vitro*. In addition, local concentrations of soluble factors in the tissue and their variations during pregnancy and between uterine cell types are poorly studied. Therefore, *in vitro* assays are usually performed with saturating levels of recombinant factors. As follows, the prime target cell of many decidual proteins remains uncertain since the respective receptors have been identified on several uterine cell types. As a consequence, opposing roles for particular factors were suggested. For example, IL10 was shown to directly impair CTB invasion, but also to abolish the adverse effects of LPS-treated macrophages on trophoblastic cell migration (119, 120). Additionally, results obtained with first trimester villous explant cultures recapitulating attachment, outgrowth and EVT migration *in vitro* (121) are often interpreted differently by authors. For example, depending on the specific analyses, outgrowth was suggested to be indicative of both increased trophoblast motility and elevated proliferative capacity.

Herein, we focus on the abundant decidual factors, cytokines, and chemokines which have been most convincingly proven to affect EVT formation and function in reliable trophoblast *in vitro* model systems. However, these studies should also be interpreted in the light of the above-mentioned limitations.

REGULATION OF EXTRAVILLOUS TROPHOBLASTS BY DECIDUAL FIBROBLASTS

During decidualization fibroblasts upregulate key markers of the pregnant endometrium of which prolactin (PRL) and insulin growth factor binding protein-1 (IGFBP-1) are amongst the most abundantly expressed proteins (122–124). Both proteins likely exert pleiotropic effects on different uterine cell types including regulation of decidualization and EVT migration (125–128). Although PRL, also involved in differentiation of the decidual glandular epithelium (129), was shown to promote motility of first trimester CTBs (130, 131), the role of IGFBP-1 is less clear due to the high complexity of the IGF/IGFBP system. Both migration-activating and -inhibiting effects were attributed to IGFBP-1 upon binding to the EVT-expressed fibronectin receptor ITGA5B1 (132–134). However, one of the main functions of IGFBP-1 could be the regulation of IGF bioavailability at the fetal-maternal interface, possibly triggered by EVT-derived IGF-II (135). Upon secretion of IGF-II from these cells decidual IGFBP-1 might get dephosphorylated and further cleaved by EVT-specific MMP-3 and MMP-9 thereby increasing unbound IGFs, the latter stimulating trophoblast migration (126, 136–139). Yet, proteolytic fragments, generated by trophoblast-derived MMPs, may also restrain trophoblast invasion. Endostatin, a cleavage product of decidual collagen XVIII, was shown to impair IGF-II-induced EVT-motility (50, 140).

Besides the prime markers IGFBP-1 and PRL, other classes of soluble DF-secreted factors were suggested to control EVT motility including chemokines, cytokines and ligands of the EGF and Wingless (WNT) signaling pathways (38, 141). Different CXCL and CCL chemokines have been identified in DFs. Their respective receptors are present on uterine leukocytes and EVTs suggesting a role in immune cell trafficking as well as trophoblast migration, respectively (142, 143). For example, CXCL14 was shown to reduce invasiveness (144), whereas CXCL12 promoted CTB migration and suppressed apoptosis of term trophoblasts through its receptor CXCR4 (145–147). CCL2, expressed by DFs, macrophages and EVTs (148, 149), may recruit T helper 17 cells into the decidua, and interleukin (IL) 17 expressed by these cells could promote trophoblast growth and invasion (150). Other interleukins, shown to stimulate CTB invasion, are IL1B (151, 152) and IL8, secreted from uterine NK cells and DFs (153, 154), whereas IL11 had inhibitory effects (155).

While EGF and heparin-binding EGF (HB-EGF), expressed by the decidua, were shown to stimulate trophoblast invasion and outgrowth from villous explants cultures, proliferation of primary EVTs and trophoblastic HTR-8/SVneo cells was unaffected (156–159). Recently, however, we could demonstrate that these factors increased proliferation of vCTBs and CCTs in villous explant cultures of early placentae (160). Moreover, in contrast to vCTBs and CCTs, EVTs largely lack the EGF/HB-EGF-specific receptors EGFR and ErbB4, and induce ErbB2 and ErbB3 during differentiation (43, 161). Heterodimers of ErbB2 and ErbB3 were shown to interact with neuregulin 1, expressed by DFs, protecting EVTs from apoptosis and thereby retaining their differentiation program (43). Therefore, upregulation of EVT invasion/differentiation by EGF/HB-EGF could largely be a consequence of increased CCT proliferation, while direct effects of these factors on EVTs might be negligible.

Like in other developing tissues WNT signaling has been suggested to play a pivotal role in placental morphogenesis and differentiation (141, 162). Activation of the pathway by secreted ligands stabilizes the key mediator of WNT signaling, β-catenin, and promotes its nuclear recruitment (163). In the nucleus β-catenin binds to DNA-binding proteins of the T-cell factor (TCF) family thereby inducing TCF-mediated gene transcription. Invasive trophoblasts, the secretory endometrium and first trimester DFs express a variety of WNT ligands suggesting autocrine as well as paracrine effects of the particular pathway (164, 165). EVT formation and differentiation is strongly associated with activation of canonical Wnt signaling and nuclear expression of β-catenin, TCF-3 and TCF-4 (40, 166). Indeed, migration and differentiation of EVTs requires TCF-4, whereas survival and proliferation of CCTs is induced by WNT5A involving non-canonical mitogen-activated protein kinase (MAPK) activity (166, 167). Moreover, canonical Wnt signaling might play a dual role in early placental development controlling both long-term expansion of vCTB progenitors and EVT differentiation (64).

IMMUNE CELL DISTRIBUTION IN THE DECIDUA

The pregnant uterus is mainly colonized by cells of the innate immune system, of which the most abundant and by far best characterized cell types are macrophages and uNK cells. Most available literature refers to numbers ranging from 50 to 70% uNK cells, 20–30 % macrophages and 10–15 % T cells of the total $CD45^{+}$ immune cells in the decidua; only 2 % account toward the less abundant leukocyte populations including dendritic cells or Tregs (30, 168–170). However, the vast majorities of comparative analyses do not consider regional differences (parietalis vs. basalis) in decidual immune distribution and may also miss certain cell populations due to pre-selective isolation methods or due to the lack of appropriate markers to distinguish certain immune cell populations from each other. Hence, before describing uNK cell and macrophage function in detail, we will shortly discuss decidual immune cell populations which in our opinion have widely been ignored in the context of reproductive biology.

Mast cells have been previously described to mainly colonize the uterine myometrium and were shown to localize around decidual vessels. Interestingly, mast cell depletion in a mouse model results in diminished spiral artery remodeling and as a consequence leads to IUGR. The same study demonstrated a close spatial distribution of mast cells and EVTs in the human decidua basalis and reported a mast cell-dependent positive effect on EVT migration (171). Another study showed a role for neutrophils in placentation and trophoblastic giant cell invasion in mice (172). Interestingly, neutrophils seem to accumulate around spiral arteries and develop a pro-angiogenic phenotype toward the second trimester of pregnancy (173). The reason for the oversight of neutrophils might be explained by methodological issues as most protocols to obtain tissue leukocytes involve density gradient centrifugation eliminating all non-mononucleated immune cells, including neutrophils. Nevertheless, it should be taken into consideration that neutrophil accumulation in the decidua may at least be partly a response to blood coagulation and tissue damage occurring during tissue collection. Although mostly ignored, some scientific papers describe the presence of B cells in human term decidua (174). Moreover, a recent study shows that term decidua basalis contains more B cells when compared to decidua parietalis tissues (175). The authors of this study further found that decidua parietalis contains a higher proportion of mature/naive B cells whereas transitional B cells were enriched in decidua basalis. Since altered B cell distributions have recently been associated with preterm labor (174), more studies are needed to determine the role of B cells during pregnancy. In addition, distribution and characterization of B cells in first trimester decidua tissues has not been studied so far. While macrophages are considered to be the main phagocytic and antigen-presenting cell type in the human decidua little is known about dendritic cell distribution and function during pregnancy. One reason for the scarce information concerning decidual dendritic cells is the lack of marker combinations, which could reliably segregate macrophages from dendritic cells, since they develop from a common myeloid progenitor and therefore express common cell surface markers (176, 177). A good example for the problem to distinguish between macrophages and dendritic cells are Langerhans cells. These cells have long been referred to as long-lived dermal dendritic cells and are now considered tissue-resident macrophages with features of dendritic cells such as T cell-stimulation in lymph nodes (178). Despite overlapping cell marker expression and functional similarities in the skin, dendritic cells have unique properties. For instance, DCs homeostatically migrate to draining lymph nodes and are much more potent in antigen cross-presentation to $CD8^{+}$ T cells (179). Consequently, DCs are likely involved in shaping host immune responses toward the invading EVTs.

PROPOSED FUNCTIONS OF UTERINE NATURAL KILLER CELLS

Unlike conventional peripheral blood (pb) NK that are efficient killers, uNK cells in rodents and humans do not normally mount cytotoxic responses against fetal or placental tissues. Instead, growing evidence highlights the importance of uNK in controlling uterine neo-angiogenesis, spiral artery remodeling, the immune response against fetal antigen, and trophoblast function (30, 180–182). However, recent work shows that aberrant inflammation in pregnancy resulting from infection or fetal-driven alloimmunity programs uNK cells to acquire cytotoxic properties that promote fetal death and/or placental dysfunction (183, 184). Therefore, a contemporary view suggests that appropriate uNK activation is important for promoting healthy placentation, where *inadequate* (not enough) or *inappropriate* (too much) uNK activity contributes to defective placentation and related disorders of pregnancy that may include recurrent miscarriage, preterm birth, and preeclampsia (185, 186). In women, uNK cell numbers rapidly expand during the progesterone-dominant luteal phase of the menstrual cycle (22). Evidence suggests that the decidual environment, enriched with factors like progesterone and transforming growth factor TGFB1, promote the differentiation of NK cell progenitors into mature uNK cells that are defined phenotypically as $CD56^{superbright}/CD16^{-}$ cells (187, 188). By contrast, the phenotype of conventional pbNK cells is predominantly $CD56^{dim}/CD16^{+}$. Other distinctive features of uNK include the expression of tissue-residency markers (i.e., CD9, CD69, CD49a) (189, 190) and cytolytic proteins (i.e., perforin, granzyme, and granulysin) (191), and the expression of a distinctive natural killer receptor repertoire (192). In particular, killer immunoglobulin-like receptor (KIR) and natural killer group 2 (NKG2) receptors are robustly expressed by uNK cells (189, 192). These and other natural killer cell receptors, are thought to modulate maternal-fetal recognition, but may also play important roles in controlling aspects of trophoblast biology.

COMMUNICATION BETWEEN INVASIVE TROPHOBLASTS AND UTERINE NATURAL KILLER CELLS

In vivo evidence shows that EVTs directly interact with uNK cells (193), indicating that by EVT- uNK cell interactions these potentially modulate each other's functions (194–196). EVTs, unlike vCTBs that do not express major histocompatibility complex (MHC) type-I molecules, express a unique combination of classical HLA-C and non-classical HLA-E, HLA-F, and HLA-G class-I ligands playing a role in immunological acceptance of the placenta/fetus (30, 197, 198). This unique MHC composition enables EVT to directly interact with and modulate uNK cell processes through specific combinations of natural killer receptors. However, hard evidence for *in vivo* or *ex vivo* natural killer cell receptor-EVT interactions has been challenging to generate, due in large part to the ethical boundaries of working with human samples of pregnancy and to the logistical hurdles of working with primary CTB cultures and uNK cells isolated from tissues of the same pregnancy. As a surrogate for primary EVTs, co-cultivation of trophoblastic HTR-8/SVneo cells with uNK cells were performed demonstrating elevated uNK cell survival and downregulation of the activating NKG2D receptor (199). However, these data have to be interpreted with caution since HTR-8/SVneo cells express a different repertoire of HLA proteins, including HLA-A and HLA-B, which are absent from EVTs (105).

MHC class-I molecules expressed on EVTs can interact with multiple natural killer receptors that transmit inhibitory or activating signals to dampen or promote uNK cytotoxicity and production of cytokines, respectively (30). Perhaps the best-studied uNK cell receptors are the family of polymorphic KIRs that are defined by the presence of either 2 (2D) or 3 (3D) immunoglobulin-like domains and long (L) or short (S) cytoplasmic tails that help initiate inhibitory (L) or activating (S) signals. Inhibitory KIRs expressed on uNK cells include KIR2DL1, KIR2DL2, and KIR2DL3, and these receptors transmit strong inhibitory signals through their immunoreceptor Tyr-based inhibitory motif (ITIM) (35). Activating uNK KIRs include KIR2DS1 and KIR2DS4 (186, 200), however the receptor KIR2DL4, an unconventional KIR that predominantly localizes to endosomes and not the cell membrane, is also capable of transmitting activating signals (104, 201, 202). KIRs bind mainly to HLA-C, expressed by multiple cell types within decidual tissue, including EVTs (203). The number of *KIR* genes in the genome of any given individual varies within the population, as does the expression of haplotypic specific HLA-C, making the immunogenic complexities of uNK cell-EVT responses unique for any given pregnancy (204).

To date, most research has examined the importance of HLA-C in controlling uNK cell-related processes through either uNK-target cell or antibody cross-linking experiments. It is important to note that, the directionality of uNK cell response to HLA-C depends largely on the epitope type, designated broadly as C1 or C2. This designation is based on a dimorphism at position 80 of the $\alpha 1$ domain of HLA-C (205). Overall, in mixed uNK cell populations that express high levels of inhibitory KIR, HLA-C challenge promotes an inhibitory signal regardless of the co-presence of activating KIRs (186). KIR-directed inhibitory signals associate with impaired or blunted degranulation (206) and reduced secretion of EVT-regulatory factors (i.e. IL8, VEGF, placental growth factor (PGF) and CXCL10, also known as IP-10) (153). In uNK cells, expressing activating KIR2DS1 or KIR2DS4, HLA-C promotes uNK cell degranulation and secretion of granulocyte-macrophage colony-stimulating factor (GM-CSF) and tumor necrosis factor (TNF) (186, 200, 207). Production of these factors potentially impacts EVT biology (discussed below). However, the direct effect of endogenous HLA-C expressed by EVTs on uNK cell processes has yet to be determined. Nonetheless, *ex vivo* EVTs physically interact with HLA-C-specific KIR2DL1 and KIR2DS1 (204), indicating that biological functions for these KIR-EVT interaction likely do exist.

HLA-E protein is present in EVTs at the 5th week of gestation but absent from these cells after the 7th week, suggesting a predominant role in implantation and/or early trophoblast development (198). Inhibitory signals elicited by HLA-E are mediated through the dimeric CD94/NKG2A receptor (208). Previous work shows that CD94/NKG2A elicits strong suppressive signals that generally override most activating inputs (209). However, whether EVT-derived HLA-E's sole purpose is to restrain uNK cell cytotoxicity in pregnancy is currently not well understood. For example, CD94 function-blocking experiments do not potentiate trophoblast killing (208), suggesting that CD94/NKG2A may serve other roles within the maternal-fetal interface that have yet to be elucidated.

The role of HLA-G in controlling uNK cells has been studied more so than other MHC class-I ligands, due in part to the relevance of its unique and restricted expression within EVT (197). Previous studies have identified two receptors expressed on uNK cells that interact with HLA-G: leukocyte immunoglobulin-like subfamily B member 1 (LILRB1) (210) and KIR2DL4 (211, 212). Interpretation of previous HLA-G-related findings necessitates caution due to the nature and design of the experimental systems used. For example, most approaches implement forced ectopic expression of HLA-G in HLA-null target cell lines, designed to synthesize either of two major HLA-G isoforms expressed by EVTs, namely membrane-bound HLA-G1 (213) or the truncated soluble HLA-G5 (211, 214). Further, many studies have interchangeably used peripheral blood NK cells or NK-like cell lines as surrogate readouts of HLA-G-uNK cell interaction within the maternal-fetal interface. These assumptions have perhaps contributed to over-interpretation of the role of HLA-G in controlling uNK cell-related processes in pregnancy. Conflicting findings have arisen from these studies, indicating that both membrane-bound and soluble HLA-G enhance the production of pro-inflammatory (IFN-γ, TNF, IL1B, IL6) and angiogenic (IL8) factors in endometrial (i.e., not decidual) (213, 215) or pbNK cells (202, 216). In support of the above findings using pbNK cells, Li et al. demonstrated that HLA-G treatment of *ex vivo*-derived uNK cells induces IL6, IL8, and TNF through processes dependent upon KIR2DL4 (212). In contrast to this, *ex vivo* uNK cells, exposed to membrane-bound HLA-G, resulted in inhibition or had marginal impact on uNK degranulation and cytokine production (214). Two recent studies, directly examining the function of HLA-G in primary EVTs and uNK cells, indicated that HLA-G does not induce cytokine secretion from uNK cells but instead dampens uNK cell activity (104, 193), a finding that is consistent with the original paradigm that HLA-G likely promotes immune cell tolerance within the fetal-maternal interface.

REGULATION OF EXTRAVILLOUS TROPHOBLASTS BY UTERINE NATURAL KILLER CELLS

Uterine NK are robust producers of cytokines and growth factors, and due to their close proximity to EVTs within the maternal-fetal interface, these cells likely play roles in regulating the diverse functions of trophoblasts. In support of this, uNK cell-generated conditioned media modifies specific biological processes of primary trophoblast, including the promotion of cell invasion (153, 154, 217). Notably, the pro-invasive effect of uNK cell-derived conditioned media is solely attributed to soluble factors produced by uNK cells harvested from later gestational age time-points within the first trimester of pregnancy (i.e., 10–13 weeks' gestation). By contrast, soluble factors produced by uNK cells from the earlier first trimester time-points do not elicit pro-invasive characteristics on EVTs, indicating that the composition of uNK cell factors is influenced by processes related to gestational age, and that the impact of uNK cells on EVT biology is relative to stage of development.

Multiple factors produced by uNK cells have been identified, and importantly, receptors for many of these substances are expressed on primary EVTs. For example, uNK cells produce high levels of IL8, TNF, interferon (INF) γ, TGFB1, CXCL10, as well as the angiogenic factors such as vascular endothelial growth factor A (VEGF-A), VEGF-C and PGF (153). Reciprocally, immunolocalization studies on implantation sites and *ex vivo* studies using primary EVTs provide evidence that invasive trophoblasts populating the maternal-fetal interface produce receptors for these ligands. For example, EVTs express CXCR1 (an IL8 receptor), CXCR3 (an CXCL10 receptor), TNFR1, as well as VEGFR-1 and VEGFR-3, the latter binding VEGF-A and VEGF-C, respectively (110, 153, 218, 219). Notably, supplementation of IL8 and CXCL10 promoted migration of primary CTBs (153). Likewise, inhibition of ligand binding to VEGFR-1 and VEGFR-3 diminished trophoblast invasion (220). Moreover, downregulation of VEGF in uNK cell-conditioned media impaired EVT outgrowth compared to controls (221). In contrast, TNF and IFN-γ inhibited trophoblast migration and invasion by increasing PAI expression and impacting MMP-directed proteolysis, respectively (222, 223). Taken together, factors produced by uNK cells do have the ability to control EVT-related processes *in vivo*. Given the interplay between promoting and restraining invasive characteristics in EVTs, uNK cells could be an important cellular component of the decidua that controls depth of EVT invasion as well as extent of trophoblast-mediated spiral artery remodeling.

CAN THE BREAKDOWN OF MATERNAL-FETAL TOLERANCE BE RELATED TO UTERINE NATURAL KILLER CELLS DYSFUNCTION?

Much research related to uNK-trophoblast interactions has centered on the possibility that uNK cells, activated by infection or inflammation, may mount cytotoxic responses toward the semi-allogeneic fetus and trophoblast, thus contributing to infection-related miscarriage and other pregnancy disorders with aberrant inflammation. Surprisingly, most well designed studies, utilizing primary syngeneic uNK cell and trophoblast co-cultures, provided convincing evidence that trophoblasts (both HLA-G- and non-HLA-G-expressing trophoblasts) are highly resistant to uNK-directed killing (193, 224). Although uNK cells do not target trophoblasts for killing, even when artificially activated, uNK still retain pro-cytotoxic features (i.e. granzyme, perforin) that enable efficient cellular immune responses against virally-infected maternal uterine stromal cells, highlighting that trophoblasts are immuno-privileged (193, 225). Nonetheless, research in mice suggests that uNK cells can adopt anti-trophoblast characteristics in the right context. For example, aberrantly activated uNK cells in response to inflammation induced by bacterial endotoxin (183) or alloimmunogenic responses (184) target fetal tissues, including the placenta, and induce fetal resorption. These uNK-driven processes lead to impairments in uterine artery remodeling and placental sufficiency, and can be reversed through genetic ablation strategies (i.e., $IL15^{-/-}$) (183) or antibody-directed inhibition of uNK cells (184). It has also been suggested that uNK cell numbers are altered in pregnancy complications such as PE and IUGR, although contradictory data have been published. Reduced numbers of uNK cells in pregnancies with IUGR have been consistently demonstrated using different methods (226–229). Some studies also suggest a decrease of uNK cells (229) or of the $CD56^{+}/CD16^{+}$ uNK subset (228) in PE compared to healthy pregnancies. In contrast, others describe an elevated number of total uNK cells or of the $CD56^{+}/CD16^{+}$ subset in PE (230, 231). More recently, research has identified pre-existing health conditions of the mother that associate with low-grade inflammation, like obesity, that potentiate uNK cell activity and modify how uNK cells interact with fetal MHC ligand (207). However, although the *in utero* environment likely shapes uNK cell processes, to date, hard evidence showing that aberrantly activated uNK cells in humans directly target trophoblasts for killing has yet to be clearly demonstrated.

REGULATION OF EXTRAVILLOUS TROPHOBLASTS BY DECIDUAL MACROPHAGES

Next to uterine natural killer cells, macrophages are thought to comprise the second largest leukocyte population within the decidua (168, 232). Besides suggested contributions to spiral artery remodeling and immune modulation (12, 233), the function of decidual macrophages, in particular their effect on EVT activity, remains largely unknown. Although historically described for their function in immune defense, inflammation, and clearance of apoptotic cells, macrophages have also been recognized to play important roles in the development, homeostasis, and repair of various tissues (234).

Macrophages are usually classified into M1, representing a classical pro-inflammatory, anti-microbial activation or into M2, referring to an anti-inflammatory phenotype promoting wound healing. A body of growing evidence however suggests that M1 and M2 rather represent two extreme poles of a broad spectrum of macrophage polarization (235). The non-exclusivity of M1 and M2 macrophage phenotypes *in vivo* has likely several reasons. Firstly, it has been shown that macrophage activation statuses are reversible when specific stimuli change. Secondly, macrophages are often exposed to opposing activating signals *in vivo* (236). For instance, the co-existence of pro-inflammatory M1 and anti-inflammatory M2 profiles has been demonstrated in various mouse models and during tumor progression (237, 238). In light of these data it is not surprising that decidual macrophages also show a unique activation status with a dominating but not exclusive M2 phenotype. While decidual macrophages express typical M2 markers such as CD209 and CD206 and secrete the anti-inflammatory cytokines IL10 and TGFB, they were also shown to secrete pro-inflammatory cytokines including IL6 and TNF and the neutrophil chemoattractant CXCL8 (IL8) (239, 240). Nevertheless, the anti-inflammatory M2-related cytokines IL10 and M-CSF were shown to be important for inducing a decidual macrophage phenotype in peripheral blood monocytes (240). In addition, decidual macrophages were able to suppress T cell activity and induce Tregs *in vitro* (194, 241), which further strengthens the notion of an M2-dominated function. Two independent studies suggested the presence of two distinct decidual macrophage subpopulations, characterized by the absence or presence of the cell surface markers CD11c and ICAM3 (239, 240). Expression of these markers may at least partly relate to immature macrophages or blood contamination, as high levels of CD11c and ICAM3 are also found in blood monocytes. More recently, a study described three decidual macrophage subtypes, based on the expression or absence of CCR2 and CD11c. Using RNA sequencing and functional assays, the authors identified distinct functional states, including differences in phagocytosis, anti-oxidative, and anti-inflammatory activities, and proximity to EVTs (242). Whether these differences indeed account for unique subpopulations or reflect cellular plasticity and thus relate to phenotypical alterations awaits further clarification.

Due to their high abundance in the decidua, it is conceivable that macrophages markedly influence the local paracrine environment and thus EVT function. As follows, it is interesting to note that decidual macrophages are more abundant at the site of implantation and accumulate at the invasive front of EVTs (243, 244). There is growing evidence for a macrophage-guided growth-promoting function in various epithelia (245–247). Interestingly, both placental and decidual macrophages could promote proximal cell column proliferation by secreting the M2-associated (248, 249) factors IL33 and Wnt5a (167, 250). These data suggest that paracrine activity of decidual macrophages could be important for the initial steps in EVT formation. Furthermore, decidual macrophages have been shown to secrete a range of factors known to alter EVT motility (239), albeit with conflicting evidence as to whether they promote or restrict EVT invasion. For instance, while IL8 (153) was described as pro-invasive factor in the context of trophoblast migration, TNF (222) and IL10 (119) have been shown to inhibit EVT motility. The net effect of these factors on EVTs may be pro-invasive, anti-invasive, or neither. In addition, it is unclear under which circumstances decidual macrophages produce these opposing cytokines in terms of macrophage polarization and EVT response. Phenotypic macrophage polarization is controlled by a complex array of soluble factors provided by the local microenvironment and even dictated by extracellular matrix-dependent cell morphology (251). Moreover, ligand distribution within tissues is limited by a wide variety of factors, including limited diffusion capacities, endocytosis, and interaction with extracellular matrix proteins. It is therefore also important to consider the spatial relationship between macrophages and EVTs.

Unfortunately, there is limited information on the difference in macrophage distribution between decidua basalis and parietalis, and especially on whether these different tissue compartments harbor specific macrophage phenotypes. Immunohistochemical studies provided evidence for an enrichment of macrophages in the decidua basalis (243, 244), which has recently been confirmed via flow cytometric analysis (175), suggesting that macrophages preferentially accumulate in the vicinity of EVTs. In a similar context, it has been shown that binding between HLA-G homodimers and macrophage-associated leukocyte immunoglobulin-like receptor B1 (LILRB1) upregulates secretion of IL6, IL8, and TNF (212). Although it is not clear whether these effects relate to membrane-bound or soluble HLA-G, the presence of EVTs likely influences the macrophage phenotype and thus could substantially influence the paracrine activity of decidual macrophages.

ARE DECIDUAL MACROPHAGES ALTERED IN COMPLICATED PREGNANCIES?

Complicated pregnancies with IUGR or early-onset PE have repeatedly been associated with compromised EVT function. Several studies have tried to decipher whether aberrations in the decidual macrophage population could mediate these EVT defects, albeit with conflicting results. Some studies suggest an increase in macrophage numbers in preeclampsia compared to healthy pregnancies (252, 253). Further, an inverse relationship between macrophage infiltration and invasion of trophoblasts into arteries, with a shift toward macrophage infiltration in preeclamptic pregnancies, was shown (252). On the contrary, other studies point toward a decrease in the number of macrophages in IUGR and PE, compared to healthy pregnancies (229, 254). Still some additional studies found no significant differences in macrophage distribution and activation patterns between preeclamptic women and preterm labor controls (255).

In addition, it is unclear whether aberrant macrophage polarization could be associated with EVT defects in

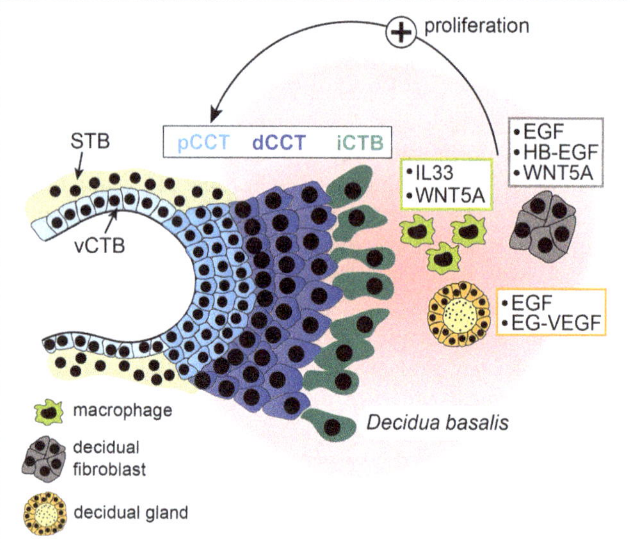

FIGURE 2 | Schematical depiction of soluble factors secreted from decidual macrophages, stromal cells, or glands. Mediators, stimulating proliferation of proximal cell column trophoblasts (pCCTs) in villous explant cultures are illustrated. dCCT, distal cell column trophoblast; STB, syncytiotrophoblast; vCTB, villous cytotrophoblast; iCTB, interstitial cytotrophoblast.

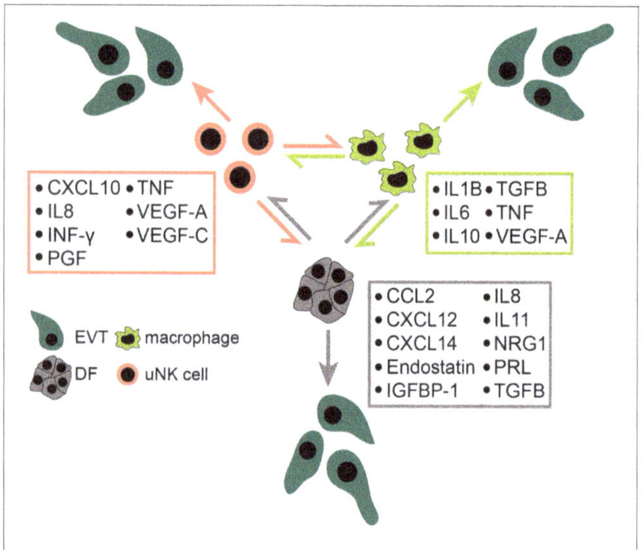

FIGURE 3 | Expression of decidual chemokines, cytokines and other soluble mediators affecting trophoblast migration and/or invasion. Some of the depicted factors likely play numerous roles at the fetal-maternal interface including activation and maturation of immune cells, as well as decidual angiogenesis and spiral artery remodeling. EVT, extravillous trophoblast; uNK cell, uterine natural killer cell; DF, decidual fibroblast.

the development of placental pathologies. In detail, some evidence exists that macrophages could display a more M1-like polarization in cases of PE, resulting in an exacerbated production of pro-inflammatory cytokines adversely affecting EVT function (256, 257). For instance, TNF has been shown to inhibit trophoblast motility in villous explant cultures (222). A study utilizing a rat model, demonstrating that systematic LPS injection results in IUGR and PE-like symptoms, also reported increased levels of TNF and exacerbated numbers of uteroplacental macrophages (258). Unfortunately, the authors did not further elucidate whether LPS-induced systemic inflammation also changes the phenotype of decidual macrophages. Nevertheless, whether a shift toward a pro-inflammatory M1-like macrophage phenotype indeed adversely affects EVT function has not been proven. As mentioned above, M2-related anti-inflammatory cytokines such as TGFB or IL10 were also reported to exert adverse effects on EVTs by restricting their migratory potential. Conversely, macrophages isolated from miscarriages showed reduced expression of IL6 and IL8, the latter with pro-invasive potential toward EVTs (153). In summary, studies investigating the functional interplay between primary macrophage and EVT cultures are scarce. Thus, the particular role of macrophages in the context of EVT function remains unclear both in healthy and complicated pregnancies. Unfortunately, there is also limited availability of suitable human *in vitro* systems to study this interaction. Immortalized monocytic cell lines, such as THP-1 cells, do not represent a useful model system for decidual macrophages due to their massive genomic rearrangements and their phenotypic and functional differences (259). It is still unclear whether the decidua-specific macrophage phenotype can be sustained in isolated primary cells or mimicked by controlled differentiation of peripheral blood monocytes *in vitro*. Moreover, more information is needed on whether macrophages change their polarization and secretory profile depending on their location within the human decidua. Finally, the long lasting paradigm of macrophage differentiation from recruited monocytes has been challenged by numerous studies demonstrating that macrophages are also maintained throughout adult life by a tissue-resident, proliferative population originating from embryonic or yolk sac-derived precursors (260, 261). In mice, tissue-resident macrophage populations, such as liver Kupffer cells (262), epidermal Langerhans cells (263), microglia (264), and pleural macrophages (265), were shown to be able to proliferate and renew independently from the bone marrow. Although very few data have been generated so far to confirm the existence of tissue-resident macrophages in humans, it is interesting to note that decidual, tissue-resident $CD34^+$ stromal cells were described to differentiate into functional $CD56^+$ uNK cells (266). Moreover, a recent study shows that continuous pregnancies induce a pregnancy-promoting memory uNK subset which differentiates from progenitors residing in the post-gravid endometrium (267). Additional studies, confirming the existence of tissue-resident NK cells and T cells in other tissues, strengthen the idea of an organ-specific immunity that is maintained independently of the bone marrow and secondary lymph nodes (268, 269). Intriguingly, several reports describe the proliferative signature of decidual macrophages (270, 271), supporting the idea that tissue-resident macrophages could be maintained in the uterus by local proliferation. On the other hand, both EVTs and decidual macrophages produce monocyte-recruiting chemokines, such as CCL2 (148, 149) or CCL4 (148, 239) suggesting a contribution of monocytes to the pool of decidual macrophages in early pregnancy. In light of these data it is still not clear whether the endometrium is continuously populated by bone marrow-derived monocytes or whether local progenitors mainly repopulate within the tissue.

SUMMARY

The influence of soluble decidual factors on trophoblast proliferation, migration and invasion has been intensively investigated using different trophoblast cell models including cell lines and primary CTBs containing a mixture of different trophoblast subtypes. However, studies about the effects of secreted proteins on cell column proliferation of the anchoring villus are scarce. Moreover, isolated primary CCTs rapidly cease proliferation in culture and undergo differentiation (57), impairing their usability for proliferation assays. Hence, only few factors were convincingly shown to promote CCT expansion using first trimester villous explant cultures (**Figure 2**). Recently however, self-renewing trophoblast stem cells and organoids have been developed (64, 272). These culture systems should allow more reliable investigations on the role of decidual growth factors in trophoblast progenitor growth, EVT formation and differentiation. Furthermore, DFs, macrophages and uNK cells express a plethora of cytokines, chemokines and soluble factors, some of which are detectable in more than one cell type (**Figure 3**). Although the majority of these proteins likely control trophoblast invasion and/or migration the prime decidual target cell of an individual factor remains elusive. Besides their presumptive role in trophoblast motility, chemokines and cytokines could regulate immune cell recruitment and mutual activation of macrophages, uNK cells and DFs as well as other less abundant immune cells of the fetal-maternal interface.

AUTHOR CONTRIBUTIONS

The manuscript was written by JP, AGB, and MK and edited by SV and JB. JP provided the graphical illustrations.

FUNDING

The present work was supported by Austrian Science Fund (grant P-28417-B30 to MK), the Austrian National Bank (grant 17613 to JP) and a Canadian Institutes of Health Research (CIHR) Open Operating Grant (201403MOP-325905-CIA-CAAA) to AGB.

REFERENCES

1. Hamilton WJ, Boyd JD. Development of the human placenta in the first three months of gestation. *J Anat* (1960) 94:297–328.
2. Castellucci M, Scheper M, Scheffen I, Celona A, Kaufmann P. The development of the human placental villous tree. *Anat Embryol.* (1990) 181:117–28. doi: 10.1007/BF00198951
3. Jones CJ, Fox H. Ultrastructure of the normal human placenta. *Electron Microsc Rev.* (1991) 4:129–78. doi: 10.1016/0892-0354(91)90019-9
4. Evain-Brion D, Malassine A. Human placenta as an endocrine organ. *Growth Horm IGF Res* (2003) 13 (Suppl. A):S34-37. doi: 10.1016/S1096-6374(03)00053-4
5. Aplin JD. Developmental cell biology of human villous trophoblast: current research problems. *Int J Dev Biol.* (2010) 54:323-9. doi: 10.1387/ijdb.082759ja
6. Burton GJ, Jauniaux E, Charnock-Jones DS. The influence of the intrauterine environment on human placental development. *Int J Dev Biol.* (2010) 54:303–12. doi: 10.1387/ijdb.082764gb
7. Pijnenborg R, Bland JM, Robertson WB, Brosens I. Uteroplacental arterial changes related to interstitial trophoblast migration in early human pregnancy. *Placenta* (1983) 4:397–413. doi: 10.1016/S0143-4004(83)80043-5
8. Pijnenborg R, Dixon G, Robertson WB, Brosens I. Trophoblastic invasion of human decidua from 8 to 18 weeks of pregnancy. *Placenta* (1980) 1:3–19. doi: 10.1016/S0143-4004(80)80012-9
9. Hustin J, Jauniaux E, Schaaps JP. Histological study of the materno-embryonic interface in spontaneous abortion. *Placenta* (1990) 11:477–86. doi: 10.1016/S0143-4004(05)80193-6
10. Brosens I, Robertson WB, Dixon HG. The physiological response of the vessels of the placental bed to normal pregnancy. *J Pathol Bacteriol.*(1967) 93:569–79. doi: 10.1002/path.1700930218
11. Pijnenborg R, Vercruysse L, Hanssens M. The uterine spiral arteries in human pregnancy: facts and controversies. *Placenta* (2006) 27:939–58. doi: 10.1016/j.placenta.2005.12.006
12. Harris LK. IFPA gabor than award lecture: transformation of the spiral arteries in human pregnancy: key events in the remodelling timeline. *Placenta* (2011) 32 (Suppl. 2):S154–8. doi: 10.1016/j.placenta.2010.11.018
13. King A, Wellings V, Gardner L, Loke YW. Immunocytochemical characterization of the unusual large granular lymphocytes in human endometrium throughout the menstrual cycle. *Hum Immunol.* (1989) 24:195–205. doi: 10.1016/0198-8859(89)90060-8
14. Smith SD, Dunk CE, Aplin JD, Harris LK, Jones RL. Evidence for immune cell involvement in decidual spiral arteriole remodeling in early human pregnancy. *Am J Pathol.* (2009) 174:1959–71. doi: 10.2353/ajpath.2009.080995
15. Zhou Y, Fisher SJ, Janatpour M, Genbacev O, Dejana E, Wheelock M, et al. Human cytotrophoblasts adopt a vascular phenotype as they differentiate. A strategy for successful endovascular invasion? *J Clin Invest.* (1997) 99:2139–51.
16. Khong TY, De Wolf F, Robertson WB, Brosens I. Inadequate maternal vascular response to placentation in pregnancies complicated by pre-eclampsia and by small-for-gestational age infants. *Br J Obstet Gynaecol.* (1986) 93:1049–59. doi: 10.1111/j.1471-0528.1986.tb07830.x
17. Pijnenborg R, Anthony J, Davey DA, Rees A, Tiltman A, Vercruysse L, et al. Placental bed spiral arteries in the hypertensive disorders of pregnancy. *Br J Obstet Gynaecol.* (1991) 98:648–55. doi: 10.1111/j.1471-0528.1991.tb13450.x
18. Romero R, Kusanovic JP, Chaiworapongsa T, Hassan SS. Placental bed disorders in preterm labor, preterm PROM, spontaneous abortion and abruptio placentae. *Best Pract Res Clin Obstet Gynaecol.* (2011) 25:313–27. doi: 10.1016/j.bpobgyn.2011.02.006
19. Fisher SJ. Why is placentation abnormal in preeclampsia? *Am J Obstet Gynecol.*(2015) 213:S115–122. doi: 10.1016/j.ajog.2015.08.042
20. Zhou Y, Damsky CH, Fisher SJ. Preeclampsia is associated with failure of human cytotrophoblasts to mimic a vascular adhesion phenotype. One cause of defective endovascular invasion in this syndrome? *J Clin Invest* (1997) 99:2152–64.
21. Zhou Y, Gormley MJ, Hunkapiller NM, Kapidzic M, Stolyarov Y, Feng V, et al. Reversal of gene dysregulation in cultured cytotrophoblasts reveals possible causes of preeclampsia. *J Clin Invest.* (2013) 123:2862–72. doi: 10.1172/JCI66966
22. Moffett A, Colucci F. Uterine NK cells: active regulators at the maternal-fetal interface. *J Clin Invest.* (2014) 124:1872–9. doi: 10.1172/JCI68107
23. Schatz F, Guzeloglu-Kayisli O, Arlier S, Kayisli UA, Lockwood CJ. The role of decidual cells in uterine hemostasis, menstruation, inflammation, adverse pregnancy outcomes and abnormal uterine bleeding. *Hum Reprod Update* (2016) 22:497–515. doi: 10.1093/humupd/dmw004

24. Burton GJ, Jauniaux E. The cytotrophoblastic shell and complications of pregnancy. *Placenta* (2017) 60:134–9. doi: 10.1016/j.placenta.2017.06.007
25. He N, van Iperen L, de Jong D, Szuhai K, Helmerhorst FM, van der Westerlaken LA, et al. Human extravillous trophoblasts penetrate decidual veins and lymphatics before remodeling spiral arteries during early pregnancy. *PLoS ONE* (2017) 12:e0169849. doi: 10.1371/journal.pone.0169849
26. Windsperger K, Dekan S, Pils S, Golletz C, Kunihs V, Fiala C, et al. Extravillous trophoblast invasion of venous as well as lymphatic vessels is altered in idiopathic, recurrent, spontaneous abortions. *Hum Reprod.* (2017) 32:1208–17. doi: 10.1093/humrep/dex058
27. Moser G, Weiss G, Sundl M, Gauster M, Siwetz M, Lang-Olip I, et al. Extravillous trophoblasts invade more than uterine arteries: evidence for the invasion of uterine veins. *Histochem Cell Biol.* (2017) 147:353–66. doi: 10.1007/s00418-016-1509-5
28. Moser G, Weiss G, Gauster M, Sundl M, Huppertz B. Evidence from the very beginning: endoglandular trophoblasts penetrate and replace uterine glands *in situ* and *in vitro*. *Hum Reprod* (2015) 30:2747–57. doi: 10.1093/humrep/dev266
29. Bulmer JN, Williams PJ, Lash GE. Immune cells in the placental bed. *Int J Dev Biol.* (2010) 54:281–94. doi: 10.1387/ijdb.082763jb
30. Wallace AE, Fraser R, Cartwright JE. Extravillous trophoblast and decidual natural killer cells: a remodelling partnership. *Hum Reprod Update* (2012) 18:458–71. doi: 10.1093/humupd/dms015
31. Hiby SE, Walker JJ, O'Shaughnessy KM, Redman CW, Carrington M, Trowsdale J, et al. Combinations of maternal KIR and fetal HLA-C genes influence the risk of preeclampsia and reproductive success. *J Exp Med.* (2004) 200:957–965. doi: 10.1084/jem.20041214
32. Hiby SE, Regan L, Lo W, Farrell L, Carrington M, Moffett A. Association of maternal killer-cell immunoglobulin-like receptors and parental HLA-C genotypes with recurrent miscarriage. *Hum Reprod.* (2008) 23:972–6. doi: 10.1093/humrep/den011
33. Hanna J, Mandelboim O. When killers become helpers. *Trends Immunol.* (2007) 28:201–6. doi: 10.1016/j.it.2007.03.005
34. Manaster I, Mandelboim O. The unique properties of uterine NK cells. *Am J Reprod Immunol.* (2010) 63:434–44. doi: 10.1111/j.1600-0897.2009.00794.x
35. Moffett A, Colucci F. Co-evolution of NK receptors and HLA ligands in humans is driven by reproduction. *Immunol Rev.* (2015) 267:283–97. doi: 10.1111/imr.12323
36. Moffett A, Chazara O, Colucci F. Maternal allo-recognition of the fetus. *Fertil Steril.* (2017) 107:1269–72. doi: 10.1016/j.fertnstert.2017.05.001
37. Knofler M. Critical growth factors and signalling pathways controlling human trophoblast invasion. *Int J Dev Biol.* (2010) 54:269–80. doi: 10.1387/ijdb.082769mk
38. Knofler M, Pollheimer J. IFPA Award in Placentology lecture: molecular regulation of human trophoblast invasion. *Placenta* (2012) 33 (Suppl.):S55–62. doi: 10.1016/j.placenta.2011.09.019
39. Kovats S, Main EK, Librach C, Stubblebine M, Fisher SJ, DeMars R. A class I antigen, HLA-G, expressed in human trophoblasts. *Science* (1990) 248:220–3. doi: 10.1126/science.2326636
40. Pollheimer J, Loregger T, Sonderegger S, Saleh L, Bauer S, Bilban M, et al. Activation of the canonical wingless/T-cell factor signaling pathway promotes invasive differentiation of human trophoblast. *Am J Pathol.* (2006) 168:1134–47. doi: 10.2353/ajpath.2006.050686
41. Damsky CH, Fitzgerald ML, Fisher SJ. Distribution patterns of extracellular matrix components and adhesion receptors are intricately modulated during first trimester cytotrophoblast differentiation along the invasive pathway, *in vivo*. *J Clin Invest.* (1992) 89:210–22. doi: 10.1172/JCI115565
42. Plessl K, Haider S, Fiala C, Pollheimer J, Knofler M. Expression pattern and function of Notch2 in different subtypes of first trimester cytotrophoblast. *Placenta* (2015) 36:365–71. doi: 10.1016/j.placenta.2015.01.009
43. Fock V, Plessl K, Draxler P, Otti GR, Fiala C, Knofler M, et al. Neuregulin-1-mediated ErbB2-ErbB3 signalling protects human trophoblasts against apoptosis to preserve differentiation. *J Cell Sci.* (2015) 128:4306–16. doi: 10.1242/jcs.176933
44. Aghababaei M, Perdu S, Irvine K, Beristain AG. A disintegrin and metalloproteinase 12 (ADAM12) localizes to invasive trophoblast, promotes cell invasion and directs column outgrowth in early placental development. *Mol Hum Reprod.* (2013) 20:235–49. doi: 10.1093/molehr/gat084
45. Biadasiewicz K, Fock V, Dekan S, Proestling K, Velicky P, Haider S, et al. Extravillous trophoblast-associated ADAM12 exerts pro-invasive properties, including induction of integrin beta 1-mediated cellular spreading. *Biol Reprod.* (2014) 90:101. doi: 10.1095/biolreprod.113.115279
46. Velicky P, Windsperger K, Petroczi K, Pils S, Reiter B, Weiss T, et al. Pregnancy-associated diamine oxidase originates from extravillous trophoblasts and is decreased in early-onset preeclampsia. *Sci Rep.* (2018) 8:6342. doi: 10.1038/s41598-018-24652-0
47. Liu Y, Fan X, Wang R, Lu X, Dang YL, Wang H, et al. Single-cell RNA-seq reveals the diversity of trophoblast subtypes and patterns of differentiation in the human placenta. *Cell Res* (2018) 28:819–32. doi: 10.1038/s41422-018-0066-y
48. Genbacev O, Jensen KD, Powlin SS, Miller RK. In vitro differentiation and ultrastructure of human extravillous trophoblast (EVT) cells. *Placenta* (1993) 14:463–75. doi: 10.1016/S0143-4004(05)80466-7
49. Vicovac L, Jones CJ, Aplin JD. Trophoblast differentiation during formation of anchoring villi in a model of the early human placenta *in vitro*. *Placenta* (1995) 16:41–56. doi: 10.1016/0143-4004(95)90080-2
50. Pollheimer J, Haslinger P, Fock V, Prast J, Saleh L, Biadasiewicz K, et al. Endostatin suppresses IGF-II-mediated signaling and invasion of human extravillous trophoblasts. *Endocrinology* (2011) 152:4431–42. doi: 10.1210/en.2011-1196
51. Lim KH, Zhou Y, Janatpour M, McMaster M, Bass K, Chun SH, et al. Human cytotrophoblast differentiation/invasion is abnormal in pre-eclampsia. *Am J Pathol.* (1997) 151:1809–18.
52. Goffin F, Munaut C, Malassine A, Evain-Brion D, Frankenne F, Fridman V, et al. Evidence of a limited contribution of feto-maternal interactions to trophoblast differentiation along the invasive pathway. *Tissue Antigens* (2003) 62:104–16. doi: 10.1034/j.1399-0039.2003.00085.x
53. Red-Horse K, Rivera J, Schanz A, Zhou Y, Winn V, Kapidzic M, et al. Cytotrophoblast induction of arterial apoptosis and lymphangiogenesis in an *in vivo* model of human placentation. *J Clin Invest.* (2006) 116:2643–52. doi: 10.1172/JCI27306
54. Bilban M, Haslinger P, Prast J, Klinglmuller F, Woelfel T, Haider S, et al. Identification of novel trophoblast invasion-related genes: heme oxygenase-1 controls motility via peroxisome proliferator-activated receptor gamma. *Endocrinology* (2009) 150:1000–13. doi: 10.1210/en.2008-0456
55. Apps R, Sharkey A, Gardner L, Male V, Trotter M, Miller N, et al. Genome-wide expression profile of first trimester villous and extravillous human trophoblast cells. *Placenta* (2011) 32:33–43. doi: 10.1016/j.placenta.2010.10.010
56. Haider S, Meinhardt G, Velicky P, Otti GR, Whitley G, Fiala C, et al. Notch signaling plays a critical role in motility and differentiation of human first-trimester cytotrophoblasts. *Endocrinology* (2014) 155:263–74. doi: 10.1210/en.2013-1455
57. Haider S, Meinhardt G, Saleh L, Fiala C, Pollheimer J, Knofler M. Notch1 controls development of the extravillous trophoblast lineage in the human placenta. *Proc Natl Acad Sci USA.* (2016) 113:E7710–E7719. doi: 10.1073/pnas.1612335113
58. Rodesch F, Simon P, Donner C, Jauniaux E. Oxygen measurements in endometrial and trophoblastic tissues during early pregnancy. *Obstet Gynecol.* (1992) 80:283–5.
59. Wakeland AK, Soncin F, Moretto-Zita M, Chang CW, Horii M, Pizzo D, et al. Hypoxia directs human extravillous trophoblast differentiation in a hypoxia-inducible factor-dependent manner. *Am J Pathol.* (2017) 187:767–80. doi: 10.1016/j.ajpath.2016.11.018
60. James JL, Stone PR, Chamley LW. The regulation of trophoblast differentiation by oxygen in the first trimester of pregnancy. *Hum Reprod Update* (2006) 12:137–44. doi: 10.1093/humupd/dmi043
61. Tuuli MG, Longtine MS, Nelson DM. Review: oxygen and trophoblast biology–a source of controversy. *Placenta* (2011) 32 (Suppl. 2):S109–18. doi: 10.1016/j.placenta.2010.12.013
62. Soares MJ, Iqbal K, Kozai K. Hypoxia and placental development. *Birth Defects Res.* (2017) 109:1309–29. doi: 10.1002/bdr2.1135
63. Chang CW, Wakeland AK, Parast MM. Trophoblast lineage specification, differentiation and their regulation by oxygen tension. *J Endocrinol.* (2018) 236:R43–56. doi: 10.1530/JOE-17-0402
64. Haider S, Meinhardt G, Saleh L, Kunihs V, Gamperl M, Kaindl U, et al. Self-renewing trophoblast organoids recapitulate the developmental

program of the early human placenta. *Stem Cell Reports* (2018) 11:537–51. doi: 10.1016/j.stemcr.2018.07.004
65. Ramsey EM, Houston ML, Harris JW. Interactions of the trophoblast and maternal tissues in three closely related primate species. *Am J Obstet Gynecol.* (1976) 124:647–52. doi: 10.1016/0002-9378(76)90068-5
66. Emera D, Romero R, Wagner G. The evolution of menstruation: a new model for genetic assimilation: explaining molecular origins of maternal responses to fetal invasiveness. *Bioessays* (2012) 34:26–35. doi: 10.1002/bies.201100099
67. Gellersen B, Brosens IA, Brosens JJ. Decidualization of the human endometrium: mechanisms, functions, and clinical perspectives. *Semin Reprod Med.* (2007) 25:445–53. doi: 10.1055/s-2007-991042
68. Burton GJ, Watson AL, Hempstock J, Skepper JN, Jauniaux E. Uterine glands provide histiotrophic nutrition for the human fetus during the first trimester of pregnancy. *J Clin Endocrinol Metab.* (2002) 87:2954–9. doi: 10.1210/jcem.87.6.8563
69. Hempstock J, Cindrova-Davies T, Jauniaux E, Burton GJ. Endometrial glands as a source of nutrients, growth factors and cytokines during the first trimester of human pregnancy: a morphological and immunohistochemical study. *Reprod Biol Endocrinol.* (2004) 2:58. doi: 10.1186/1477-7827-2-58
70. Burton GJ, Jauniaux E, Charnock-Jones DS. Human early placental development: potential roles of the endometrial glands. *Placenta* (2007) 28 (Suppl. A):S64–69. doi: 10.1016/j.placenta.2007.01.007
71. Charnock-Jones DS, Sharkey AM, Fenwick P, Smith SK. Leukaemia inhibitory factor mRNA concentration peaks in human endometrium at the time of implantation and the blastocyst contains mRNA for the receptor at this time. *J Reprod Fertil.* (1994) 101:421–6. doi: 10.1530/jrf.0.1010421
72. Cullinan EB, Abbondanzo SJ, Anderson PS, Pollard JW, Lessey BA, Stewart CL. Leukemia inhibitory factor (LIF) and LIF receptor expression in human endometrium suggests a potential autocrine/paracrine function in regulating embryo implantation. *Proc Natl Acad Sci U S A* (1996) 93:3115–20. doi: 10.1073/pnas.93.7.3115
73. Hornung D, Lebovic DI, Shifren JL, Vigne JL, Taylor RN. Vectorial secretion of vascular endothelial growth factor by polarized human endometrial epithelial cells. *Fertil Steril.* (1998) 69:909–15. doi: 10.1016/S0015-0282(98)00044-2
74. Ngan ES, Lee KY, Yeung WS, Ngan HY, Ng EH, Ho PC. Endocrine gland-derived vascular endothelial growth factor is expressed in human peri-implantation endometrium, but not in endometrial carcinoma. *Endocrinology* (2006) 147:88–95. doi: 10.1210/en.2005-0543
75. Brouillet S, Murthi P, Hoffmann P, Salomon A, Sergent F, De Mazancourt P, et al. EG-VEGF controls placental growth and survival in normal and pathological pregnancies: case of fetal growth restriction (FGR). *Cell Mol Life Sci.* (2013) 70:511–25. doi: 10.1007/s00018-012-1141-z
76. Athanassiades A, Hamilton GS, Lala PK. Vascular endothelial growth factor stimulates proliferation but not migration or invasiveness in human extravillous trophoblast. *Biol Reprod.* (1998) 59:643–54. doi: 10.1095/biolreprod59.3.643
77. Bischof P, Haenggeli L, Campana A. Effect of leukemia inhibitory factor on human cytotrophoblast differentiation along the invasive pathway. *Am J Reprod Immunol.* (1995) 34:225–30. doi: 10.1111/j.1600-0897.1995.tb00945.x
78. Nachtigall MJ, Kliman HJ, Feinberg RF, Olive DL, Engin O, Arici A. The effect of leukemia inhibitory factor (LIF) on trophoblast differentiation: a potential role in human implantation. *J Clin Endocrinol Metab.* (1996) 81:801–6.
79. Paiva P, Menkhorst E, Salamonsen L, Dimitriadis E. Leukemia inhibitory factor and interleukin-11: critical regulators in the establishment of pregnancy. *Cytokine Growth Factor Rev.* (2009) 20:319–28. doi: 10.1016/j.cytogfr.2009.07.001
80. Gellersen B, Brosens JJ. Cyclic decidualization of the human endometrium in reproductive health and failure. *Endocr Rev.* (2014) 35:851–905. doi: 10.1210/er.2014-1045
81. Kajihara T, Jones M, Fusi L, Takano M, Feroze-Zaidi F, Pirianov G, et al. Differential expression of FOXO1 and FOXO3a confers resistance to oxidative cell death upon endometrial decidualization. *Mol Endocrinol.* (2006) 20:2444–55. doi: 10.1210/me.2006-0118
82. Kajihara T, Uchino S, Suzuki M, Itakura A, Brosens JJ, Ishihara O. Human chorionic gonadotropin confers resistance to oxidative stress-induced apoptosis in decidualizing human endometrial stromal cells. *Fertil Steril.* (2011) 95:1302–7. doi: 10.1016/j.fertnstert.2010.05.048
83. Aplin JD, Charlton AK, Ayad S. An immunohistochemical study of human endometrial extracellular matrix during the menstrual cycle and first trimester of pregnancy. *Cell Tissue Res.* (1988) 253:231–40. doi: 10.1007/BF00221758
84. Church HJ, Vicovac LM, Williams JD, Hey NA, Aplin JD. Laminins 2 and 4 are expressed by human decidual cells. *Lab Invest.* (1996) 74:21–32.
85. Xu G, Guimond MJ, Chakraborty C, Lala PK. Control of proliferation, migration, and invasiveness of human extravillous trophoblast by decorin, a decidual product. *Biol Reprod.* (2002) 67:681–9. doi: 10.1095/biolreprod67.2.681
86. Winship A, Cuman C, Rainczuk K, Dimitriadis E. Fibulin-5 is upregulated in decidualized human endometrial stromal cells and promotes primary human extravillous trophoblast outgrowth. *Placenta* (2015) 36:1405–11. doi: 10.1016/j.placenta.2015.10.008
87. Harris LK, Jones CJ, Aplin JD. Adhesion molecules in human trophoblast - a review. II extravillous trophoblast. *Placenta* (2009) 30:299–304. doi: 10.1016/j.placenta.2008.12.003
88. Tantbirojn P, Crum CP, Parast MM. Pathophysiology of placenta creta: the role of decidua and extravillous trophoblast. *Placenta* (2008) 29:639–45. doi: 10.1016/j.placenta.2008.04.008
89. Hannon T, Innes BA, Lash GE, Bulmer JN, Robson SC. Effects of local decidua on trophoblast invasion and spiral artery remodeling in focal placenta creta - an immunohistochemical study. *Placenta* (2012) 33:998–1004. doi: 10.1016/j.placenta.2012.09.004
90. Lala PK, Graham CH. Mechanisms of trophoblast invasiveness and their control: the role of proteases and protease inhibitors. *Cancer Metastasis Rev.* (1990) 9:369–79. doi: 10.1007/BF00049525
91. Bischof P, Meisser A, Campana A. Paracrine and autocrine regulators of trophoblast invasion–a review. *Placenta* (2000) 21 (Suppl. A):S55–60. doi: 10.1053/plac.2000.0521
92. Queenan JTJr, Kao LC, Arboleda CE, Ulloa-Aguirre A, Golos TG, Cines DB, et al. Regulation of urokinase-type plasminogen activator production by cultured human cytotrophoblasts. *J Biol Chem* (1987) 262:10903–6.
93. Feinberg RF, Kao LC, Haimowitz JE, Queenan JT Jr, Wun TC, Strauss JF III, et al. Plasminogen activator inhibitor types 1 and 2 in human trophoblasts. PAI-1 is an immunocytochemical marker of invading trophoblasts. *Lab Invest.* (1989) 61:20–6.
94. Fisher SJ, Cui TY, Zhang L, Hartman L, Grahl K, Zhang GY, et al. Adhesive and degradative properties of human placental cytotrophoblast cells *in vitro*. *J Cell Biol* (1989) 109:891–902. doi: 10.1083/jcb.109.2.891
95. Zini JM, Murray SC, Graham CH, Lala PK, Kariko K, Barnathan ES, et al. Characterization of urokinase receptor expression by human placental trophoblasts. *Blood* (1992) 79:2917–29.
96. Schatz F, Lockwood CJ. Progestin regulation of plasminogen activator inhibitor type 1 in primary cultures of endometrial stromal and decidual cells. *J Clin Endocrinol Metab.* (1993) 77:621–5.
97. Bogic LV, Ohira RH, Yamamoto SY, Okazaki KJ, Millar K, Bryant-Greenwood GD. Tissue plasminogen activator and its receptor in the human amnion, chorion, and decidua at preterm and term. *Biol Reprod.* (1999) 60:1006–12. doi: 10.1095/biolreprod60.4.1006
98. Plaisier M, Koolwijk P, Willems F, Helmerhorst FM, van Hinsbergh VW. Pericellular-acting proteases in human first trimester decidua. *Mol Hum Reprod.* (2008) 14:41–51. doi: 10.1093/molehr/gam085
99. Chen CP, Bajoria R, Aplin JD. Decreased vascularization and cell proliferation in placentas of intrauterine growth-restricted fetuses with abnormal umbilical artery flow velocity waveforms. *Am J Obstet Gynecol.* (2002) 187:764–9. doi: 10.1067/mob.2002.125243
100. Lopez-Mejia IC, De Toledo M, Della Seta F, Fafet P, Rebouissou C, Deleuze V, et al. Tissue-specific and SRSF1-dependent splicing of fibronectin, a matrix protein that controls host cell invasion. *Mol Biol Cell* (2013) 24:3164–76. doi: 10.1091/mbc.e13-03-0142
101. Weimar CH, Macklon NS, Post Uiterweer ED, Brosens JJ, Gellersen B. The motile and invasive capacity of human endometrial stromal cells: implications for normal and impaired reproductive function. *Hum Reprod Update* (2013) 19:542–57. doi: 10.1093/humupd/dmt025

102. Schwenke M, Knofler M, Velicky P, Weimar CH, Kruse M, Samalecos A, et al. Control of human endometrial stromal cell motility by PDGF-BB, HB-EGF and trophoblast-secreted factors. *PLoS ONE* (2013) 8:e54336. doi: 10.1371/journal.pone.0054336
103. Hess AP, Hamilton AE, Talbi S, Dosiou C, Nyegaard M, Nayak N, et al. Decidual stromal cell response to paracrine signals from the trophoblast: amplification of immune and angiogenic modulators. *Biol Reprod.* (2007) 76:102–17. doi: 10.1095/biolreprod.106.054791
104. Tilburgs T, Crespo AC, van der Zwan A, Rybalov B, Raj T, Stranger B, et al. Human HLA-G+ extravillous trophoblasts: Immune-activating cells that interact with decidual leukocytes. *Proc Natl Acad Sci USA* (2015) 112:7219–24. doi: 10.1073/pnas.1507977112
105. Apps R, Murphy SP, Fernando R, Gardner L, Ahad T, Moffett A. Human leucocyte antigen (HLA) expression of primary trophoblast cells and placental cell lines, determined using single antigen beads to characterize allotype specificities of anti-HLA antibodies. *Immunology* (2009) 127:26–39. doi: 10.1111/j.1365-2567.2008.03019.x
106. Bilban M, Tauber S, Haslinger P, Pollheimer J, Saleh L, Pehamberger H, et al. Trophoblast invasion: assessment of cellular models using gene expression signatures. *Placenta* (2010) 31:989–96. doi: 10.1016/j.placenta.2010.08.011
107. Genbacev O, Joslin R, Damsky CH, Polliotti BM, Fisher SJ. Hypoxia alters early gestation human cytotrophoblast differentiation/invasion *in vitro* and models the placental defects that occur in preeclampsia. *J Clin Invest.* (1996) 97:540–50. doi: 10.1172/JCI118447
108. Lash GE, Hornbuckle J, Brunt A, Kirkley M, Searle RF, Robson SC, et al. Effect of low oxygen concentrations on trophoblast-like cell line invasion. *Placenta* (2007) 28:390–8. doi: 10.1016/j.placenta.2006.06.001
109. Selick CE, Horowitz GM, Gratch M, Scott RTJr, Navot D, Hofmann GE. Immunohistochemical localization of transforming growth factor-beta in human implantation sites. *J Clin Endocrinol Metab.* (1994) 78:592–6.
110. Lash GE, Schiessl B, Kirkley M, Innes BA, Cooper A, Searle RF, et al. Expression of angiogenic growth factors by uterine natural killer cells during early pregnancy. *J Leukoc Biol.* (2006) 80:572–80. doi: 10.1189/jlb.0406250
111. Graham CH, Lysiak JJ, McCrae KR, Lala PK. Localization of transforming growth factor-beta at the human fetal-maternal interface: role in trophoblast growth and differentiation. *Biol Reprod.* (1992) 46:561–72. doi: 10.1095/biolreprod46.4.561
112. Forbes K, Souquet B, Garside R, Aplin JD, Westwood M. Transforming growth factor-{beta} (TGF{beta}) receptors I/II differentially regulate TGF{beta}1 and IGF-binding protein-3 mitogenic effects in the human placenta. *Endocrinology* (2010) 151:1723–31. doi: 10.1210/en.2009-0896
113. Cheng JC, Chang HM, Leung PC. Transforming growth factor-beta1 inhibits trophoblast cell invasion by inducing Snail-mediated down-regulation of vascular endothelial-cadherin protein. *J Biol Chem.* (2013) 288:33181–92. doi: 10.1074/jbc.M113.488866
114. Prossler J, Chen Q, Chamley L, James JL. The relationship between TGFbeta, low oxygen and the outgrowth of extravillous trophoblasts from anchoring villi during the first trimester of pregnancy. *Cytokine* (2014) 68:9–15. doi: 10.1016/j.cyto.2014.03.001
115. Xu J, Sivasubramaniyam T, Yinon Y, Tagliaferro A, Ray J, Nevo O, et al. Aberrant TGFbeta signaling contributes to altered trophoblast differentiation in preeclampsia. *Endocrinology* (2016) 157:883–99. doi: 10.1210/en.2015-1696
116. Wolf K, Te Lindert M, Krause M, Alexander S, Te Riet J, Willis AL, et al. Physical limits of cell migration: control by ECM space and nuclear deformation and tuning by proteolysis and traction force. *J Cell Biol.* (2013) 201:1069–84. doi: 10.1083/jcb.201210152
117. Zybina TG, Kaufmann P, Frank HG, Freed J, Kadyrov M, Biesterfeld S. Genome multiplication of extravillous trophoblast cells in human placenta in the course of differentiation and invasion into endometrium and myometrium. I Dynamics of polyploidization. *Tsitologiia* (2002) 44:1058–67.
118. Zybina TG, Frank HG, Biesterfeld S, Kaufmann P. Genome multiplication of extravillous trophoblast cells in human placenta in the course of differentiation and invasion into endometrium and myometrium. II Mechanisms of polyploidization. *Tsitologiia* (2004) 46:640–8.
119. Roth I, Fisher SJ. IL-10 is an autocrine inhibitor of human placental cytotrophoblast MMP-9 production and invasion. *Dev Biol.* (1999) 205:194–204. doi: 10.1006/dbio.1998.9122
120. Renaud SJ, Macdonald-Goodfellow SK, Graham CH. Coordinated regulation of human trophoblast invasiveness by macrophages and interleukin 10. *Biol Reprod.* (2007) 76:448–54. doi: 10.1095/biolreprod.106.055376
121. Genbacev O, Schubach SA, Miller RK. Villous culture of first trimester human placenta–model to study extravillous trophoblast (EVT) differentiation. *Placenta* (1992) 13:439–61. doi: 10.1016/0143-4004(92)90051-T
122. Riddick DH, Luciano AA, Kusmik WF, Maslar IA. De novo synthesis of prolactin by human decidua. *Life Sci.* (1978) 23:1913–21. doi: 10.1016/0024-3205(78)90557-X
123. Golander A, Hurley T, Barrett J, Handwerger S. Synthesis of prolactin by human decidua *in vitro*. *J Endocrinol.* (1979) 82:263–7. doi: 10.1677/joe.0.0820263
124. Rutanen EM, Koistinen R, Wahlstrom T, Bohn H, Ranta T, Seppala M. Synthesis of placental protein 12 by human decidua. *Endocrinology* (1985) 116:1304–9. doi: 10.1210/endo-116-4-1304
125. Giudice LC, Mark SP, Irwin JC. Paracrine actions of insulin-like growth factors and IGF binding protein-1 in non-pregnant human endometrium and at the decidual-trophoblast interface. *J Reprod Immunol.* (1998) 39:133–48. doi: 10.1016/S0165-0378(98)00018-7
126. Gibson JM, Aplin JD, White A, Westwood M. Regulation of IGF bioavailability in pregnancy. *Mol Hum Reprod.* (2001) 7:79–87. doi: 10.1093/molehr/7.1.79
127. Jabbour HN, Critchley HO. Potential roles of decidual prolactin in early pregnancy. *Reproduction* (2001) 121:197–205. doi: 10.1530/rep.0.1210197
128. Marano RJ, Ben-Jonathan N. Minireview: extrapituitary prolactin: an update on the distribution, regulation, and functions. *Mol Endocrinol.* (2014) 28:622–33. doi: 10.1210/me.2013-1349
129. Turco MY, Gardner L, Hughes J, Cindrova-Davies T, Gomez MJ, Farrell L, et al. Long-term, hormone-responsive organoid cultures of human endometrium in a chemically defined medium. *Nat Cell Biol.* (2017) 19:568–77. doi: 10.1038/ncb3516
130. Stefanoska I, Jovanovic Krivokuca M, Vasilijic S, Cujic D, Vicovac L. Prolactin stimulates cell migration and invasion by human trophoblast *in vitro*. *Placenta* (2013) 34:775–83. doi: 10.1016/j.placenta.2013.06.305
131. Garrido-Gomez T, Dominguez F, Quinonero A, Diaz-Gimeno P, Kapidzic M, Gormley M, et al. Defective decidualization during and after severe preeclampsia reveals a possible maternal contribution to the etiology. *Proc Natl Acad Sci USA* (2017) 114:E8468–E8477. doi: 10.1073/pnas.1706546114
132. Irwin JC, Giudice LC. Insulin-like growth factor binding protein-1 binds to placental cytotrophoblast alpha5beta1 integrin and inhibits cytotrophoblast invasion into decidualized endometrial stromal cultures. *Growth Horm IGF Res.* (1998) 8:21–31. doi: 10.1016/S1096-6374(98)80318-3
133. Gleeson LM, Chakraborty C, McKinnon T, Lala PK. Insulin-like growth factor-binding protein 1 stimulates human trophoblast migration by signaling through alpha 5 beta 1 integrin via mitogen-activated protein Kinase pathway. *J Clin Endocrinol Metab.* (2001) 86:2484–93. doi: 10.1210/jcem.86.6.7532
134. Tanaka K, Sakai K, Matsushima M, Matsuzawa Y, Izawa T, Nagashima T, et al. Branched-chain amino acids regulate insulin-like growth factor-binding protein 1 (IGFBP1) production by decidua and influence trophoblast migration through IGFBP1. *Mol Hum Reprod.* (2016) 22:890–9. doi: 10.1093/molehr/gaw032
135. Han VK, Bassett N, Walton J, Challis JR. The expression of insulin-like growth factor (IGF) and IGF-binding protein (IGFBP) genes in the human placenta and membranes: evidence for IGF-IGFBP interactions at the feto-maternal interface. *J Clin Endocrinol Metab.* (1996) 81:2680–93.
136. Hamilton GS, Lysiak JJ, Han VK, Lala PK. Autocrine-paracrine regulation of human trophoblast invasiveness by insulin-like growth factor (IGF)-II and IGF-binding protein (IGFBP)-1. *Exp Cell Res.* (1998) 244:147–56. doi: 10.1006/excr.1998.4195
137. Lacey H, Haigh T, Westwood M, Aplin JD. Mesenchymally-derived insulin-like growth factor 1 provides a paracrine stimulus for trophoblast migration. *BMC Dev Biol.* (2002) 2:5. doi: 10.1186/1471-213X-2-5
138. Coppock HA, White A, Aplin JD, Westwood M. Matrix metalloprotease-3 and−9 proteolyze insulin-like growth factor-binding protein-1. *Biol Reprod.* (2004) 71:438–43. doi: 10.1095/biolreprod.103.023101

139. Husslein H, Haider S, Meinhardt G, Prast J, Sonderegger S, Knofler M. Expression, regulation and functional characterization of matrix metalloproteinase-3 of human trophoblast. *Placenta* (2009) 30:284–91. doi: 10.1016/j.placenta.2008.12.002
140. Pollheimer J, Husslein P, Knofler M. Invasive trophoblasts generate regulatory collagen XVIII cleavage products. *Placenta* (2005) 26 (Suppl. A):S42–45. doi: 10.1016/j.placenta.2004.12.005
141. Knofler M, Pollheimer J. Human placental trophoblast invasion and differentiation: a particular focus on Wnt signaling. *Front Genet.* (2013) 4:190. doi: 10.3389/fgene.2013.00190
142. Red-Horse K, Drake PM, Gunn MD, Fisher SJ. Chemokine ligand and receptor expression in the pregnant uterus: reciprocal patterns in complementary cell subsets suggest functional roles. *Am J Pathol.* (2001) 159:2199–213. doi: 10.1016/S0002-9440(10)63071-4
143. Red-Horse K, Drake PM, Fisher SJ. Human pregnancy: the role of chemokine networks at the fetal-maternal interface. *Expert Rev Mol Med.* (2004) 6:1–14. doi: 10.1017/S1462399404007720
144. Kuang H, Chen Q, Zhang Y, Zhang L, Peng H, Ning L, et al. The cytokine gene CXCL14 restricts human trophoblast cell invasion by suppressing gelatinase activity. *Endocrinology* (2009) 150:5596–605. doi: 10.1210/en.2009-0570
145. Hanna J, Wald O, Goldman-Wohl D, Prus D, Markel G, Gazit R, et al. CXCL12 expression by invasive trophoblasts induces the specific migration of CD16- human natural killer cells. *Blood* (2003) 102:1569–77. doi: 10.1182/blood-2003-02-0517
146. Jaleel MA, Tsai AC, Sarkar S, Freedman PV, Rubin LP. Stromal cell-derived factor-1 (SDF-1) signalling regulates human placental trophoblast cell survival. *Mol Hum Reprod.* (2004) 10:901–9. doi: 10.1093/molehr/gah118
147. Zhou WH, Du MR, Dong L, Yu J, Li DJ. Chemokine CXCL12 promotes the cross-talk between trophoblasts and decidual stromal cells in human first-trimester pregnancy. *Hum Reprod.* (2008) 23:2669–79. doi: 10.1093/humrep/den308
148. Svensson-Arvelund J, Mehta RB, Lindau R, Mirrasekhian E, Rodriguez-Martinez H, Berg G, et al. The human fetal placenta promotes tolerance against the semiallogeneic fetus by inducing regulatory T cells and homeostatic M2 macrophages. *J Immunol.* (2015) 194:1534–44. doi: 10.4049/jimmunol.1401536
149. Choudhury RH, Dunk CE, Lye SJ, Aplin JD, Harris LK, Jones RL. Extravillous trophoblast and endothelial cell crosstalk mediates leukocyte infiltration to the early remodeling decidual spiral arteriole wall. *J Immunol.* (2017) 198:4115–28. doi: 10.4049/jimmunol.1601175
150. Wu HX, Jin LP, Xu B, Liang SS, Li DJ. Decidual stromal cells recruit Th17 cells into decidua to promote proliferation and invasion of human trophoblast cells by secreting IL-17. *Cell Mol Immunol.* (2014) 11:253–62. doi: 10.1038/cmi.2013.67
151. Librach CL, Feigenbaum SL, Bass KE, Cui TY, Verastas N, Sadovsky Y, et al. Interleukin-1 beta regulates human cytotrophoblast metalloproteinase activity and invasion *in vitro*. *J Biol Chem.* (1994) 269:17125–31.
152. Prutsch N, Fock V, Haslinger P, Haider S, Fiala C, Pollheimer J, et al. The role of interleukin-1beta in human trophoblast motility. *Placenta* (2012) 33:696–703. doi: 10.1016/j.placenta.2012.05.008
153. Hanna J, Goldman-Wohl D, Hamani Y, Avraham I, Greenfield C, Natanson-Yaron S, et al. Decidual NK cells regulate key developmental processes at the human fetal-maternal interface. *Nat Med.* (2006) 12:1065–74. doi: 10.1038/nm1452
154. De Oliveira LG, Lash GE, Murray-Dunning C, Bulmer JN, Innes BA, Searle RF, et al. Role of interleukin 8 in uterine natural killer cell regulation of extravillous trophoblast cell invasion. *Placenta* (2010) 31:595–601. doi: 10.1016/j.placenta.2010.04.012
155. Paiva P, Salamonsen LA, Manuelpillai U, Dimitriadis E. Interleukin 11 inhibits human trophoblast invasion indicating a likely role in the decidual restraint of trophoblast invasion during placentation. *Biol Reprod.* (2009) 80:302–10. doi: 10.1095/biolreprod.108.071415
156. Maruo T, Matsuo H, Murata K, Mochizuki M. Gestational age-dependent dual action of epidermal growth factor on human placenta early in gestation. *J Clin Endocrinol Metab* (1992) 75:1362–7.
157. Bass KE, Morrish D, Roth I, Bhardwaj D, Taylor R, Zhou Y, et al. Human cytotrophoblast invasion is up-regulated by epidermal growth factor: evidence that paracrine factors modify this process. *Dev Biol.* (1994) 164:550–61. doi: 10.1006/dbio.1994.1223
158. Leach RE, Kilburn B, Wang J, Liu Z, Romero R, Armant DR. Heparin-binding EGF-like growth factor regulates human extravillous cytotrophoblast development during conversion to the invasive phenotype. *Dev Biol.* (2004) 266:223–37. doi: 10.1016/j.ydbio.2003.09.026
159. Biadasiewicz K, Sonderegger S, Haslinger P, Haider S, Saleh L, Fiala C, et al. Transcription factor AP-2alpha promotes EGF-dependent invasion of human trophoblast. *Endocrinology* (2011) 152:1458–69. doi: 10.1210/en.2010-0936
160. Fock V, Plessl K, Fuchs R, Dekan S, Milla SK, Haider S, et al. Trophoblast subtype-specific EGFR/ERBB4 expression correlates with cell cycle progression and hyperplasia in complete hydatidiform moles. *Hum Reprod.* (2015) 30:789–99. doi: 10.1093/humrep/dev027
161. Wright JK, Dunk CE, Amsalem H, Maxwell C, Keating S, Lye SJ. HER1 signaling mediates extravillous trophoblast differentiation in humans. *Biol Reprod.* (2010) 83:1036–45. doi: 10.1095/biolreprod.109.083246
162. Sonderegger S, Pollheimer J, Knofler M. Wnt signalling in implantation, decidualisation and placental differentiation–review. *Placenta* (2010) 31:839–47. doi: 10.1016/j.placenta.2010.07.011
163. Gordon MD, Nusse R. Wnt signaling: multiple pathways, multiple receptors, and multiple transcription factors. *J Biol Chem.* (2006) 281:22429–33. doi: 10.1074/jbc.R600015200
164. Tulac S, Nayak NR, Kao LC, Van Waes M, Huang J, Lobo S, et al. Identification, characterization, and regulation of the canonical Wnt signaling pathway in human endometrium. *J Clin Endocrinol Metab.* (2003) 88:3860–6. doi: 10.1210/jc.2003-030494
165. Sonderegger S, Husslein H, Leisser C, Knofler M. Complex expression pattern of Wnt ligands and frizzled receptors in human placenta and its trophoblast subtypes. *Placenta* (2007) 28 (Suppl. A):S97–102. doi: 10.1016/j.placenta.2006.11.003
166. Meinhardt G, Haider S, Haslinger P, Proestling K, Fiala C, Pollheimer J, et al. Wnt-dependent T-cell factor-4 controls human etravillous trophoblast motility. *Endocrinology* (2014) 155:1908–20. doi: 10.1210/en.2013-2042
167. Meinhardt G, Saleh L, Otti GR, Haider S, Velicky P, Fiala C, et al. Wingless ligand 5a is a critical regulator of placental growth and survival. *Sci Rep.* (2016) 6:28127. doi: 10.1038/srep28127
168. Bulmer JN, Johnson PM. Macrophage populations in the human placenta and amniochorion. *Clin Exp Immunol.* (1984) 57:393–403.
169. Heikkinen J, Mottonen M, Alanen A, Lassila O. Phenotypic characterization of regulatory T cells in the human decidua. *Clin Exp Immunol.* (2004) 136:373–8. doi: 10.1111/j.1365-2249.2004.02441.x
170. Tilburgs T, Claas FH, Scherjon SA. Elsevier trophoblast research award lecture: unique properties of decidual T cells and their role in immune regulation during human pregnancy. *Placenta* (2010) 31 (Suppl.) S82–6. doi: 10.1016/j.placenta.2010.01.007
171. Meyer N, Woidacki K, Knofler M, Meinhardt G, Nowak D, Velicky P, et al. Chymase-producing cells of the innate immune system are required for decidual vascular remodeling and fetal growth. *Sci Rep.* (2017) 7:45106. doi: 10.1038/srep45106
172. Nadkarni S, Smith J, Sferruzzi-Perri AN, Ledwozyw A, Kishore M, Haas R, et al. Neutrophils induce proangiogenic T cells with a regulatory phenotype in pregnancy. *Proc Natl Acad Sci USA.* (2016) 113:E8415–E8424. doi: 10.1073/pnas.1611944114
173. Amsalem H, Kwan M, Hazan A, Zhang J, Jones RL, Whittle W, et al. Identification of a novel neutrophil population: proangiogenic granulocytes in second-trimester human decidua. *J Immunol.* (2014) 193:3070–9. doi: 10.4049/jimmunol.1303117
174. Huang B, Faucette AN, Pawlitz MD, Pei B, Goyert JW, Zhou JZ, et al. Interleukin-33-induced expression of PIBF1 by decidual B cells protects against preterm labor. *Nat Med.* (2017) 23:128–35. doi: 10.1038/nm.4244
175. Solders M, Gorchs L, Gidlof S, Tiblad E, Lundell AC, Kaipe H. Maternal adaptive immune cells in decidua parietalis display a more activated and coinhibitory phenotype compared to decidua basalis. *Stem Cells Int.* (2017) 2017:8010961. doi: 10.1155/2017/8010961
176. Hume DA. Macrophages as APC and the dendritic cell myth. *J Immunol.* (2008) 181:5829–35. doi: 10.4049/jimmunol.181.9.5829

177. Murray PJ, Wynn TA. Protective and pathogenic functions of macrophage subsets. *Nat Rev Immunol.* (2011) 11:723–37. doi: 10.1038/nri3073
178. Doebel T, Voisin B, Nagao K. Langerhans cells - the macrophage in dendritic cell clothing. *Trends Immunol.* (2017) 38:817–28. doi: 10.1016/j.it.2017.06.008
179. Hashimoto D, Miller J, Merad M. Dendritic cell and macrophage heterogeneity *in vivo*. *Immunity* (2011) 35:323–35. doi: 10.1016/j.immuni.2011.09.007
180. Chakraborty D, Rumi MA, Konno T, Soares MJ. Natural killer cells direct hemochorial placentation by regulating hypoxia-inducible factor dependent trophoblast lineage decisions. *Proc Natl Acad Sci USA.* (2011) 108:16295–300. doi: 10.1073/pnas.1109478108
181. Lima PD, Zhang J, Dunk C, Lye SJ, Croy BA. Leukocyte driven-decidual angiogenesis in early pregnancy. *Cell Mol Immunol.* (2014) 11:522–37. doi: 10.1038/cmi.2014.63
182. Sharkey AM, Xiong S, Kennedy PR, Gardner L, Farrell LE, Chazara O, et al. Tissue-specific education of decidual NK cells. *J Immunol.* (2015) 195:3026–32. doi: 10.4049/jimmunol.1501229
183. Lee AJ, Kandiah N, Karimi K, Clark DA, Ashkar AA. Interleukin-15 is required for maximal lipopolysaccharide-induced abortion. *J Leukoc Biol.* (2013) 93:905–12. doi: 10.1189/jlb.0912442
184. Yougbare I, Tai WS, Zdravic D, Oswald BE, Lang S, Zhu G, et al. Activated NK cells cause placental dysfunction and miscarriages in fetal alloimmune thrombocytopenia. *Nat Commun.* (2017) 8:224. doi: 10.1038/s41467-017-00269-1
185. Ball E, Bulmer JN, Ayis S, Lyall F, Robson SC. Late sporadic miscarriage is associated with abnormalities in spiral artery transformation and trophoblast invasion. *J Pathol.* (2006) 208:535–42. doi: 10.1002/path.1927
186. Xiong S, Sharkey AM, Kennedy PR, Gardner L, Farrell LE, Chazara O, et al. Maternal uterine NK cell-activating receptor KIR2DS1 enhances placentation. *J Clin Invest.* (2013) 123:4264–72. doi: 10.1172/JCI68991
187. Eriksson M, Meadows SK, Wira CR, Sentman CL. Unique phenotype of human uterine NK cells and their regulation by endogenous TGF-beta. *J Leukoc Biol.* (2004) 76:667–75. doi: 10.1189/jlb.0204090
188. Male V, Sharkey A, Masters L, Kennedy PR, Farrell LE, Moffett A. The effect of pregnancy on the uterine NK cell KIR repertoire. *Eur J Immunol.* (2011) 41:3017–27. doi: 10.1002/eji.201141445
189. Cerdeira AS, Rajakumar A, Royle CM, Lo A, Husain Z, Thadhani RI, et al. Conversion of peripheral blood NK cells to a decidual NK-like phenotype by a cocktail of defined factors. *J Immunol.* (2013) 190:3939–48. doi: 10.4049/jimmunol.1202582
190. Montaldo E, Vacca P, Chiossone L, Croxatto D, Loiacono F, Martini S, et al. Unique Eomes(+) NK cell subsets are present in uterus and decidua during early pregnancy. *Front Immunol.* (2015) 6:646. doi: 10.3389/fimmu.2015.00646
191. King A, Wooding P, Gardner L, Loke YW. Expression of perforin, granzyme A and TIA-1 by human uterine CD56+ NK cells implies they are activated and capable of effector functions. *Hum Reprod.* (1993) 8:2061–7. doi: 10.1093/oxfordjournals.humrep.a137982
192. Chazara O, Xiong S, Moffett A. Maternal KIR and fetal HLA-C: a fine balance. *J Leukoc Biol.* (2011) 90:703–16. doi: 10.1189/jlb.0511227
193. Tilburgs T, Evans JH, Crespo AC, Strominger JL. The HLA-G cycle provides for both NK tolerance and immunity at the maternal-fetal interface. *Proc Natl Acad Sci USA* (2015) 112:13312–7. doi: 10.1073/pnas.1517724112
194. Vacca P, Cantoni C, Vitale M, Prato C, Canegallo F, Fenoglio D, et al. Crosstalk between decidual NK and CD14+ myelomonocytic cells results in induction of Tregs and immunosuppression. *Proc Natl Acad Sci USA.* (2010) 107:11918–23. doi: 10.1073/pnas.1001749107
195. Co EC, Gormley M, Kapidzic M, Rosen DB, Scott MA, Stolp HA, et al. Maternal decidual macrophages inhibit NK cell killing of invasive cytotrophoblasts during human pregnancy. *Biol Reprod.* (2013) 88:155. doi: 10.1095/biolreprod.112.099465
196. Gaynor LM, Colucci F. Uterine natural killer cells: functional distinctions and influence on pregnancy in humans and mice. *Front Immunol.* (2017) 8:467. doi: 10.3389/fimmu.2017.00467
197. Lee CQ, Gardner L, Turco M, Zhao N, Murray MJ, Coleman N, et al. What is trophoblast? a combination of criteria define human first-trimester trophoblast. *Stem Cell Rep.* (2016) 6:257–72. doi: 10.1016/j.stemcr.2016.01.006
198. Hackmon R, Pinnaduwage L, Zhang J, Lye SJ, Geraghty DE, Dunk CE. Definitive class I human leukocyte antigen expression in gestational placentation: HLA-F, HLA-E, HLA-C, and HLA-G in extravillous trophoblast invasion on placentation, pregnancy, and parturition. *Am J Reprod Immunol.* (2017) 77:e12643. doi: 10.1111/aji.12643
199. Zhang J, Dunk CE, Kwan M, Jones RL, Harris LK, Keating S, et al. Human dNK cell function is differentially regulated by extrinsic cellular engagement and intrinsic activating receptors in first and second trimester pregnancy. *Cell Mol Immunol.* (2017) 14:203–13. doi: 10.1038/cmi.2015.66
200. Kennedy PR, Chazara O, Gardner L, Ivarsson MA, Farrell LE, Xiong S, et al. Activating KIR2DS4 is expressed by uterine NK cells and contributes to successful pregnancy. *J Immunol.* (2016) 197:4292–300. doi: 10.4049/jimmunol.1601279
201. Rajagopalan S, Long EO. KIR2DL4 (CD158d): An activation receptor for HLA-G. *Front Immunol.* (2012) 3:258. . doi: 10.3389/fimmu.2012.00258
202. Rajagopalan S, Long EO. Cellular senescence induced by CD158d reprograms natural killer cells to promote vascular remodeling. *Proc Natl Acad Sci U S A* (2012) 109:20596–601. doi: 10.1073/pnas.1208248109
203. Sharkey AM, Gardner L, Hiby S, Farrell L, Apps R, Masters L, et al. Killer Ig-like receptor expression in uterine NK cells is biased toward recognition of HLA-C and alters with gestational age. *J Immunol.* (2008) 181:39–46. doi: 10.4049/jimmunol.181.1.39
204. Hiby SE, Apps R, Sharkey AM, Farrell LE, Gardner L, Mulder A, et al. Maternal activating KIRs protect against human reproductive failure mediated by fetal HLA-C2. *J Clin Invest.* (2010) 120:4102–10. doi: 10.1172/JCI43998
205. Apps R, Gardner L, Hiby SE, Sharkey AM, Moffett A. Conformation of human leucocyte antigen-C molecules at the surface of human trophoblast cells. *Immunology* (2008) 124:322–8. doi: 10.1111/j.1365-2567.2007.02789.x
206. Crespo AC, Strominger JL, Tilburgs T. Expression of KIR2DS1 by decidual natural killer cells increases their ability to control placental HCMV infection. *Proc Natl Acad Sci USA.* (2016) 113:15072–7. doi: 10.1073/pnas.1617927114
207. Castellana B, Perdu S, Kim Y, Chan K, Atif J, Marziali M, et al. Maternal obesity alters uterine NK activity through a functional KIR2DL1/S1 imbalance. *Immunol Cell Biol.* (2018). doi: 10.1111/imcb.12041
208. King A, Allan DS, Bowen M, Powis SJ, Joseph S, Verma S, et al. HLA-E is expressed on trophoblast and interacts with CD94/NKG2 receptors on decidual NK cells. *Eur J Immunol.* (2000) 30:1623–31. doi: 10.1002/1521-4141(200006)30:6<1623::AID-IMMU1623>3.0.CO;2-M
209. El Costa H, Casemayou A, Aguerre-Girr M, Rabot M, Berrebi A, Parant O, et al. Critical and differential roles of NKp46- and NKp30-activating receptors expressed by uterine NK cells in early pregnancy. *J Immunol.* (2008) 181:3009–17. doi: 10.4049/jimmunol.181.5.3009
210. Apps R, Gardner L, Sharkey AM, Holmes N, Moffett A. A homodimeric complex of HLA-G on normal trophoblast cells modulates antigen-presenting cells via LILRB1. *Eur J Immunol.* (2007) 37:1924–37. doi: 10.1002/eji.200737089
211. Rajagopalan S, Long EO. A human histocompatibility leukocyte antigen (HLA)-G-specific receptor expressed on all natural killer cells. *J Exp Med.* (1999) 189:1093–100. doi: 10.1084/jem.189.7.1093
212. Li C, Houser BL, Nicotra ML, Strominger JL. HLA-G homodimer-induced cytokine secretion through HLA-G receptors on human decidual macrophages and natural killer cells. *Proc Natl Acad Sci USA.* (2009) 106:5767–72. doi: 10.1073/pnas.0901173106
213. van der Meer A, Lukassen HG, van Lierop MJ, Wijnands F, Mosselman S, Braat DD, et al. Membrane-bound HLA-G activates proliferation and interferon-gamma production by uterine natural killer cells. *Mol Hum Reprod.* (2004) 10:189–95. doi: 10.1093/molehr/gah032
214. Apps R, Sharkey A, Gardner L, Male V, Kennedy P, Masters L, et al. *Ex vivo* functional responses to HLA-G differ between blood and decidual NK cells. *Mol Hum Reprod.* (2011) 17:577–86. doi: 10.1093/molehr/gar022
215. van der Meer A, Lukassen HG, van Cranenbroek B, Weiss EH, Braat DD, van Lierop MJ, et al. Soluble HLA-G promotes Th1-type cytokine production by cytokine-activated uterine and peripheral natural killer cells. *Mol Hum Reprod.* (2007) 13:123–33. doi: 10.1093/molehr/gal100

216. Rajagopalan S, Bryceson YT, Kuppusamy SP, Geraghty DE, van der Meer A, Joosten I, et al. Activation of NK cells by an endocytosed receptor for soluble HLA-G. *PLoS Biol* (2006) 4:e9. doi: 10.1371/journal.pbio.0040009
217. Lash GE, Otun HA, Innes BA, Bulmer JN, Searle RF, Robson SC. Inhibition of trophoblast cell invasion by TGFB1:2, and 3 is associated with a decrease in active proteases. *Biol Reprod.* (2005) 73:374–81. doi: 10.1095/biolreprod.105.040337
218. Athanassiades A, Lala PK. Role of placenta growth factor (PIGF) in human extravillous trophoblast proliferation, migration and invasiveness. *Placenta* (1998) 19:465–73. doi: 10.1016/S0143-4004(98)91039-6
219. Knofler M, Mosl B, Bauer S, Griesinger G, Husslein P. TNF-alpha/TNFRI in primary and immortalized first trimester cytotrophoblasts. *Placenta* (2000) 21:525–35. doi: 10.1053/plac.1999.0501
220. Zhou Y, McMaster M, Woo K, Janatpour M, Perry J, Karpanen T, et al. Vascular endothelial growth factor ligands and receptors that regulate human cytotrophoblast survival are dysregulated in severe preeclampsia and hemolysis, elevated liver enzymes, and low platelets syndrome. *Am J Pathol.* (2002) 160:1405–23. doi: 10.1016/S0002-9440(10)62567-9
221. Zhang J, Dunk CE, Lye SJ. Sphingosine signalling regulates decidual NK cell angiogenic phenotype and trophoblast migration. *Hum Reprod.* (2013) 28:3026–37. doi: 10.1093/humrep/det339
222. Bauer S, Pollheimer J, Hartmann J, Husslein P, Aplin JD, Knofler M. Tumor necrosis factor-alpha inhibits trophoblast migration through elevation of plasminogen activator inhibitor-1 in first-trimester villous explant cultures. *J Clin Endocrinol Metab.* (2004) 89:812–22. doi: 10.1210/jc.2003-031351
223. Lash GE, Otun HA, Innes BA, Kirkley M, De Oliveira L, Searle RF, et al. Interferon-gamma inhibits extravillous trophoblast cell invasion by a mechanism that involves both changes in apoptosis and protease levels. *FASEB J.* (2006) 20:2512–8. doi: 10.1096/fj.06-6616com
224. Kopcow HD, Allan DS, Chen X, Rybalov B, Andzelm MM, Ge B, et al. Human decidual NK cells form immature activating synapses and are not cytotoxic. *Proc Natl Acad Sci USA.* (2005) 102:15563–8. doi: 10.1073/pnas.0507835102
225. Crespo AC, van der Zwan A, Ramalho-Santos J, Strominger JL, Tilburgs T. Cytotoxic potential of decidual NK cells and CD8+ T cells awakened by infections. *J Reprod Immunol.* (2017) 119:85–90. doi: 10.1016/j.jri.2016.08.001
226. Stallmach T, Hebisch G, Orban P, Lu X. Aberrant positioning of trophoblast and lymphocytes in the feto-maternal interface with pre-eclampsia. *Virchows Arch.* (1999) 434:207–11. doi: 10.1007/s004280050329
227. Eide IP, Rolfseng T, Isaksen CV, Mecsei R, Roald B, Lydersen S, et al. Serious foetal growth restriction is associated with reduced proportions of natural killer cells in decidua basalis. *Virchows Arch.* (2006) 448:269–76. doi: 10.1007/s00428-005-0107-z
228. Rieger L, Segerer S, Bernar T, Kapp M, Majic M, Morr AK, et al. Specific subsets of immune cells in human decidua differ between normal pregnancy and preeclampsia–a prospective observational study. *Reprod Biol Endocrinol.* (2009) 7:132. doi: 10.1186/1477-7827-7-132
229. Williams PJ, Bulmer JN, Searle RF, Innes BA, Robson SC. Altered decidual leucocyte populations in the placental bed in pre-eclampsia and foetal growth restriction: a comparison with late normal pregnancy. *Reproduction* (2009) 138:177–84. doi: 10.1530/REP-09-0007
230. Wilczynski JR, Tchorzewski H, Banasik M, Glowacka E, Wieczorek A, Lewkowicz P, et al. Lymphocyte subset distribution and cytokine secretion in third trimester decidua in normal pregnancy and preeclampsia. *Eur J Obstet Gynecol Reprod Biol.* (2003) 109:8–15. doi: 10.1016/S0301-2115(02)00350-0
231. Bachmayer N, Rafik Hamad R, Liszka L, Bremme K, Sverremark-Ekstrom E. Aberrant uterine natural killer (NK)-cell expression and altered placental and serum levels of the NK-cell promoting cytokine interleukin-12 in pre-eclampsia. *Am J Reprod Immunol.* (2006) 56:292–301. doi: 10.1111/j.1600-0897.2006.00429.x
232. Lessin DL, Hunt JS, King CR, Wood GW. Antigen expression by cells near the maternal-fetal interface. *Am J Reprod Immunol Microbiol.* (1988) 16:1–7. doi: 10.1111/j.1600-0897.1988.tb00169.x
233. Ning F, Liu H, Lash GE. The role of decidual macrophages during normal and pathological pregnancy. *Am J Reprod Immunol.* (2016) 75:298–309. doi: 10.1111/aji.12477
234. Okabe Y, Medzhitov R. Tissue biology perspective on macrophages. *Nat Immunol.* (2016) 17:9–17. doi: 10.1038/ni.3320
235. Mosser DM, Edwards JP. Exploring the full spectrum of macrophage activation. *Nat Rev Immunol.* (2008) 8:958–69. doi: 10.1038/nri2448
236. Piccolo V, Curina A, Genua M, Ghisletti S, Simonatto M, Sabo A, et al. Opposing macrophage polarization programs show extensive epigenomic and transcriptional cross-talk. *Nat Immunol.* (2017) 18:530–40. doi: 10.1038/ni.3710
237. Helm O, Held-Feindt J, Grage-Griebenow E, Reiling N, Ungefroren H, Vogel I, et al. Tumor-associated macrophages exhibit pro- and anti-inflammatory properties by which they impact on pancreatic tumorigenesis. *Int J Cancer* (2014) 135:843–61. doi: 10.1002/ijc.28736
238. Kratochvill F, Neale G, Haverkamp JM, Van de Velde LA, Smith AM, Kawauchi D, et al. TNF Counterbalances the Emergence of M2 Tumor Macrophages. *Cell Rep.* (2015) 12:1902–14. doi: 10.1016/j.celrep.2015.08.033
239. Houser BL, Tilburgs T, Hill J, Nicotra ML, Strominger JL. Two unique human decidual macrophage populations. *J Immunol.*(2011) 186:2633–42. doi: 10.4049/jimmunol.1003153
240. Svensson J, Jenmalm MC, Matussek A, Geffers R, Berg G, Ernerudh J. Macrophages at the fetal-maternal interface express markers of alternative activation and are induced by M-CSF and IL-10. *J Immunol.* (2011) 187:3671–82. doi: 10.4049/jimmunol.1100130
241. Sayama S, Nagamatsu T, Schust DJ, Itaoka N, Ichikawa M, Kawana K, et al. Human decidual macrophages suppress IFN-gamma production by T cells through costimulatory B7-H1:PD-1 signaling in early pregnancy. *J Reprod Immunol.* (2013) 100:109–17. doi: 10.1016/j.jri.2013.08.001
242. Jiang X, Du MR, Li M, Wang H. Three macrophage subsets are identified in the uterus during early human pregnancy. *Cell Mol Immunol.* (2018). doi: 10.1038/s41423-018-0008-0. [Epub ahead of print].
243. Kabawat SE, Mostoufi-Zadeh M, Driscoll SG, Bhan AK. Implantation site in normal pregnancy. A study with monoclonal antibodies. *Am J Pathol.*(1985) 118:76–84.
244. Helige C, Ahammer H, Moser G, Hammer A, Dohr G, Huppertz B, et al. Distribution of decidual natural killer cells and macrophages in the neighbourhood of the trophoblast invasion front: a quantitative evaluation. *Hum Reprod.* (2014) 29:8–17. doi: 10.1093/humrep/det353
245. Pull SL, Doherty JM, Mills JC, Gordon JI, Stappenbeck TS. Activated macrophages are an adaptive element of the colonic epithelial progenitor niche necessary for regenerative responses to injury. *Proc Natl Acad Sci USA* (2005) 102:99–104. doi: 10.1073/pnas.0405979102
246. Mussar K, Tucker A, McLennan L, Gearhart A, Jimenez-Caliani AJ, Cirulli V, et al. Macrophage/epithelium cross-talk regulates cell cycle progression and migration in pancreatic progenitors. *PLoS ONE* (2014) 9:e89492. doi: 10.1371/journal.pone.0089492
247. Dang T, Liou GY. Macrophage cytokines enhance cell proliferation of normal prostate epithelial cells through activation of ERK and Akt. *Sci Rep.* (2018) 8:7718. doi: 10.1038/s41598-018-26143-8
248. Bergenfelz C, Medrek C, Ekstrom E, Jirstrom K, Janols H, Wullt M, et al. Wnt5a induces a tolerogenic phenotype of macrophages in sepsis and breast cancer patients. *J Immunol.* (2012) 188:5448–58. doi: 10.4049/jimmunol.1103378
249. Seo DH, Che X, Kwak MS, Kim S, Kim JH, Ma HW, et al. Interleukin-33 regulates intestinal inflammation by modulating macrophages in inflammatory bowel disease. *Sci Rep.* (2017) 7:851. doi: 10.1038/s41598-017-00840-2
250. Fock V, Mairhofer M, Otti GR, Hiden U, Spittler A, Zeisler H, et al. Macrophage-derived IL-33 is a critical factor for placental growth. *J Immunol* (2013) 191:3734–43. doi: 10.4049/jimmunol.1300490
251. McWhorter FY, Wang T, Nguyen P, Chung T, Liu WF. Modulation of macrophage phenotype by cell shape. *Proc Natl Acad Sci USA* (2013) 110:17253–8. doi: 10.1073/pnas.1308887110
252. Reister F, Frank HG, Heyl W, Kosanke G, Huppertz B, Schroder W, et al. The distribution of macrophages in spiral arteries of the placental bed in pre-eclampsia differs from that in healthy patients. *Placenta* (1999) 20:229–33. doi: 10.1053/plac.1998.0373
253. Schonkeren D, van der Hoorn ML, Khedoe P, Swings G, van Beelen E, Claas F, et al. Differential distribution and phenotype of decidual macrophages in

preeclamptic versus control pregnancies. *Am J Pathol.* (2011) 178:709–17. doi: 10.1016/j.ajpath.2010.10.011
254. Burk MR, Troeger C, Brinkhaus R, Holzgreve W, Hahn S. Severely reduced presence of tissue macrophages in the basal plate of pre-eclamptic placentae. *Placenta* (2001) 22:309–16. doi: 10.1053/plac.2001.0624
255. Kim JS, Romero R, Cushenberry E, Kim YM, Erez O, Nien JK, et al. Distribution of CD14+ and CD68+ macrophages in the placental bed and basal plate of women with preeclampsia and preterm labor. *Placenta* (2007) 28:571–6. doi: 10.1016/j.placenta.2006.07.007
256. Saito S, Umekage H, Sakamoto Y, Sakai M, Tanebe K, Sasaki Y, et al. Increased T-helper-1-type immunity and decreased T-helper-2-type immunity in patients with preeclampsia. *Am J Reprod Immunol.* (1999) 41:297–306. doi: 10.1111/j.1600-0897.1999.tb00442.x
257. Wilczynski JR, Tchorzewski H, Glowacka E, Banasik M, Lewkowicz P, Szpakowski M, et al. Cytokine secretion by decidual lymphocytes in transient hypertension of pregnancy and pre-eclampsia. *Mediators Inflamm.* (2002) 11:105–11. doi: 10.1080/09629350220131962
258. Cotechini T, Komisarenko M, Sperou A, Macdonald-Goodfellow S, Adams MA, Graham CH. Inflammation in rat pregnancy inhibits spiral artery remodeling leading to fetal growth restriction and features of preeclampsia. *J Exp Med.* (2014) 211:165–79. doi: 10.1084/jem.201630295
259. Odero MD, Zeleznik-Le NJ, Chinwalla V, and Rowley JD. Cytogenetic and molecular analysis of the acute monocytic leukemia cell line THP-1 with an MLL-AF9 translocation. *Genes Chromosomes Cancer* (2000) 29:333–8. doi: 10.1002/1098-2264(2000)9999:9999<::AID-GCC1040>3.0.CO;2-Z
260. Gomez Perdiguero E, Klapproth K, Schulz C, Busch K, Azzoni E, Crozet L, et al. Tissue-resident macrophages originate from yolk-sac-derived erythro-myeloid progenitors. *Nature* (2015) 518:547–51. doi: 10.1038/nature13989
261. Ginhoux F, Guilliams M. Tissue-resident macrophage ontogeny and homeostasis. *Immunity* (2016) 44:439–49. doi: 10.1016/j.immuni.2016.02.024
262. Klein I, Cornejo JC, Polakos NK, John B, Wuensch SA, Topham DJ, et al. Kupffer cell heterogeneity: functional properties of bone marrow derived and sessile hepatic macrophages. *Blood* (2007) 110:4077–85. doi: 10.1182/blood-2007-02-073841
263. Merad M, Manz MG, Karsunky H, Wagers A, Peters W, Charo I, et al. Langerhans cells renew in the skin throughout life under steady-state conditions. *Nat Immunol.* (2002) 3:1135–41. doi: 10.1038/ni852
264. Ginhoux F, Greter M, Leboeuf M, Nandi S, See P, Gokhan S, et al. Fate mapping analysis reveals that adult microglia derive from primitive macrophages. *Science* (2010) 330:841–5. doi: 10.1126/science.1194637
265. Jenkins SJ, Ruckerl D, Cook PC, Jones LH, Finkelman FD, van Rooijen N, et al. Local macrophage proliferation, rather than recruitment from the blood, is a signature of TH2 inflammation. *Science* (2011) 332:1284–8. doi: 10.1126/science.1204351
266. Vacca P, Vitale C, Montaldo E, Conte R, Cantoni C, Fulcheri E, et al. CD34+ hematopoietic precursors are present in human decidua and differentiate into natural killer cells upon interaction with stromal cells. *Proc Natl Acad Sci USA* (2011) 108:2402–7. doi: 10.1073/pnas.1016257108
267. Gamliel M, Goldman-Wohl D, Isaacson B, Gur C, Stein N, Yamin R, et al. Trained memory of human uterine NK cells enhances their function in subsequent pregnancies. *Immunity* (2018) 48:951–62 e955. doi: 10.1016/j.immuni.2018.03.030
268. Carbone FR. Tissue-resident memory T cells and fixed immune surveillance in nonlymphoid organs. *J Immunol.* (2015) 195:17–22. doi: 10.4049/jimmunol.1500515
269. Bjorkstrom NK, Ljunggren HG, Michaelsson J. Emerging insights into natural killer cells in human peripheral tissues. *Nat Rev Immunol.* (2016) 16:310–20. doi: 10.1038/nri.2016.34
270. Kammerer U, Eggert AO, Kapp M, McLellan AD, Geijtenbeek TB, Dietl J, et al. Unique appearance of proliferating antigen-presenting cells expressing DC-SIGN (CD209) in the decidua of early human pregnancy. *Am J Pathol* (2003) 162:887–96. doi: 10.1016/S0002-9440(10)63884-9
271. Gustafsson C, Mjosberg J, Matussek A, Geffers R, Matthiesen L, Berg G, et al. Gene expression profiling of human decidual macrophages: evidence for immunosuppressive phenotype. *PLoS ONE* (2008) 3:e2078. doi: 10.1371/journal.pone.0002078
272. Okae H, Toh H, Sato T, Hiura H, Takahashi S, Shirane K, et al. Derivation of human trophoblast stem cells. *Cell Stem Cell* (2018) 22:50–63 e56. doi: 10.1016/j.stem.2017.11.004

14

Hofbauer Cells: Their Role in Healthy and Complicated Pregnancy

Leticia Reyes[1*] *and Thaddeus G. Golos*[2]

[1] *Department of Pathobiological Sciences, School of Veterinary Medicine, University of Wisconsin-Madison, Madison, WI, United States,* [2] *Department of Comparative Biosciences, Wisconsin National Primate Research Center, School of Veterinary Medicine, University of Wisconsin-Madison, Madison, WI, United States*

Correspondence:
Leticia Reyes
lreyes2@wisc.edu

Hofbauer cells are placental villous macrophages of fetal origin that are present throughout pregnancy. Although Hofbauer cell populations are antigenically and morphologically heterogeneous, their epigenetic, antigenic, and functional profiles most closely resemble alternatively activated macrophages or what are referred to as M2a, M2b, M2c, and M2d polarity subtypes. Consistent with an M2-like profile, these cells play an important role in placental development including vasculogenesis and angiogenesis. During placental inflammation Hofbauer cells may produce pro-inflammatory cytokines or mediators that damage the villous cell barrier, and induce fibrotic responses within the villi as a continuum of chronic inflammation. However, to date, there is no evidence that Hofbauer cells become classically activated or adopt an M1 polarity phenotype that is able to kill microbes. To the contrary, their predominant M2 like qualities may be why these cells are ineffective in controlling most TORCH infections. Moreover, Hofbauer cells may contribute to vertical transmission of various pathogens to the fetus since they can harbor live virus and serve as reservoirs within the placenta. The goal of this review is to summarize what is currently known about the role of Hofbauer cells in normal and complicated pregnancies that involve immunologic disorders, inflammation, and/or infection.

Keywords: Hofbauer cells, placental macrophages, preeclampsia, villitis, chorioamnionitis, Zika, TORCH

HOFBAUER CELLS IN NORMAL PREGNANCY

Hofbauer Cell Location and Proposed Function

Hofbauer cells (HBC) originally referred to round to ovoid placental macrophages with a small nucleus and abundant vacuolated cytoplasm that could be identified by light microscopy (1). Subsequent ultrastructural studies further identified placental macrophages that were spindle or stellate shaped (2, 3) and that these cells are of fetal origin (4). HBC is now often used to describe any fetal derived placental macrophage that resides within the placental villous core, amnion, and chorionic lavae (5). HBCs are found in human placental tissue as early as 18 days post-conception (6) and remain throughout gestation (1).

HBCs are presumed to play a role in placental morphogenesis and homeostasis. HBCs are typically in apposition to endothelium and trophoblasts where they can mediate the function of these cells through paracrine signals or possibly cell-to-cell crosstalk (7–9). HBCs are pro-angiogenic in that they express large amounts of vascular endothelial growth factor (VEGF) (10, 11), and Sprouty (Spry) proteins Spry 1, 2, and 3 that modulate branching morphogenesis of placental villi (12). It has been suggested that HBC may participate in vasoregulation of placental blood vessels since they have the capacity to produce prostaglandin E_2 and thromboxane *in vitro* (13).

Phenotypic Diversity of HBCs

As is typical of macrophages, HBCs exhibit plasticity and their pleomorphism is likely a reflection of the complex and shifting microenvironment in which they reside (14–16). This has been verified through a variety of techniques including electron microscopy, immunohistochemistry, and flow cytometry. Initial descriptions of HBC pleomorphism came from ultrastructural observations that reported 4 types of macrophages based on their shape (3). Histochemical studies have further classified HBC subtypes by their expression of major histocompatibility complex (MHC) type II, complement receptors, lectins, lipopolysaccharide co-receptor (CD14), and CD68 that vary based on HBC location within the placenta as well as gestational stage (5, 15–19). Using multi-parameter flow cytometry coupled with serial gating of first trimester macaque HBCs, we previously identified two HBC subsets based on whether or not they expressed CD68 (14). To further illustrate this point we reanalyzed the dataset and added additional samples from late second trimester (gestation day 100), and near term (gestation day 160) (20, 21). We specifically measured the expression of HLA-DR, CD14, DC-SIGN, CD68, CD64, and CD163 in HBC by flow cytometry (**Figure 1**; **Table 1**, workflow detailed in **Supplementary Material**). Although our panel was not comprehensive, it included markers previously validated in rhesus macaque HBCs (18), some of which indicate innate immune activation, such as CD14 (23), or immune modulation (DC-SIGN, HLA-DR, CD68) (1, 15, 18, 24). In order to better capture the spectrum of HBC diversity, we used an unbiased approach to analyze the high-dimensional flow cytometric data. Raw flow cytometry data files were first processed with FlowJo, LLC version 10 software (Ashland, OR). Processed datasets from first ($n = 2$), second ($n = 2$), and third ($n = 1$) trimester pregnancies were then imported into Cytofkit (https://bioconductor.org/packages/cytofkit/), normalized, and analyzed with the DensVM computational clustering tool (22). t-Distributed Stochastic Neighbor Embedding (t-SNE) was used to created 2-dimensional maps of all HBC subsets generated by DensVM (**Figure 1**).

With this approach we identified 10 HBC subsets within macaque placental tissues (**Figure 1**; **Table 1**). The 10 HBC subsets were subsequently validated by serial manual gating (**Table 2**). Both first and third trimester HBC populations were more diverse than the second trimester (8 vs. 5 clusters, respectively). This is not unusual given the physiological events that occur during these stages of pregnancy. For example, during the first trimester, HBCs are thought to participate in placental villous growth and tissue remodeling (13). At the same time HBCs in the vicinity of the placental bed may be affected by the inflammatory processes necessary for decidualization and embryo implantation (25). During the latter part of the third trimester, HBCs scattered through the placenta are exposed to various products released from senescent trophoblasts (26), necrotic cell debris associated with fibrinoid deposits within aging placental villi (13), and inflammatory mediators produced during parturition (27). These may promote the development of specialized subsets of HBCs in response to their microenvironment. Alternatively, they may represent different populations of fetal monocytes that are trafficking to the placenta across gestation.

In order to assess gestation dependent changes in HBC subsets, marker expression heatmaps specific to each gestational stage were generated (**Figure 2**). We found that both CD163 and CD64 appeared to be constitutively expressed in all HBC subsets throughout pregnancy, indicating that these markers may be well-suited for the identification of HBCs in general. However, CD68 which is often used as a single marker to identify HBCs had variable expression over time. Namely, the intensity of CD68 expression peaked in the second trimester and significantly dropped as pregnancy progressed. This temporal expression pattern is similar to previous studies that described human HBC populations as changing in density as pregnancy progressed (1, 24).

As expected (5), there was at least one population of HBC that was negative for HLA-DR (cluster 5). Of the HBC subsets that were positive, HLA-DR expression followed a similar pattern to CD68 in that peak expression was observed in second trimester placenta. However, contrary to human studies (5), we found the proportion of HLA-DR positive cells in first trimester placenta to be greater than third trimester tissue. This may be due to timing of sampling since human studies evaluated tissues collected during 8–10 weeks gestation (5) whereas we examined tissues collected at a later gestational time point that developmentally would be equivalent to 17–18 weeks in human gestation.

DC-SIGN positive HBCs were present in all 3 stages of pregnancy; albeit with varying degrees of DC-SIGN expression. Consistent with Yang et al. (28) we found that DC-SIGN positive third trimester macaque HBCs co-expressed CD14, CD68, and CD163. In contrast to Bockle et al (29), we detected a large population of DC-SIGN positive HBC in third trimester placenta that co-expressed HLA-DR (23% in cluster 6). One caveat is that these cells had dim expression of both markers, which may explain why these cells may not be readily detected by immunofluorescent histology.

Of all the markers that we studied, the proportion of CD14 positive cells and their level of CD14 expression was the most diverse. Midgestation placenta, which is characterized by immune tolerance, had the greatest proportion of $CD14^{Hi}$ positive HBCs that were also $CD163^{Hi}$ (cluster 10). Although increased CD14 expression has been linked to pro-inflammatory HBCs (23), in normal pregnancy CD14 expression may represent an immune suppressed phenotype. $CD14^{Hi}/CD163^{Hi}$ expression as seen in cluster 10, is characteristic of immunosuppressive M2d or tumor associated macrophages (TAM) (30). CD14 positive HBCs also express anti-inflammatory TGF-β and IL-10 (31).

Even though this was a pilot experiment with a small sample size, our results demonstrate the potential of utilizing computational methods to analyze multidimensional data from HBCs. For instance, we obtained a global perspective on how HBC subsets change during pregnancy. Moreover, we gained insights into which macrophage markers may or may not be suitable for the general identification of HBCs by flow cytometric or immunohistochemical approaches.

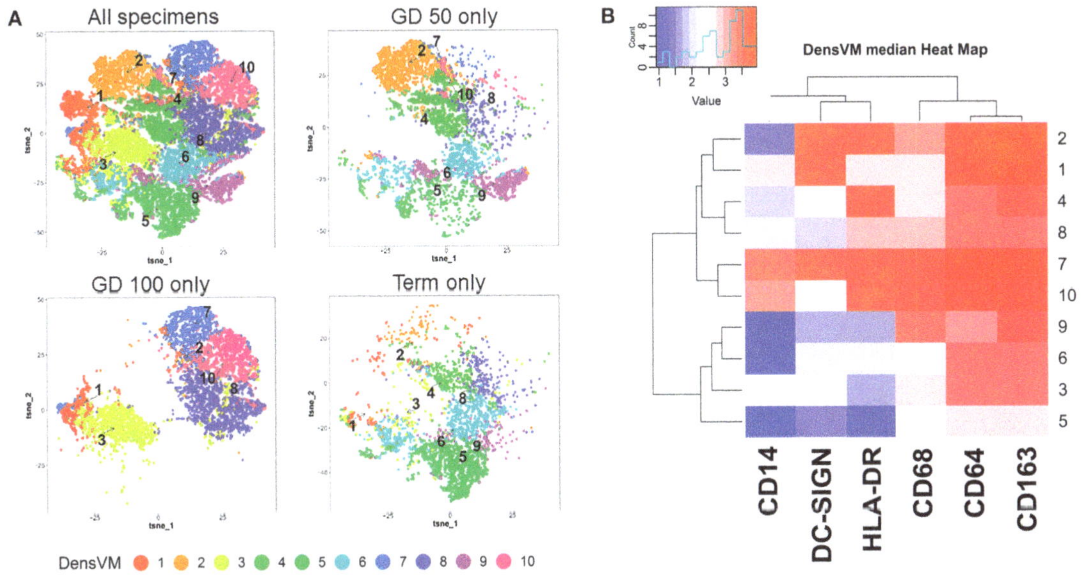

FIGURE 1 | Marker defined HBC subsets within macaque placenta collected at different stages of gestation: Gestation day (GD) 50 ± 2 days ($n = 2$), GD100 ± 2 days ($n = 2$), and Term. **(A)** *t*-SNE visualization of DensVM generated HBC clusters of combined flow cytometry data from all gestation stages (All specimens) and by each individual gestation stage. **(B)** Marker and cluster specific DensVM median heatmap generated with flow cytometry data from all gestation stages. Clustering was ranked by both HBC cluster group (designated by row) and marker median expression (column). Images were created with Cytofkit ShinyAPP (22).

TABLE 1 | Marker profiles of HBC subsets generated with DensVM clustering algorithm (22).

Cluster	1st[a]	2nd[a]	3rd	Marker profile
1	–	5 ± 4	3	CD163^{Hi}/CD64^{Hi}/CD68^{Lo}/HLA-DR^{+}/DC-SIGN^{Hi}/CD14^{Hi}
2	23 ± 22	–	3	CD163^{Hi}/CD64^{Hi}/CD68^{Med}/HLA-DR^{Hi}/DC-SIGN^{Hi}/CD14^{Lo}
3	–	24 ± 18	4	CD163^{Med}/CD64^{Med}/CD68^{Lo}/HLA-DR^{Lo}/DC-SIGN^{Med}/CD14^{Lo}
4	17 ± 1	–	10	CD163^{Med}/CD64^{Med}/CD68^{Lo}/HLA-DR^{Hi}/DC-SIGN^{Med}/CD14^{Lo}
5	8 ± 6	–	48	CD163^{Lo}/CD64^{Lo}/CD68^{Lo}/HLA-DR^{-}/DC-SIGN^{Lo}/CD14^{-}
6	11 ± 4	–	23	CD163^{Med}/CD64^{Med}/CD68^{Lo}/HLA-DR^{Med}/DC-SIGN^{Med}/CD14^{-}
7	2 ± 0.1	16 ± 5	–	CD163^{Hi}/CD64^{Hi}/CD68^{Hi}/HLA-DR^{Hi}/DC-SIGN^{Hi}/CD14^{Hi}
8	3 ± 1	24 ± 21	6	CD163^{Med}/CD64^{Med}/CD68^{Med}/HLA-DR^{Med}/DC-SIGN^{Med}/CD14^{Lo}
9	12 ± 3	–	3	CD163^{Med}/CD64^{Lo}/CD68^{Hi}/HLA-DR^{Lo}/DC-SIGN^{Lo}/CD14^{-}
10	2 ± 2	20 ± 2	–	CD163^{+}/CD64^{Hi}/CD68^{Hi}/HLA-DR^{Hi}/DC-SIGN^{Med}/CD14^{Hi}

[a] *Values represent the mean ± SD% positive cells per group ($n = 2$) per gestation group.*

TABLE 2 | Marker profiles of HBC subsets generated by manual gating using FlowJo Software.

Cluster	1st[a]	2nd[a]	3rd	Marker profile
1	–	1.3 ± 0.4	8	CD163^{Hi}/CD64^{Hi}/CD68^{Lo}/HLA-DR^{+}/DC-SIGN^{Hi}/CD14^{Hi}
2	11 ± 11	–	1	CD163^{Hi}/CD64^{Hi}/CD68^{Med}/HLA-DR^{Hi}/DC-SIGN^{Hi}/CD14^{Lo}
3	–	20 ± 24	6	CD163^{Med}/CD64^{Med}/CD68^{Lo}/HLA-DR^{Lo}/DC-SIGN^{Med}/CD14^{Lo}
4	19 ± 4	–	3	CD163^{Med}/CD64^{Med}/CD68^{Lo}/HLA-DR^{Hi}/DC-SIGN^{Med}/CD14^{Lo}
5	8 ± 1	–	52	CD163^{Lo}/CD64^{Lo}/CD68^{Lo}/HLA-DR^{-}/DC-SIGN^{Lo}/CD14^{-}
6	9 ± 4	–	17	CD163^{Med}/CD64^{Med}/CD68^{Lo}/HLA-DR^{Med}/DC-SIGN^{Med}/CD14^{-}
7	1.8 ± 0.4	6 ± 3	–	CD163^{Hi}/CD64^{Hi}/CD68^{Hi}/HLA-DR^{Hi}/DC-SIGN^{Hi}/CD14^{Hi}
8	2.3 ± 1	17 ± 19	3.2	CD163^{Med}/CD64^{Med}/CD68^{Med}/HLA-DR^{Med}/DC-SIGN^{Med}/CD14^{Lo}
9	6 ± 4	–	2.5	CD163^{Med}/CD64^{Lo}/CD68^{Hi}/HLA-DR^{Lo}/DC-SIGN^{Lo}/CD14^{-}
10	0.5 ± 0.7	8 ± 7	–	CD163^{+}/CD64^{Hi}/CD68^{Hi}/HLA-DR^{Hi}/DC-SIGN^{Med}/CD14^{Hi}

[a] *Values represent the mean ± SD% positive cells per group ($n = 2$) per gestation group.*

TABLE 3 | General features of macrophage polarity pertinent to HBC (30, 33, 34).

	M1	M2a	M2b	M2c	M2d
Stimulus	IFN-γ + LPS IFN-γ + TNF GM-CSF	IL-4 IL-13 Fungal and parasitic infections	Immune complexes IL-1R	IL-10 TGF-β Glucocorticoids	IL-6 LIF M-CSF Adenosine
Surface markers	CD80 MHC II	CD163 IL-1R MHC II CD206 IL-RN DC-SIGN	CD86 MHC II	CD163 TLR1 TLR8 CD206 CD14	CD163 CD14 CD85
Secreted factors	TNF IL-1β IL-6 IL-12 IL-23 CCL10 CCL11 CCL5 CCL8 CCL9 CCL2 CCL3 CCL4	IL-10 TGF-β IL-1ra	IL-1 IL-6 IL-10 TNF-α CCL1	IL-10 TGF-β CCR2 Pentraxin 3	VEGF MMP-9 IDO IL-10 IL-12 TNF-α TGF-β CCL5 CXCL10 CXCL16
Biological effects	TH1 responses Killing intracellular pathogens Tumor resistance	TH2 responses Killing of extracellular responses	TH2 activation Immune regulation	Immune regulation Matrix deposition and tissue remodeling	Immune suppression Angiogenesis

Functional Diversity of HBCs

Mills et al. (32) were the first to introduce the concept that macrophage function could be polarized based on how the cell metabolized arginine. Arginine conversion to nitric oxide was linked to a macrophage that produced IFN-γ and inhibited wound healing, which was labeled as M1. Arginine conversion to ornithine was linked to a macrophage that produced TGF-β and promoted wound healing, this phenotype was labeled as M2. Over the years, the criteria for defining a macrophage as M1 has expanded (**Table 2**) to include microbicidal activity, and the production of pro-inflammatory cytokines and chemokines that promote cell mediated (TH1 type) responses. M2 polarity phenotype has been divided subsequently into M2a, M2b, M2c, and M2d subcategories (reviewed by Martinez et al. (33)), which are based on their responses to various agonists (**Table 3**). Collectively, M2 subtypes are linked by a dominant TH2 response profile, their development in response to fungal or helminth infections, and their role in tissue remodeling. However, M2b polarized macrophages share some qualities in M1 in that they can be pro-inflammatory by producing TNF, IL-1, and IL-6 along with IL-10, but they lack microbicidal activity.

Since HBC are macrophages, it has been assumed that these cells protect the placenta and fetus from infection (13), which would be consistent with an M1 phenotype. However, there is no experimental evidence that HBCs within the placenta are capable of killing microbes (discussed in the next section of this review). Pro-M1 genes in HBC, such as TLR9, IL1B, IL12RB2, CD48, and FGR are silenced by methylation (35). On the other hand, pro-M2 genes, such as CCL2, CCL13, CCL14, CD209, and A2M are hypomethylated in HBCs and thus available for transcription (35). Collectively, HBCs isolated from term human placenta display M2a, M2b, and M2c characteristics based on cell surface marker profiles and cytokine expression (19, 31, 36). HBCs also share some features with M2d phenotype in that they are immune suppressive, pro-angiogenic, and co-express CD163 and CD14 (7, 10, 12, 36). Moreover, HBCs form multinucleated giant cells that express matrix metalloproteinase genes along with VEGF-C (37), which are also features of M2d. Hypothetically, a normal pregnancy has a balanced blend of HBC subtypes that functionally complement each other in providing optimal vascular development, villous growth and immune tolerance. Conversely, an imbalance in HBC subtypes may bring about or exacerbate pathologic pregnancy.

THE ROLE OF HBCS IN PREGNANCY COMPLICATIONS

Villitis

Villitis is a histopathologic diagnosis with multiple underlying etiologies (38). It can be a consequence of hematogenous infection of the placenta by TORCH organisms that include

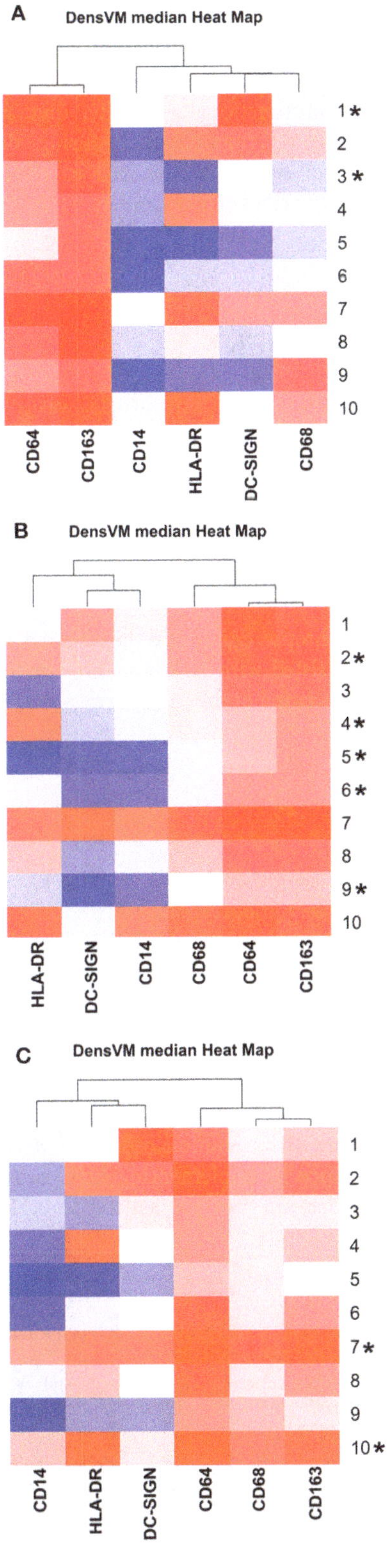

FIGURE 2 | DensVM median heatmaps specific to each gestation stage. **(A)** GD50 ± 2 days, **(B)** GD100 ± 2 days ($n = 2$), and **(C)** Term ($n = 1$). Heatmaps were clustered by median expression of each marker (column). *Denotes HBC clusters that contained 1% of cells for that specific gestation stage. Images were created with Cytofkit ShinyAPP (22).

Toxoplasma, Others (syphilis, varicella-zoster, parvovirus B19), Rubella, Cytomegalovirus (CMV), and Herpes infections (38, 39). However, most cases of villitis are not associated with infection, but may be immune mediated (40, 41). Acute villitis is usually caused by infection and it characterized by polymorphonuclear leukocytic infiltration of the villi with or without necrosis. *Listeria monocytogenes* infection during pregnancy is one of the most common causes of acute villitis (13, 42). Placental infection with *Treponema pallidin* (syphilis) may also present as acute villitis, but chronic villitis is more characteristic of congenital syphilis (43, 44). On the other hand chronic villitis is characterized by infiltration of the tissue by lymphocytes and macrophages. It may be accompanied by cellular proliferation and fibrosis of the villi. Most cases of villitis are multifocal and asymptomatic, but the lesion can be more extensive leading to preterm birth or miscarriage.

Perturbed HBC function is a common occurrence in chronic villitis. HBC hyperplasia or proliferation is seen in chronic villitis caused by infection with CMV, Zika, Herpes virus, Coxsackie, and villitis of unknown etiology (VUE) (38, 45–47). Regardless of the underlying cause, HBCs in chronic villitis exhibit an inflammatory phenotype. Satosar and colleagues showed an increase in the number of TNF positive HBCs with a concomitant decrease in SOCS-1 (suppressors of cytokine signaling) positive HBCs in villitis placentas positive for viral and bacterial infection (45). A similar response is also evident in VUE, which is now recognized to be an immune mediated process that resembles maternal anti-fetal rejection and placental graft vs. host disease (40). In VUE, hyperplastic HBCs are intermixed with infiltrating maternal macrophages and $CD8^{+}$ T cells with an inflammatory transcriptome that is similar to the biological processes that occur during antigen presentation and immune response (40). In particular, HBCs in VUE are positive for CXCL9, CXCL10, CXCL11, and CXCL13 (40, 45). In this scenario HBCs are thought to be contributing to placental damage. In the case of TORCH infections, it is unknown whether HBCs are contributing to placental damage, or controlling infection. The presence of viral inclusions (CMV, Herpes Simplex, Coxsackie) or parasites (*Toxoplasma* and *Leishmania*) can certainly be found in HBCs, but it is unknown if these organisms are live and replication, or dying within the cell. HBCs are harboring live organisms these organisms are viable in these cells (38, 39).

HBC hyperplasia without villitis has also been observed with placental Zika virus infection (48, 49). This lesion is characterized by enlarged, hydropic chorionic villi, hyperplasia and focal proliferation of HBC, without necrosis or lymphocytic infiltration of the affected villi (48, 49). Some of the proliferating HBCs were found to contain Zika virus (49). Since Zika has been shown to replicate in HBCs (50–52), it has been proposed by several investigators that these cells may serve as a source of infection to the fetus (48, 53). However, the significance of HBCs in releasing infectious Zika virions is questionable since by Gavegnano and colleagues showed that Zika virions released from HBCs were incapable of infecting susceptible Vero cells (54). Whether antiviral responses in HBC are effective or compromised *in vivo* is yet to be determined. Regardless, perturbations in HBCs during placental infection with Zika suggest that these cells have altered function that may be detrimental to placental morphogenesis.

Preterm Delivery

There are a limited number of studies concerning HBCs in preterm delivery. These have been limited to chorioamnionitis-induced spontaneous preterm birth, severe preeclampsia, and HELLP syndrome. Two independent studies have shown that the density of CD68$^+$ HBCs are significantly reduced in chorioamnionitis (24, 37). The underlying mechanism for a decrease in HBCs during chorioamnionitis is unknown but it has been speculated that these cells may be undergoing apoptosis (37). HBC function, particularly multinucleated giant cells, is altered in placentas with chorioamnionitis. Namely, these cells exhibited decreased tolerogenic activity compared to the same cells retrieved from normal pregnancies (37). The application of high dimensional flow cytometry may allow discernment of the significance of a decrease in the density of CD68$^+$ cells: is CD68 selectively lost from a subset of cells? Does a different population of HBCs arise in these placentas?

Although a subset of preeclampsia patients develop HELLP, HELLP is considered a separate syndrome. Preeclampsia and HELLP have different clinical presentations (55, 56). Classical preeclampsia is characterized by hypertension and proteinuria, whereas HELLP involves activation of the coagulation system (55). Pathologic features within the placenta also differ between preeclampsia and HELLP. Infarction, intervillous thrombosis, and abruption is more common in placentas from preeclampsia patients than patients with HELLP (55). Furthermore, HBC numbers, and their expression of DC-SIGN and IL-10 are significantly reduced in patients with severe preeclampsia (28, 57). It has been suggested that the reduction of HBCs in preeclampsia may be promoting inflammatory damage due to the loss of tolerance-promoting HBCs (28). In contrast to preeclampsia, patients with HELLP exhibit increased numbers of CD68$^+$ HBCs, and it was concluded that this may be due to increased inflammation or an adaptive response (56).

CONCLUDING REMARKS

Our understanding of the role of HBCs in pregnancy is still rudimentary, but current evidence provides a compelling argument that these cells are important in placental development and homeostasis. At least in some pregnancy complications, such as VUE and chorioamnionitis, HBC dysfunction may be contributing to disease pathogenesis. Since HBCs exhibit functional plasticity, they may be ideal targets for therapeutic manipulation during disease states. However, additional studies are needed to better define the functional role of various HBC subsets in both health and disease.

ETHICS STATEMENT

Macaque data presented in this article was obtained with approval from the University of Wisconsin Institutional Animal Care and Use Committee.

AUTHOR CONTRIBUTIONS

LR conceived of the topic, conducted the research, and wrote the manuscript. TG assisted with non-human primate studies, and contributed to the writing of the manuscript.

FUNDING

This work was supported by award number R21AI136014-01. The content is solely the responsibility of the authors and does not necessarily represent the official views of the National Institutes of Health.

ACKNOWLEDGMENTS

The authors thank Aleks Stanic-Kostic and Bryce Wolfe for advice and assistance in implementing high-dimensional flow cytometry, and Xiao-jun Wu for assistance in Hofbauer cell isolation.

REFERENCES

1. Ingman K, Cookson VJKW, Jones CJP, Aplin JD. Characterisation of Hofbauer cells in first and second trimester placenta: incidence, phenotype, survival *in vitro* and motility. *Placenta* (2010) 31:535–44. doi: 10.1016/j.placenta.2010.03.003
2. Castellucci M, Schweikhart G, Kaufmann P, Zaccheo D. The stromal architecture of the immature intermediate villus of the human placenta. Functional and clinical implications. *Gynecol Obstet Invest.* (1984) 18:95–99.
3. Castellucci M, Zaccheo D, Pescetto G. A three-dimensional study of the normal human placental villous core. I. The Hofbauer cells. *Cell Tissue Res.* (1980) 210:235–47.
4. Kim JS, Romero R, Kim MR, Kim YM, Friel L, Espinoza J, et al. Involvement of Hofbauer cells and maternal T cells in villitis of unknown aetiology. *Histopathology* (2008) 52:457–64. doi: 10.1111/j.1365-2559.2008.02964.x
5. Bulmer JN, Johnson PM. Macrophage populations in the human placenta and amniochorion. *Clin Exp Immunol.* (1984) 57:393–403.
6. Kurt B. The human placenta. J. D. Boyd and W. J. Hamilton. Heffer, Cambridge, 365 pp. 1970. *Teratology* (1973) 8:77–8. doi: 10.1002/tera.1420080118
7. Cervar M, Blaschitz A, Dohr G, Desoye G. Paracrine regulation of distinct trophoblast functions *in vitro* by placental macrophages. *Cell Tissue Res.* (1999) 295:297–305.
8. Seval Y, Korgun ET, Demir R. Hofbauer cells in early human placenta: possible implications in vasculogenesis and angiogenesis. *Placenta* (2007) 28:841–5. doi: 10.1016/j.placenta.2007.01.010
9. Khan S, Katabuchi H, Araki M, Nishimura R, Okamura H. Human villous macrophage-conditioned media enhance human trophoblast growth and differentiation *in vitro*. *Biol Reprod.* (2000) 62:1075–83. doi: 10.1095/biolreprod62.4.1075

10. Demir R, Kayisli UA, Seval Y, Celik-Ozenci C, Korgun ET, Demir-Weusten AY, et al. Sequential expression of VEGF and its receptors in human placental villi during very early pregnancy: differences between placental vasculogenesis and angiogenesis. *Placenta* (2004) 25:560–72. doi: 10.1016/j.placenta.2003.11.011
11. Ahmed A, Li XF, Dunk C, Whittle MJ, Rushton DI, Rollason T. Colocalisation of vascular endothelial growth factor and its Flt-1 receptor in human placenta. *Growth Factors* (1995) 12:235–43.
12. Anteby EY, Natanson-Yaron S, Greenfield C, Goldman-Wohl D, Haimov-Kochman R, Holzer H, et al. Human placental Hofbauer cells express sprouty proteins: a possible modulating mechanism of villous branching. *Placenta* (2005) 26:476–83. doi: 10.1016/j.placenta.2004.08.008
13. Benirschke K, Burton, Graham J, Baergen, Rebecca N. *Pathology of the Human Placenta* Berlin Heidelberg: Springer-Verlag Berlin Heidelberg (2012). 941 p.
14. Reyes L, Wolfe B, Golos T. Hofbauer cells: placental macrophages of fetal origin. *Results Probl Cell Differ.* (2017) 62:45–60. doi: 10.1007/978-3-319-54090-0_3
15. Goldstein J, Braverman M, Salafia C, Buckley P. The phenotype of human placental macrophages and its variation with gestational age. *Am J Pathol.* (1988) 133:648–59.
16. Bulmer JN, Morrison L, Smith JC. Expression of class II MHC gene products by macrophages in human uteroplacental tissue. *Immunology* (1988) 63:707–14.
17. Sutton L, Mason DY, Redman CW. HLA-DR positive cells in the human placenta. *Immunology* (1983) 49:103–12.
18. Breburda EE, Dambaeva SV, Slukvin, II, Golos TG. Selective distribution and pregnancy-specific expression of DC-SIGN at the maternal-fetal interface in the rhesus macaque: DC-SIGN is a putative marker of the recognition of pregnancy. *Placenta* (2006) 27:11–21. doi: 10.1016/j.placenta.2004.11.006
19. Schliefsteiner C, Peinhaupt M, Kopp S, Logl J, Lang-Olip I, Hiden U, et al. Human placental Hofbauer cells maintain an anti-inflammatory M2 phenotype despite the presence of gestational diabetes mellitus. *Front Immunol.* (2017) 8:888. doi: 10.3389/fimmu.2017.00888
20. de Rijk EPCT, Van Esch E. The macaque placenta—a mini-review. *Toxicol Pathol.* (2008) 36(7_Suppl.):108S–18S. doi: 10.1177/01926233083 26095
21. Patrick LW. The fine structure of the placental villi of the rhesus monkey (Macaca mulatta). *Anat Rec.* (1970) 167:141–63. doi: 10.1002/ar.1091670203
22. Chen H, Lau MC, Wong MT, Newell EW, Poidinger M, Chen J. Cytofkit: a bioconductor package for an integrated mass cytometry data analysis pipeline. *PLOS Comput Biol.* (2016) 12:e1005112. doi: 10.1371/journal.pcbi.1005112
23. Young OM, Tang Z, Niven-Fairchild T, Tadesse S, Krikun G, Norwitz ER, et al. Toll-like receptor-mediated responses by placental Hofbauer cells (HBCs): a potential pro-inflammatory role for fetal M2 macrophages. *Am J Reprod Immunol.* (2015) 73:22–35. doi: 10.1111/aji.12336
24. Vinnars MT, Rindsjo E, Ghazi S, Sundberg A, Papadogiannakis N. The number of CD68(+) (Hofbauer) cells is decreased in placentas with chorioamnionitis and with advancing gestational age. *Pediatr Dev Pathol.* (2010) 13:300–4. doi: 10.2350/09-03-0632-OA.1
25. Dekel N, Gnainsky Y, Granot I, Racicot K, Mor G. The role of inflammation for a successful implantation. *Am J Reprod Immunol.* (2014) 72:141–7. doi: 10.1111/aji.12266
26. Sultana Z, Maiti K, Dedman L, Smith R. Is there a role for placental senescence in the genesis of obstetric complications and fetal growth restriction? *Am J Obstet Gynecol.* (2018) 218(2 Supplement):S762–73. doi: 10.1016/j.ajog.2017.11.567
27. Romero R, Espinoza J, Goncalves LF, Kusanovic JP, Friel LA, Nien JK. Inflammation in preterm and term labour and delivery. *Semin Fetal Neonatal Med.* (2006) 11:317–26. doi: 10.1016/j.siny.2006.05.001
28. Yang SW, Cho EH, Choi SY, Lee YK, Park JH, Kim MK, et al. DC-SIGN expression in Hofbauer cells may play an important role in immune tolerance in fetal chorionic villi during the development of preeclampsia. *J Reprod Immunol.* (2017) 124:30–7. doi: 10.1016/j.jri.2017.09.012
29. Bockle BC, Solder E, Kind S, Romani N, Sepp NT. DC-sign+ $CD163^+$ macrophages expressing hyaluronan receptor LYVE-1 are located within chorion villi of the placenta. *Placenta* (2008) 29:187–92. doi: 10.1016/j.placenta.2007.11.003
30. Duluc D, Delneste Y, Tan F, Moles MP, Grimaud L, Lenoir J, et al. Tumor-associated leukemia inhibitory factor and IL-6 skew monocyte differentiation into tumor-associated macrophage-like cells. *Blood* (2007) 110:4319–30. doi: 10.1182/blood-2007-02-072587
31. Johnson EL, Chakraborty R. Placental Hofbauer cells limit HIV-1 replication and potentially offset mother to child transmission (MTCT) by induction of immunoregulatory cytokines. *Retrovirology* (2012) 9:101. doi: 10.1186/1742-4690-9-101
32. Mills CD, Kincaid K, Alt JM, Heilman MJ, Hill AM. M-1/M-2 Macrophages and the Th1/Th2 Paradigm. *J Immunol.* (2000) 164:6166–73. doi: 10.4049/jimmunol.164.12.6166
33. Martinez FO, Sica A, Mantovani A, Locati M. Macrophage activation and polarization. *Front Biosci.* (2008) 13:2692. doi: 10.2741/2692
34. Roszer T. Understanding the mysterious M2 macrophage through activation markers and effector mechanisms. *Mediators Inflamm.* (2015) 2015:816460. doi: 10.1155/2015/816460
35. Kim SY, Romero R, Tarca AL, Bhatti G, Kim CJ, Lee J, et al. Methylome of fetal and maternal monocytes and macrophages at the feto-maternal interface. *Am J Reprod Immunol.* (2012) 68:8–27. doi: 10.1111/j.1600-0897.2012.01108.x
36. Loegl J, Hiden U, Nussbaumer E, Schliefsteiner C, Cvitic S, Lang I, et al. Hofbauer cells of M2a, M2b and M2c polarization may regulate feto-placental angiogenesis. *Reproduction* (2016) 152:447–55. doi: 10.1530/rep-16-0159
37. Ben Amara A, Gorvel L, Baulan K, Derain-Court J, Buffat C, Verollet C, et al. Placental macrophages are impaired in chorioamnionitis, an infectious pathology of the placenta. *J Immunol.* (2013) 191:5501–14. doi: 10.4049/jimmunol.1300988
38. Bittencourt AL, Garcia AG. The placenta in hematogenous infections. *Pediatr Pathol Mol Med.* (2002) 21:401–32. doi: 10.1080/152279502760157768
39. Faye-Petersen OM. The placenta in preterm birth. *J Clin Pathol.* (2008) 61:1261–75. doi: 10.1136/jcp.2008.055244
40. Kim MJ, Romero R, Kim CJ, Tarca AL, Chhauy S, LaJeunesse C, et al. Villitis of unknown etiology is associated with a distinct pattern of chemokine up-regulation in the feto-maternal and placental compartments: implications for conjoint maternal allograft rejection and maternal anti-fetal graft-versus-host disease. *J Immunol.* (2009) 182:3919–27. doi: 10.4049/jimmunol.0803834
41. Tamblyn JA, Lissauer DM, Powell R, Cox P, Kilby MD. The immunological basis of villitis of unknown etiology–review. *Placenta* (2013) 34:846–55. doi: 10.1016/j.placenta.2013.07.002
42. Wolfe B, Wiepz GJ, Schotzko M, Bondarenko GI, Durning M, Simmons HA, et al. Acute fetal demise with first trimester maternal infection resulting from listeria monocytogenes in a nonhuman primate model. *mBio* (2017) 8:e01938-16. doi: 10.1128/mBio.01938-16
43. Qureshi F, Jacques SM, Reyes MP. Placental histopathology in syphilis. *Hum Pathol.* (1993) 24:779–84.
44. Genest DR, Choi-Hong SR, Tate JE, Qureshi F, Jacques SM, Crum C. Diagnosis of congenital syphilis from placental examination: comparison of histopathology, Steiner stain, and polymerase chain reaction for Treponema pallidum DNA. *Hum Pathol.* (1996) 27:366–72.
45. Satosar A, Ramirez NC, Bartholomew D, Davis J, Nuovo GJ. Histologic correlates of viral and bacterial infection of the placenta associated with severe morbidity and mortality in the newborn. *Hum Pathol.* (2004) 35:536–45. doi: 10.1016/j.humpath.2004.01.015
46. Schwartz DA, Khan R, Stoll B. Characterization of the fetal inflammatory response to cytomegalovirus placentitis. An immunohistochemical study. *Arch Pathol Lab Med.* (1992) 116:21–7.
47. Noronha L, Zanluca C, Azevedo ML, Luz KG, Santos CN. Zika virus damages the human placental barrier and presents marked fetal neurotropism. *Mem Inst Oswaldo Cruz* (2016) 111:287–93. doi: 10.1590/0074-02760 160085
48. Schwartz DA. Viral infection, proliferation, and hyperplasia of Hofbauer cells and absence of inflammation characterize the placental pathology of fetuses with congenital Zika virus infection. *Arch Gynecol Obstet.* (2017) 295:1361–8. doi: 10.1007/s00404-017-4361-5
49. Rosenberg AZ, Yu W, Hill DA, Reyes CA, Schwartz DA. Placental pathology of Zika virus: viral infection of the placenta induces villous stromal macrophage (Hofbauer cell) proliferation and hyperplasia. *Arch Pathol Lab Med.* (2017) 141:43–8. doi: 10.5858/arpa.2016-0401-OA
50. Jurado KA, Simoni MK, Tang Z, Uraki R, Hwang J, Householder S, et al. Zika virus productively infects primary human placenta-specific macrophages. *JCI Insight* (2016) 1:88461. doi: 10.1172/jci.insight.88461

51. Quicke KM, Bowen JR, Johnson EL, McDonald CE, Ma H, O'Neal JT, et al. Zika virus infects human placental macrophages. *Cell Host Microbe* (2016) 20:83–90. doi: 10.1016/j.chom.2016.05.015
52. Tabata T, Petitt M, Puerta-Guardo H, Michlmayr D, Wang C, Fang-Hoover J, et al. Zika virus targets different primary human placental cells, suggesting two routes for vertical transmission. *Cell Host Microbe* (2016) 20:155–66. doi: 10.1016/j.chom.2016.07.002
53. Simoni MK, Jurado KA, Abrahams VM, Fikrig E, Guller S. Zika virus infection of Hofbauer cells. *Am J Reprod Immunol.* (2016) 77:e12613. doi: 10.1111/aji.12613
54. Gavegnano C, Bassit LC, Cox BD, Hsiao HM, Johnson EL, Suthar M, et al. Jak inhibitors modulate production of replication-competent Zika virus in human Hofbauer, trophoblasts, and neuroblastoma cells. *Pathog Immun.* (2017) 2:199–218. doi: 10.20411/pai.v2i2.190
55. Vinnars MT, Wijnaendts LC, Westgren M, Bolte AC, Papadogiannakis N, Nasiell J. Severe preeclampsia with and without HELLP differ with regard to placental pathology. *Hypertension* (2008) 51:1295–9. doi: 10.1161/HYPERTENSIONAHA.107.104844
56. Evsen MS, Kalkanli S, Deveci E, Sak ME, Ozler A, Baran O, et al. Human placental macrophages (Hofbauer cells) in severe preeclampsia complicated by HELLP syndrome:v immunohistochemistry of chorionic villi. *Anal Quant Cytopathol Histpathol.* (2013) 35:283–8.
57. Tang Z, Buhimschi IA, Buhimschi CS, Tadesse S, Norwitz E, Niven-Fairchild T, et al. Decreased levels of folate receptor-beta and reduced numbers of fetal macrophages (Hofbauer cells) in placentas from pregnancies with severe preeclampsia. *Am J Reprod Immunol.* (2013) 70:104–15. doi: 10.1111/aji.12112

15

Prenatal Immune and Endocrine Modulators of Offspring's Brain Development and Cognitive Functions Later in Life

Steven Schepanski [1,2]***, Claudia Buss*** [3,4]***, Ileana L. Hanganu-Opatz*** [2†] ***and Petra C. Arck*** [1*†]

[1] Laboratory of Experimental Feto-Maternal Medicine, Department of Obstetrics and Fetal Medicine, University Medical Center Hamburg-Eppendorf, Hamburg, Germany, [2] Developmental Neurophysiology, Institute of Neuroanatomy, University Medical Center Hamburg-Eppendorf, Hamburg, Germany, [3] Institute of Medical Psychology, Berlin Institute of Health, Charité-Universitätsmedizin Berlin, Corporate Member of Freie Universität Berlin, Humboldt-Universität zu Berlin, Berlin, Germany, [4] Development, Health, and Disease Research Program, University of California, Irvine, Orange, CA, United States

***Correspondence:**
Petra C. Arck
p.arck@uke.de

Milestones of brain development in mammals are completed before birth, which provide the prerequisite for cognitive and intellectual performances of the offspring. Prenatal challenges, such as maternal stress experience or infections, have been linked to impaired cognitive development, poor intellectual performances as well as neurodevelopmental and psychiatric disorders in the offspring later in life. Fetal microglial cells may be the target of such challenges and could be functionally modified by maternal markers. Maternal markers can cross the placenta and reach the fetus, a phenomenon commonly referred to as "vertical transfer." These maternal markers include hormones, such as glucocorticoids, and also maternal immune cells and cytokines, all of which can be altered in response to prenatal challenges. Whilst it is difficult to discriminate between the maternal or fetal origin of glucocorticoids and cytokines in the offspring, immune cells of maternal origin—although low in frequency—can be clearly set apart from offspring's cells in the fetal and adult brain. To date, insights into the functional role of these cells are limited, but it is emergingly recognized that these maternal microchimeric cells may affect fetal brain development, as well as post-natal cognitive performances and behavior. Moreover, the inheritance of vertically transferred cells across generations has been proposed, yielding to the presence of a microchiome in individuals. Hence, it will be one of the scientific challenges in the field of neuroimmunology to identify the functional role of maternal microchimeric cells as well as the brain microchiome. Maternal microchimeric cells, along with hormones and cytokines, may induce epigenetic changes in the fetal brain. Recent data underpin that brain development in response to prenatal stress challenges can be altered across several generations, independent of a genetic predisposition, supporting an epigenetic inheritance. We here discuss how fetal brain development and offspring's cognitive functions later in life is modulated in the turnstile of prenatal challenges by introducing novel and recently emerging pathway, involving maternal hormones and immune markers.

Keywords: pregnancy, fetal brain development, prenatal infection, maternal distress, maternal microchimeric cells, cytokines, glucocorticoids (GC), epigenetic aberrations

INTRODUCTION

The vertical transmission of maternal immune and endocrine markers is increasingly recognized to modulate fetal neurodevelopment and future mental health of the offspring. Emerging evidence arising from observational studies in humans reveals that prenatal environmental challenges such as maternal distress perception and infections are associated with an impaired fetal neurodevelopment and increased risk for neurological or psychiatric disorders later in life (1–6). Insights into the underlying mechanisms and pathogenesis of prenatally programmed poor mental health are increasingly emerging. It is well known that neurodevelopment results from the interaction of genetic, epigenetic and environmental factors, through which proliferation, migration of neural progenitor cells and establishment of neuronal circuits are modulated. Disruptions of these neurodevelopmental pathways may subsequently affect future brain function, as reflected by cognitive and intellectual impairment and increased the risk for neurodevelopmental and psychiatric disorders later in life (7).

Here, we compile the currently available evidence arising from observational studies supporting the concept of a developmental origin of brain disorders. We further outline cornerstones of brain development in mice and humans and discuss the effect of prenatal challenges, primarily maternal distress and infections, on maternal immune-endocrine adaptation to pregnancy. Lastly, we introduce novel concepts on how an altered maternal immune-endocrine adaptation to pregnancy can impact on offspring's brain development and subsequent mental health.

Developmental Origin of Neurological Dysfunctions and Psychiatric Disorders

Pregnancy is characterized by significant adaptational processes of the maternal immune and endocrine system in order to ensure its progression until term, which is required for adequate fetal development. These adaptational processes are highly responsive and vulnerable to challenges, such as high maternal stress perception or maternal infections. In this context, chronic stress states (e.g., depression or anxiety) affect approx. 10–15% of pregnant women worldwide (8). Moreover, negative life events may pose a significant threat to maternal wellbeing during pregnancy. **Table 1** provides a comprehensive overview of published evidence largely arising from observational studies that reveal a significant association between various types of maternal distress perception to which the mother was exposed to at specific gestational periods and the risk for psychiatric disorders in the offspring later in life, i.e., during childhood or adolescence. Disorders observed in the offspring include autism spectrum disorder (ASD) (9), depressive symptoms (10–12), anxiety, borderline personality disorder, eating disorders (23) and attention-deficit/hyperactivity disorder (ADHD) (3, 14–20, 22, 45). Interestingly, whilst a sex-specific risk is well known for psychiatric disorders, only very few studies paid attention whether prenatal stress perception skews the risk for such disorders in a sex-specific way. One study describes a sex-bias for ADHD upon prenatal stress, mirrored by a higher risk in daughters (20). Moreover, the timing of the prenatal challenge may be pivotal, as the risk for neurodevelopmental diseases appears to be differentially affected by the trimester of exposure (**Table 1**). In fact, surges of maternal IL-6 levels during the third trimester—which may result from distress or infections—showed a strongest impact on working memory performance in children. These behavioral changes were associated with alterations of brain regions tightly associated with working memory, as identified by functional MRI (46).

Besides high stress perception, maternal infection during pregnancy can interfere with fetal neurodevelopment and increase the risk for neurological dysfunctions and psychiatric disorders in the offspring (**Table 2**). Here, most of the studies focus on the distinct pathogens that have led to maternal infection during pregnancy (1, 35, 37, 42, 43). For example, maternal infection with influenza A or B virus has been associated with an increased risk for developing schizophrenia, although findings between studies are highly ambiguous and hence, hotly debated. Some studies report that influenza infection during the first trimester may trigger the risk for schizophrenia, whilst such effect could not be confirmed in studies focusing on infection at mid to late pregnancy (29–31, 47). The latter includes observations arising from Scandinavian registry analyses, where the query for prenatal influenza infection was solidly based on International Classification of Diseases (ICD)-coded diagnoses (48, 49). A recent meta-analysis confirms that evidence is insufficient to support gestational influenza as a risk factor for schizophrenia and bipolar disorder in the offspring (50). Besides these viral infections, also bacterial infections during pregnancy have been linked to an increased risk for schizophrenia in the offspring in adulthood (36, 44). For instance, 13% of all children surviving the maternal listeria monocytogenes infection were suffering from meningitis in early childhood (38) and this in return is significantly associated with developing schizophrenia and psychotic episodes later in life (39).

Milestones of Brain Development in Mice and Humans

Given that some of the observational studies summarized above highlight that the time point at which challenges occur prenatally may be crucial to trigger changes in fetal neurodevelopment, we here provide a brief summary of key aspects of fetal brain development that commence or are completed at distinct periods of gestation. We also include the brain development of mice, as mouse models have become pivotal in understanding how prenatal challenges affect neurodevelopment and brain functions later in life, as outlined in the subsequent paragraphs.

In humans and mice, brain development shows similar developmental processes (**Figure 1**). Noteworthy, sex-specific differences occur as a result of a faster cerebral maturation in girls (55), which leaves boys at higher risk for challenges-induced disruptions due to the greater window of vulnerability. Some developmental steps continue after birth in mice, which are already completed at birth in humans. This reduces the time window in mice during which vertically transferred maternal biological mediators can impact on offspring's brain development, a confounder which should be considered when

TABLE 1 | Summary of human studies examining the effect of prenatal maternal distress on offspring's mental health.

Proxy for prenatal maternal distress	Offspring's age at outcome evaluation	Offspring's outcome	Reference
INCIDENCE DURING THE FIRST TRIMESTER			
Exposure to a natural disaster	Childhood-preadolescence	ASD symptoms	(9)
Questionnaires-based evaluation of stress perception	Adolescence-adulthood	Internalizing and externalizing problems Depressive symptoms	(10–12)
Self-reported stressful events	Birth-adulthood	No risk for psychosis	(13)
INCIDENCE DURING THE SECOND TRIMESTER			
Exposure to a natural disaster	Childhood-preadolescence	ASD symptoms	(9)
Questionnaires-based evaluation of depression	Childhood-adolescence	Internalizing and externalizing problems Anxiety symptoms Depressive symptoms Hyperactivity Borderline personality disorder	(3, 14–18)
Self-reported stressful events	Childhood-adolescence	Internalizing problems Depressive symptoms ADHD symptoms No association to total psychiatric problems No risk for psychosis	(13, 19–21)
Questionnaires-based assessment of anxiety	Child-preadolescence	Total psychiatric problems Internalizing and externalizing problems Anxiety symptoms Depressive symptoms Hyperactivity	(14, 22)
Saliva cortisol	Preadolescence	ADHD symptoms especially in boys	(21)
INCIDENCE DURING THE THIRD TRIMESTER			
Exposure to a natural disaster	Childhood-preadolescence	ASD symptoms Eating disorder symptoms	(9, 23)
Questionnaires-based evaluation of depression	Preadolescence-adolescence	Externalizing problems Hyperactivity	(18, 24)
Self-reported stressful events	Birth–adulthood	ADHD symptoms No association to total psychiatric problems No risk for psychosis	(13, 20, 21)
Questionnaires-based assessment of anxiety	Childhood-adolescence	Internalizing problems Depressive symptoms Hyperactivity	(3, 14, 15)
Saliva cortisol	Preadolescence	ADHD symptoms especially in girls	(21)
Physician-based diagnoses of depression	Childhood-adulthood	Depressive symptoms ADHD symptoms	(6, 25)
ICD-based diagnoses of anxiety	Childhood	ADHD symptoms	(6)
INCIDENCE DURING PREGNANCY WITHOUT FURTHER TRIMESTER SPECIFICATION			
Self-reported stressful events	Childhood-adulthood	Eating disorders ASD symptoms Schizophrenia in male offspring	(26–28)

discussing the biological relevance of findings on prenatal challenges in mice. Hence, when evaluating the impact of maternal markers on fetal development in mice, research endeavor should focus on milestones that are completed prior to birth, such as neurulation, neuronal migration and microglia invasion, as well as synaptogenesis and neurogenesis, the latter being largely completed at birth.

Effect of Prenatal Challenges on Maternal Immune-Endocrine Adaptation to Pregnancy

In mice and humans, healthy brain development is crucially dependent on an endocrine and immunological homeostasis of the mother-fetus dyad. Here, the balance between pro- and anti-inflammatory cytokines is crucial, as neurogenesis, migration, differentiation and apoptosis are well known to be responsive to cytokine challenges (**Table 3**). Besides cytokines, chemokines are also important in modulating neurodevelopment and the risk for psychiatric diseases. Since these interactions have been addressed in recent reviews (80–82), we refrain from including them here. Similarly, glucocorticoids, which are initially largely maternally derived during gestation in the fetus, can interfere with fetal brain development in mice and humans. Moreover, additional factors such as maternal immune cells can affect fetal brain development. Prenatal stimuli and challenges, including maternal stress perception and infection, have been show to interfere with the

TABLE 2 | Overview of studies examining the effects prenatal infection and related maternal immune activation on offspring's mental health in human.

Gestational time point of infection	Proxy used to identify prenatal infection	Offspring's age at evaluation	Offspring's outcome	Reference
VIRAL INFECTIONS DURING PREGNANCY				
Each trimester	Maternal antibodies against Influenza virus A and B	Adulthood	Increased risk for schizophrenia	(29–31)
End of pregnancy	Maternal antibodies against cytomegalovirus, rubella virus, human parvovirus B19, herpes simplex virus 1 and 2	Lifetime	Increased risk for schizophrenia Increased risk for psychosis	(32, 33)
Newborn's blood (5–7 days old)	Maternal antibodies against herpes simplex virus 2	Lifetime	Increased risk for schizophrenia	(34)
Pregnancy	Retrospective estimation infection	2–5 years	Maternal fever, but not influenza, increases the risk for schizophrenia	(35)
BACTERIAL INFECTIONS DURING PREGNANCY				
End of pregnancy	Maternal antibodies against chlamydia trachomatis	Lifetime	Increase risk for schizophrenia	(32)
Pregnancy	Retrospective estimation	32–34 and 45–47 years	Increased risk for schizophrenia	(36)
Pregnancy	Maternal C-reactive protein	ASD diagnosis	Increased risk for ASD	(37)
Pregnancy	ICD-based registry queries	–	Increased risk for schizophrenia and psychotic episodes via meningitis in childhood	(38, 39)
PARASITIC INFECTIONS DURING PREGNANCY				
Each trimester	Maternal antibodies against toxoplasma gondii	24–30 years	Increased risk for schizophrenia	(30, 40)
End of pregnancy	Maternal antibodies against toxoplasma gondii	Lifetime	Increased risk for schizophrenia	(41)
NON-CLASSIFIED PRENATAL INFECTIONS				
Pregnancy	ICD-based registry queries	Lifetime	Increased risk for ASD Increased severity of ASD symptoms compared to non-infected ASD offspring	(1, 42, 43)
Pregnancy	ICD-based registry queries	Lifetime	Maternal infection before and after pregnancy increased the risk for schizophrenia	(44)

endocrine and immunological hemostasis in the mother. This includes the activation of the sympathetic nervous system and the hypothalamus-pituitary-adrenal (HPA) axis, subsequently leading to an excess secretion and availability of free, biologically active glucocorticoids (83, 84). Pregnancy itself is considered to be a state of "hypercortisolism," which is an essential requirement to meet the maternal demand for increased metabolism and energy generation. The fetus is also critically dependent on the transfer of maternal glucocorticoids, which is controlled for by placental enzymes such as 11ß-Hydroxysteroid-Dehydrogenase (11ß-HSD)-1 and -2 (83, 84). Maternal glucocorticoids ensure structural and functional development of fetal organs, as the fetus is not capable of producing glucocorticoids until late in development. However, elevated glucocorticoid concentrations in the context of maternal stress may negatively impact on fetal brain development (83).

Besides the effect of prenatal challenges on maternal glucocorticoid levels, the maternal immune response may also be skewed toward inflammation in the context of stress in human pregnancy or infection (85, 86). Similarly in mice, maternal stress challenges have been shown to increase levels of pro-inflammatory cytokines in dams (87) and decrease tolerogenic markers such as $CD4^{+}$ regulatory T cells (88). Similarly, prenatal infection e.g., with influenza A virus in mice leads to an increased type 1 response, along with an increased production of pro-inflammatory cytokines, compared to non-infected pregnant mice (89). Equally, the use of "danger signals" such as lipopolysaccharide to induce an inflammatory response in pregnant mice resulted in a collapse of immune tolerance toward the fetus (90).

Maternal cytokines, glucocorticoids as well as maternal immune cells can cross the placenta. Whilst it is difficult to determine if cytokines are maternally derived or produced by the fetus, maternal immune cells can be clearly identified in the offspring. These maternal microchimeric cells can persist in the offspring long after birth (91). Hence, opposed to the vertical transfer of maternal cytokines and glucocorticoids, maternal microchimeric cells may be capable to continuously modulate brain function in the offspring even after birth.

Impact of Altered Maternal Immune-Endocrine Adaptation to Pregnancy and Offspring's Brain Development and Mental Health

The vertical transfer of maternal immune and endocrine markers is increasingly recognized to modulate fetal neurodevelopment and future mental health of the offspring. As mentioned above,

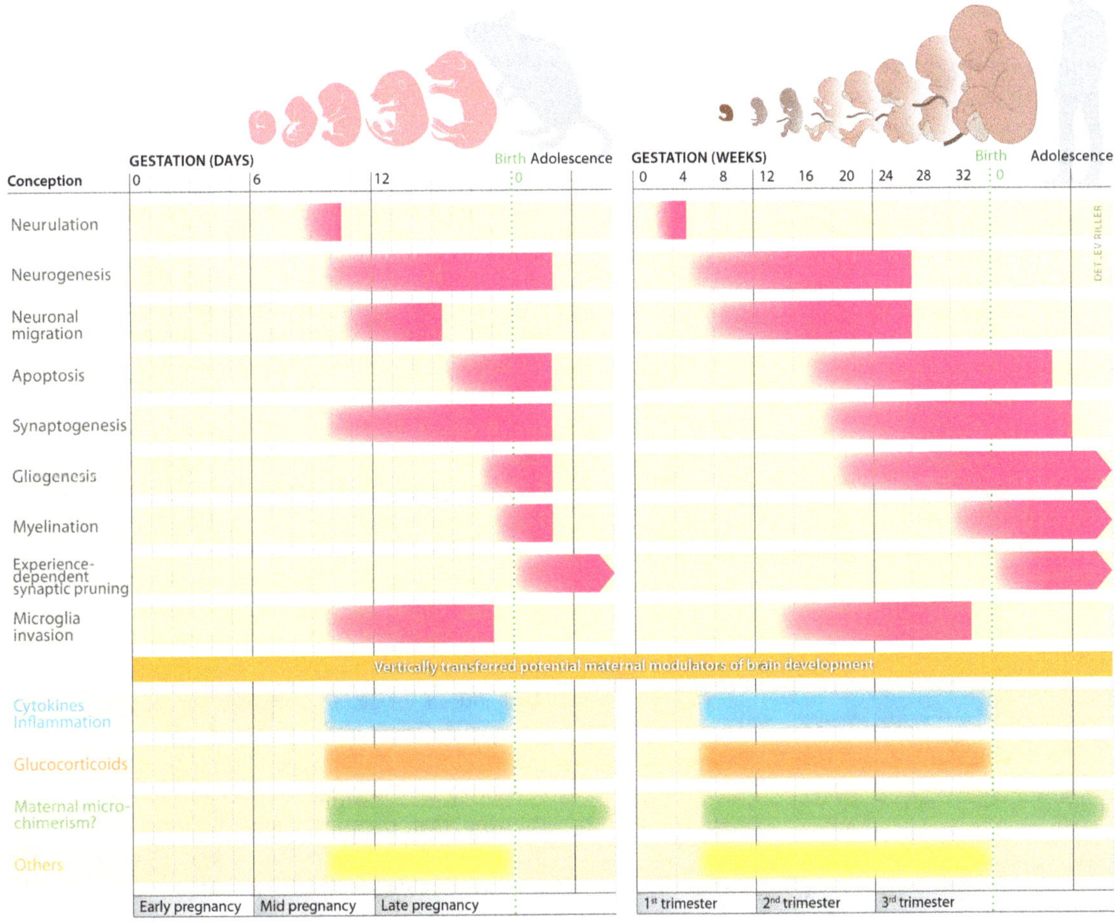

FIGURE 1 | Milestones of brain development in mice and humans. In **both species,** brain development commences with neurulation, a process creating the neural tube. This provides the prerequisite for the subsequent production of neuron from neural stem cells, a process defined as neurogenesis. Early during human development, at gestation week 4, the anterior part of the neural tube begins to form into distinct regions. The forebrain, midbrain and hindbrain are defined as the anterior part; the spinal cord is located at the posterior part. Two weeks later, the neural tube can be clearly divided into the brain regions that are present at birth. Some of the previously produced neurons now start to migrate to distinct brain regions, a process that continues until approx. week 26. Earlier by week 11, the cerebrum has developed—more rapidly than other structures—and largely covers the entire brain, except cerebellum and medulla oblongata. Due to its progressive development within the cranium, the cerebrum is forced to convolve itself resulting in gyri and sulci (51). During the second trimester of pregnancy, several processes start to define brain connectivity. These include synaptogenesis, gliogenesis, and apoptosis. Simultaneously, microglial cells invasion begins. By mid-third trimester, the fine-tuning of neuronal connectivity starts with proliferation of myelin sheaths throughout the neurons of the central nervous system (52). Shortly after birth, the previously established neuronal connections are reduced based on neuronal activity, meaning a reduction of neuronal connections to the ones often used. Since murine gestation is much shorter compared to human pregnancy, some developmental steps continue to proceed after birth. In mice, neural development begins during mid-pregnancy, followed by neurulation and formation of the neural tube (53). Subsequently, production of neurons, their migration and the formation of synapses occur almost simultaneously. Also, yolk sac-derived microglial cells invade the fetus starting on day 9 of pregnancy (54). The developmental milestones underlying brain development in mice and humans are highly susceptible to challenges and can be modulated by maternal markers vertically transferred during pregnancy. Hereby, the time point and intensity of the challenges clearly determine the impact and damage they may cause.

the impact of cytokines on fetal brain development has been well studied and it is widely accepted that milestones of physiological fetal brain development are modulated by cytokines (**Table 3**). Hence, exposure to an imbalanced cytokine response during fetal life may disturb fetal brain development, thereby increasing the risk for neurodevelopmental disorders (92).

In mice, fetal exposure to an altered, pro-inflammatory maternal cytokine response can affect brain morphology, mirrored by e.g., an increased pyramidal cell density or reduced neurogenesis (93–96). Similarly, prenatal maternal treatment with the immunostimulant polyinosinic:polycytidylic acid (poly I:C) to mirror some effects of a viral infection has been shown to result in reduced axonal size, myelin thickness and cortical volume of the hippocampus and amygdala in rodent offspring (97, 98). A general maternal immune activation during pregnancy has also been shown to cause presynaptic deficits in hippocampus (99), pro-inflammatory activation in hippocampal microglia (100) or an increase of microglial cell frequencies in the fetal brain (101). Hence, a wealth of studies has shown that maternal immune activation during pregnancy adversely affects

TABLE 3 | Key cytokines influencing neural cell development.

Cytokine	Functional outcome	Reference
IL-1α	Supports astrocyte lineage commitment	(56)
	Increases neurogenesis	(57)
	Increases microglia activity	(58)
IL-1β	Inhibition of neurogenesis	(59–61)
	Supports astrocyte lineage commitment	(58, 59)
IL-6	Supports establishment synaptic connectivity	(62, 63)
	Suppresses astrocyte development	(64)
TNF-α	Inhibition of neural progenitor cell proliferation and differentiation (via TNF receptor 1)	(65)
	Supports cell survival (via TNF receptor 2)	(65)
	Neuroprotective functions	(66)
IL-2	Increases differentiation of neural progenitor cells	(67)
	Increases neurogenesis	(68)
IFN-γ	Supports differentiation, migration and neuronal outgrowth (via microglia activation)	(69)
IL-10	Increases neural progenitor cell survival, differentiation and neuronal myelination	(70)
	Supports oligodendroglia progenitor cell survival Increases neural progenitor cell migration	(71) (72)
IL-4	Neuroprotection (via microglia activation)	(69)
TGF-β	Excessive concentration leads to declined neurogenesis	(73)
LIF	Promotion of cell growth (via inhibition of differentiation)	(74)
	Supports neural stem cell self-renewal	(75, 76)
IL-17	Inhibition of adult neurogenesis and synaptic function, decreases neural stem cell numbers, proliferation and differentiation	(77–79)

fetal brain development on multiple levels. Yet, it is difficult to comprehensively pinpoint distinct pathways, as the studies performed to date have been rather diverse with regard to the species, the gestational time point or the cause of maternal immune activation (102). In humans, a great deal of research focused on the role of maternal levels of interleukin-6 as a proxy for a prenatal inflammatory challenge. Key observations include that maternal IL-6 levels affects offspring's structural and functional connectivity already at the time of birth (103), delaying the development of sensory and cognitive processing (46, 104).

Similar to cytokines, fetal exposure to elevated concentrations of maternal glucocorticoids has been proposed to exert long-lasting, partly sex-specific effects on offspring's brain morphology and function in rodents but also in humans. This includes decreased dendritic morphology and neuronal volume in hippocampi of both sexes in mice, whereas an increased dendritic branching has been detected only in females (105). Another study using mouse models reports an increased spine density, dendritic length and other morphological features in pyramidal neurons of prenatally stressed males, which was decreased in females (106).

In humans, elevated maternal cortisol concentrations in early pregnancy have been associated with larger amygdala volumes, an altered neural connectivity, along with affective symptoms and internalizing problems in girls (107). Interestingly, moderately elevated maternal cortisol levels in late pregnancy could be associated with greater cortical thickness primarily in frontal regions and enhanced cognitive performance in children (108). These findings point to the importance of considering the moderating role of sex and timing of exposure to glucocorticoids during pregnancy.

Since the experimental or study designs differ with regard to stress paradigms/glucocorticoids applications, time point of prenatal interventions or postnatal analyses, species and read-out parameter (109–111), it is not yet possible to comprehensively summarize the outcome of these studies beyond the statement that prenatal stress and related glucocorticoid surges induce sex- and brain area-specific differences in neuronal complexity and neurogenesis. This may subsequently lead to altered cognitive functions later in life.

Microglial cells, which are the resident macrophages of the CNS, have also been extensively studied in response to prenatal stress or prenatal glucocorticoid application. Due to their phagocytic phenotype, microglia have a functional role in remodeling, shaping and pruning of synapses (112). And indeed, prenatal corticosterone application increased the microglial density in the embryonic brain overall and promoted their amoeboid phenotype (113). Interestingly, this result was supported by isolating and culturing P1-2 microglial cells, showing that they are more likely to acquire an amoeboid phenotype (114). At postnatal age, stress increased the total glia cell number in the hippocampus of female but not male offspring (115). One study showed an increased number of microglia cells in the dentate gyrus, suggesting an adverse effect on neurogenesis and simultaneously no changes in the CA1 of the hippocampus (116, 117). The early stress exposure seems to support phagocytic microglia function in the early brain and potentially stimulate their activity throughout early murine lifetime. Their role as a potential mediator between prenatal stress and early neurobiological changes remains vague, especially in other important brain areas such like the PFC.

The barrier between periphery and the brain is an essential interface for communication between both compartments. Even though the blood brain barrier is supposed to be well established during early development, its function in stress and cytokine-related diseases is poorly investigated. However, its permeability is a key component in how maternal markers may influence the offspring's brain development. This topic is excellently described in an comprehensive review elsewhere [see review, (118)] and thus not explained here.

In **Figure 2**, we depict key effects of cytokines/inflammation and glucocorticoids on microglia cells and neurons in the prefrontal cortex, hippocampus and amygdala of the fetal brain. We deliberately focused on these specific brain regions due to their specific relevance for the mental health problems that have been described in the context of maternal stress and infection (122).

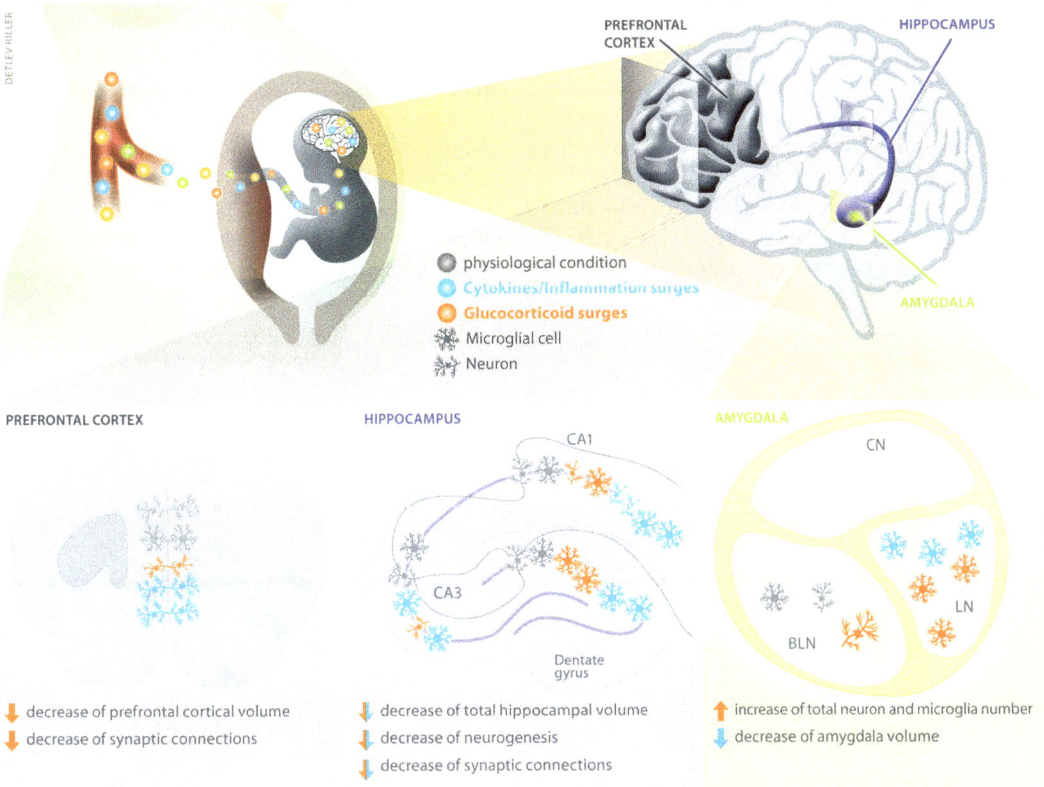

FIGURE 2 | Consequences of cytokine and glucocorticoid surges on distinct areas of the offspring's brain. Maternal cytokines and glucocorticoids can transplacentally cross into the fetus and differentially affect offspring's brain development by interfering with e.g., cell differentiation, axonal growth, and synaptic connectivity. The brain regions depicted here are of pivotal relevance for mental health due to their involvement in cognitive functions. Compared to physiological conditions, prenatal surges of maternal cytokines increase the number of neuronal connections in a subdivision of the prefrontal cortex, whereas glucocorticoids decreases them (105, 119). Additionally, prenatal glucocorticoid exposure decreases prefrontal cortical volume. In the hippocampus, an increase of cytokines is known to increase the number of microglial cells in the corn ammonis area 1 (CA1), whilst simultaneously reducing dendritic arborizations and neuronal complexity (111). Similarly, in the CA3 and dentate gyrus (DG) of the hippocampus, the microglia density increases after cytokine exposure. Also glucocorticoid surges deteriorate the neuronal complexity in CA1 and CA3 (109, 110) and have been shown to increases the number of microglia in DG. Both, cytokines and glucocorticoids can decrease total hippocampal volume, neurogenesis and synaptic connections. Prenatal cytokine surges can also decrease the amygdala volume, whereas glucocorticoids have been shown to increase the number of neurons and microglia. There is no evidence that the central nucleus (CN) of the amygdala is affected, but an increased microglia density after prenatal cytokine and glucocorticoid exposure has been detected in the lateral nucleus (LN) (120, 121). Contrarily, an increased number of neuronal connections and microglia was detectable upon glucocorticoid challenge in the basolateral nucleus (BLN).

Besides the effect of glucocorticoids and cytokines on neurogenesis, synaptogenesis, axon growth etc., these mediators can also exert indirect effects on these fundamental processes of fetal brain development, i.e., by altering the concentration or availability of neurotransmitters. The primary excitatory neurochemical in the central nervous system, glutamate, which acts through different types of metabotropic glutamate receptors (mGluR) has been investigated in a number of studies (123–125). Indeed, a variant of the Kozak sequence of exon 1 of the mGluR 3 could be associated with e.g., bipolar affective disorder (126). Moreover, a reduced expression of mGluR receptors in the hippocampus has been observed in response to prenatal stress (127–129). Brain functions such as mood, satiety, sleep, body temperature and nociception are also critically dependent on the serotonergic system, and prenatal challenges have been shown to interfere with the rate of serotonin synthesis (130), the number of serotonin positive cells (131) and its receptor density (132) in the offspring's brain. Further, the cholinergic system is important in regulating brain function (e.g., learning and short-term memory) (133) that has been shown to be impacted in the offspring in the context of maternal stress and infection during pregnancy. Some evidence from rodent models support the notion that prenatal stress challenges interfere with the release of cholinergic factors in the offspring, such as acetylcholine (134), whereby changes of behavior have not been evaluated in this study.

Introducing a Novel Pathway in the Developmental Origin of Neurocognitive Functions and Psychiatric Disorders: the Impact of Maternal Microchimeric Cells

Maternal microchimeric cells, which are vertically transferred from mother to fetus during pregnancy and—at least in part—during lactation (135–137), can be detected in the offspring's brain during fetal and adult life. Hence, maternal microchimeric cells have the potential to modulate brain development and the risk for neurodevelopmental disorders. To date, no insights are available on the role of maternal microchimeric cells in brain development and their potential ability to tailor the nervous system individually. Moreover, brain structures where maternal microchimeric cells may abundantly populate have not yet been identified. However, since maternal microchimeric cells have been identified as maternal immune cells of the innate and adaptive immune response, they hold the strong potential to shape neurons by acquiring a phagocytic phenotype, akin to offspring's microglial cells. Future studies should aim at elucidating the functional role of maternal microchimeric cells on the developing brain and to understand whether they may modulate the risk for brain-related disorders.

Given the plethora of mediators that may be functionally involved in shaping brain development and subsequent function, whilst being altered upon maternal stress, infection and other

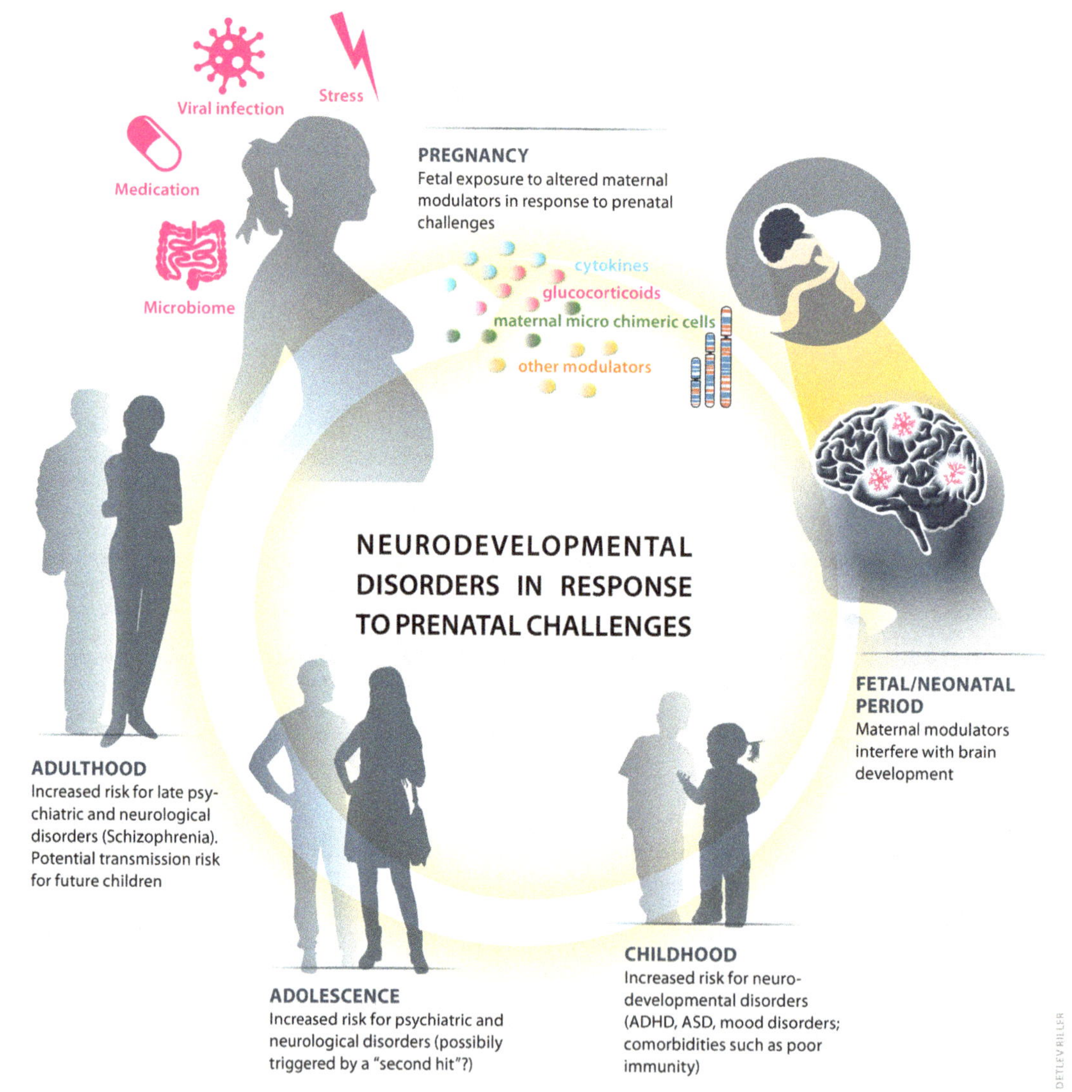

FIGURE 3 | Prenatal challenges and related alterations of immune and endocrine markers can prime postnatal neurodevelopmental disorders. Maternal well-being and health can be challenged during pregnancy, e.g., by distress or infection. This subsequently leads to increased cytokines and glucocorticoids levels and potentially to altered frequencies or phenotypes of maternal microchimeric cells in the offspring. Upon entering the fetal brain, such vertically transferred maternal modulators can significantly interfere with physiologically occurring brain development. A combination of genetic susceptibility and disturbed brain development can subsequently increase the risk for neurodevelopmental disorders in childhood. Subsequent postnatal environmental challenges —drug abuse, trauma, infection, others—may perpetuate such prenatally triggered risk for neurodevelopmental disorders, psychiatric and neurological diseases during adolescence and adulthood, which can also be passed on to the next generation.

prenatal conditions (138), it is not surprising that we are far from fully understanding the developmental origin of neurocognitive functions and brain disorders. Also, it seems unlikely that single mediators determine a clear-cut "good or bad" outcome. It is more likely that the mediators we here proposed act synergistically in modulating brain development and subsequent function with an advantageous or disadvantageous outcome. Hypothetically, this synergistic cross talk could involve the expression of glucocorticoid receptor on maternal microchimeric cells or the release of cytokines from maternal microchimeric cells entering the fetal brain. The longevity of such cells would surpass the short-term effect that could result from the potential transplacental transfer of cytokines itself, as cytokines are rapidly metabolized.

Functional Impact of Vertically Transferred Maternal Markers on the Developing Brain

In response the environmental challenges, altered levels of maternal markers that cross the placental barrier may affect the developing brain by inducing epigenetic alterations of somatic cells (139–142) Persistent epigenetic differences triggered by the prenatal exposure to stress challenges in humans include increased and decreased methylation of insulin-like growth factor 2 or the glucocorticoid receptor gene (NR3C1) in brain cells, depending on the timing of exposure (143, 144). Prenatal distress has been associated with hyper- as well as demethylation of specific regulatory sites in key genes involved in stress processing, such as the glucocorticoid receptor (144–146). Similarly, findings arising from mouse models on maternal immune activation during pregnancy include the observations of a hypoacetlyation of e.g., genes modulating neuronal development, synaptic transmission and immune signaling in the cortex region in exposed offspring (147), as well as sex-specific DNA hypomethylation in the hypothalamus of females (148), specifically affecting the promoter region of methyl CpG-binding protein 2, which is associated with neurodevelopmental disorders (149). Interestingly, prenatal immune activation in mice could be linked to hypermethylation of glutamic acid decarboxylase 1 and 2 in the brain (150), associated with altered behavior.

Strikingly, mouse models have revealed that alterations of brain function can be passed on to the next generations (151), suggesting that underlying epigenetic alterations triggered by prenatal challenges may be intergenerationally inherited. This notion could provide an explanation for the increasing incidence of behavioral disorders (152). Moreover, it implies that exposure of the mother to environmental challenges during pregnancy may not only directly interfere with fetal brain development, but also affects fetal primordial germ cells (153), which may subsequently interfere with brain development in the generation of grandchildren. Primordial germ cells undergo sequential epigenetic events, which are distinct from fetal somatic cells, hereby preserving the plasticity required for the generation of gametes (154–157). Once the offspring reaches adulthood and such oocytes are fertilized, the resulting zygote again undergoes significant epigenetic reprogramming, which includes the demethylation of the maternal and paternal genome, followed by a genome-wide *de novo* methylation (158).

Animal data indicate the possibility of transmission of behavioral traits mediated by epigenetic modifications through the maternal, as well as paternal germ line (159–162), implying the generation of oocytes and sperm may be equally affected. Intriguingly, how epigenetic changes induced by environmental challenges can be maintained throughout the multiple epigenetic reprogramming events physiologically occurring during reprogramming of primordial germ cells and the zygote is still largely elusive. Insights from mouse studies provide a first glimpse, as they reveal that certain regions of the genome, i.e., differentially methylated regions, are resistant to zygotic reprogramming (158). However, future research is required to identify pathways of intergeneration epigenetic inheritance of altered brain function in the offspring, aiming also to differentiate between *de novo* acquired epigenetic alterations from those inherited through the germ line. Besides such intergenerational inheritance of epigenetic marks, the possibility of transgenerational inheritance of epigenetic changes to one further generation of descent, the great-grand generation, has been considered. The primordial germ cells of the forth generation would not have been directly exposed to the environmental challenges or mediators released by the great-grandmother during pregnancy. However, to date, convincing evidence of transgenerational inheritance of epigenetic marks is only available from botany research using plants, whilst confirmation in mammals is somewhat elusive (163).

Besides such epigenetic pathways, the brain as target tissue for prenatal challenges may be affected in its electrical synchrony, which is defined as the coordinated oscillatory activity and neural firing rate between connected brain areas. These links are a prerequisite to execute cognitive tasks (164, 165). Interestingly, prenatal exposure to maternal inflammation or stress impairs oscillatory synchronicity (166), which commenced already during developmental stages in a mouse model of neuropsychiatric disorders (167–169) and affected spatial memory tasks (170, 171).

Outlook

Higher cognitive functions such as planning, self-regulation, memory, learning, and emotional processes result from a complex, tailored, and precisely shaped large-scale communication of neuronal networks (172). These neuronal networks begins to develop prenatally and disturbances of such developing neural systems during pregnancy can disrupt brain development via the vertical transfer of maternal markers, such as cytokines, glucocorticoids or microchimeric cells of the maternal immune system. Subsequently, the risk for mental disorders and diseases can increase in the offspring (**Figure 3**). As most of the studies are correlative, future research should aim to investigate causalities between maternal factors and children's health outcome. Clearly, adverse postnatal childhood experiences can further aggravate such cognitive and behavioral dysfunctions (173–178) and thus, should be considered in experimental designs and observational studies.

AUTHOR CONTRIBUTIONS

SS and PA developed the structure of the review article, SS provided the first draft, which was amended by CB on aspects including prenatal cytokines and epigenetic pathways, by IH-O by insights on brain development and by PA on issues related to maternal immune adaptation to pregnancy. All authors have been involved in the interpretation of published evidence, critically revised the manuscript and gave their final approval of the version to be published.

ACKNOWLEDGMENTS

Writing of this review and reference to the authors' own work were made possible through funding by the Deutsche Forschungsgemeinschaft (KFO296, AR232/26-2 to PA and SFB 936 B5, SPP 1665 Ha4466/12-1 to IH-O) and ERC Consolidator Grant 681577 to IH-O and R01 MH-105538, 5UG3OD023349 and ERC Starting grant 639766 to CB.

REFERENCES

1. Christian MA, Samms-Vaughan M, Lee M, Bressler J, Hessabi M, Grove ML, et al. Maternal exposures associated with autism spectrum disorder in jamaican children. *J Autism Dev Disord.* (2018) 48:2766–78. doi: 10.1007/s10803-018-3537-6
2. Dimitrova N, Turpin H, Borghini A, Harari MM, Urben S, Müller-Nix C, Perinatal stress moderates the link between early and later emotional skills in very preterm-born children: an 11-year-long longitudinal study. *Early Hum Dev.* (2018) 121:8–14. doi: 10.1016/j.earlhumdev.2018.04.015
3. Glynn LM, Howland MA, Sandman CA, Davis EP, Phelan M, Baram TZ, et al. Prenatal maternal mood patterns predict child temperament and adolescent mental health. *J Affect Disord.* (2018) 228:83–90. doi: 10.1016/j.jad.2017.11.065
4. Laplante DP, Hart KJ, O'Hara MW, Brunet A, and King S. Prenatal maternal stress is associated with toddler cognitive functioning: the Iowa flood study. *Early Hum Dev.* (2018) 116:84–92. doi: 10.1016/j.earlhumdev.2017.11.012
5. Nolvi S, Pesonen H, Bridgett DJ, Korja R, Kataja EL, Karlsson H, et al. Infant sex moderates the effects of maternal pre-and postnatal stress on executive functioning at 8 months of age. *Infancy* (2018) 23:194–210. doi: 10.1111/infa.12206
6. Vizzini L, Popovic M, Zugna D, Vitiello B, Trevisan M, Pizzi C, et al. Maternal anxiety, depression and sleep disorders before and during pregnancy, and preschool ADHD symptoms in the NINFEA birth cohort study. *Epidemiol Psychiatric Sci.* 2018:1–11. doi: 10.1017/S2045796018000185
7. Bale TL, Baram TZ, Brown AS, Goldstein JM, Insel TR, McCarthy MM, et al. Early life programming and neurodevelopmental disorders. *Biol Psychiatry* (2010) 68:314–9. doi: 10.1016/j.biopsych.2010.05.028
8. Fisher J, Cabral de Mello M, Patel V, Rahman A, Tran T, Holton S, et al. Prevalence and determinants of common perinatal mental disorders in women in low- and lower-middle-income countries: a systematic review. *Bull World Health Organ.* (2012) 90:139G–49G. doi: 10.2471/BLT.11.091850
9. Walder DJ, Laplante DP, Sousa-Pires A, Veru F, Brunet A, and King S. Prenatal maternal stress predicts autism traits in 6½ year-old children: Project Ice Storm. *Psychiatry Res.* (2014) 219:353–60. doi: 10.1016/j.psychres.2014.04.034
10. Betts KS, Williams GM, Najman JM, Alati R. Maternal depressive, anxious, and stress symptoms during pregnancy predict internalizing problems in adolescence. *Depress Anxiety* (2014) 31:9–18. doi: 10.1002/da.22210
11. Betts KS, Williams GM, Najman JM, Alati R. The relationship between maternal depressive, anxious, and stress symptoms during pregnancy and adult offspring behavioral and emotional problems. *Depress Anxiety* (2015) 32:82–90. doi: 10.1002/da.22272
12. Kingsbury M, Weeks M, MacKinnon N, Evans J, Mahedy L, Dykxhoorn J, et al. Stressful life events during pregnancy and offspring depression: evidence from a prospective cohort study. *J Am Acad Child Adolesc Psychiatry* (2016) 55:709–716e2. doi: 10.1016/j.jaac.2016.05.014
13. Abel KM, Heuvelman HP, Jorgensen L, Magnusson C, Wicks S, Susser E, et al. Severe bereavement stress during the prenatal and childhood periods and risk of psychosis in later life: population based cohort study. *BMJ* (2014) 348:f7679. doi: 10.1136/bmj.f7679
14. O'Donnell KJ, Glover V, Holbrook JD, O'Connor TG. Maternal prenatal anxiety and child brain-derived neurotrophic factor (BDNF) genotype: effects on internalizing symptoms from 4 to 15 years of age. *Dev Psychopathol.* (2014). 26(4 Pt 2):1255–66. doi: 10.1017/S095457941400100X
15. O'Donnell KJ, Glover V, Barker ED, O'Connor TG. The persisting effect of maternal mood in pregnancy on childhood psychopathology. *Dev Psychopathol.* (2014) 26:393–403. doi: 10.1017/S0954579414000029
16. Capron LE, Glover V, Pearson RM, Evans J, O'Connor TG, Stein A, et al. Associations of maternal and paternal antenatal mood with offspring anxiety disorder at age 18 years. *J Affect Disord.* (2015) 187:20–6. doi: 10.1016/j.jad.2015.08.012
17. Winsper C, Wolke D, Lereya T. Prospective associations between prenatal adversities and borderline personality disorder at 11-12 years. *Psychol Med.* (2015) 45:1025–37. doi: 10.1017/S0033291714002128
18. Leis JA, Heron J, Stuart EA, and Mendelson T. Associations between maternal mental health and child emotional and behavioral problems: does prenatal mental health matter? *J Abnormal Child Psychol.* (2014). 42:161–71. doi: 10.1007/s10802-013-9766-4
19. Tearne JE, Allen KL, Herbison CE, Lawrence D, Whitehouse AJ, Sawyer MG, et al. The association between prenatal environment and children's mental health trajectories from 2 to 14 years. *Eur Child Adolesc Psychiatry* (2015) 24:1015–24. doi: 10.1007/s00787-014-0651-7
20. Zhu P, Hao JH, Tao RX, Huang K, Jiang XM, Zhu YD, et al. Sex-specific and time-dependent effects of prenatal stress on the early behavioral symptoms of ADHD: a longitudinal study in China. *Eur Child Adolesc Psychiatry* (2015) 24:1139–47. doi: 10.1007/s00787-015-0701-9
21. Isaksson J, Lindblad F, Valladares E, Hogberg U. High maternal cortisol levels during pregnancy are associated with more psychiatric symptoms in offspring at age of nine - A prospective study from Nicaragua. *J Psychiatr Res.* (2015) 71:97–102. doi: 10.1016/j.jpsychires.2015.09.016
22. Pickles A, Sharp H, Hellier J, and Hill J. Prenatal anxiety, maternal stroking in infancy, and symptoms of emotional and behavioral disorders at 3.5 years. *Eur Child Adolesc Psychiatry* (2017) 26:325–34. doi: 10.1007/s00787-016-0886-6
23. St-Hilaire A, Steiger H, Liu A, Laplante DP, Thaler L, Magill T, et al. A prospective study of effects of prenatal maternal stress on later eating-disorder manifestations in affected offspring: preliminary indications based on the Project Ice Storm cohort. *Int J Eat Disord.* (2015) 48:512–6. doi: 10.1002/eat.22391
24. Korhonen M, Luoma I, Salmelin R, Tamminen T. Maternal depressive symptoms: associations with adolescents' internalizing and externalizing problems and social competence. *Nord J Psychiatry* (2014) 68:323–32. doi: 10.3109/08039488.2013.838804
25. Plant DT, Pariante CM, Sharp D, Pawlby S. Maternal depression during pregnancy and offspring depression in adulthood: role of child maltreatment. *Br J Psychiatry* (2015) 207:213–20. doi: 10.1192/bjp.bp.114.156620
26. Fineberg AM, Ellman LM, Schaefer CA, Maxwell SD, Shen L, H Chaudhury N, et al. Fetal exposure to maternal stress and risk for schizophrenia spectrum disorders among offspring: differential influences of fetal sex. *Psychiatry Res.* (2016). 236:91–7. doi: 10.1016/j.psychres.2015.12.026

27. Rijlaarsdam J, van IMH, Verhulst FC, Jaddoe VW, Felix JF, Tiemeier H, et al. Prenatal stress exposure, oxytocin receptor gene (OXTR) methylation, and child autistic traits: the moderating role of OXTR rs53576 genotype. *Autism Res.* (2017) 10:430–8. doi: 10.1002/aur.1681
28. Su X, Xu B, Liang H, Olsen J, Yuan W, Cnattingius S, et al. Prenatal maternal bereavement and risk of eating disorders in infants and toddlers: a population-based cohort study. *BMC Psychiatry* (2015) 15:229. doi: 10.1186/s12888-015-0612-9
29. Brown AS, Begg MD, Gravenstein S, Schaefer CA, Wyatt RJ, Bresnahan M, et al. Serologic evidence of prenatal influenza in the etiology of schizophrenia. *Arch Gen Psychiatry* (2004) 61:774–80. doi: 10.1001/archpsyc.61.8.774
30. Brown AS, Vinogradov S, Kremen WS, Poole JH, Deicken RF, Penner JD, et al. Prenatal exposure to maternal infection and executive dysfunction in adult schizophrenia. *Am J Psychiatry* (2009) 166:683–90. doi: 10.1176/appi.ajp.2008.08010089
31. Ellman LM, Yolken RH, Buka SL, Torrey EF, Cannon TD. Cognitive functioning prior to the onset of psychosis: the role of fetal exposure to serologically determined influenza infection. *Biol Psychiatry* (2009) 65:1040–7. doi: 10.1016/j.biopsych.2008.12.015
32. Buka SL, Tsuang MT, Torrey EF, Klebanoff MA, Bernstein D, Yolken RH. Maternal infections and subsequent psychosis among offspring. *Arch Gen Psychiatry* (2001) 58:1032–7. doi: 10.1001/archpsyc.58.11.1032
33. Buka SL, Cannon TD, Torrey EF, Yolken RH, Collaborative Study Group on the Perinatal Origins of Severe Psychiatric D. Maternal exposure to herpes simplex virus and risk of psychosis among adult offspring. *Biol Psychiatry* (2008) 63:809–15. doi: 10.1016/j.biopsych.2007.09.022
34. Mortensen PB, Pedersen CB, Hougaard DM, Norgaard-Petersen B, Mors O, Borglum AD, et al. A Danish national birth cohort study of maternal HSV-2 antibodies as a risk factor for schizophrenia in their offspring. *Schizophr Res.* (2010) 122:257–63. doi: 10.1016/j.schres.2010.06.010
35. Zerbo O, Iosif AM, Walker C, Ozonoff S, Hansen RL, Hertz-Picciotto I. Is maternal influenza or fever during pregnancy associated with autism or developmental delays? Results from the CHARGE (CHildhood Autism Risks from Genetics and Environment) study. *J Autism Dev Disord.* (2013). 43:25–33. doi: 10.1007/s10803-012-1540-x
36. Sørensen HJ, Mortensen EL, Reinisch JM, Mednick SA. Association between prenatal exposure to bacterial infection and risk of schizophrenia. *Schizophrenia Bull.* (2008) 35:631–7. doi: 10.1093/schbul/sbn121
37. Brown AS, Sourander A, Hinkka-Yli-Salomaki S, McKeague IW, Sundvall J, Surcel HM. Elevated maternal C-reactive protein and autism in a national birth cohort. *Mol Psychiatry* (2014) 19:259–64. doi: 10.1038/mp.2012.197
38. Smith B, Kemp M, Ethelberg S, Schiellerup P, Bruun BG, Gerner-Smidt P, et al. Listeria monocytogenes: maternal-foetal infections in Denmark 1994-2005. *Scand J Infect Dis.* (2009). 41:21–5. doi: 10.1080/00365540802468094
39. Abrahao AL, Focaccia R, Gattaz WF. Childhood meningitis increases the risk for adult schizophrenia. *World J Biol Psychiatry* (2005). 6(Suppl 2):44–8. doi: 10.1080/15622970510030063
40. Brown AS, Schaefer CA, Quesenberry CP Jr, Liu L, Babulas VP, Susser ES. Maternal exposure to toxoplasmosis and risk of schizophrenia in adult offspring. *Am J Psychiatry* (2005) 162:767–73. doi: 10.1176/appi.ajp.162.4.767
41. Xiao J, Buka SL, Cannon TD, Suzuki Y, Viscidi RP, Torrey EF, et al. Serological pattern consistent with infection with type I Toxoplasma gondii in mothers and risk of psychosis among adult offspring. *Microbes Infect.* (2009) 11:1011–8. doi: 10.1016/j.micinf.2009.07.007
42. Atladottir HO, Thorsen P, Ostergaard L, Schendel DE, Lemcke S, Abdallah M, et al. Maternal infection requiring hospitalization during pregnancy and autism spectrum disorders. *J Autism Dev Disord.* (2010) 40:1423–30. doi: 10.1007/s10803-010-1006-y
43. Patel S, Masi A, Dale RC, Whitehouse AJO, Pokorski I, Alvares GA, et al. Social impairments in autism spectrum disorder are related to maternal immune history profile. *Mol Psychiatry* (2017). doi: 10.1038/mp.2017.201. [Epub ahead of print].
44. Nielsen PR, Laursen TM, Mortensen PB. Association between parental hospital-treated infection and the risk of schizophrenia in adolescence and early adulthood. *Schizophrenia Bull.* (2011) 39:230–7. doi: 10.1093/schbul/sbr149
45. Polanczyk G, de Lima MS, Horta BL, Biederman J, Rohde LA. The worldwide prevalence of ADHD: a systematic review and metaregression analysis. *Am J Psychiatry* (2007) 164:942–8. doi: 10.1176/ajp.2007.164.6.942
46. Rudolph MD, Graham AM, Feczko E, Miranda-Dominguez O, Rasmussen JM, Nardos R, et al. Maternal IL-6 during pregnancy can be estimated from newborn brain connectivity and predicts future working memory in offspring. *Nat Neurosci.* (2018) 21:765–72. doi: 10.1038/s41593-018-0128-y
47. Brown AS, Hooton J, Schaefer CA, Zhang H, Petkova E, Babulas V, et al. Elevated maternal interleukin-8 levels and risk of schizophrenia in adult offspring. *Am J Psychiatry* (2004) 161:889–95. doi: 10.1176/appi.ajp.161.5.889
48. Blomstrom A, Karlsson H, Gardner R, Jorgensen L, Magnusson C, Dalman C. Associations between maternal infection during pregnancy, childhood infections, and the risk of subsequent psychotic disorder–a Swedish cohort study of nearly 2 million individuals. *Schizophr Bull.* (2016) 42:125–33. doi: 10.1093/schbul/sbv112
49. Selten JP, Frissen A, Lensvelt-Mulders G, Morgan VA. Schizophrenia and 1957 pandemic of influenza: meta-analysis. *Schizophr Bull.* (2010) 36:219–28. doi: 10.1093/schbul/sbp147
50. Selten JP, Termorshuizen F. The serological evidence for maternal influenza as risk factor for psychosis in offspring is insufficient: critical review and meta-analysis. *Schizophr Res.* (2017) 183:2–9. doi: 10.1016/j.schres.2016.11.006
51. Andersen SL. Trajectories of brain development: point of vulnerability or window of opportunity? *Neurosci Biobehav Rev.* (2003) 27:3–18. doi: 10.1016/S0149-7634(03)00005-8
52. Knuesel I, Chicha L, Britschgi M, Schobel SA, Bodmer M, Hellings JA, et al. Maternal immune activation and abnormal brain development across CNS disorders. *Nat Rev Neurol.* (2014) 10:643–60. doi: 10.1038/nrneurol.2014.187
53. Molnár Z, Price DJ. Brain development. In: Baldock R, Bard J, Davidson DR, Morriss-Kay G, editors. *Kaufman's Atlas of Mouse Development Supplement.* Amsterdam: Academic Press (2015). p. 239–52.
54. Ginhoux F, Greter M, Leboeuf M, Nandi S, See P, Gokhan S, et al. Fate mapping analysis reveals that adult microglia derive from primitive macrophages. *Science* (2010) 330:841–5. doi: 10.1126/science.1194637
55. Taylor DC, Differential rates of cerebral maturation between sexes and between hemispheres. Evidence from epilepsy. *Lancet* (1969) 2:140–2. doi: 10.1016/S0140-6736(69)92445-3
56. Ajmone-Cat MA, Cacci E, Ragazzoni Y, Minghetti L, Biagioni S. Pro-gliogenic effect of IL-1alpha in the differentiation of embryonic neural precursor cells *in vitro*. *J Neurochem.* (2010) 113:1060–72. doi: 10.1111/j.1471-4159.2010.06670.x
57. Ling ZD, Potter ED, Lipton JW, Carvey PM. Differentiation of mesencephalic progenitor cells into dopaminergic neurons by cytokines. *Exp Neurol.* (1998) 149:411–23. doi: 10.1006/exnr.1998.6715
58. Monje ML, Toda H, Palmer TD. Inflammatory blockade restores adult hippocampal neurogenesis. *Science* (2003) 302:1760–5. doi: 10.1126/science.1088417
59. Koo JW, Duman RS. IL-1beta is an essential mediator of the antineurogenic and anhedonic effects of stress. *Proc Natl Acad Sci USA.* (2008) 105:751–6. doi: 10.1073/pnas.0708092105
60. Crampton SJ, Collins LM, Toulouse A, Nolan YM, O'Keeffe GW. Exposure of foetal neural progenitor cells to IL-1beta impairs their proliferation and alters their differentiation-a role for maternal inflammation? *J Neurochem.* (2012) 120:964–73. doi: 10.1111/j.1471-4159.2011.07634.x
61. Wang X, Fu S, Wang Y, Yu P, Hu J, Gu W, et al. Interleukin-1beta mediates proliferation and differentiation of multipotent neural precursor cells through the activation of SAPK/JNK pathway. *Mol Cell Neurosci.* (2007) 36:343–54. doi: 10.1016/j.mcn.2007.07.005
62. Chucair-Elliott AJ, Conrady C, Zheng M, Kroll CM, Lane TE, Carr DJ. Microglia-induced IL-6 protects against neuronal loss following HSV-1 infection of neural progenitor cells. *Glia* (2014) 62:1418–34. doi: 10.1002/glia.22689
63. Yang P, Wen H, Ou S, Cui J, Fan D. IL-6 promotes regeneration and functional recovery after cortical spinal tract injury by reactivating intrinsic growth program of neurons and enhancing synapse formation. *Exp Neurol.* (2012) 236:19–27. doi: 10.1016/j.expneurol.2012.03.019
64. Oh J, McCloskey MA, Blong CC, Bendickson L, Nilsen-Hamilton M, Sakaguchi DS. Astrocyte-derived interleukin-6 promotes specific neuronal

differentiation of neural progenitor cells from adult hippocampus. *J Neurosci Res.* (2010) 88:2798–809. doi: 10.1002/jnr.22447
65. Iosif RE, Ekdahl CT, Ahlenius H, Pronk CJ, Bonde S, Kokaia Z, et al. Tumor necrosis factor receptor 1 is a negative regulator of progenitor proliferation in adult hippocampal neurogenesis. *J Neurosci.* (2006) 26:9703–12. doi: 10.1523/JNEUROSCI.2723-06.2006
66. Bruce AJ, Boling W, Kindy MS, Peschon J, Kraemer PJ, Carpenter MK, et al. Altered neuronal and microglial responses to excitotoxic and ischemic brain injury in mice lacking TNF receptors. *Nat Med.* (1996) 2:788–94. doi: 10.1038/nm0796-788
67. Sarder M, Abe K, Saito H, Nishiyama N. Comparative effect of IL-2 and IL-6 on morphology of cultured hippocampal neurons from fetal rat brain. *Brain Res.* (1996) 715:9–16. doi: 10.1016/0006-8993(95)01291-5
68. Beck RD Jr, Wasserfall C, Ha GK, Cushman JD, Huang Z, Atkinson MA, et al. Changes in hippocampal IL-15, related cytokines, and neurogenesis in IL-2 deficient mice. *Brain Res.* (2005) 1041:223–30. doi: 10.1016/j.brainres.2005.02.010
69. Butovsky O, Ziv Y, Schwartz A, Landa G, Talpalar AE, Pluchino S, et al. Microglia activated by IL-4 or IFN-gamma differentially induce neurogenesis and oligodendrogenesis from adult stem/progenitor cells. *Mol Cell Neurosci.* (2006) 31:149–60. doi: 10.1016/j.mcn.2005.10.006
70. Yang J, Jiang Z, Fitzgerald DC, Ma C, Yu S, Li H, et al. Adult neural stem cells expressing IL-10 confer potent immunomodulation and remyelination in experimental autoimmune encephalitis. *J Clin Invest.* (2009) 119:3678–91. doi: 10.1172/JCI37914
71. Molina-Holgado E, Vela JM, Arevalo-Martin A, Guaza C. LPS/IFN-gamma cytotoxicity in oligodendroglial cells: role of nitric oxide and protection by the anti-inflammatory cytokine IL-10. *Eur J Neurosci.* (2001) 13:493–502. doi: 10.1046/j.0953-816x.2000.01412.x
72. Guan Y, Jiang Z, Ciric B, Rostami AM, Zhang GX. Upregulation of chemokine receptor expression by IL-10/IL-4 in adult neural stem cells. *Exp Mol Pathol.* (2008) 85:232–6. doi: 10.1016/j.yexmp.2008.07.003
73. Buckwalter MS, Yamane M, Coleman BS, Ormerod BK, Chin JT, Palmer T, et al. Chronically increased transforming growth factor-beta1 strongly inhibits hippocampal neurogenesis in aged mice. *Am J Pathol.* (2006) 169:154–64. doi: 10.2353/ajpath.2006.051272
74. Ikeda K, Iwasaki Y, Shiojima T, Kinoshita M. Neuroprotective effect of various cytokines on developing spinal motoneurons following axotomy. *J Neurol Sci.* (1996) 135:109–13. doi: 10.1016/0022-510X(95)00263-2
75. Bauer S, Patterson PH. Leukemia inhibitory factor promotes neural stem cell self-renewal in the adult brain. *J Neurosci.* (2006) 26:12089–99. doi: 10.1523/JNEUROSCI.3047-06.2006
76. Deverman BE, Patterson PH. Cytokines and CNS development. *Neuron* (2009) 64:61–78. doi: 10.1016/j.neuron.2009.09.002
77. Li Z, Li K, Zhu L, Kan Q, Yan Y, Kumar P, et al. Inhibitory effect of IL-17 on neural stem cell proliferation and neural cell differentiation. *BMC Immunol.* (2013) 14:20. doi: 10.1186/1471-2172-14-20
78. Liu Q, Xin W, He P, Turner D, Yin J, Gan Y, et al. Interleukin-17 inhibits adult hippocampal neurogenesis. *Sci Rep.* (2014) 4:7554. doi: 10.1038/srep07554
79. Wong H, Hoeffer C. Maternal IL-17A in autism. *Exp Neurol.* (2018) 299(Pt A):228–40. doi: 10.1016/j.expneurol.2017.04.010
80. Guyon A. CXCL12 chemokine and its receptors as major players in the interactions between immune and nervous systems. *Front Cell Neurosci.* (2014) 8:65. doi: 10.3389/fncel.2014.00065
81. Stuart MJ, Singhal G, Baune BT. Systematic review of the neurobiological relevance of chemokines to psychiatric disorders. *Front Cell Neurosci.* (2015) 9:357. doi: 10.3389/fncel.2015.00357
82. Tran PB, Miller RJ. Chemokine receptors: signposts to brain development and disease. *Nat Rev Neurosci.* (2003) 4:444–55. doi: 10.1038/nrn1116
83. Solano ME, Holmes MC, Mittelstadt PR, Chapman KE, Tolosa E. Antenatal endogenous and exogenous glucocorticoids and their impact on immune ontogeny and long-term immunity. *Semin Immunopathol.* (2016) 38:739–63. doi: 10.1007/s00281-016-0575-z
84. Sandman CA, Davis EP, Buss C, Glynn LM. Prenatal programming of human neurological function. *Int J Pept.* (2011) 2011:837596. doi: 10.1155/2011/837596
85. Arck PC, Rose M, Hertwig K, Hagen E, Hildebrandt M, Klapp BF. Stress and immune mediators in miscarriage. *Hum Reprod.* (2001) 16:1505–11. doi: 10.1093/humrep/16.7.1505
86. Christian LM, Glaser R, Porter K, Iams JD. Stress-induced inflammatory responses in women: effects of race and pregnancy. *Psychosom Med.* (2013) 75:658–69. doi: 10.1097/PSY.0b013e31829bbc89
87. Solano ME, Kowal MK, O'Rourke GE, Horst AK, Modest K, Plosch T, et al. Progesterone and HMOX-1 promote fetal growth by CD8+ T cell modulation. *J Clin Invest.* (2015) 125:1726–38. doi: 10.1172/JCI68140
88. Blois SM, Ilarregui JM, Tometten M, Garcia M, Orsal AS, Cordo-Russo R, et al. A pivotal role for galectin-1 in fetomaternal tolerance. *Nat Med.* (2007) 13:1450–7. doi: 10.1038/nm1680
89. Engels G, Hierweger AM, Hoffmann J, Thieme R, Thiele S, Bertram S, et al. Pregnancy-related immune adaptation promotes the emergence of highly virulent H1N1 influenza virus strains in allogenically pregnant mice. *Cell Host Microbe* (2017) 21:321–33. doi: 10.1016/j.chom.2017.02.020
90. Friebe A, Douglas AJ, Solano E, Blois SM, Hagen E, Klapp BF, et al. Neutralization of LPS or blockage of TLR4 signaling prevents stress-triggered fetal loss in murine pregnancy. *J Mol Med.* (2011) 89:689–99. doi: 10.1007/s00109-011-0743-5
91. Kinder JM, Stelzer IA, Arck PC, Way SS. Immunological implications of pregnancy-induced microchimerism. *Nat Rev Immunol.* (2017) 17:483–94. doi: 10.1038/nri.2017.38
92. Bauer S, Kerr BJ, Patterson PH. The neuropoietic cytokine family in development, plasticity, disease and injury. *Nat Rev Neurosci.* (2007) 8:221–32. doi: 10.1038/nrn2054
93. Fatemi SH, Earle J, Kanodia R, Kist D, Emamian ES, Patterson PH, et al. Prenatal viral infection leads to pyramidal cell atrophy and macrocephaly in adulthood: implications for genesis of autism and schizophrenia. *Cell Mol Neurobiol.* (2002) 22:25–33. doi: 10.1023/A:1015337611258
94. Baharnoori M, Brake WG, Srivastava LK. Prenatal immune challenge induces developmental changes in the morphology of pyramidal neurons of the prefrontal cortex and hippocampus in rats. *Schizophr Res.* (2009) 107:99–109. doi: 10.1016/j.schres.2008.10.003
95. Cui K, Ashdown H, Luheshi GN, Boksa P. Effects of prenatal immune activation on hippocampal neurogenesis in the rat. *Schizophr Res.* (2009) 113:288–97. doi: 10.1016/j.schres.2009.05.003
96. Meyer U, Nyffeler M, Engler A, Urwyler A, Schedlowski M, Knuesel I, et al. The time of prenatal immune challenge determines the specificity of inflammation-mediated brain and behavioral pathology. *J Neurosci.* (2006) 26:4752–62. doi: 10.1523/JNEUROSCI.0099-06.2006
97. Makinodan M, Tatsumi K, Manabe T, Yamauchi T, Makinodan E, Matsuyoshi H, et al. Maternal immune activation in mice delays myelination and axonal development in the hippocampus of the offspring. *J Neurosci Res.* (2008) 86:2190–200. doi: 10.1002/jnr.21673
98. Fernandez de Cossio L, Guzman A, van der Veldt S, Luheshi GN. Prenatal infection leads to ASD-like behavior and altered synaptic pruning in the mouse offspring. *Brain Behav Immun.* (2017) 63:88–98. doi: 10.1016/j.bbi.2016.09.028
99. Giovanoli S, Weber-Stadlbauer U, Schedlowski M, Meyer U, Engler H. Prenatal immune activation causes hippocampal synaptic deficits in the absence of overt microglia anomalies. *Brain Behav Immun.* (2016) 55:25–38. doi: 10.1016/j.bbi.2015.09.015
100. Schaafsma W, Basterra LB, Jacobs S, Brouwer N, Meerlo P, Schaafsma A, et al. Maternal inflammation induces immune activation of fetal microglia and leads to disrupted microglia immune responses, behavior, and learning performance in adulthood. *Neurobiol Dis.* (2017) 106:291–300. doi: 10.1016/j.nbd.2017.07.017
101. Hui CW, St-Pierre A, El Hajj H, Remy Y, Hebert SS, Luheshi GN, et al. Prenatal immune challenge in mice leads to partly sex-dependent behavioral, microglial, and molecular abnormalities associated with schizophrenia. *Front Mol Neurosci.* (2018) 11:13. doi: 10.3389/fnmol.2018.00013
102. Bilbo SD, Schwarz JM. Early-life programming of later-life brain and behavior: a critical role for the immune system. *Front Behav Neurosci.* (2009) 3:14. doi: 10.3389/neuro.08.014.2009
103. Graham AM, Rasmussen JM, Rudolph MD, Heim CM, Gilmore JH, Styner M, et al. Maternal systemic interleukin-6 during pregnancy is associated with

newborn amygdala phenotypes and subsequent behavior at 2 years of age. *Biol Psychiatry* (2018) 83:109–19. doi: 10.1016/j.biopsych.2017.05.027
104. Graham AM, Buss C, Rasmussen JM, Rudolph MD, Demeter DV, Gilmore JH, et al. Implications of newborn amygdala connectivity for fear and cognitive development at 6-months-of-age. *Dev Cogn Neurosci.* (2016) 18:12–25. doi: 10.1016/j.dcn.2015.09.006
105. Mychasiuk R, Gibb R, Kolb B. Prenatal stress alters dendritic morphology and synaptic connectivity in the prefrontal cortex and hippocampus of developing offspring. *Synapse* (2012) 66:308–14. doi: 10.1002/syn.21512
106. Bock J, Murmu MS, Biala Y, Weinstock M, Braun K. Prenatal stress and neonatal handling induce sex-specific changes in dendritic complexity and dendritic spine density in hippocampal subregions of prepubertal rats. *Neuroscience* (2011) 193:34–43. doi: 10.1016/j.neuroscience.2011.07.048
107. Buss C, Davis EP, Shahbaba B, Pruessner JC, Head K, Sandman CA. Maternal cortisol over the course of pregnancy and subsequent child amygdala and hippocampus volumes and affective problems. *Proc Natl Acad Sci USA.* (2012) 109:E1312-9. doi: 10.1073/pnas.1201295109
108. Davis EP, Head K, Buss C, Sandman CA. Prenatal maternal cortisol concentrations predict neurodevelopment in middle childhood. *Psychoneuroendocrinology* (2017) 75:56–63. doi: 10.1016/j.psyneuen.2016.10.005
109. Lemaire V, Koehl M, Le Moal M, Abrous DN. Prenatal stress produces learning deficits associated with an inhibition of neurogenesis in the hippocampus. *Proc Natl Acad Sci USA.* (2000) 97:11032–7. doi: 10.1073/pnas.97.20.11032
110. Jia N, Yang K, Sun Q, Cai Q, Li H, Cheng D, et al. Prenatal stress causes dendritic atrophy of pyramidal neurons in hippocampal CA3 region by glutamate in offspring rats. *Dev Neurobiol.* (2010) 70:114–25. doi: 10.1002/dneu.20766
111. Hayashi A, Nagaoka M, Yamada K, Ichitani Y, Miake Y, Okado N. Maternal stress induces synaptic loss and developmental disabilities of offspring. *Int J Dev Neurosci.* (1998) 16:209–16. doi: 10.1016/S0736-5748(98)00028-8
112. Schafer DP, Lehrman EK, Kautzman AG, Koyama R, Mardinly AR, Yamasaki R, et al. Microglia sculpt postnatal neural circuits in an activity and complement-dependent manner. *Neuron* (2012) 74:691–705. doi: 10.1016/j.neuron.2012.03.026
113. Bittle J, Stevens HE. The role of glucocorticoid, interleukin-1beta, and antioxidants in prenatal stress effects on embryonic microglia. *J Neuroinflammation* (2018) 15:44. doi: 10.1186/s12974-018-1079-7
114. Slusarczyk J, Trojan E, Glombik K, Budziszewska B, Kubera M, Lason W, et al. Prenatal stress is a vulnerability factor for altered morphology and biological activity of microglia cells. *Front Cell Neurosci.* (2015) 9:82. doi: 10.3389/fncel.2015.00082
115. Behan AT, van den Hove DL, Mueller L, Jetten MJ, Steinbusch HW, Cotter DR, et al. Evidence of female-specific glial deficits in the hippocampus in a mouse model of prenatal stress. *Eur Neuropsychopharmacol.* (2011) 21:71–9. doi: 10.1016/j.euroneuro.2010.07.004
116. Diz-Chaves Y, Astiz M, Bellini MJ, Garcia-Segura LM. Prenatal stress increases the expression of proinflammatory cytokines and exacerbates the inflammatory response to LPS in the hippocampal formation of adult male mice. *Brain Behav Immun.* (2013) 28:196–206. doi: 10.1016/j.bbi.2012.11.013
117. Diz-Chaves Y, Pernia O, Carrero P, Garcia-Segura LM. Prenatal stress causes alterations in the morphology of microglia and the inflammatory response of the hippocampus of adult female mice. *J Neuroinflammation* (2012) 9:71. doi: 10.1186/1742-2094-9-71
118. Stolp HB, Liddelow SA, Sá-Pereira I, Dziegielewska KM, Saunders NR. Immune responses at brain barriers and implications for brain development and neurological function in later life. *Front Integr Neurosci.* (2013) 7:61. doi: 10.3389/fnint.2013.00061
119. Murmu MS, Salomon S, Biala Y, Weinstock M, Braun K, Bock J. Changes of spine density and dendritic complexity in the prefrontal cortex in offspring of mothers exposed to stress during pregnancy. *Eur J Neurosci.* (2006) 24:1477–87. doi: 10.1111/j.1460-9568.2006.05024.x
120. Salm AK, Pavelko M, Krouse EM, Webster W, Kraszpulski M, Birkle DL. Lateral amygdaloid nucleus expansion in adult rats is associated with exposure to prenatal stress. *Brain Res Dev Brain Res.* (2004) 148:159–67. doi: 10.1016/j.devbrainres.2003.11.005
121. Ancatén González C, Gutiérrez-Rojas C, Bustamante Valdés C. Maternal exercise reverses morphologic changes in amygdala neurons produced by prenatal stress. *Neurology Psychiatry Brain Res.* (2017) 24:36–42. doi: 10.1016/j.npbr.2017.04.004
122. McEwen BS, Nasca C, Gray JD. Stress effects on neuronal structure: hippocampus, amygdala, and prefrontal cortex. *Neuropsychopharmacology* (2016) 41:3–23. doi: 10.1038/npp.2015.171
123. Shigemoto R, Kinoshita A, Wada E, Nomura S, Ohishi H, Takada M, et al. Differential presynaptic localization of metabotropic glutamate receptor subtypes in the rat hippocampus. *J Neurosci.* (1997) 17:7503–22. doi: 10.1523/JNEUROSCI.17-19-07503.1997
124. Skeberdis VA, Lan J, Opitz T, Zheng X, Bennett MV, Zukin RS. mGluR1-mediated potentiation of NMDA receptors involves a rise in intracellular calcium and activation of protein kinaseC. *Neuropharmacology C* (2001) 40:856–65. doi: 10.1016/S0028-3908(01)00005-3
125. Ambrosini A, Bresciani L, Fracchia S, Brunello N, Racagni G. Metabotropic glutamate receptors negatively coupled to adenylate cyclase inhibit N-methyl-D-aspartate receptor activity and prevent neurotoxicity in mesencephalic neurons *in vitro*. *Mol Pharmacol.* (1995) 47:1057–64.
126. Kandaswamy R, McQuillin A, Sharp SI, Fiorentino A, Anjorin A, Blizard RA, et al. Genetic association, mutation screening, and functional analysis of a Kozak sequence variant in the metabotropic glutamate receptor 3 gene in bipolar disorder. *JAMA Psychiatry* (2013) 70:591–8. doi: 10.1001/jamapsychiatry.2013.38
127. Laloux C, Mairesse J, Van Camp G, Giovine A, Branchi I, Bouret S, et al. Anxiety-like behaviour and associated neurochemical and endocrinological alterations in male pups exposed to prenatal stress. *Psychoneuroendocrinology* (2012) 37:1646–58. doi: 10.1016/j.psyneuen.2012.02.010
128. Zuena AR, Mairesse J, Casolini P, Cinque C, Alema GS, Morley-Fletcher S, et al. Prenatal restraint stress generates two distinct behavioral and neurochemical profiles in male and female rats. *PLoS ONE* (2008) 3:e2170. doi: 10.1371/journal.pone.0002170
129. Yaka R, Salomon S, Matzner H, Weinstock M. Effect of varied gestational stress on acquisition of spatial memory, hippocampal LTP and synaptic proteins in juvenile male rats. *Behav Brain Res.* (2007) 179:126–32. doi: 10.1016/j.bbr.2007.01.018
130. Muneoka K, Mikuni M, Ogawa T, Kitera K, Kamei K, Takigawa M, et al. Prenatal dexamethasone exposure alters brain monoamine metabolism and adrenocortical response in rat offspring. *Am J Physiol.* (1997) 273(5 Pt 2):R1669–75. doi: 10.1152/ajpregu.1997.273.5.R1669
131. Van den Hove DL, Leibold NK, Strackx E, Martinez-Claros M, Lesch KP, Steinbusch HW, et al. Prenatal stress and subsequent exposure to chronic mild stress in rats; interdependent effects on emotional behavior and the serotonergic system. *Eur Neuropsychopharmacol.* (2014) 24:595–607. doi: 10.1016/j.euroneuro.2013.09.006
132. Ramboz S, Oosting R, Amara DA, Kung HF, Blier P, Mendelsohn M, et al. Serotonin receptor 1A knockout: an animal model of anxiety-related disorder. *Proc Natl Acad Sci USA.* (1998) 95:14476–81. doi: 10.1073/pnas.95.24.14476
133. Giocomo LM, Hasselmo ME. Nicotinic modulation of glutamatergic synaptic transmission in region CA3 of the hippocampus. *Eur J Neurosci.* (2005) 22:1349–56. doi: 10.1111/j.1460-9568.2005.04316.x
134. Day JC, Koehl M, Deroche V, Le Moal M, Maccari S. Prenatal stress enhances stress- and corticotropin-releasing factor-induced stimulation of hippocampal acetylcholine release in adult rats. *J Neurosci.* (1998) 18:1886–92. doi: 10.1523/JNEUROSCI.18-05-01886.1998
135. Nelson JL. The otherness of self: microchimerism in health and disease. *Trends Immunol.* (2012) 33:421–7. doi: 10.1016/j.it.2012.03.002
136. Vernochet C, Caucheteux SM, Kanellopoulos-Langevin C. Bi-directional cell trafficking between mother and fetus in mouse placenta. *Placenta* (2007) 28:639–49. doi: 10.1016/j.placenta.2006.10.006
137. Stelzer IA, Thiele K, Solano ME. Maternal microchimerism: lessons learned from murine models. *J Reprod Immunol.* (2015) 108:12–25. doi: 10.1016/j.jri.2014.12.007

138. Buss C, Entringer S, Wadhwa PD. Fetal programming of brain development: intrauterine stress and susceptibility to psychopathology. *Sci Signal.* (2012) 5(245):pt7. doi: 10.1126/scisignal.2003406
139. Palma-Gudiel H, Córdova-Palomera A, Leza JC, Fananás L. Glucocorticoid receptor gene (NR3C1) methylation processes as mediators of early adversity in stress-related disorders causality: a critical review. *Neurosci Biobehav Rev.* (2015) 55:520–35. doi: 10.1016/j.neubiorev.2015.05.016
140. Bale TL. Epigenetic and transgenerational reprogramming of brain development. *Nat Rev Neurosci.* (2015) 16:332. doi: 10.1038/nrn3818
141. Bock C. Epigenetic biomarker development. *Epigenomics* (2009) 1:99–110. doi: 10.2217/epi.09.6
142. Teh AL, Pan H, Chen L, Ong, ML, Dogra S, Wong J, et al. The effect of genotype and in utero environment on inter-individual variation in neonate DNA methylomes. *Genome Res.* (2014) 24:1064–74. doi: 10.1101/gr.171439.113
143. Heijmans BT, Tobi EW, Stein AD, Putter H, Blauw GJ, Susser ES, et al. Persistent epigenetic differences associated with prenatal exposure to famine in humans. *Proc Natl Acad Sci USA.* (2008) 105:17046–9. doi: 10.1073/pnas.0806560105
144. Oberlander TF, Weinberg J, Papsdorf M, Grunau R, Misri S, Devlin AM. Prenatal exposure to maternal depression, neonatal methylation of human glucocorticoid receptor gene (NR3C1) and infant cortisol stress responses. *Epigenetics* (2008) 3:97–106. doi: 10.4161/epi.3.2.6034
145. Braithwaite EC, Kundakovic M, Ramchandani PG, Murphy SE, Champagne FA. Maternal prenatal depressive symptoms predict infant NR3C1 1F and BDNF IV DNA methylation. *Epigenetics* (2015) 10:408–17. doi: 10.1080/15592294.2015.1039221
146. Radtke KM, Ruf M, Gunter HM, Dohrmann K, Schauer M, Meyer A, et al. Transgenerational impact of intimate partner violence on methylation in the promoter of the glucocorticoid receptor. *Transl Psychiatry* (2011) 1:e21. doi: 10.1038/tp.2011.21
147. Tang B, Jia H, Kast RJ, Thomas EA. Epigenetic changes at gene promoters in response to immune activation *in utero*. *Brain Behav Immun.* (2013) 30:168–75. doi: 10.1016/j.bbi.2013.01.086
148. Basil P, Li Q, Dempster EL, Mill J, Sham PC, Wong CC, et al. Prenatal maternal immune activation causes epigenetic differences in adolescent mouse brain. *Transl Psychiatry* (2014) 4:e434. doi: 10.1038/tp.2014.80
149. Chahrour M, Jung SY, Shaw C, Zhou X, Wong ST, Qin J, et al. MeCP2, a key contributor to neurological disease, activates and represses transcription. *Science* (2008) 320:1224–9. doi: 10.1126/science.1153252
150. Labouesse MA, Dong E, Grayson DR, Guidotti A, Meyer U. Maternal immune activation induces GAD1 and GAD2 promoter remodeling in the offspring prefrontal cortex. *Epigenetics* (2015) 10:1143–55. doi: 10.1080/15592294.2015.1114202
151. Bohacek J, Gapp K, Saab BJ, Mansuy IM. Transgenerational epigenetic effects on brain functions. *Biol Psychiatry* (2013) 73:313–20. doi: 10.1016/j.biopsych.2012.08.019
152. Buss C, Entringer S, Moog NK, Toepfer P, Fair DA, Simhan HN, et al. Intergenerational transmission of maternal childhood maltreatment exposure: implications for fetal brain development. *J Am Acad Child Adolesc Psychiatry* (2017) 56:373–82. doi: 10.1016/j.jaac.2017.03.001
153. Skinner MK. Role of epigenetics in developmental biology and transgenerational inheritance. *Birth Defects Res C Embryo Today* (2011) 93:51–5. doi: 10.1002/bdrc.20199
154. Cowley M, Oakey RJ. Resetting for the next generation. *Mol Cell.* (2012) 48:819–21. doi: 10.1016/j.molcel.2012.12.007
155. Hackett JA, Zylicz JJ, Surani MA. Parallel mechanisms of epigenetic reprogramming in the germline. *Trends Genet.* (2012) 28:164–74. doi: 10.1016/j.tig.2012.01.005
156. Seisenberger S, Andrews S, Krueger F, Arand J, Walter J, Santos F, et al. The dynamics of genome-wide DNA methylation reprogramming in mouse primordial germ cells. *Mol Cell.* (2012) 48:849–62. doi: 10.1016/j.molcel.2012.11.001
157. Smallwood SA, Tomizawa S, Krueger F, Ruf N, Carli N, Segonds-Pichon A, et al. Dynamic CpG island methylation landscape in oocytes and preimplantation embryos. *Nat Genet.* (2011) 43:811–4. doi: 10.1038/ng.864
158. Smith ZD, Chan MM, Mikkelsen TS, Gu H, Gnirke A, Regev A, et al. A unique regulatory phase of DNA methylation in the early mammalian embryo. *Nature* (2012) 84:339–44. doi: 10.1038/nature10960
159. Gapp K, Jawaid A, Sarkies P, Bohacek J, Pelczar P, Prados J, et al. Implication of sperm RNAs in transgenerational inheritance of the effects of early trauma in mice. *Nat Neurosci.* (2014) 17:667–9. doi: 10.1038/nn.3695
160. Franklin TB, Russig H, Weiss IC, Graff J, Linder N, Michalon A, et al. Epigenetic transmission of the impact of early stress across generations. *Biol Psychiatry* (2010) 68:408–15. doi: 10.1016/j.biopsych.2010.05.036
161. Pang S, Curran SP. Longevity and the long arm of epigenetics: acquired parental marks influence lifespan across several generations. *Bioessays* (2012) 34:652–4. doi: 10.1002/bies.201200046
162. Rodgers AB, Morgan CP, Leu NA, Bale TL. Transgenerational epigenetic programming via sperm microRNA recapitulates effects of paternal stress. *Proc Natl Acad Sci USA.* (2015) 112:13699–704. doi: 10.1073/pnas.1508347112
163. Heard E, Martienssen RA. Transgenerational epigenetic inheritance: myths and mechanisms. *Cell* (2014) 157:95–109. doi: 10.1016/j.cell.2014.02.045
164. Cenquizca LA, Swanson LW. Spatial organization of direct hippocampal field CA1 axonal projections to the rest of the cerebral cortex. *Brain Res Rev.* (2007) 56:1–26. doi: 10.1016/j.brainresrev.2007.05.002
165. Jones MW, Wilson MA. Theta rhythms coordinate hippocampal-prefrontal interactions in a spatial memory task. *PLoS Biol.* (2005) 3:e402. doi: 10.1371/journal.pbio.0030402
166. Dickerson DD, Wolff AR, Bilkey DK. Abnormal long-range neural synchrony in a maternal immune activation animal model of schizophrenia. *J Neurosci.* (2010) 30:12424–31. doi: 10.1523/JNEUROSCI.3046-10.2010
167. Bitzenhofer SH, Sieben K, Siebert KD, Spehr M, Hanganu-Opatz IL. Oscillatory activity in developing prefrontal networks results from theta-gamma-modulated synaptic inputs. *Cell Rep.* (2015) 11:486–97. doi: 10.1016/j.celrep.2015.03.031
168. Zheng C, Quan M, Zhang T. Decreased thalamo-cortical connectivity by alteration of neural information flow in theta oscillation in depression-model rats. *J Comput Neurosci.* (2012) 33:547–58. doi: 10.1007/s10827-012-0400-1
169. Quan M, Zheng C, Zhang N, Han D, Tian Y, Zhang T, et al. Impairments of behavior, information flow between thalamus and cortex, and prefrontal cortical synaptic plasticity in an animal model of depression. *Brain Res Bull.* (2011) 85:109–16. doi: 10.1016/j.brainresbull.2011.03.002
170. Oliveira JF, Dias NS, Correia M, Gama-Pereira F, Sardinha VM, Lima A, et al. Chronic stress disrupts neural coherence between cortico-limbic structures. *Front Neural Circuits* (2013) 7:10. doi: 10.3389/fncir.2013.00010
171. Jacinto LR, Reis JS, Dias NS, Cerqueira JJ, Correia JH, Sousa N. Stress affects theta activity in limbic networks and impairs novelty-induced exploration and familiarization. *Front Behav Neurosci.* (2013) 7:127. doi: 10.3389/fnbeh.2013.00127
172. Kirischuk S, Sinning A, Blanquie O, Yang JW, Luhmann HJ, Kilb W. Modulation of neocortical development by early neuronal activity: physiology and pathophysiology. *Front Cell Neurosci.* (2017) 11:379. doi: 10.3389/fncel.2017.00379
173. Biedermann SV, Meliss S, Simmons C, Nothling J, Suliman S, Seedat S. Sexual abuse but not posttraumatic stress disorder is associated with neurocognitive deficits in South African traumatized adolescents. *Child Abuse Negl.* (2018) 80:257–67. doi: 10.1016/j.chiabu.2018.04.003
174. Teicher MH, Anderson CM, Ohashi K, Khan A, McGreenery CE, Bolger EA, et al. Differential effects of childhood neglect and abuse during sensitive exposure periods on male and female hippocampus. *Neuroimage* (2018) 169:443–52. doi: 10.1016/j.neuroimage.2017.12.055
175. Anda RF, Felitti VJ, Bremner JD, Walker JD, Whitfield C, Perry BD, et al. The enduring effects of abuse and related adverse experiences in childhood. A convergence of evidence from neurobiology and epidemiology. *Eur Arch Psychiatry Clin Neurosci.* (2006) 256:174–86. doi: 10.1007/s00406-005-0624-4
176. Danese A, Moffitt TE, Harrington H, Milne BJ, Polanczyk G, Pariante CM, et al. Adverse childhood experiences and adult risk factors for age-related disease: depression, inflammation, and clustering of

metabolic risk markers. *Arch Pediatr Adolesc Med.* (2009) 163:1135–43. doi: 10.1001/archpediatrics.2009.214

177. Dube SR, Felitti VJ, Dong M, Giles WH, Anda RF. The impact of adverse childhood experiences on health problems: evidence from four birth cohorts dating back to 1900. *Prev Med.* (2003) 37:268–77. doi: 10.1016/S0091-7435(03)00123-3
178. Heim C, Plotsky PM, Nemeroff CB. Importance of studying the contributions of early adverse experience to neurobiological findings in depression. *Neuropsychopharmacology* (2004) 29:641–8. doi: 10.1038/sj.npp.1300397

16

The Immunogenetic Conundrum of Preeclampsia

A. Inkeri Lokki [1,2], Jenni K. Heikkinen-Eloranta [3] and Hannele Laivuori [4,5,6,7]*

[1] Research Programs Unit, Immunobiology Research Program, University of Helsinki, Helsinki, Finland, [2] Bacteriology and Immunology, University of Helsinki and Helsinki University Hospital, Helsinki, Finland, [3] Obstetrics and Gynecology, University of Helsinki and Helsinki University Hospital, Helsinki, Finland, [4] Medical and Clinical genetics, University of Helsinki and Helsinki University Hospital, Helsinki, Finland, [5] Institute for Molecular Medicine Finland, Helsinki Institute of Life Science, University of Helsinki, Helsinki, Finland, [6] Faculty of Medicine and Life Sciences, University of Tampere, Tampere, Finland, [7] Department of Obstetrics and Gynecology, Tampere University Hospital, Tampere, Finland

***Correspondence:**
A. Inkeri Lokki
inkeri.lokki@helsinki.fi

Pregnancy is an immunological challenge to the mother. The fetal tissues including the placenta must be protected from activation of the maternal immune system. On the other hand, the placental tissue sheds into the maternal circulation and must be adequately identified and phagocytized by the maternal immune system. During a healthy pregnancy, numerous immunosuppressive processes take place that allow the allograft fetus to thrive under exposure to humoral and cellular components of the maternal immune system. Breakdown of immune tolerance may result in sterile inflammation and cause adverse pregnancy outcomes such as preeclampsia, a vascular disease of the pregnancy with unpredictable course and symptoms from several organs. Immunological incompatibility between mother and fetus is strongly indicated in preeclampsia. Recently, genetic factors linking immunological pathways to predisposition to preeclampsia have been identified. In this mini-review genetic variation in immunological factors are discussed in the context of preeclampsia. Specifically, we explore immunogenetic and immunomodulary mechanisms contributing to loss of tolerance, inflammation, and autoimmunity in preeclampsia.

Keywords: preeclampsia, genetics, complement, major histocompatibility complex, FLT1, autoimmunity, pregnancy

INTRODUCTION

Preeclampsia is a heterogeneous vascular disease of the human pregnancy that presents in a previously normotensive woman during the second half of the pregnancy with hypertension and proteinuria, or preeclampsia-associated signs in the absence of proteinuria (1, 2). Preeclampsia occurs in 3% of pregnancies (3), and it is one of the most important causes of maternal and fetal morbidity and mortality worldwide. The etiology of preeclampsia is incompletely understood, but it has its origins in early pregnancy and delivery of the placenta is the only cure (4). Two distinct subtypes has been frequently used in the literature based on the timing of the disease onset/delivery: early-onset $<34 + 0$ and late-onset ≥ 34 weeks of gestation. However, better understanding of the etiology and different subtypes is needed for early recognition and preventive measures.

Preeclampsia is considered a two stage-disease in which poorly perfused placenta produces factor(s) leading to systemic vascular disease and the clinical manifestations of preeclampsia (5).

At 8 weeks of gestation, the trophoblast cells invade from the placenta into the maternal tissue and into the uterine arteries. These endovascular trophoblast cells facilitate the remodeling of spiral uterine arteries, which is essential for a healthy pregnancy. In order for the placentation process to be sufficient to support a healthy pregnancy, the extravillous trophoblast cells must avoid detection by the alternative pathway, subsequent complement activation, and immune response ((4, 6); **Figure 1**). Immunogenetic susceptibility to preeclampsia may have effect in the early stages of pregnancy whereby through loss of maternal tolerance toward the fetal components, the process of placentation is impaired. On the other hand, during the third trimester, underlying immunogenetic predisposition may aggravate sterile inflammation, which is exacerbated by systemic endothelial dysfunction in the mother's vasculature and result in progression of preeclampsia ((10) **Figure 2A**).

Data from epidemiological studies suggest that maternal and paternal genes through fetus affect the risk of preeclampsia, and its genetic basis is polygenic. Heritability of preeclampsia has estimated 55% with greater maternal (35%) than fetal (20%) contribution (12). Genes coding for components of the immune system are among the more important candidates in the quest to pinpoint clinically relevant genetic association. This is also evidenced by numerous non-genetic studies and observations involving components of the immune system (13–15). Activation of alternative pathway of complement activation has been shown to coincide with the critical weeks of placentation (16, 17). The role of decidual monocyte populations in healthy and pathological pregnancies have been reviewed elsewhere (18).

Genetic risk profile for preeclampsia is currently poorly characterized. The genetic studies have suffered from non-reproducibility and been lacking functional validation. Recently, in a large genome wide association study of preeclampsia a first robust association in the fetal genome was found in the common variant near Fms related tyrosine kinase gene (*FLT1*) encoding anti-angiogenic factor Fms-like tyrosine kinase 1 (FLT1) (19). Our group has published protective maternal low-frequency variants in the same gene (20).

In this mini-review we explore the immunogenetic role of *FLT1* in preeclampsia and selected genetic studies implicating loss of immune tolerance in early pregnancy or late pregnancy inflammation in preeclampsia. Dysregulation of complement system and autoimmunity are discussed in detail as potential causes of loss of maternal tolerance, while obesity is considered a possible cause of inflammation.

IMMUNOGENIC FLT1? AN EVOLUTIONARY PERSPECTIVE

The anti-angiogenic factor, soluble FLT1 is also known to have an anti-inflammatory function (21). FLT1 is expressed on inflammatory cells in addition to endothelial and trophoblast cells (22). In areas of Africa, where *Plasmodium falciparum* malaria is endemic, first pregnancies share a particular risk of not only preeclampsia but also of placental malaria (23). In placental malaria, the fetal tissue will express an excess of sFLT1 apparently in an attempt to regulate the maternal inflammatory response thereby reducing the rate of spontaneous abortions (24). Consequently, positive selection on a genetic variant with capacity to resist placental malaria by increasing sFLT concentration may have influenced *FLT1* allele frequencies within the general population enough to introduce a novel risk to preeclampsia (25).

Soluble FLT1 is conserved across vertebrates. The human FLT1 protein contains two tyrosine kinase catalytic (TyrKc) domains, three domains from the immunoglobulin (Ig) cell adhesion molecule (cam) subfamily (Igcam), one Ig-like domain, and one true Ig domain (26). In a detailed molecular evolutionary analysis, in contrast to other related proteins, in FLT1, only the TyrKc domains located at amino acids 819-933 and 991-1157 were found to be conserved across vertebrates (26). Large degree of variance between related proteins may be a reflection of recent evolutionary selection pressure on the FLT1. Malaria is known to be a potent source of immunological selection. Together this evidence is in support of possible thus far poorly understood immunological roles of the FLT1.

The major contributor to sFLT1 load in human pregnancy is the recently evolved isoform sFLT1-e15 (27). Overexpression of the primate specific isoform sFLT1-e15a is also associated with preeclampsia suggesting, that this novel isoform harbors thus far unexplained fitness advantages (27, 28). Assuming that sFLT1 is pathogenic, it is thereby possible that in non-primate mammals' conditions that lead to pregnancy-associated pathological rise in sFLT1 do not exist. On the other hand, it is also possible that the sFLT1 in humans has evolved specific functions, patterns of expression, or regulatory mechanisms that are essential for development of preeclampsia (25).

Further evidence of the immunological interactions of FLT1 is derived from a murine model, where increase in complement activation resulted in increased levels of FLT1 (29). Monocytes can be stimulated to express an excess of FLT1 when exposed to complement activation products C3a and C5a *in vitro* (29). Additionally, nuclear factor of activated T-cells (NFAT) transcription factors are involved in expression of mRNA of inflammatory cytokines, sFLT1-e15, and FLT1, as well as, and secretion of sFLT1 from primary human cytotrophoblasts (30). NFAT transcription factors may in further studies prove to be another link between FLT1 and immune response. Furthermore, angiogenic dysregulation may play a role in activation of the classical pathway in the kidney in a murine model of preeclampsia as evidenced by C4 deposition in the tissue in presence of excess sFLT1 (31).

FLT1 3'UTR dinucleotide repeat polymorphism have been shown to influence the expression of FLT1 and fetal outcome in the context of placental malaria with possible immunomodulatory effect (23). As far as we know, the distribution of these repeat polymorphisms in preeclampsia has not been explored.

TOLERATING OFFSPRING: DUAL ROLE OF COMPLEMENT SYSTEM IN RECOGNIZING AND CLEARING OF FETAL MATERIAL

Complement system is an ancient part of innate immunity, which consists of cell surface-bound and freely circulating

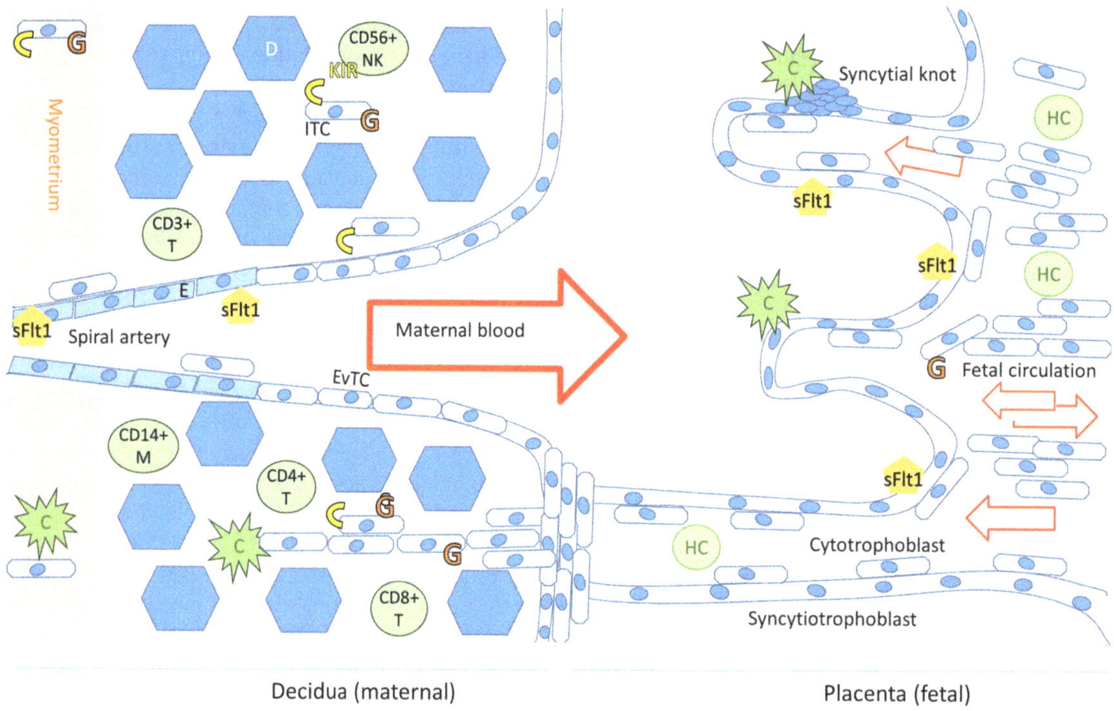

FIGURE 1 | Schematic representation of the maternal-fetal interface and its immunologicalplayers. Trophoblast cells (fetal) and endothelial cells (maternal) express sFlt1. The placental villi are shown in the right side of the image and decidua on the left. Invading trophoblast cells will encounter maternal complement system (C) in the decidua and in the intervillous space. Invading extravillous trophoblasts express HLA-C and HLA-G receptors (in yellow and orange, respectively), expression of HLA-G by villous trophoblast cells in the placenta decreases during the course of the pregnancy (7). Successful trophoblast invasion will extend to the vascular layers of myometrium and invade the uterine spiral arteries, where endovascular trophoblast cells (EvTC) will replace endothelial cells (E) causing remodulation and relaxation of the spiral artery to allow for non-turbulent high volume low pressure circulation into the intervillous space. Interstitial trophoblast cells (ITC) will remain in the maternal tissue creating tolerance of the fetal tissue in the maternal immune system. Hofbauer cells (HC) are the predominant immune cell population in the villi throughout placental development. The decidual immune cell population consists of macrophages (M), natural killer cells (NK), and populations of T-cells (T). Tolerance inducing Treg and Breg cells in particular are essential for a healthy pregnancy (8). Figure adapted from Lokki 2017 PhD thesis (9).

proteins that interact in a cascade of activation and regulation. Complement system has the capacity to discriminate between self- and non-self-cells and particles, and thereby maintain tolerance, or activate adaptive immunity. Complement activation can lead to inflammation, cell death, and tissue destruction. However, complement system also has a crucial role as a facilitator of phagocytosis thereby clearing debris and altered cells, in addition to removing pathogens. To protect own tissues from complement-mediated destruction and death, pathways of complement activation must be carefully regulated. Complement system has been studied extensively in preeclampsia, but genetic association studies linking components of the complement system to preeclampsia are not as plentiful.

Preeclampsia has previously been likened to thrombotic microangiopathies (TMA), which are caused by inadequate regulation of the complement system. In TMA, complement attacks against endogenous tissue structures such as endothelial cells and blood cells causing vascular damage and kidney failure. Pregnancy can act as a trigger of TMA syndromes. Atypical hemolytic uremic syndrome (aHUS) is a complement disease of the kidney with a TMA mechanism (32). Dysregulation of alternative pathway of complement system is indicated in aHUS (33). Similarly, most preeclampsia associations in complement system are found in the alternative pathway (34, 35).

The component C3 is in the core of the complement system. It can be activated by three different pathways. C3 can also become spontaneously activated in the human serum (32). Via the alternative pathway of complement activation, C3 is spontaneously activated and cleaved into activation products C3a and C3b in the absence of complement regulators. According to the sequence context, a haplotype spanning the active domains of C3 may predispose or protect from severe preeclampsia in a Finnish population (36, 37). We found a haplotype of 16 SNPs spanning the functionally critical sections in the middle of the gene. In this haplotype, three SNPs have most robust independent associations to severe preeclampsia further supporting its functional significance (36).

The results of this and other studies indicate that parallel to mice, C3 also plays a central role in the healthy human pregnancy (38, 39). The mechanism of haplotype association to severe preeclampsia is unclear but the effect may be due to functional or regulatory attributes of this region. For example, functional effect may affect the extravillous trophoblasts' capacity to evade complement activation by C3 binding, thereby

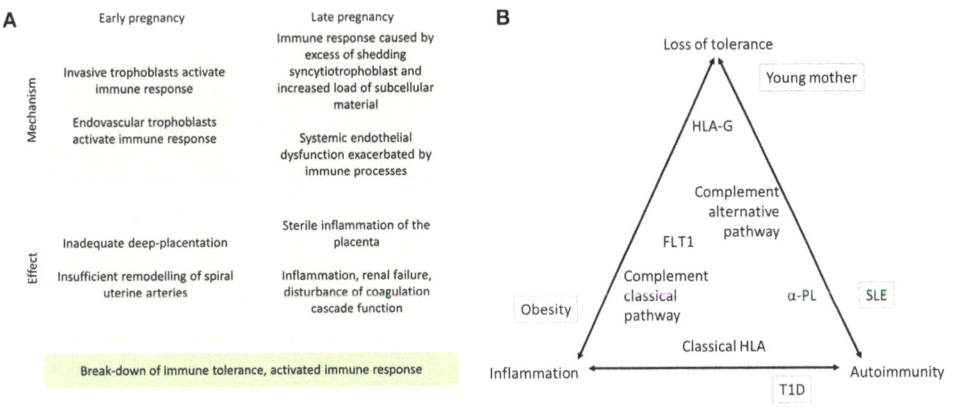

FIGURE 2 | (A) The proposed mechanisms of immune response in the etiology of preeclampsia. Immune mechanisms contribute to preeclampsia in early and late stages of the pregnancy. Specifically, if alternative pathway (AP) of complement system fails to recognize the invading trophoblast cells at the placental bed or in the uterine arteries, placentation may remain superficial and maternal uterine spiral artery remodeling may be compromised. In later stages of the pregnancy, complement activation aiming to facilitate phagosytosis of excess syncytiotrophoblast debris may induce sterile inflammation of the placenta locally. Concurrently, systemic endothelial dysfunction including disturbed coagulation function may be aggravated by immune activation and result in inflammation and shifting of Th2 to Th1 helper cell as well as disturbance of Treg and Th17 cell balances thereby further contributing to activation of the maternal immune response including erroneous antigen presenting in patients with applicable HLA alleles (11). **(B)** The triad of immune mechanisms in preeclampsia. The placement of contributing factors represents their suggested role in contributing to loss of tolerance, inflammation, and autoimmunity. Environmental risk factors outside in boxes, and the immunogenetic factors discussed in this review are inside the triangle. α-PL, anti-phospholipid antibodies; HLA, human leukocyte antigen; FLT1, Fms-like tyrosine kinase 1; T1D, type 1 diabetes.

compromising deep placentation and spiral artery remodeling in early pregnancy. Inflammation caused by excess complement activation may also be involved in a later stage of preeclampsia influencing severity of symptoms such as hypertension (40).

Immune complexes or opsonisation of the target surface by C1 complex triggers the activation of the classical pathway of complement system. Clearance of placenta-derived particles is crucial when preeclampsia symptoms develop in later pregnancy. Classical pathway activation results in cleavage of C4, which is a homolog of C3. C4 is present in two proteins, C4A and C4B, which are coded by usually two copies of each gene. While copy number variation of both *C4* is common, zero copies of both resulting in complete *C4* deficiency are very rare (41). Results of a pilot study conducted on mother-infant pairs with early-onset (delivery < 34 weeks of gestation) or late-onset (delivery ≥ 34 weeks of gestation) preeclampsia and non-preeclamptic controls suggest that deficiencies in *C4* may predispose to preeclampsia (14). *C4A* or *C4B* deficiencies were found almost twice as often in women with early-onset preeclampsia than in healthy controls. *C4A* deficiencies are observed in 16% of general population in Finland (42). In preeclampsia, *C4A* deficiencies were found in 40% (2/5) of women with late-onset preeclampsia and in 43% (3/7) of women with early-onset preeclampsia. None were observed in controls ($n = 7$). The copy number of *C4* seems to decrease with the severity of preeclamptic symptoms (14). *C4A* deficiencies have previously been linked to autoimmune diseases (43). The patients in the preeclampsia study did not suffer from autoimmune diseases. The high incidence of *C4A* deficiency in preeclampsia supports the importance of classical pathway of complement system in preeclampsia.

Membrane co-factor protein (MCP, CD46) has the capacity to regulate both alternative and classical pathways of complement activation by binding to C3b or C4b and acting as a co-factor to the inactivator enzyme Factor I. MCP is a widely expressed type 1 membrane bound protein. aHUS, can be caused by mutations in *MCP* (44–47). Proteinuria is one of the cornerstone symptoms of preeclampsia, but its degree varies between patients. Renal dysfunction due to uncontrolled complement activation has been suspected to be the underlying link between preeclampsia and kidney diseases. To investigate whether sequence variants in the *CD46* might predispose to preeclampsia, we sequenced the *MCP* gene in preeclamptic women with severe proteinuria and in non-preeclamptic controls (37, 48). The results of this study do not corroborate the previously reported association of A304V to severe preeclampsia in a cohort of autoimmune pregnancies (49). We observed similar minor allele frequency (MAF) of ~6% in cases and controls. We also found one control woman, who was homozygous to 304*V allele. Heterozygosity for another functional single nucleotide polymorphism (SNP) K32N (rs150429980) was found in one preeclamptic woman and one control. Thereby results are inconclusive. It is possible, however, that MCP plays a part in a particular subtype of preeclampsia, due to the heterogenous nature of the disease.

The complement co-factor I (coded by *CFI*) is a serine protease that inactivates C3b and C4b in the presence of a co-factor protein, such as complement factor H (FH) and MCP. In the PROMISSE cohort consisting of patients with anti-phospholipid antibodies or systemic lupus erythematosus (SLE), two severe preeclamptic patients with a history of complicated pregnancies were found to carry the loss-of-function mutation I398L in *CFI* (49). Furthermore, a mutation in the *CFH* the gene coding for FH with unknown functional consequence was found in another patient (49). While FH is mainly effective in inhibition of the alternative pathway, MCP and factor I have the capacity to regulate both alternative and classical pathways of complement activation.

IMMUNOGENETIC PREDISPOSITION FOR COMPROMISED TOLERANCE

Major histocompatibility (MHC) in chromosome 6 (6p21.3), is the most polymorphic region of the human genome as a result of diverse and shifting immunological selection pressures. Many of the genes in the MHC code for proteins with immunological function. Genes coding for C4A and C4B are located in the MHC as are the genes coding for human leukocyte antigen (HLA) receptors.

At least two autoimmune diseases exist that harbor an increased susceptibility to preeclampsia. Among other immunological defects, aberrant NK cell biology has also been implicated in both, SLE and Type 1 Diabetes. Together these observations might shed light to the disease mechanisms in pregnancy complications.

The proportion of natural killer (NK) cells increases markedly in the uterus/endometrium during implantation and they likely have an important function during early stages of placentation (50, 51). Accordingly, genotypes of KIR receptors on the NK cells in combination with genotypes of their ligands, HLA-C on fetal trophoblast cells have been under investigation in preeclampsia (52–54).

SLE is characterized by a diminished number of NK cells with variety of functional abnormalities (55). SLE shares many symptoms with preeclampsia, including hypertension, proteinuria, and thrombocytopenia. SLE carries a 2- to 4-fold increase in risk of preeclampsia during pregnancy. In a Swedish population-based registry study, the risk for severe preeclampsia in SLE patients was 4.3% (56). Among the MHC loci, the HLA-DRB1*15:01, one of the strongest susceptibility loci for SLE in European-descent populations, is also associated to reproductive failure, i.e., recurrent pregnancy loss and secondary recurrent pregnancy loss (57, 58).

Among pregnant women with Type 1 diabetes (T1D), 15–20% develop preeclampsia (59), and nephropathy further increases the risk of preeclampsia to up to 42–52% (60), which raises questions of shared pathologies. NK cells have a crucial role in trophoblast invasion and spiral artery remodeling in the early stages of pregnancy, as well as in the recognition of the allograft fetal cells. Diverse aberrations of NK cell function are widely evidenced in T1D [reviewed in (61)]. It has been shown, that during the diabetic pregnancy, NK cells adhering to normal decidual endothelium are diminished in comparison to the non-diabetic control pregnancies suggested reduced number of NK cells homing to decidua in the diabetic pregnancy (62). Furthermore, the peripheral blood CD56bright NK cells from pregnant T1D patients expressed very low levels of selectin L (SELL) and alpha 4 integrin (ITGA4), which are important receptors for homing to the uterus (63). CXCL10 and CXCL12 chemokines are produced by the decidua. Their receptors CXCR3 and CXCR4, respectively, were expressed in lower levels on NK cells from T1D patients (63). Furthermore, the expression of activating receptor CD335 in the NK cell is increased during pregnancy in T1D patients. Aberrant NK cell function may result in the increased Th1/Th2 ratio and enhanced activation of intermediate and non-classical monocytes (64), both of which have been observed in preeclampsia, as well as T1D. This may contribute to the underlying mechanism of higher incidence of preeclampsia in T1D patients.

While the villous trophoblasts in the placenta are HLA null, the invasive extravillous trophoblasts (EVT) express genes belonging to the MHC, namely HLA-E, -F, -G, and -C genes (**Figure 1**). Trophoblast cells do not express HLA class II on the placental surface but syncytiotrophoblast, the outer most layer of placental villi, contains intracellular HLA class II antigens (65). Therefore, compatibility of maternal and fetal HLA genotypes may also influence the immune response in late pregnancy when fetal components are released from the disintegrating placenta. In this context, HLA-A, -B, -DR, and -DQ gene groups may also be relevant in preeclampsia, but thus far, this hypothesis has received little attention.

HLA-G is considered to be protective and tolerogenic during pregnancy. HLA-G is present in semen, which suggests that immune tolerance induction starts already before conception. There are several studies suggesting low or reduced levels of sHLA-G in preeclampsia patients and reduced levels of HLA-G mRNA has been observed in placentas of preeclamptic women (66–69). In a study of genetic polymorphisms, a 14-bp ins/del polymorphism in the 3'UTR of exon 8 of the HLA-G gene was associated with mRNA stability and overall HLA-G production (70). The role of HLA-G polymorphism in preeclampsia is still unresolved.

ANTIANGIOGENIC SFLT1 AND INCREASED INFLAMMATORY RESPONSE IN ESTABLISHED PREECLAMPSIA

Inappropriate maternal immune responses to trophoblast in early pregnancy may lead to abnormal placentation and set the stage for clinical preeclampsia later in pregnancy. Established preeclampsia is characterized by endothelial dysfunction and systemic inflammatory response to placental oxidative stress [**Figure 2A**; (71)].

It has been suggested that antiangiogenic sFLT1 sensitizes endothelial cells to pro-inflammatory factors (72). The first genome wide association study of offspring from preeclamptic pregnancies reported that common variants near *FLT1* on chromosome 13 were associated with preeclampsia (19). Incidence of preeclampsia is known to be increased in pregnancies with fetal Trisomy 13 (73) suggesting that increased placental production of sFLT1 has a role in preeclampsia susceptibility. Furthermore, the importance of the *FLT1* in the disease is evidenced by the recently discovered protective variants in the gene (20).

Normal third-trimester pregnancy is characterized by activation of peripheral blood leukocytes, which is further increased in preeclampsia (74). Increase in the maternal circulating levels of proinflammatory cytokines tumor necrosis factor alpha (TNF α), interleukin (IL)-6, and also the anti-inflammatory cytokine IL-10 in the third trimester of pregnancy in women affected by preeclampsia have been demonstrated in a meta-analysis (75).

Obesity increases the risk of preeclampsia 2- to 3-fold (76–78), but the underlying mechanisms are not fully understood. Obesity is a state of uncontrolled inflammatory responses leading to systemic low-grade inflammation and increased insulin resistance (79). Even modestly overweight women have vascular endothelial dysfunction assessed by brachial artery ultrasound flow-mediated vasodilation (80). The secretion of pro-inflammatory cytokines including TNFα and IL-6 is increased in hypertrophic adipocytes (79). Herse and coworkers have also shown that TNFα decreased sFLT1 expression in mature adipocytes (81). We and others have found lower concentration of sFLT1 in obese compared to normal-weight preeclamptic women, but not in respective normotensive pregnant women (82, 83). Associations between maternal body mass index and proinflammatory cytokines TNFα and MCP-1 in maternal plasma have been demonstrated (84). Thus, the production of sFLT1 and proinflammatory cytokines by placenta and extraplacental sources may be different in obese and normal-weight women during pregnancy and in normal and complicated pregnancies.

CONCLUSION

The mechanisms regulating the immune response are central in normal pregnancy and the development of preeclampsia (**Figure 2A**). Mechanisms of autoimmunity, loss of tolerance, and inflammation in preeclampsia are evidenced in this mini-review (**Figure 2B**). Angiogenic proteins, continuous subclinical inflammation, and insulin resistance in preeclamptic women have been suggested to result in increased cardiovascular risk that with additional risk factors may result in cardiovascular disease (85–87). Thus far, investigation into the genetic background of the immunological pathogenesis of preeclampsia has mostly concentrated on the genes coding complement components and MHC. While both pathways are relevant to the early pregnancy and later clinical manifestations of preeclampsia, studies addressing other immunological mechanisms will be a welcome contribution to increase our understanding of the complex immunological interactions in the disease.

AUTHOR CONTRIBUTIONS

All authors listed have made a substantial, direct and intellectual contribution to the work, and approved it for publication.

ACKNOWLEDGMENTS

Figure 1 is adapted from Ph.D. thesis by AL, University of Helsinki 2017, available at https://helda.helsinki.fi/handle/10138/228534 reprinted with permission of University of Helsinki.

REFERENCES

1. Tranquilli AL, Dekker G, Magee L, Roberts J, Sibai BM, Steyn W, et al. The classification, diagnosis and management of the hypertensive disorders of pregnancy: a revised statement from the ISSHP. *Pregnancy Hypertens* (2014) 4:97–104. doi: 10.1016/j.preghy.2014.02.001
2. American College of Obstetricians and Gynecologists, Task Force on Hypertension in Pregnancy. Hypertension in pregnancy. Report of the American College of Obstetricians and Gynecologists' Task Force on Hypertension in Pregnancy. *Obstet Gynecol.* (2013) 122:1122–31. doi: 10.1097/01.AOG.0000437382.03963.88
3. Lisonkova S, Joseph KS. Incidence of preeclampsia: risk factors and outcomes associated with early- versus late-onset disease. *Am J Obstet Gynecol.* (2013) 209:544.e1–12. doi: 10.1016/j.ajog.2013.08.019
4. Redman CW, Sargent IL. Latest advances in understanding preeclampsia. *Science* (2005) 308:1592–4. doi: 10.1126/science.1111726
5. Roberts JM, Hubel CA. The two stage model of preeclampsia: variations on the theme. *Placenta* (2009) 30 (Suppl. A):S32–7. doi: 10.1016/j.placenta.2008.11.009
6. Regal JF, Burwick RM, Fleming SD. The complement system and preeclampsia. *Curr Hypertens Rep.* (2017) 19:87. doi: 10.1007/s11906-017-0784-4
7. Kovats S, Main EK, Librach C, Stubblebine M, Fisher SJ, DeMars R. A class I antigen, HLA-G, expressed in human trophoblasts. *Science* (1990) 248:220–3.
8. Ghaebi M, Nouri M, Ghasemzadeh A, Farzadi L, Jadidi-Niaragh F, Ahmadi M, et al. Immune regulatory network in successful pregnancy and reproductive failures. *Biomed Pharmacother.* (2017) 88:61–73. doi: 10.1016/j.biopha.2017.01.016
9. Lokki AI. *The Conundrum of Pre-eclampsia – From Candidate Genes to Complement System.* PhD-thesis, University of Helsinki, Helsinki, Finland (2017).
10. Lynch AM, Salmon JE. Dysregulated complement activation as a common pathway of injury in preeclampsia and other pregnancy complications. *Placenta* (2010) 31:561–7. doi: 10.1016/j.placenta.2010.03.010
11. Darmochwal-Kolarz D, Kludka-Sternik M, Tabarkiewicz J, Kolarz B, Rolinski J, Leszczynska-Gorzelak B, et al. The predominance of Th17 lymphocytes and decreased number and function of Treg cells in preeclampsia. *J Reprod Immunol.* (2012) 93:75–81. doi: 10.1016/j.jri.2012.01.006
12. Cnattingius S, Reilly M, Pawitan Y, Lichtenstein P. Maternal and fetal genetic factors account for most of familial aggregation of preeclampsia: a population-based Swedish cohort study. *Am J Med Genet A.* (2004) 130A:365–71. doi: 10.1002/ajmg.a.30257
13. He Y, Xu B, Song D, Yu F, Chen Q, Zhao M. Expression of the complement system's activation factors in plasma of patients with early/late-onset severe pre-eclampsia. *Am J Reprod Immunol.* (2016) 76:205–211. doi: 10.1111/aji.12541
14. Lokki AI, Heikkinen-Eloranta J, Jarva H, Saisto T, Lokki ML, Laivuori H, et al. Complement activation and regulation in preeclamptic placenta. *Front Immunol.* (2014) 5:312. doi: 10.3389/fimmu.2014.00312
15. Banadakoppa M, Vidaeff AC, Yallampalli U, Ramin SM, Belfort MA, Yallampalli C. Complement split products in amniotic fluid in pregnancies subsequently developing early-onset preeclampsia. *Dis Markers* (2015) 2015:263109. doi: 10.1155/2015/263109
16. Lynch AM, Murphy JR, Byers T, Gibbs RS, Neville MC, Giclas PC, et al. Alternative complement pathway activation fragment Bb in early pregnancy as a predictor of preeclampsia. *Am J Obstet Gynecol.* (2008) 198:385.e1–9. doi: 10.1016/j.ajog.2007.10.793

17. Lynch AM, Wagner BD, Giclas PC, West NA, Gibbs RS, Holers VM. The relationship of longitudinal levels of complement Bb during pregnancy with preeclampsia. *Am J Reprod Immunol.* (2016) 75:104–11. doi: 10.1111/aji.12439
18. Ning F, Liu H, Lash GE. The role of decidual macrophages during normal and pathological pregnancy. *Am J Reprod Immunol.* (2016) 75:298-309. doi: 10.1111/aji.12477
19. McGinnis R, Steinthorsdottir V, Williams NO, Thorleifsson G, Shooter S, Hjartardottir S, et al. Variants in the fetal genome near FLT1 are associated with risk of preeclampsia. *Nat Genet.* (2017) 49:1255–60. doi: 10.1038/ng.3895
20. Lokki AI, Daly E, Triebwasser M, Kurki MI, Roberson EDO, Happola P, et al. Protective low-frequency variants for preeclampsia in the fms related tyrosine kinase 1 gene in the Finnish population. *Hypertension* (2017) 70:365–71. doi: 10.1161/HYPERTENSIONAHA.117.09406
21. Yano K, Liaw PC, Mullington JM, Shih SC, Okada H, Bodyak N, et al. Vascular endothelial growth factor is an important determinant of sepsis morbidity and mortality. *J Exp Med.* (2006) 203:1447–58. doi: 10.1084/jem.20060375
22. Luttun A, Tjwa M, Moons L, Wu Y, Angelillo-Scherrer A, Liao F, et al. Revascularization of ischemic tissues by PlGF treatment, and inhibition of tumor angiogenesis, arthritis and atherosclerosis by anti-Flt1. *Nat Med.* (2002) 8:831–40. doi: 10.1038/nm731
23. Muehlenbachs A, Fried M, Lachowitzer J, Mutabingwa TK, Duffy PE. Natural selection of FLT1 alleles and their association with malaria resistance in *utero. Proc Natl Acad Sci USA.* (2008) 105:14488–491. doi: 10.1073/pnas.0803657105
24. Muehlenbachs A, Mutabingwa TK, Edmonds S, Fried M, Duffy PE. Hypertension and maternal-fetal conflict during placental malaria. *PLoS Med.* (2006) 3:e446. doi: 10.1371/journal.pmed.0030446
25. Brown EA, Ruvolo M, Sabeti PC. Many ways to die, one way to arrive: how selection acts through pregnancy. *Trends Genet.* (2013) 29:585–92. doi: 10.1016/j.tig.2013.03.001
26. Dormer A, Beck G. Evolutionary analysis of human vascular endothelial growth factor, angiopoietin, and tyrosine endothelial kinase involved in angiogenesis and immunity. *In Silico Biol.* (2005) 5:323–39.
27. Palmer KR, Tong S, Kaitu'u-Lino TJ. Placental-specific sFLT-1: role in pre-eclamptic pathophysiology and its translational possibilities for clinical prediction and diagnosis. *Mol Hum Reprod.* (2017) 23:69–78. doi: 10.1093/molehr/gaw077
28. Thomas CP, Andrews JI, Raikwar NS, Kelley EA, Herse F, Dechend R, et al. A recently evolved novel trophoblast-enriched secreted form of fms-like tyrosine kinase-1 variant is up-regulated in hypoxia and preeclampsia. *J Clin Endocrinol Metab.* (2009) 94:2524–30. doi: 10.1210/jc.2009-0017
29. Girardi G, Yarilin D, Thurman JM, Holers VM, Salmon JE. Complement activation induces dysregulation of angiogenic factors and causes fetal rejection and growth restriction. *J Exp Med.* (2006) 203:2165–75. doi: 10.1084/jem.20061022
30. Ye L, Gratton A, Hannan NJ, Cannon P, Deo M, Palmer KR, et al. Nuclear factor of activated T-cells (NFAT) regulates soluble fms-like tyrosine kinase-1 secretion (sFlt-1) from human placenta. *Placenta* (2016) 48:110–18. doi: 10.1016/j.placenta.2016.10.013
31. Penning M, Chua JS, van Kooten C, Zandbergen M, Buurma A, Schutte J, et al. Classical complement pathway activation in the kidneys of women with preeclampsia. *Hypertension* (2015) 66:117–25. doi: 10.1161/HYPERTENSIONAHA.115.05484
32. Meri S. Complement activation in diseases presenting with thrombotic microangiopathy. *Eur J Intern Med.* (2013) 24:496–502. doi: 10.1016/j.ejim.2013.05.009
33. Sridharan M, Go RS, Willrich MAV. Atypical hemolytic uremic syndrome: review of clinical presentation, diagnosis and management. *J Immunol Methods* (2018). 461:15–22. doi: 10.1016/j.jim.2018.07.006
34. Alrahmani L, Willrich MAV. The complement alternative pathway and preeclampsia. *Curr Hypertens Rep.* (2018) 20:40. doi: 10.1007/s11906-018-0836-4
35. Lokki AI, Triebwasser M, Daly E, Auro K, Perola M, FINNPEC, et al. Rare mutations in factor H predispose to severe preeclampsia. *Mol Immunol.* (2018) 102:184–85. doi: 10.1016/j.molimm.2018.06.147
36. Lokki AI, Kaartokallio T, Holmberg V, Onkamo P, Koskinen LLE, Saavalainen P, et al. Analysis of complement C3 gene reveals susceptibility to severe preeclampsia. *Front Immunol.* (2017) 8:589. doi: 10.3389/fimmu.2017.00589
37. Jääskeläinen T, Heinonen S, Kajantie E, Kere J, Kivinen K, Pouta A, et al. Cohort profile: the finnish genetics of pre-eclampsia consortium (FINNPEC). *BMJ Open* (2016) 6:e013148 doi: 10.1136/bmjopen-2016-013148
38. Xu C, Mao D, Holers VM, Palanca B, Cheng AM, Molina H. A critical role for murine complement regulator crry in fetomaternal tolerance. *Science* (2000) 287:498–501. doi: 10.1126/science.287.5452.498
39. Mohlin FC, Gros P, Mercier E, Gris JR, Blom AM. Analysis of C3 Gene variants in patients with idiopathic recurrent spontaneous pregnancy loss. *Front Immunol.* (2018) 9:1813. doi: 10.3389/fimmu.2018.01813
40. Lillegard KE, Johnson AC, Lojovich SJ, Bauer AJ, Marsh HC, Gilbert JS, et al. Complement activation is critical for placental ischemia-induced hypertension in the rat. *Mol Immunol.* (2013) 56:91–7. doi: 10.1016/j.molimm.2013.04.009
41. Lokki ML, Colten HR. Genetic deficiencies of complement. *Ann Med.* (1995) 27:451–9. doi: 10.3109/07853899709002453
42. Wennerstrom A, Vlachopoulou E, Lahtela LE, Paakkanen R, Eronen KT, Seppanen M, et al. Diversity of extended HLA-DRB1 haplotypes in the Finnish population. *PLoS ONE* (2013) 8:e79690. doi: 10.1371/journal.pone.0079690
43. Samano ES, Ribeiro Lde M, Gorescu RG, Rocha KC, Grumach AS. Involvement of C4 allotypes in the pathogenesis of human diseases. *Rev Hosp Clin Fac Med Sao Paulo* (2004) 59:138–44. doi: 10.1590/S0041-87812004000300009
44. Manchester M, Valsamakis A, Kaufman R, Liszewski MK, Alvarez J, Atkinson JP, et al. Measles virus and C3 binding sites are distinct on membrane cofactor protein (CD46). *Proc Nat Acad Sci USA.* (1995) 92:2303–7.
45. Richards A, Kemp EJ, Liszewski MK, Goodship JA, Lampe AK, Decorte R, et al. Mutations in human complement regulator, membrane cofactor protein (CD46), predispose to development of familial hemolytic uremic syndrome. *Proc Nat Acad Sci USA.* (2003) 100:12966–71. doi: 10.1073/pnas.2135497100
46. Fremeaux-Bacchi V, Moulton EA, Kavanagh D, Dragon-Durey M, Blouin J, Caudy A, et al. Genetic and functional analyses of membrane cofactor protein (CD46) mutations in atypical hemolytic uremic syndrome. *J Am Soc Nephrol.* (2006) 17:2017–25. doi: 10.1681/ASN.2005101051
47. Fang CJ, Fremeaux-Bacchi V, Liszewski MK, Pianetti G, Noris M, Goodship THJ, et al. Membrane cofactor protein mutations in atypical hemolytic uremic syndrome (aHUS), fatal Stx-HUS, C3 glomerulonephritis, and the HELLP syndrome. *Blood* (2008) 111:624–32. doi: 10.1182/blood-2007-04-084533
48. Lokki AI, Aalto-Viljakainen T, Meri S, Laivuori H. Genetic analysis of membrane cofactor protein (CD46) of the complement system in women with and without preeclamptic pregnancies. *PLoS ONE* (2015) 10:e0117840. doi: 10.1371/journal.pone.0117840
49. Salmon JE, Heuser C, Triebwasser M, Liszewski MK, Kavanagh D, Roumenina L, et al. Mutations in complement regulatory proteins predispose to preeclampsia: a genetic analysis of the PROMISSE cohort. *PLoS Med.* (2011) 8:e1001013. doi: 10.1371/journal.pmed.1001013
50. Ashkar AA, Di Santo JP, Croy BA. Interferon gamma contributes to initiation of uterine vascular modification, decidual integrity, and uterine natural killer cell maturation during normal murine pregnancy. *J Exp Med.* (2000) 192:259–70. doi: 10.1084/jem.192.2.259
51. Bulmer JN, Williams PJ, Lash GE. Immune cells in the placental bed. *Int J Dev Biol.* (2010) 54:281–94. doi: 10.1387/ijdb.082763jb
52. Hiby SE, Walker JJ, O'Shaughnessy KM, Redman CWG, Carrington M, Trowsdale J, et al. Combinations of maternal KIR and fetal HLA-C genes influence the risk of preeclampsia and reproductive success. *J Exp Med.* (2004) 200:957–65. doi: 10.1084/jem.20041214
53. Saito S, Takeda Y, Sakai M, Nakabayahi M, Hayakawa S. The incidence of pre-eclampsia among couples consisting of Japanese women and Caucasian men. *J Reprod Immunol.* (2006) 70:93–8. doi: 10.1016/j.jri.2005.12.005
54. Hiby SE, Apps R, Chazara O, Farrell LE, Magnus P, Trogstad L, et al. Maternal KIR in combination with paternal HLA-C2 regulate human birth weight. *J Immunol.* (2014) 192:5069–73. doi: 10.4049/jimmunol.1400577
55. Spada R, Rojas JM, Barber DF. Recent findings on the role of natural killer cells in the pathogenesis of systemic lupus erythematosus. *J Leukoc Biol.* (2015) 98:479–87. doi: 10.1189/jlb.4RU0315-081RR
56. Simard JF, Arkema EV, Nguyen C, Svenungsson E, Wikstrom AK, Palmsten K, et al. Early-onset preeclampsia in lupus pregnancy. *Paediatr Perinat Epidemiol.* (2017) 31:29–36. doi: 10.1111/ppe.12332

57. Kolte AM, Steffensen R, Christiansen OB, Nielsen HS. Maternal HY-restricting HLA class II alleles are associated with poor long-term outcome in recurrent pregnancy loss after a boy. *Am J Reprod Immunol.* (2016) 76:400–5. doi: 10.1111/aji.12561
58. Gambino CM, Di Bona D, Aiello A, Carru C, Duro G, Guggino G, et al. HLA-C1 ligands are associated with increased susceptibility to systemic lupus erythematosus. *Hum Immunol.* (2018) 79:172–7. doi: 10.1016/j.humimm.2018.01.005
59. Weissgerber TL, Mudd LM. Preeclampsia and diabetes. *Curr Diab Rep.* (2015) 15:3–9. doi: 10.1007/s11892-015-0579-4
60. Klemetti MM, Laivuori H, Tikkanen M, Nuutila M, Hiilesmaa V, Teramo K. Obstetric and perinatal outcome in type 1 diabetes patients with diabetic nephropathy during 1988 2011. *Diabetologia* (2015) 58.678–86. doi: 10.1007/s00125-014-3488-1
61. Marca V, Gianchecchi E, Fierabracci A. Type 1 diabetes and its multi-factorial pathogenesis: the putative role of NK cells. *Int J Mol Sci.* (2018) 19:E794. doi: 10.3390/ijms19030794
62. Seaward AV, Burke SD, Ramshaw H, Smith GN, Croy BA. Circulating CD56+ cells of diabetic women show deviated homing potential for specific tissues during and following pregnancy. *Hum Reprod.* (2011) 26:1675–84. doi: 10.1093/humrep/der114
63. Burke SD, Seaward AV, Ramshaw H, Smith GN, Virani S, Croy BA, et al. Homing receptor expression is deviated on CD56+ blood lymphocytes during pregnancy in Type 1 diabetic women. *PLoS ONE* (2015) 10:e0119526. doi: 10.1371/journal.pone.0119526
64. Groen B, van der Wijk AE, van den Berg PP, Lefrandt JD, van den Berg G, Sollie KM, et al. Immunological adaptations to pregnancy in women with type 1 diabetes. *Sci Rep.* (2015) 5:13618. doi: 10.1038/srep13618
65. Ranella A, Vassiliadis S, Mastora C, Valentina M, Dionyssopoulou E, Athanassakis I. Constitutive intracellular expression of human leukocyte antigen (HLA)-DO and HLA-DR but not HLA-DM in trophoblast cells. *Hum Immunol.* (2005) 66:43–55. doi: 10.1016/j.humimm.2004.10.002
66. Yie SM, Taylor RN, Librach C. Low plasma HLA-G protein concentrations in early gestation indicate the development of preeclampsia later in pregnancy. *Am J Obstet Gynecol.* (2005) 193:204–08. doi: 10.1016/j.ajog.2004.11.062
67. Hackmon R, Koifman A, Hyodo H, Glickman H, Sheiner E, Geraghty DE. Reduced third-trimester levels of soluble human leukocyte antigen G protein in severe preeclampsia. *Am J Obstet Gynecol.* (2007) 197:255.e1-255.e5. doi: 10.1016/j.ajog.2007.06.033
68. He Y, Chen S, Huang H, Chen Q. Association between decreased plasma levels of soluble human leukocyte antigen-G and severe pre-eclampsia. *J Perinat Med.* (2016) 44:283–90. doi: 10.1515/jpm-2015-0062
69. Marozio L, Garofalo A, Berchialla P, Tavella AM, Salton L, Cavallo F, et al. Low expression of soluble human leukocyte antigen G in early gestation and subsequent placenta-mediated complications of pregnancy. *J Obstet Gynaecol Res.* (2017) 43:1391–6. doi: 10.1111/jog.13377
70. Lynge Nilsson L, Djurisic S, Hviid TV. Controlling the immunological crosstalk during conception and pregnancy: HLA-G in reproduction. *Front Immunol.* (2014) 5:198. doi: 10.3389/fimmu.2014.00198
71. Redman CW, Sargent IL. Immunology of pre-eclampsia. *Am J Reprod Immunol.* (2010) 63:534–43. doi: 10.1111/j.1600-0897.2010.00831.x
72. Cindrova-Davies T, Sanders DA, Burton GJ, Charnock-Jones DS. Soluble FLT1 sensitizes endothelial cells to inflammatory cytokines by antagonizing VEGF receptor-mediated signalling. *Cardiovasc Res.* (2011) 89:671–9. doi: 10.1093/cvr/cvq346
73. Bdolah Y, Palomaki GE, Yaron Y, Bdolah-Abram T, Goldman M, Levine RJ, et al. Circulating angiogenic proteins in trisomy 13. *Am J Obstet Gynecol.* (2006) 194:239–45. doi: 10.1016/j.ajog.2005.06.031
74. Sacks GP, Studena K, Sargent K, Redman CW. Normal pregnancy and preeclampsia both produce inflammatory changesin peripheral blood leukocytes akin to those of sepsis. *Am J Obstet Gynecol.* (1998) 179:80–6. doi: 10.1016/S0002-9378(98)70254-6
75. Lau SY, Guild SJ, Barrett CJ, Chen Q, McCowan L, Jordan V, et al. Tumor necrosis factor-alpha, interleukin-6, and interleukin-10 levels are altered in preeclampsia: a systematic review and meta-analysis. *Am J Reprod Immunol.* (2013) 70:412–27. doi: 10.1111/aji.12138
76. Bodnar LM, Ness RB, Markovic N, Roberts JM. The risk of preeclampsia rises with increasing prepregnancy body mass index. *Ann Epidemiol.* (2005) 15:475–82. doi: 10.1016/j.annepidem.2004.12.008
77. Duckitt K, Harrington D. Risk factors for pre-eclampsia at antenatal booking: systematic review of controlled studies. *BMJ* (2005) 330:565. doi: 10.1136/bmj.38380.674340.E0
78. Jeyabalan A. Epidemiology of preeclampsia: impact of obesity. *Nutr Rev.* (2013) 71 (Suppl. 1):S18–25. doi: 10.1111/nure.12055
79. Choe SS, Huh JY, Hwang IJ, Kim JI, Kim JB. Adipose tissue remodeling: its role in energy metabolism and metabolic disorders. *Front Endocrinol.* (2016) 7:30. doi: 10.3389/fendo.2016.00030
80. Patel AR, Hui H, Kuvin JT, Pandian NG, Karas RH. Modestly overweight women have vascular endothelial dysfunction. *Clin Cardiol.* (2009) 32:269–73. doi: 10.1002/clc.20451
81. Herse F, Fain JN, Janke J, Engeli S, Kuhn C, Frey N, et al. Adipose tissue-derived soluble fms-like tyrosine kinase 1 is an obesity-relevant endogenous paracrine adipokine. *Hypertension* (2011) 58:37–42. doi: 10.1161/HYPERTENSIONAHA.111.171322
82. Suwaki N, Masuyama H, Nakatsukasa H, Masumoto A, Sumida Y, Takamoto N, et al. Hypoadiponectinemia and circulating angiogenic factors in overweight patients complicated with pre-eclampsia. *Am J Obstet Gynecol.* (2006) 195:1687–92. doi: 10.1016/j.ajog.2006.04.003
83. Jääskeläinen T, Heinonen S, Hämäläinen E, Pulkki K, Romppanen J, Laivuori H, FINNPEC. Impact of obesity on angiogenic and inflammatory markers in the Finnish Genetics of Pre-eclampsia Consortium (FINNPEC) cohort. *Int J Obes.* (2018). doi: 10.1038/s41366-018-0217-8. [Epub ahead of print].
84. Aye IL, Lager S, Ramirez VI, Gaccioli F, Dudley DJ, Jansson T, et al. Increasing maternal body mass index is associated with systemic inflammation in the mother and the activation of distinct placental inflammatory pathways. *Biol Reprod.* (2014) 90:129. doi: 10.1095/biolreprod.113.116186
85. Sattar N, Greer IA. Pregnancy complications and maternal cardiovascular risk: opportunities for intervention and screening? *BMJ* (2002) 325:157–60. doi: 10.1136/bmj.325.7356.157
86. Kvehaugen AS, Dechend R, Ramstad HB, Troisi R, Fugelseth D, Staff AC. Endothelial function and circulating biomarkers are disturbed in women and children after preeclampsia. *Hypertension* (2011) 58:63–9. doi: 10.1161/HYPERTENSIONAHA.111.172387
87. Wolf M, Hubel CA, Lam C, Sampson M, Ecker JL, Ness RB, et al. Preeclampsia and future cardiovascular disease: potential role of altered angiogenesis and insulin resistance. *J Clin Endocrinol Metab.* (2004) 89:6239–43. doi: 10.1210/jc.2004-0548

17

The Role of Extracellular Vesicles and PIBF in Embryo-Maternal Immune-Interactions

Julia Szekeres-Bartho [1,2,3,4]*, *Sandra Šućurović* [5] *and Biserka Mulac-Jeričević* [5]

[1] Department of Medical Biology and Central Electron Microscope Laboratory, Medical School, Pécs University, Pécs, Hungary, [2] János Szentágothai Research Centre, Pécs University, Pécs, Hungary, [3] Endocrine Studies, Centre of Excellence, Pécs University, Pécs, Hungary, [4] MTA-PTE Human Reproduction Research Group, Pécs, Hungary, [5] Department of Physiology and Immunology, Faculty of Medicine, University of Rijeka, Rijeka, Croatia

***Correspondence:**
Julia Szekeres-Bartho
Szekeres.julia@pte.hu

Pregnancy represents a unique immunological situation. Though paternal antigens expressed by the conceptus are recognized by the immune system of the mother, the immune response does not harm the fetus. Progesterone and a progesterone induced protein; PIBF are important players in re-adjusting the functioning of the maternal immune system during pregnancy. PIBF expressed by peripheral pregnancy lymphocytes, and other cell types, participates in the feto-maternal communication, partly, by mediating the immunological actions of progesterone. Several splice variants of PIBF were identified with different physiological activity. The full length 90 kD PIBF protein plays a role in cell cycle regulation, while shorter splice variants are secreted and act as cytokines. Aberrant production of PIBF isoforms lead to the loss of immune-regulatory functions, resulting in and pregnancy failure. By up regulating Th2 type cytokine production and by down-regulating NK activity, PIBF contributes to the altered attitude of the maternal immune system. Normal pregnancy is characterized by a Th2-dominant cytokine balance, which is partly due to the action of the smaller PIBF isoforms. These bind to a novel form of the IL-4 receptor, and induce increased production of IL-3, IL-4, and IL-10. The communication between the conceptus and the mother is established via extracellular vesicles (EVs). Pre-implantation embryos produce EVs both *in vitro*, and *in vivo*. PIBF transported by the EVs from the embryo to maternal lymphocytes induces increased IL-10 production by the latter, this way contributing to the Th2 dominant immune responses described during pregnancy.

Keywords: pregnancy, progesterone, PIBF, NK cells, cytokines, extracellular vesicles

INTRODUCTION

Fifty per cent of the antigens expressed by the fetus originate from the father. Therefore, they are recognized as foreign and should be "rejected," yet in spite of all odds, the maternal immune system does not attack the fetus.

The immune system of the mother must comply with two conflicting requirements, i.e., while creating a favorable environment for the developing fetus, it has to be prepared to control possible emerging infections. By establishing a delicate balance, the foeto-maternal unit is able to satisfy the interests of both the mother and the fetus. Progesterone, and its mediator the progesterone-induced blocking factor (PIBF) are important players in this process. In addition to its endocrine effects, progesterone also acts as an "immunosteroid" (1). Progesterone induces Th2 differentiation of established T cell clones (2) and regulates the homing and activity of uterine NK cells (3), among others, by upregulating HLA-G gene expression (4), which is the ligand for both NK inhibitory and activating receptors. Many of the immunological effects of progesterone are mediated by PIBF.

This review aims to give an overview on the diverse roles of progesterone and PIBF in re-setting the functions of the maternal immune system, and on extracellular vesicles (EVs) as means of establishing the communication between the two sides of the feto-maternal unit.

PROGESTERONE RECEPTORS

The biological activity of progesterone is mediated by genomic and non-genomic pathways. The former depends on two nuclear progesterone receptor (PR) isoforms, PRA, and PRB (5, 6). Both isoforms are the products of the same gene, but their transcription is controlled by two distinct promoters (7).

Mice lacking PRA are infertile (8, 9), while the PRB isoform mediates the effects of progesterone on mammary gland development (10). The reproductive tissue responses to progesterone depend on the relative expression of the two isoforms (11). Progesterone can also signal through membrane-bound PRs or via the MAPK or PI3K/Akt pathway. The latter entirely bypasses the classical PR pathway, signaling either through the JNK pathway or by increasing cAMP (12).

Studies on PR knock out mice revealed, that PRs are required not only for endometrial receptivity and decidualization (13), but also for establishing an appropriate immune environment in the endometrium (14) (**Figure 1**). Several studies using nuclear and cytosol binding assays and immunohistochemistry—indicate, that in certain conditions lymphoid cells might express PRs (15–20).

Peripheral lymphocytes of pregnant women, but not those of non-pregnant individuals express PRs (21, 22). Earlier we demonstrated an inverse relationship between progesterone binding capacity and cytotoxic activity of peripheral human lymphocytes (23). The cytotoxic activity of pregnancy lymphocytes was significantly reduced by progesterone at concentrations comparable to those, present in pregnancy serum, while 100-fold higher progesterone concentrations were required to alter the cytotoxic activity of lymphocytes from non-pregnant individuals (24). These findings already suggested that pregnancy lymphocytes might contain progesterone binding sites, which enable them to respond to progesterone.

The number of PR positive cells increases throughout normal gestation. In women with recurrent miscarriage, or in those, showing clinical symptoms of threatened pre-term delivery, the % of PR expressing cells among peripheral lymphocytes, is significantly lower than in women with uneventful pregnancies (21, 22). These findings suggest, that the presence of PR positive lymphocytes is required for a normally progressing pregnancy.

PR expression in peripheral lymphocytes or lymphoid cell lines has been confirmed by several studies (15–17, 25, 26). Both classical PR isoforms are present in peripheral blood NK cells (18), however, PR expression in decidual NK cells is controversial. Van den Heuvel et al. (3) demonstrated PRs in murine decidual NK cells, while Henderson et al. (27) failed to detect of PRs in purified decidual NK cells. Nevertheless, the majority of decidual NK cells are PIBF positive (28).

Both *in vitro* and *in vivo* activation of human non-pregnancy lymphocytes result in increased PR expression (29, 30). Paternal leukocyte immunization of women with recurrent miscarriage also increases the number of PR expressing lymphocytes (31).

These data indicate that PR expression is a characteristic feature of activated immune cells (**Figure 2**).

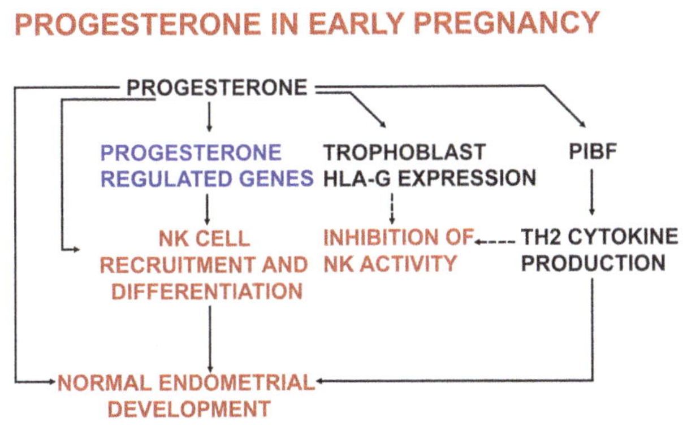

FIGURE 1 | The effects of progesterone on endometrial development and on the immune system in early pregnancy.

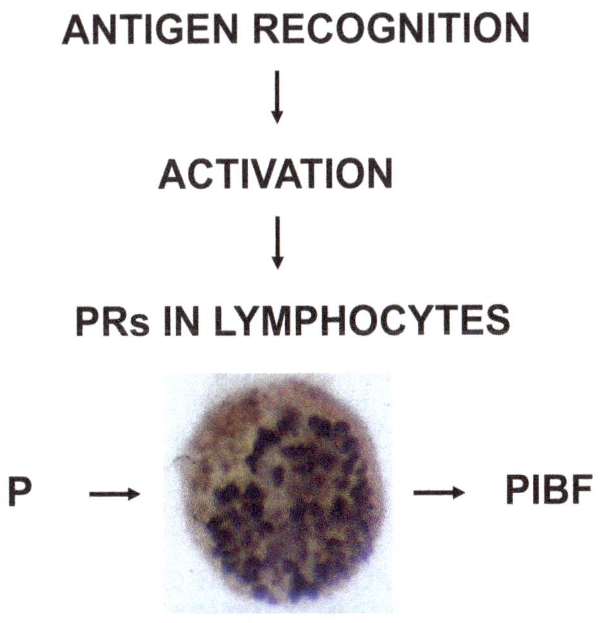

FIGURE 2 | The induction and biological significance of lymphocyte progesterone receptors. Following recognition of fetal antigens, maternal lymphocytes become activated and express progesterone receptors (PR). The presence of PRs enables the cells, to respond to progesterone (P), e.g., by PIBF production.

PROGESTERONE-REGULATED GENES

Among the progesterone-regulated genes, the transcription factors Hox-A10, Hox-A11, and the glican binding protein galectin-1 (Gal-1) are the most relevant for the feto- maternal immunological interaction (32). Hox-A10 deficient mice are characterized by a polyclonal T cell proliferation (33), and impaired decidual NK cell differentiation (24, 25, 34, 35).

Gal-1 expression in the female reproductive system was described in the nineties, and recently, many functional aspects of this lectin during pregnancy have been discovered (36–38). Gal-1 gene expression in the mouse uterine tissues has been shown to be regulated by ovarian steroids during implantation (39). In line with this, Than et al. (40) identified an estrogen response element in the Gal-1 gene.

Altered Gal-1 expression in the placenta has been implicated in several pregnancy pathologies.

Proteomic studies showed that Gal-1 expression is reduced in placental villous tissues from patients with spontaneous miscarriages (41). On the other hand, placental Gal-1 expression was found to be increased in severe preeclampsia (42) as well as in chorioamnionitis (43), possibly representing a fetal response to an exaggerated systemic maternal inflammation.

In pregnant mice, stress-induced Gal-1-deficiency results in an increased rate of fetal loss, which is corrected by progesterone exposure. Gal-1 treatment on the other hand, prevents the stress-induced decrease of progesterone as well as PIBF levels, and restores the resorption rates to a normal level (44). These data suggest a cross-regulation between progesterone and Gal-1 at the foeto-maternal interface.

PIBF is another progesterone-regulated gene. The mouse PIBF1 gene, is transcribed to 16 different mRNAs, the longest of which is 3,677 bp long and includes 18 exons. The predicted protein is a 90 kDa molecule, composed of 756 amino acids (45). The full-length PIBF protein shows a peri-nuclear localization, (46) and has been identified as a component of the peri-centriolar satellite (47), suggesting its role in cell cycle regulation. Alternative splicing produces several smaller isoforms, which are localized in the cytoplasm (45) and are accountable for the immunological effects of PIBF.

In murine pregnancy, embryo resorption as well as term delivery are associated with the absence or lower expression of the N terminal PIBF exons, which might have important functional consequences (48).

The loss of the N-terminal exons results in a significantly reduced production of the full length protein, and also prevents the synthesis of the smaller protein isoforms, which act on the cytokine pattern and NK activity (45).

THE IMMUNO-MODULATING EFFECTS OF PIBF AND THE MAINTENANCE OF PREGNANCY

PIBF was first described as a 34 kDa protein produced by activated pregnancy lymphocytes (30). It has become evident since, that PIBF might be expressed by various reproductive tissues as well as malignant tumors (49–51). A human study illustrated that trophoblast cells in the placenta could express PIBF proteins of 30, 50, and 90 kDa in first trimester (52).

Several human studies suggest an association between PIBF levels and the outcome of pregnancy. In a prospective cohort study attempting to identify early risk factors for miscarriage, PIBF was one of the factors showing a strong association with miscarriage risk (53). In normal human pregnancy, both serum-and urinary PIBF concentrations increase during gestation, while in women, with miscarriage, or preterm labor, urinary PIBF levels fail to increase (54). Preterm birth was predictable by lower than normal pregnancy PIBF values mesaured at 24–28gestational week (55), but not at 11–13 weeks of gestation (56), suggesting, that predictive value of PIBF determination depends on the interval, between sampling and the onset of labor. In line with this, progestogen-treatment of women with threatened miscarriage corrected the initially low PIBF levels, and in parallel, reduced the miscarriage rate to a similar level of healthy controls (57).

While the full length PIBF has been shown to regulate trophoblast and tumor cell invasiveness (58–60), the smaller isoforms are secreted, bind to the PIBF receptor (39, 61) and via their cytokine-like functions, play a role in the materno-fetal relationship, both in animal models and in humans.

Some of the immunological effects of progesterone, e.g., that on NK activity and cytokine balance, are mediated by PIBF.

Earlier studies showed that in mice PIBF protects pregnancy by controlling NK activity (62). Anti-PIBF treatment of pregnant mice results in increased resorption, which are corrected by simultaneously neutralizing NK activity with anti-NK antibodies (62).

Decidual NK cells, are functionally different from their circulating counterparts. Though decidual NK cells selectively overexpress perforin and granzymes A and B (41, 63), their cytotoxic activity is low. In normal pregnancy decidual NK cells contribute to creating a favorable environment for placentation, implantation and embryo development (64), yet they are equipped with cytotoxic molecules, to fight intrauterine infections (65, 66).

In the day 12 mouse decidua, there is an abundance of PIBF positive granulated cells. These cells are missing from the deciduae of alymphoid mice, but when alymphoid mice are reconstituted of with bone marrow from male BALB/c mice, the PIBF positive granulated cells re-appear in the decidua. These data suggest that the PIBF+ cells belong to the lymphoid lineage, and based on their DBA lectin reactivity, to the group of NK cells.

PIBF+ NK cells contain perforin, which co-localizes with PIBF in the cytoplasmic granules. In day 12.5 normal mouse pregnancy only 54% of the PIBF + decidual NK cells contain perforin, whereas in PIBF deficient mice of the same gestational age, not only do most of the PIBF + NK cells disappear, but all of the remaining ones are perforin positive (28).

This implies that in mice PIBF exerts a pregnancy protective effect by keeping NK activity under restraint.

The local mechanism of the protective action of PIBF is less easily studied in humans, than in animal models. Nevertheless, a recent study showed that the otherwise scarcely studied decidual B cells produce PIBF under the effect of IL-33, and that these PIBF + B cells are missing from the choriodecidual area of women with pre-term labor (67) (Nature).

In spite of their high perforin content, spontaneous cytotoxic activity of human decidual NK cells is moderate (68). Progesterone inhibits human NK cytolytic activity *in vitro* (19), and upregulates HLA-G gene expression (4). Because HLA-G is a ligand for NK inhibitory and activating receptors, upregulation of HLA-G by progesterone might be one of the pathways accounting for the low cytotoxic activity of decidual NK cells.

Decidual NK activity appears to be affected by PIBF. PIBF inhibits upregulation of perforin expression in activated human decidual NK cells and prevents degranulation (69, 70).

Though there is no evidence that NK cells directly attack the trophoblast, recurrent miscarriage is often accompanied by increased decidual NK activity (71–75), suggesting that this mechanism might be a factor in the underlying pathology of repeated pregnancy loss.

It is well-established, that while normally progressing pregnancies are characterized by a Th2 dominant cytokine pattern, an excess of Th1-associated cytokines leads to pregnancy termination (76, 77). In humans, recurrent miscarriages are associated with a Thl-dominant peripheral cytokine profile (78–82).

Both progesterone and PIBF play a role in the induction of the Th2 biased cytokine balance. In the presence of progesterone resting human peripheral blood T cells differentiate into Th2-like clones, furthermore, progesterone treatment of Th1-like T cell clones shifts the cytokine production of these cells toward Th2 (2). Neutralization of endogenous PIBF activity in pregnant mice by specific anti-PIBF antibody terminates pregnancy, reduces the synthesis of IL-10, and increases that of IFN-γ (83).

The PIBF receptor is a glycosylphosphatidylinositol (GPI)-anchored protein, which, for signaling, temporarily associates with the alpha chain of the IL-4 receptor (39, 61). Engagement of the PIBF receptor results in immediate STAT6 activation, whereas, a 24 h incubation with progesterone is needed to phosphorylate STAT6, indicating, that the effect of progesterone on Th2 cytokine production is mediated by PIBF (61) (**Figure 3**).

By signaling via this novel form of the IL-4 receptor (39, 61), PIBF induces increased production of IL-3, IL-4, and IL-10 by activated murine lymphocytes (84).

Raghupathy et al. (78, 79) investigated the production of Thl and Th2 cytokines by progesterone treated peripheral blood lymphocytes isolated from women with recurrent miscarriage. They showed that progestogen induced PIBF production down-regulates the production of Thl-type cytokines and stimulates the production of Th2-type cytokines. Furthermore, progestogen treatment of women with pre-term delivery induces a Th2 dominant cytokine pattern (78, 79).

Taken together, these data suggest, that by up regulating Th2 type cytokine production and by down-regulating NK activity PIBF affects the immune response in a way, which might have an impact on the foeto-maternal relationship.

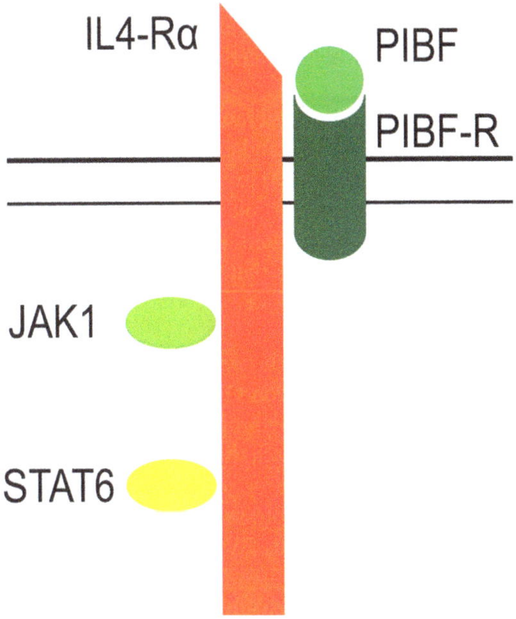

FIGURE 3 | The structure of the PIBF receptor. The receptor for PIBF is a GPI anchored protein. After PIBF binding the receptor associates with the alpha chain of the IL-4 receptor. This initiates intracellular signaling, via the Jak/STAT pathway.

THE PERI-IMPLANTATION EMBRYO COMMUNICATES WITH THE MATERNAL IMMUNE SYSTEM VIA EXTRACELLULAR VESICLES

Earlier studies described a communication between the embryo and the maternal immune system. Embryo culture media were shown to exert an immunosuppressive activity (84). In line with this, incubation of human peripheral lymphocytes with the culture media of fertilized eggs, but not with follicular fluid resulted in increased IL-10 mRNA expression by the lymphocytes (85).

These data suggest that embryo derived signals, can influence the maternal immune response, however, the mechanism of signal transport has not been thoroughly investigated.

In recent years EVs have received much attention. These membrane-coated structures may express phosphatidylserine (PS) in their membrane (86), which reacts with Annexin V. EVs are categorized by their origin and size (87). Exosomes are 30–100 nm, and originate from internalized endocytic vesicles. Microvesicles (100 nm^{-1} μm in diameter), are shed from the plasma membrane by budding, and apoptotic vesicles (1–5 μm in diameter) are released from cells undergoing apoptosis (88).

All types of cells produce EVs which transport various cargos, (including proteins, nucleic acids, and lipids) from one cell to the other. Proteins, e.g., cytokines carried and released by EVs could initiate signaling pathways, and thus alter the biological functions of the target cells (89, 90).

EVs might be considered as candidates for conveying the information from the embryo to the mother. The message carried by EVs has been shown to affect the reproductive process at different points.

EVs have been demonstrated in mouse oocytes (91) as well as in the follicular fluid (92–96) and extra villous trophoblast (97). The tetraspanins CD9 and CD81 expressed by oocyte derived EVs have been suggested to play a role in sperm-oocyte membrane fusion (98–100). Follicular fluid exosomes contain miRNAs, some of them targeting genes that regulate oocyte growth (95) as well as different pathways of reproduction, and endocrine functions (94).

EV—mediated interactions between the endometrium and the blastocyst promote implantation (101). In sheep endometrium, EV production is controlled by progesterone, and endometrium derived EVs were shown to reach the embryo, (102).

EVs from a human uterine epithelial cells express the extracellular matrix metalloprotease inducer (103) which induces the expression of MMPs, thus EVs might also play a role in endometrial remodeling (101, 103, 104).

EVs can be produced by virtually all cell types, however it has been debated, whether a single embryo would be able to produce a detectable amount of EVs. The more so, because the culture medium contains serum or serum albumin, both of which could also be a source of EVs. In a review Tannetta et al. (105) points out the difficulty of measuring EVs in embryo culture medium.

Now there is evidence, that pre-implantation embryos produce EVs both *in vitro* and *in vivo* (106).

Earlier we showed that spent media of *in vitro* cultured human embryos contain a significantly higher number of EVs, than empty media, and the number of nucleic acid containing EVs in day 5 human embryo culture media, might serve as an indicator of embryo competence (106). Other groups have also reported the presence of EVs in embryo culture medium. It is now obvious that embryos release EVs, which are taken up by close by cells (90). Giacomini et al. (107) characterized HLA-G containing EVs isolated from conditioned media from *in vitro* cultured human embryos. EVs were demonstrated in the culture medium of bovine blastocyst and the characteristics of these EVs varied depending on embryo competence (108). Qu et al. (109) showed that the negative effects of culture media replacement during embryo culture are due to the loss of embryo derived EVs, and can be corrected by exosome supplementation. This suggests, that embryo derived EVs do indeed carry molecules that promote normal embryo development.

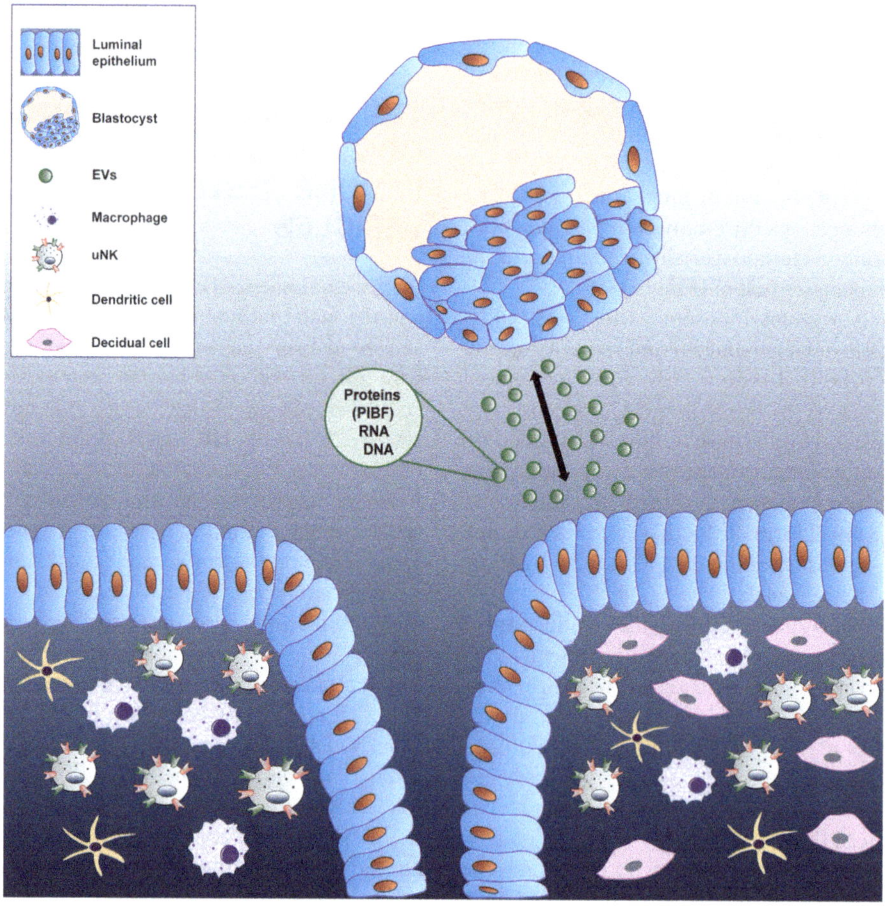

FIGURE 4 | Communication between the embryo and the maternal immune system via extracellular vesicles.

Embryo-derived EVs might also communicate with the maternal immune system by presenting antigens (110, 111), carrying MHC molecules (112–115), or cytokines (116–121). HLA-G-positive EVs isolated from the plasma from healthy term pregnant women have been reported to bind to T lymphocytes (122), and moderately decrease peripheral T lymphocyte STAT3 phosphorylation (122). EVs at the same time can induce pro-inflammatory cytokines and chemokines in primary macrophage cultures (123, 124).

EVs bind to CD8+ and–though to a lesser degree to CD4+ lymphocytes-, via the phosphatidylserine—phosphatidylserine receptor interaction (125). CD4+ and CD8+ cells express similar numbers of phosphatidylserine receptors, therefore, it is likely, that in addition to the phosphatidylserine—phosphatidylserine receptor interaction, other, yet unidentified mechanisms might also be involved in binding of EVs to CD8+ cells. With immuno-electron microscopy we identified PIBF in embryo-derived EVs, and showed that these PIBF containing EVs might affect the immune response (125).

Incubation of murine spleen cells with embryo-derived EVs, increased the number of IL-10+ cells among peripheral CD8+ cells, but not in the CD4+ population. IL-10 producing CD8+ T lymphocytes might moderate antigen-induced inflammatory responses, since these cells have been shown to control influenza virus induced inflammation in the foet (126), and to prevent liver damage during chronic hepatitis C virus infection (127).

Pre-treatment of EVs with an anti-PIBF antibody abrogates the above described effect of the EVs. These data suggest that PIBF transported by the EVs from the embryo to maternal lymphocytes might induce increased IL-10 production by the latter, this way contributing to the Th2 dominant immune responses described during pregnancy. The finding is in line with our earlier data, (83) showing increased IL-10 production of murine spleen cells in the presence of PIBF.

This pathway might have its significance in reproduction. Because embryo derived EVs transport various molecules, - PIBF, among others-, it cannot be ruled out, that these structures act as means of feto-maternal or materno-fetal communication in the peri-implantation period (**Figure 4**).

AUTHOR CONTRIBUTIONS

JS-B wrote the paper. BM-J, SŠ, and JS-B designed and performed the experiments.

ACKNOWLEDGMENTS

This work was supported by GINOP-2.3.2-15-201600021, PTE ÁOK-KA 2017–22 EFOP-3.6.1.-16-2016-00004, EFOP-3.6.3-VEKOP-16-2017-00009 to JS-B, and Croatian science foundation (HRZZ 3432) BM-J and a grant from the University of Rijeka, Croatia 13.06.1.1.08 BM-J.

REFERENCES

1. Siiteri PK, Febres F, Clemens LE, Chang RJ, Gondos B, Stites DP. Progesterone and the maintenance of pregnancy: is progesterone nature's immunosuppressant? *Ann NY Acad Sci.* (1997) 286:384–97. doi: 10.1111/j.1749-6632.1977.tb29431.x
2. Piccinni MP, Giudizi MG, Biagiotti R, Beloni L, Giannarini L, Sampognaro S, et al. Progesterone favors the development of human T helper cells producing Th2-type cytokines and promotes both IL-4 production and membrane CD30 expression in established Th1 cells clones. *J Immunol.* (1995) 155:128–33.
3. Van den Heuvel MJ, Chantakru S, Xumei X, Evans EE, Tekpetey F, Mote PA, et al. Trafficking of circulating pro-NK cells to the decidualizing uterus: regulatory mechanisms in the mouse and human. *Immunol Invest.* (2005). 34:273–93. doi: 10.1081/IMM-200064488
4. Yie SM, Xiao R, Librach CL. Progesterone regulates HLA-G gene expression through a novel progesterone response element *Hum Reprod.* (2006) 21:2538–44. doi: 10.1093/humrep/del126
5. Li X, Lonard DM, O'Malley BW. A contemporary understanding of progesterone receptor function. *Mech Ageing Dev.* (2004) 125:669–78. doi: 10.1016/j.mad.2004.04.007
6. Mulac-Jericevic B, Conneely OM. Reproductive tissue selective actions of progesterone receptors. *Reproduction* (2004) 128:139–46. doi: 10.1530/rep.1.00189
7. Li X, O'Malley BW. Unfolding the action of progesterone receptor. *J Biol Chem.* (2003) 278:39261–4. doi: 10.1074/jbc.R300024200
8. Mulac-Jericevic B, Mullinax RA, DeMayo FJ, Lydon JP, Conneely OM. Subgroup of reproductive functions of progesterone mediated by progesterone receptor-B isoform. *Science* (2000) 289:1751–4. doi: 10.1126/science.289.5485.1751
9. Mulac-Jericevic B, Lydon JP, DeMayo FJ, Conneely OM. Defective mammary gland morphogenesis in mice lacking the progesterone receptor B isoform. *Proc Natl Acad Sci USA.* (2003) 100:9744–9. doi: 10.1073/pnas.1732707100
10. Conneely OM, Jericevic BM, Lydon JP. Progesterone receptors in mammary gland development and tumorigenesis. *J Mammary Gland Biol Neoplasia.* (2003) 8:205–14. doi: 10.1023/A:1025952924864
11. Fernandez-Valdivia R, Mukherjee A, Mulac-Jericevic B, Conneely OM, DeMayo FJ, Amato P, et al. Revealing progesterone's role in uterine and mammary gland biology: insights from the mouse. *Semin Reprod Med.* (2005) 23:22–37. doi: 10.1055/s-2005-864031
12. Gellersen B, Fernandes MS, Brosens JJ. Non-genomic progesterone actions in female reproduction. *Hum Reprod Update* (2009) 15:119–38. doi: 10.1093/humupd/dmn044
13. Lydon JP, DeMayo FJ, Funk CR, Mani SK, Hughes AR, Montgomery CA, et al. Mice lacking progesterone receptor exhibit pleiotropic reproductive abnormalities. *Genes Dev.* (1995) 9:2266–78. doi: 10.1101/gad.9.18.2266
14. Tibbetts TA, Conneely OM, O'Malley BW. Progesterone via its receptor antagonizes the pro-inflammatory activity of estrogen in the mouse uterus. *Biol Reprod.* (1999) 60:1158–65. doi: 10.1095/biolreprod60.5.1158
15. Kimoto Y. A single human cell expresses all messenger ribonucleic acids: the arrow of time in a cell. *Mol Gen Genet.* (1998) 258:233–9. doi: 10.1007/s004380050727
16. Daniel L, Vincent C, Rousset F, Klein B, Bataille R, Flacher M, et al. Estrogen and progesterone receptors in some human myeloma cell lines and murine hybridomas. *J Steroid Biochem.* (1988) 30:363–7. doi: 10.1016/0022-4731(88)90124-0
17. Pasanen S, Ylikomi T, Palojoki E, Syvala H, Pelto-Huikko M, Tuohimaa P. Progesterone receptor in chicken bursa of Fabricius and thymus: evidence for expression in B-lymphocytes. *Mol Cell Endocrinol.* (1998) 141:119–28. doi: 10.1016/S0303-7207(98)00086-0
18. Arruvito L, Giulianelli S, Flores AC, Paladino N, Barboza M, Lanari C, et al. NK cells expressing a progesterone receptor are susceptible

to progesterone-induced apoptosis. *J Immunol.* (2008) 180:5746–53. doi: 10.4049/jimmunol.180.8.5746
19. Hansen KA, Opsahl MS, Nieman LK, Baker JR Jr, Klein TA. Natural killer cell activity from pregnant subjects is modulated by RU 486. *Am J Obstetr Gynecol.* (1992) 166:87–90. doi: 10.1016/0002-9378(92)91835-X
20. Roussev RG, Higgins NG, McIntyre JA. Phenotypic characterization of normal human placental mononuclear cells. *J Reprod Immunol.* (1993) 25:15–29. doi: 10.1016/0165-0378(93)90039-K
21. Szekeres-Bartho J, Szekeres GY, Debre P, Autran B, Chaouat G. Reactivity of lymphocytes to a progesterone receptor-specific monoclonal antibody. *Cell Immunol.* (1990) 125:273–83. doi: 10.1016/0008-8749(90)90083-4
22. Szekeres-Bartho J, Reznikoff-Etievant MF, Varga P, Varga Z, Chaouat G. Lymphocytic progesterone receptors in human pregnancy. *J Reprod Immunol.* (1989) 16:239–47. doi: 10.1016/0165-0378(89)90053-3
23. Szekeres-Bartho J, Csernus V, Hadnagy J, Pacsa AS. Immunosuppressive effect of serum progesterone during pregnancy depends on the progesterone binding capacity of the lymphocytes. *J Reprod Immunol.* (1983) 5:81–8. doi: 10.1016/0165-0378(83)90003-7
24. Szekeres-Bartho J, Hadnagy J, Pacsa AS. The suppressive effect of progesterone on lymphocyte cytotoxicity: unique progesterone sensitivity of pregnancy lymphocytes. *J Reprod Immunol.* (1985) 7:121–8. doi: 10.1016/0165-0378(85)90066-X
25. Szekeres-Bartho J, Barakonyi A, Polgar B, Par G, Faust Z, Palkovics T, et al. The role of g/d T cells in progesterone-mediated immunomodulation during pregnancy: a review. *Am J Reprod Immunol.* (1999) 42:44–8. doi: 10.1111/j.1600-0897.1999.tb00464.x
26. Barakonyi A, Kovacs KT, Miko E, Szereday L, Varga P, Szekeres-Bartho J, et al. Recognition of nonclassical HLA class I antigens by gamma delta T cells during pregnancy. *J Immunol.* (2002) 168:2683–8. doi: 10.4049/jimmunol.168.6.2683
27. Henderson TA, Saunders PT, Moffet-King A, Grrome NO, Critchley HO. Steroid receptor expression in uterine natural killer cells. *J Clin Endocrinol Metabol.* (2003) 88:440–9. doi: 10.1210/jc.2002-021174
28. Bogdan A, Berta G, Szekeres-Bartho J. PIBF positive uterine NK cells in the mouse decidua. *J Reprod Immunol.* (2017) 119:38–43. doi: 10.1016/j.jri.2016.12.001
29. Paldi A, d'Auriol L, Misrahi M, Bakos AM, Chaouat G, Szekeres-Bartho J. Expression of the gene coding for the progesterone receptor in activated human lymphocytes. *Endocrine* J. (1994) 2:317–321.
30. Szekeres-Bartho J, Weill BJ, Mike G, Houssin D, Chaouat G. Progesterone receptors in lymphocytes of liver-transplanted and transfused patients. *Immunol Lett.* (1989) 22:259–61. doi: 10.1016/0165-2478(89)90162-4
31. Chiu L, Nishimura M, Ishi Y, Nieda M, Maeshima M, Takedani Y, et al. Enhancement of the expression of progesterone receptor on progesterone -treated lymphocytes after immunotherapy in unexplained recurrent spontaneous abortion. *Am J Reprod Immunol.* (1996) 35:552–7. doi: 10.1111/j.1600-0897.1996.tb00056.x
32. Choe YS, Shim C, Choi D, Lee CS, Lee KK, Kim K. Expression of galectin-1 mRNA in the mouse uterus is under the control of ovarian steroids during blastocyst implantation. *Mol Reprod Dev.* (1997) 48:261–66.
33. Yao MW, Lim H, Schust DJ, Choe SE, Farago A, Ding Y, et al. Gene expression profiling reveals progesterone-mediated cell cycle and immunoregulatory roles of Hoxa-10 in the preimplantation uterus. *Mol Endocrinol.* (2003) 17:610–27. doi: 10.1210/me.2002-0290
34. Rahman MA, Li M, Li P, Wang H, Dey SK, Das SK. Hoxa-10 deficiency alters region-specific gene expression and perturbs differentiation of natural killer cells during decidualization. *Dev Biol.* (2006) 290:105–17. doi: 10.1016/j.ydbio.2005.11.016
35. Daftary GS, Taylor HS. Endocrine regulation of HOX genes. *Endocrine Rev.* (2006) 27:331–55. doi: 10.1210/er.2005-0018
36. Phillips B, Knisley K, Weitlauf KD, Dorsett J, Lee V, Weitlauf H. Differential expression of two beta-galactoside-binding lectins in the reproductive tracts of pregnant mice. *Biol Reprod.* (1996) 55:548–58. doi: 10.1095/biolreprod55.3.548
37. Maquoi E, van den Brûle FA, Castronovo V, Foidart JM. Changes in the distribution pattern of galectin-1 and galectin-3 in human placenta correlates with the differentiation pathways of trophoblasts. *Placenta* (1997) 18:433–9.
38. Barrientos G, Freitag N, Tirado-González I, Unverdorben L, Jeschke U, Thijssen VL, et al. Involvement of galectin-1 in reproduction: past, present and future. *Hum Reprod Update.* (2014) 20:175–93. doi: 10.1093/humupd/dmt040
39. Choe YS, Shim C, Choi D, Lee CS, Lee KK, Kim K. Expression of galectin-1 mRNA in the mouse uterus is under the control of ovarian steroids during blastocyst implantation. *Mol Reprod Dev.* (1997) 48:261–6.
40. Than NG, Romero R, Erez O, Weckle A, Tarca AL, Hotra J, et al. Emergence of hormonal and redox regulation of galectin-1 in placental mammals: implication in maternal-fetal immune tolerance. *Proc Natl Acad Sci USA.* (2008) 14:105. doi: 10.1073/pnas.0807606105
41. Liu AX, Jin F, Zhang WW, Zhou TH, Zhou CY, Yao WM, et al. Proteomic analysis on the alteration of protein expression in the placental villous tissue of early pregnancy loss. *Biol Reprod.* (2006) 75:414–20. doi: 10.1095/biolreprod.105.049379
42. Than NG, Erez O, Wildman DE, Tarca AL, Edwin SS, Abbas A, et al. Severe preeclampsia is characterized by increased placental expression of galectin-1. *J Matern Fetal Neonatal Med.* (2008) 21:429–42. doi: 10.1080/14767050802041961
43. Than NG, Kim SS, Abbas A, Han YM, Hotra J, Tarca AL, et al. Chorioamnionitis and increased galectin-1 expression in PPROM -an anti-inflammatory response in the fetal membranes? *Am J Reprod Immunol.* (2008) 60:298–311. doi: 10.1111/j.1600-0897.2008.00624.x
44. Blois S, Ilarregui JM, Tometten M, Garcia M, Orsal AF, Toscano M, et al. A pivotal role for galectin-1 in fetal tolerance. *Nat Med.* (2007) 13:1450–7. doi: 10.1038/nm1680
45. Polgar B, Kispal G, Lachmann M, Paar C, Nagy E, Csere P, et al. Molecular cloning and immunologic characterization of a novel cDNA coding for progesterone-induced blocking factor. *J Immunol.* (2003) 171:5956–63. doi: 10.4049/jimmunol.171.11.5956
46. Lachmann M, Gelbmann D, Kálmán E, Polgár B, Buschle M, von Gabain A, et al. PIBF (progesterone induced blocking factor) is overexpressed in highly proliferating cells and associated with the centrosome. *Int J of Cancer* (2004) 112:51–60. doi: 10.1002/ijc.20326
47. Kim K, Rhee K. The pericentriolar satellite protein CEP90 is crucial for integrity of the mitotic spindle pole. *J Cell Sci.* (2011) 124:338–47. doi: 10.1242/jcs.078329
48. Bogdan A, Polgar B, Szekeres-Bartho J. Progesterone induced blocking factor isoforms in normal and failed murine pregnancies. *Am J Reprod Immunol.* (2014) 71:131–6. doi: 10.1111/aji.12183
49. Srivastava MD, Thomas A, Srivastava BI, Check JH. Expression and modulation of progesterone induced blocking factor (PIBF) and innate immune factors in human leukemia cell lines by progesterone and mifepristone. *Leuk Lymphoma.* (2007) 48:1610–7. doi: 10.1080/10428190701471999
50. Kyurkchiev D, Naydenov E, Tumangelova-Yuzeir K, Ivanova-Todorova E, Belemezova K, Bochev I, et al. Cells isolated from human glioblastoma multiforme express progesterone-induced blocking factor (PIBF). *Cell Mol Neurobiol.* (2014) 34:479–89. doi: 10.1007/s10571-014-0031-3
51. Gutiérrez-Rodríguez A, Hansberg-Pastor V, Camacho-Arroyo I. Proliferative and invasive effects of progesterone-induced blocking factor in human glioblastoma cells. *Biomed Res Int.* (2017) 2017:1295087. doi: 10.1155/2017/1295087
52. Anderle C, Hammer A, Polgar B, Hartmann M, Wintersteiger R, Blaschitz A, et al. Human trophoblast cells express the immunomodulator progesterone-induced blocking factor. *J Reprod Immunol.* (2008) 79:26–36. doi: 10.1016/j.jri.2008.06.002
53. Nakamura K, Sheps S, Arck PC. Stress and reproductive failure: past notions, present insights and future directions. *J Assist Reprod Genet.* (2008) 25:47–62. doi: 10.1007/s10815-008-9206-5
54. Polgár B, Nagy E, Mikó E, Varga P, Szekeres-Bartho J. Urinary progesterone-induced blocking factor concentration is related to pregnancy outcome. *Biol Reprod.* (2004) 71:1699–705. doi: 10.1095/biolreprod.104.030437
55. Hudić I, Szekeres-Bartho J, Stray-Pedersen B, Fatušić Z, Polgar B, et al. Lower urinary and serum progesterone-induced blocking factor in women with preterm birth. *J Reprod Immunol.* (2016) 117:66–69. doi: 10.1016/j.jri.2016.07.003
56. Beta J, Szekeres-Bartho J, Skyfta E, Akolekar R, Nicolaides KH. Maternal serum progesterone-induced blocking factor at 11-13 weeks' gestation in spontaneous early preterm delivery. *Fetal Diagn Ther.* (2011) 29:197–200. doi: 10.1159/000322388

57. Kalinka J, Szekeres-Bartho J. The impact of dydrogesterone supplementation on hormonal profile and progesterone-induced blocking factor concentrations in women with threatened abortion. *Am J Reprod Immunol.* (2005) 53:166–71. doi: 10.1111/j.1600-0897.2005.00261.x
58. Miko E, Halasz M, Jericevic-Mulac B, Wicherek L, Arck P, Arató, G. Progesterone-induced blocking factor (PIBF) and trophoblast invasiveness. *J Reprod Immunol.* (2011) 90:50–7. doi: 10.1016/j.jri.2011.03.005
59. Halasz M, Polgar B, Berta G, Czimbalek L, Szekeres-Bartho J. Progesterone-induced blocking factor differentially regulates trophoblast and tumor invasion by altering matrix metalloproteinase activity. *Cell Mol Life Sci.* (2013) 70:4617–30. doi: 10.1007/s00018-013-1404-3
60. Balassa T, Berta G, Jakab L, Bohonyi N, Szekeres-Bartho J. The effect of the progesterone-induced blocking factor (PIBF) on E-cadherin expression, cell motility and invasion of primary tumour cell lines. *J Reprod Immunol.* (2018) 125:8–15. doi: 10.1016/j.jri.2017.10.047
61. Kozma N, Halasz M, Polgar B, Poehlmann TG, Markert UR, Palkovics T, et al. Progesterone-induced blocking factor activates STAT6 via binding to a novel IL-4 receptor. *J Immunol.* (2006) 176:819–26. doi: 10.4049/jimmunol.176.2.819
62. Szekeres-Bartho J, Par G, Dombay GY, Smart YC, Volgyi Z. The antiabortive effect of progesterone-induced blocking factor in mice is manifested by modulating NK activity. *Cell Immunol.* (1997) 177:194–99. doi: 10.1006/cimm.1997.1090
63. Koopman LA, Kopcow HD, Rybalov B, Boyson JE, Orange JS, Schatz F, et al. Human decidual natural killer cells are a unique NK cell subset with immunomodulatory potential. *J Exp Med.* (2003) 198:1201–12. doi: 10.1084/jem.20030305
64. Redhead ML, Portilho NA, Felker AM, Mohammad S, Mara DL, Croy BA. The Transcription Factor NFIL3 is essential for normal placental and embryonic development but not for uterine natural killer (UNK) cell differentiation in mice. *Biol Reprod.* (2016) 94:101. doi: 10.1095/biolreprod.116.138495
65. Quillay H, El Costa H, Duriez M, Marlin R, Cannou C, Madec Y, et al. NK cells control HIV-1 infection of macrophages through soluble factors and cellular contacts in the human decidua. *Retrovirology.* (2016) 13:39. doi: 10.1186/s12977-016-0271-z
66. Barel MT, Ressing M, Pizzato N, van Leeuwen D, Le Bouteiller P, Lenfant F, et al. Human cytomegalovirus-encoded US2 differentially affects surface expression of MHC class I locus products and targets membrane-bound, but not soluble HLA-G1 for degradation. *J Immunol.* (2003) 171:6757–65. doi: 10.4049/jimmunol.171.12.6757
67. Huang B, Faucette AN, Pawlitz MD, Pei B, Goyert JW, Zhou JZ, et al. Interleukin-33-induced expression of PIBF1 by decidual B cells protects against preterm labor. *Nat Med.* (2017) 23:128–35. doi: 10.1038/nm.4244
68. Crncic TB, Laskarin G, Frankovic KJ, Tokmadzic VS, Strobo N, Bedenicki I, et al. Early pregnancy decidual lymphocytes beside perforin use Fas ligand (FasL) mediated cytotoxicity. *J Reprod Immunol.* (2007) 73:108–17. doi: 10.1016/j.jri.2006.07.001
69. Faust Z, Laskarin G, Rukavina D, Szekeres-Bartho J. Progesterone-induced blocking factor inhibits degranulation of natural killer cells. *Am J Reprod Immunol.* (1999) 42:71–5.
70. Laskarin G, Strbo N, Sotosek V, Rukavina D, Faust Z, Szekeres-Bartho J, et al. Progesterone directly and indirectly affects perforin expression in cytolytic cells. *Am J Reprod Immunol.* (1999) 42:312–20. doi: 10.1111/j.1600-0897.1999.tb00107.x
71. Quenby S, Farquharson R. Uterine natural killer cells, implantation failure and recurrent miscarriage. *Reprod Biomed Online* (2006) 13:24–8. doi: 10.1016/S1472-6483(10)62012-3
72. Veljkovic Vujaklija D, Dominovic M, Gulic T, Mahmutefendic H, Haller H, Saito S, et al. Granulysin expression and the interplay of granulysin and perforin at the maternal-fetal interface. *J Reprod Immunol.* (2013) 97:186–96. doi: 10.1016/j.jri.2012.11.003
73. Yamada H, Kato EH, Kobashi G, Ebina Y, Shimada S, Morikawa M, et al. High NK cell activity in early pregnancy correlates with subsequent abortion with normal chromosomes in women with recurrent abortion. *Am J Reprod Immunol.* (2001) 46:132–6. doi: 10.1111/j.8755-8920.2001.460203.x
74. Quenby S, Nik H, Innes B, Lash G, Turner M, Drury J, et al. Uterine natural killer cells and angiogenesis in recurrent reproductive failure. *Hum Reprod.* (2009) 24:45–54. doi: 10.1093/humrep/den348
75. Lachapelle MH, Miron P, Hemmings R, Roy DC. Endometrial TB, and NK cells in patients with recurrent spontaneous abortion. Altered profile and pregnancy outcome. *J Immunol.* (1996) 156:4027–34.
76. Wegmann TG, Lin H, Guilbert L, Mosmann TR. Bidirectional cytokine interactions in the maternal-fetal relationship: is successful pregnancy a TH2 phenomenon? *Immunol Today* (1993) 14:353–6. doi: 10.1016/0167-5699(93)90235-D
77. Raghupathy R. Th1-type immunity is incompatible with successful pregnancy. *Immunol Today* (1997) 18:478–82.
78. Raghupathy R, Al Mutawa E, Makhseed M, Azizieh F, Szekeres-Bartho J. Modulation of cytokine production by dydrogesterone in lymphocytes from women with recurrent abortion. *Brit J Ob Gyn.* (2005) 112:1096–01. doi: 10.1111/j.1471-0528.2005.00633.x
79. Raghupathy R, Al-Mutawa E, Al-Azemi M, Makhseed M, Azizieh F, Szekeres-Bartho J. The progesterone-induced blocking factor (PIBF) modulates cytokine production by lymphocytes from women with recurrent miscarriage and with preterm delivery. *J Reprod Immunol.* (2009) 80:91–9. doi: 10.1016/j.jri.2009.01.004
80. Rezaei A, Dabbagh A. T-helper (1) cytokines increase during early pregnancy in women with a history of recurrent spontaneous abortion. *Med Sci Monit.* (2002) 8:CR607–10.
81. Hossein H, Mahroo M, Abbas A, Firouzeh A, Nadia H. Cytokine production by peripheral blood mononuclear cells in RM. *Cytokine* (2004) 28:83–6. doi: 10.1016/j.cyto.2004.07.002
82. Wilson B, Moor J, Jenkins C, Miller H, Walker JJ, McLean MA, et al. Abnormal first trimester serum interleukin 18 levels are associated with a poor outcome in women with a history of RM. *Am J Reprod Immunol.* (2004) 51:156–9. doi: 10.1046/j.8755-8920.2003.00126.x
83. Szekeres-Bartho J, Faust Z, Varga P, Szereday L, Kelemen K. The immunological pregnancy protective effect of progesterone is manifested via controlling cytokine production. *Am J Reprod Immunol.* (1996) 35:348–51. doi: 10.1111/j.1600-0897.1996.tb00492.x
84. Szekeres-Bartho J, Wegmann TG. A progesterne-dependent immuno-modulatory protein alters the Th1/Th2 balance *J. Reprod Immunol.* (1996) 31:81–95. doi: 10.1016/0165-0378(96)00964-3
85. Daya S, Clark DA. Immunosuppressive factor (or factors) produced by human embryos *in vitro*. *N Engl. J Med.* (1986) 24:1551–2.
86. Kelemen K, Paldi A, Tinneberg H, Torok A, Szekeres-Bartho J. Early recognition of pregnancy by the maternal immune system. *Am J Reprod Immunol.* (1998) 39:351–5. doi: 10.1111/j.1600-0897.1998.tb00368.x
87. Morel O, Jesel L, Freyssinet J-M, Toti F. Cellular mechanisms underlying the formation of circulating microparticles. *Arterioscler Thromb Vasc Biol.* (2011) 31:15–26. doi: 10.1161/ATVBAHA.109.200956
88. Raposo G, Stoorvogel W. Extracellular vesicles: exosomes, microvesicles, and friends. *J Cell Biol.* (2013) 200:373–83. doi: 10.1083/jcb.201211138
89. Desrochers LM, Bordeleau F, Reinhart-King CA, Cerione RA, Antonyak MA. Microvesicles provide a mechanism for intercellular communication by embryonic stem cells during embryo implantation. *Nat Commun.* (2016) 7:11958. doi: 10.1038/ncomms11958
90. Saadeldin IM, Kim SJ, Choi YB, Lee BC. Improvement of cloned embryos development by co-culturing with parthenotes: a possible role of exosomes/microvesicles for embryos paracrine communication. *Cell Reprogr.* (2014) 16:223e234. doi: 10.1089/cell.2014.0003
91. Barraud-Lange V, Chalas Boissonnas C, Serres C, Auer J, Schmitt A, Lefevre B, et al. Membrane transfer from oocyte to sperm occurs in two CD9-independent ways that do not supply the fertilising ability of Cd9-deleted oocytes. *Reproduction* (2012) 144:53–66. doi: 10.1530/REP-12-0040
92. da Silveira JC, Veeramachaneni DN, Winger QA, Carnevale EM, Bouma GJ. Cell-secreted vesicles in equine ovarian follicular fluid contain miRNAs and proteins: a possible new form of cell communication within the ovarian follicle. *Biol Reprod.* (2012) 86:71. doi: 10.1095/biolreprod.111.093252
93. Diez-Fraile A, Lammens T, Tilleman K, Witkowski W, Verhasselt B, de Sutter P, et al. Age-associated differential microRNA levels in human follicular fluid reveal pathways potentially determining fertility and success of in vitro fertilization. *Hum Fertil.* (2014) 17:90–8. doi: 10.3109/14647273.2014.897006

94. Sang Q, Yao Z, Wang H, Feng R, Zhao X, Xing Q, et al. Identification of microRNAs in human follicular fluid: characterization of microRNAs that govern steroidogenesis in vitro and are associated with polycystic ovary syndrome *in vivo*. *J Clin Endocrinol Metab.* (2013) 98:3068–79. doi: 10.1210/jc.2013-1715
95. Sohel MM, Hoelker M, Noferesti SS, Salilew-Wondim D, Tholen E, Looft C, et al. Exosomal and non-exosomal transport of extra-cellular microRNAs in follicular fluid: implications for bovine oocyte developmental competence. *PLoS ONE* (2013) 8:e78505. doi: 10.1371/journal.pone.0078505
96. Burns G, Brooks K, Wildung M, Navakanitworakul R, Christenson LK, Spencer TE. Extracellular vesicles in luminal fluid of the ovine uterus. *PLoS ONE* (2014) 9:e90913. doi: 10.1371/journal.pone.0090913
97. Atay S, Gercel-Taylor C, Kesimer M, Taylor DD. Morphologic and proteomic characterization of exosomes released by cultured extravillous trophoblast cells. *Exp Cell Res.* (2011) 317:1192–202. doi: 10.1016/j.yexcr.2011.01.014
98. Rubinstein E, Ziyyat A, Prenant M, Wrobel E, Wolf JP, Levy S, et al. Reduced fertility of female mice lacking CD81. *Dev Biol.* (2006) 290:351–8. doi: 10.1016/j.ydbio.2005.11.031
99. Tanigawa M, Miyamoto K, Kobayashi S, Sato M, Akutsu H, Okabe M, et al. Possible involvement of CD81 in acrosome reaction of sperm in mice. *Mol Reprod Dev.* (2008) 75:150–5. doi: 10.1002/mrd.20709
100. Ohnami N, Nakamura A, Miyado M, Sato M, Kawano N, Yoshida K, et al. CD81 and CD9 work independently as extracellular components upon fusion of sperm and oocyte. *Biol Open* (2012) 1:640–7. doi: 10.1242/bio.20121420
101. Ng YH, Rome S, Jalabert A, Forterre A, Singh H, Hincks CL, et al. Endometrial exosomes/microvesicles in the uterine microenvironment: a new paradigm for embryo-endometrial crosstalk at implantation. *PLoS ONE* (2013) 8:e58502. doi: 10.1371/journal.pone.0058502
102. Burns GW, Brooks KE, O'Neil EV, Hagen DE, Behura SK, Spencer TE. Progesterone effects on extracellular vesicles in the sheep uterus. *Biol Reprod.* (2018) 98:612–22. doi: 10.1093/biolre/ioy011
103. Braundmeier AG, Dayger CA, Mehrotra P, Belton RJ Jr, Nowak RA. EMMPRIN is secreted by human uterine epithelial cells in microvesicles and stimulates metalloproteinase production by human uterine fibroblast cells. *Reprod Sci.* (2012) 19:1292–301. doi: 10.1177/1933719112450332
104. Burnett LA, Light MM, Mehrotra P, Nowak RA. Stimulation of GPR30 increases release of EMMPRIN-containing microvesicles in human uterine epithelial cells. *J Clin Endocrinol Metab.* (2012) 97:4613–22. doi: 10.1210/jc.2012-2098
105. Tannetta D, Dragovic R, Alyahyaei Z, Southcombe J. Extracellular vesicles and reproduction-promotion of successful pregnancy. *Cell Mol Immunol.* (2014) 11:548–63. doi: 10.1038/cmi.2014.42
106. Pallinger E, Bognar Z, Bodis J, Csabai T, Farkas N, Godony K, et al. A simple and rapid flow cytometry-based assay to identify a competent embryo prior to embryo transfer. *Sci Rep.* (2017) 6:39927. doi: 10.1038/srep39927
107. Giacomini E, Vago R, Sanchez AM, Podini P, Zarovni N, Murdica V, et al. Secretome of *in vitro* cultured human embryos contains extracellular vesicles that are uptaken by the maternal side. *Sci Rep.* (2017) 7:5210. doi: 10.1038/s41598-017-05549-w
108. Mellisho EA, Velásquez AE, Nuñez MJ, Cabezas JG, Cueto JA, Fader C, et al. Identification and characteristics of extracellular vesicles from bovine blastocysts produced *in vitro*. *PLoS ONE* (2017) 12:e0178306. doi: 10.1371/journal.pone.0178306
109. Qu P, Qing S, Liu R, Qin H, Wang W, Qiao F, et al. Effects of embryo-derived exosomes on the development of bovine cloned embryos. *PLoS ONE* (2017). 12:e0174535. doi: 10.1371/journal.pone.0174535
110. Montecalvo A, Shufesky WJ, Stolz DB, Sullivan MG, Wang Z, Divito SJ, et al. Exosomes as a short-range mechanism to spread alloantigen between dendritic cells during T cell allorecognition. *J Immunol.* (2008) 180:3081–90. doi: 10.4049/jimmunol.180.5.3081
111. Raposo G, Nijman HW, Stoorvogel W, Liejendekker R, Harding CV, Melief CJ, et al. B lymphocytes secrete antigen-presenting vesicles. *J Exp Med.* (1996) 183:1161–72. doi: 10.1084/jem.183.3.1161
112. Nolte-'t Hoen EN, Buschow SI, Anderton SM, Stoorvogel W, Wauben MH. Activated T cells recruit exosomes secreted by dendritic cells via LFA-1. *Blood* (2009) 113:1977–81. doi: 10.1182/blood-2008-08-174094
113. Zitvogel L, Regnault A, Lozier A, Wolfers J, Flament C, Tenza D, et al. Eradication of established murine tumors using a novel cell-free vaccine: dendritic cell-derived exosomes. *Nat Med.* (1998) 4:594–600. doi: 10.1038/nm0598-594
114. Admyre C, Bohle B, Johansson SM, Focke-Tejkl M, Valenta R, Scheynius A, et al. B cell-derived exosomes can present allergen peptides and activate allergen-specific T cells to proliferate and produce TH2-like cytokines. *J Allergy Clin Immunol.* (2007) 120:1418–24. doi: 10.1016/j.jaci.2007.06.040
115. Wakim LM, Bevan MJ. Cross-dressed dendritic cells drive memory CD8+ T-cell activation after viral infection. *Nature* (2011) 471:629–32. doi: 10.1038/nature09863
116. MacKenzie A, Wilson HL, Kiss-Toth E, Dower SK, North RA, Surprenant A. Rapid secretion of interleukin-1beta by microvesicle shedding. *Immunity* (2001) 15:825–35. doi: 10.1016/S1074-7613(01)00229-1
117. Pizzirani C, Ferrari D, Chiozzi P, Adinolfi E, Sandonà D, Savaglio E, et al. Stimulation of P2 receptors causes release of IL-1beta-loaded microvesicles from human dendritic cells. *Blood* (2007) 109:3856–64. doi: 10.1182/blood-2005-06-031377
118. Qu Y, Franchi L, Nunez G, Dubyak GR. Nonclassical IL-1 beta secretion stimulated by P2X7 receptors is dependent on inflammasome activation and correlated with exosome release in murine macrophages. *J Immunol.* (2007) 179:1913–25. doi: 10.4049/jimmunol.179.3.1913
119. Xiang X, Liu Y, Zhuang X, Zhang S, Michalek S, Taylor DD, et al. TLR2-mediated expansion of MDSCs is dependent on the source of tumor exosomes. *Am J Pathol.* (2010) 177:1606–10. doi: 10.2353/ajpath.2010.100245
120. Chalmin F, Ladoire S, Mignot G, Vincent J, Bruchard M, Remy-Martin JP, et al. Membrane-associated Hsp72 from tumor-derived exosomes mediates STAT3-dependent immunosuppressive function of mouse and human myeloid-derived suppressor cells. *J Clin Invest.* (2010) 120:457–71. doi: 10.1172/JCI40483
121. Liu Y, Xiang X, Zhuang X, Zhang S, Liu C, Cheng Z, et al. Contribution of MyD88 to the tumor exosome-mediated induction of myeloid derived suppressor cells. *Am J Pathol.* (2010) 176:2490–9. doi: 10.2353/ajpath.2010.090777
122. Pap E, Pallinger E, Falus A, Kiss AA, Kittel A, Kovacs P, et al. T lymphocytes are targets for platelet- and trophoblast-derived microvesicles during pregnancy. *Placenta* (2008) 29:826–32. doi: 10.1016/j.placenta.2008.06.006
123. Atay S, Gercel-Taylor C, Suttles J, Mor G, Taylor DD. Trophoblast derived exosomes mediate monocyte recruitment and differentiation. *Am J Reprod Immunol.* (2011) 65:65–77. doi: 10.1111/j.1600-0897.2010.00880.x
124. Atay S, Gercel-Taylor C, Taylor DD. Human trophoblast-derived exosomal fibronectin induces pro-inflammatory IL-1beta production by macrophages. *Am J Reprod Immunol.* (2011) 66:259–69. doi: 10.1111/j.1600-0897.2011.00995.x
125. Pallinger E, Bognar Z, Bogdan A, Csabai T, Abraham H, Szekeres-Bartho J. PIBF+ extracellular vesicles from mouse embryos affect IL-10 production by CD8+ cells. *Sci Rep.* (2018) 8:4662. doi: 10.1038/s41598-018-23112-z
126. Sun J, Madan R, Karp CL, Braciale TJ. Effector T cells control lung inflammation during acute influenza virus infection by producing IL-10 Nature *Medicine* (2009) 15:277–84. doi: 10.1038/nm.1929
127. Abel M, Sène D, Pol S, Bourlière M, Poynard T, Charlotte F, et al. Intrahepatic virus-specific IL-10-producing CD8 T cells prevent liver damage during chronic hepatitis C virus infection. *Hepatology* (2006) 44:1607–16. doi: 10.1002/hep.21438

Permissions

All chapters in this book were first published by Frontiers; hereby published with permission under the Creative Commons Attribution License or equivalent. Every chapter published in this book has been scrutinized by our experts. Their significance has been extensively debated. The topics covered herein carry significant findings which will fuel the growth of the discipline. They may even be implemented as practical applications or may be referred to as a beginning point for another development.

The contributors of this book come from diverse backgrounds, making this book a truly international effort. This book will bring forth new frontiers with its revolutionizing research information and detailed analysis of the nascent developments around the world.

We would like to thank all the contributing authors for lending their expertise to make the book truly unique. They have played a crucial role in the development of this book. Without their invaluable contributions this book wouldn't have been possible. They have made vital efforts to compile up to date information on the varied aspects of this subject to make this book a valuable addition to the collection of many professionals and students.

This book was conceptualized with the vision of imparting up-to-date information and advanced data in this field. To ensure the same, a matchless editorial board was set up. Every individual on the board went through rigorous rounds of assessment to prove their worth. After which they invested a large part of their time researching and compiling the most relevant data for our readers.

The editorial board has been involved in producing this book since its inception. They have spent rigorous hours researching and exploring the diverse topics which have resulted in the successful publishing of this book. They have passed on their knowledge of decades through this book. To expedite this challenging task, the publisher supported the team at every step. A small team of assistant editors was also appointed to further simplify the editing procedure and attain best results for the readers.

Apart from the editorial board, the designing team has also invested a significant amount of their time in understanding the subject and creating the most relevant covers. They scrutinized every image to scout for the most suitable representation of the subject and create an appropriate cover for the book.

The publishing team has been an ardent support to the editorial, designing and production team. Their endless efforts to recruit the best for this project, has resulted in the accomplishment of this book. They are a veteran in the field of academics and their pool of knowledge is as vast as their experience in printing. Their expertise and guidance has proved useful at every step. Their uncompromising quality standards have made this book an exceptional effort. Their encouragement from time to time has been an inspiration for everyone.

The publisher and the editorial board hope that this book will prove to be a valuable piece of knowledge for researchers, students, practitioners and scholars across the globe.

List of Contributors

Sinuhe Hahn, Lenka Vokalova and Simona W. Rossi
Department of Biomedicine, University Hospital Basel, Basel, Switzerland

Paul Hasler
Division of Rheumatology, Medical University Department, Kantonsspital Aarau, Aarau, Switzerland

Shane Vontelin van Breda
Department of Biomedicine, University Hospital Basel, Basel, Switzerland
Division of Rheumatology, Medical University Department, Kantonsspital Aahrau, Aarau, Switzerland

Irene Mathilde Hoesli and Olav Lapaire
Department of Obstetrics, University Women's Hospital Basel, Basel, Switzerland

Elizabeth A. Scheef, Lesli M. Sprehe, Dawn Szeltner, Dollnovan Tran and Marissa Fahlberg
Division of Immunology, Tulane National Primate Research Center, Covington, LA, United States

Matilda J. Moström and Amitinder Kaur
Division of Immunology, Tulane National Primate Research Center, Covington, LA, United States
Department of Microbiology and Immunology, Tulane School of Medicine, New Orleans, LA, United States

Jon D. Hennebold and Victoria H. J. Roberts
Division of Reproductive and Developmental Sciences, Oregon National Primate Research Center, Beaverton, OR, United States

Nicholas J. Maness
Department of Microbiology and Immunology, Tulane School of Medicine, New Orleans, LA, United States
Division of Microbiology, Tulane National Primate Research Center, Covington, LA, United States

Tom E. C. Kieffer, Sicco A. Scherjon and Jelmer R. Prins
Department of Obstetrics and Gynecology, University Medical Center Groningen, University of Groningen, Groningen, Netherlands

Anne Laskewitz and Marijke M. Faas
Division of Medical Biology, Department of Pathology and Medical Biology, University Medical Center Groningen, University of Groningen, Groningen, Netherlands

Christina M. Newman, Jenna R. Rosinski and Dawn M. Dudley
Pathology and Laboratory Medicine, University of Wisconsin-Madison, Madison, WI, United States

David H. O'Connor
Pathology and Laboratory Medicine, University of Wisconsin-Madison, Madison, WI, United States
Wisconsin National Primate Research Center, University of Wisconsin-Madison, Madison, WI, United States

Alice F. Tarantal and Michele L. Martinez
Pediatrics, Cell Biology and Human Anatomy, School of Medicine, University of California, Davis, CA, United States
California National Primate Research Center, University of California, Davis, CA, United States

Heather A. Simmons
Wisconsin National Primate Research Center, University of Wisconsin-Madison, Madison, WI, United States

Terry K. Morgan
Pathology, Oregon Health and Sciences University, Portland, OR, United States

Xiankun Zeng
Pathology Division, United States Army Medical Research Institute of Infectious Diseases, Frederick, MD, United States

Mason I. Bliss and Thomas C. Friedrich
Pathobiological Sciences, University of Wisconsin-Madison, Madison, WI, United States

Ellie K. Bohm and Matthew T. Aliota
Veterinary and Biomedical Sciences, University of Minnesota, Saint Paul, MN, United States

Christopher J. Miller
California National Primate Research Center, University of California, Davis, CA, United States
Pathology, Microbiology, and Immunology, School of Veterinary Medicine, Center for Immunology and Infectious Diseases, University of California, Davis, CA, United States

Ranjith Kamity and Nazeeh Hanna
Women and Children Research Laboratory, Division of Neonatology, Department of Pediatrics, NYU Winthrop Hospital, Mineola, NY, United States

Surendra Sharma
Department of Pediatrics, Women and Infants Hospital, Warren Alpert Medical School of Brown University, Providence, RI, United States

Omayma Amin, Jenna Powers and Katherine M. Bricker
Department of Pediatrics, Emory University School of Medicine, Atlanta, GA, United States

Ann Chahroudi
Department of Pediatrics, Emory University School of Medicine, Atlanta, GA, United States
Center for Childhood Infections and Vaccines of Children's Healthcare of Atlanta and Emory University, Atlanta, GA, United States

Eva Miko, Matyas Meggyes, Katalin Doba, Aliz Barakonyi and Laszlo Szereday
Department of Medical Microbiology and Immunology, Medical School, University of Pécs, Pécs, Hungary
Janos Szentagothai Research Centre, Pécs, Hungary

Patricia Zadorosnei Rebutini, Daniele Margarita Marani Prá, André Luiz Parmegiani de Oliveira, Felipe da Silva Dezidé rio, Viviane Maria de Carvalho Hessel Dias and Lucia de Noronha
Postgraduate Program of Health Sciences, School of Medicine, Pontifícia Universidade Católica do Paraná -PUCPR, Curitiba, Brazil

Aline Cristina Zanchettin, Aline Simoneti Fonseca and Cleber Machado-Souza
Postgraduate Program in Biotechnology Applied in Health of Children and Adolescent, Pelé Pequeno Príncipe, Research Institute, Faculdades Pequeno Príncipe, Curitiba, Brazil

Emanuele Therezinha Schueda Stonoga, Júlio César Honório Dagostini, Elisa Carolina Hlatchuk and Ana Paula Percicote
Department of Medical Pathology, Clinical Hospital, Universidade Federal do Paraná-UFPR, Curitiba, Brazil

Isabella Naomi Furuie and Jessica da Silva Longo
Department of Tocogynecology, Clinical Hospital, Universidade Federal do Paraná, UFPR, Curitiba, Brazil

Bárbara Maria Cavalli, Carolina Lumi Tanaka Dino and Newton Sergio de Carvalho
Postgraduate Program of Tocogynecology and Women's Health, Clinical Hospital, Universidade Federal do Paraná-UFPR, Curitiba, Brazil

Sonia Mara Raboni
Department of Infectious Disease, Clinical Hospital, Universidade Federal do Paraná-UFPR, Curitiba, Brazil

Meri Bordignon Nogueira
Postgraduate Program of Tocogynecology and Women's Health, Clinical Hospital, Universidade Federal do Paraná-UFPR, Curitiba, Brazil
Virology Laboratory, Clinical Hospital, Universidade Federal do Paraná-UFPR, Curitiba, Brazil

Sandra M. Blois
Reproductive Medicine Research Group, Division of General Internal and Psychosomatic Medicine, Berlin Institute of Health, Charité – Universitätsmedizin Berlin, Corporate Member of Freie Universität Berlin, Humboldt-Universität zu Berlin, Berlin, Germany
Experimental and Clinical Research Center, a Cooperation Between the Max Delbrück Center for Molecular Medicine in the Helmholtz Association, and Charité - Universitätsmedizin Berlin, Berlin, Germany

Nancy Freitag
Experimental and Clinical Research Center, a Cooperation Between the Max Delbrück Center for Molecular Medicine in the Helmholtz Association, and Charité - Universitätsmedizin Berlin, Berlin, Germany

Gabriela Dveksler
Department of Pathology, Uniformed Services University of the Health Sciences, Bethesda, MD, United States

Gerardo R. Vasta
Department of Microbiology and Immunology, Institute of Marine and Environmental Technology, University of Maryland School of Medicine, UMB, Baltimore, MD, United States

Véronique Blanchard
Berlin Institute of Health, Institute of Laboratory Medicine, Clinical Chemistry and Pathobiochemistry, Charité – Universitätsmedizin Berlin, Corporate Member of Freie Universität Berlin, Humboldt-Universität zu Berlin, Berlin, Germany

Gabriela Barrientos
Laboratory of Experimental Medicine, Hospital Alemán, School of Medicine, University of Buenos Aires, CONICET, Buenos Aires, Argentina

Jessica Badolato-Corrêa, Iury Amancio Paiva, Débora Familiar-Macedo, Helver Gonçalves Dias, Caroline Fernandes-Santos, Monique da Rocha Queiroz Lima, Elzinandes Leal de Azeredo and Luzia Maria de-Oliveira-Pinto
Laboratory of Viral Immunology, Fundação Oswaldo Cruz, Rio de Janeiro, Brazil

Fabiana Rabe Carvalho and Andréa Alice Silva
Multiuser Laboratory for Research in Nephrology and Medical Science, School of Medicine, Universidade Federal Fluminense, Niterói, Brazil

Alex Pauvolid-Corrêa
Department of Veterinary Integrative Biosciences, Texas A&M University, College Station, TX, United States
Laboratory of Respiratory Viruses and Measles, Fiocruz, Rio de Janeiro, Brazil

Mariana Gandini
Laboratory of Cellular Microbiology, Fundação Oswaldo Cruz, Rio de Janeiro, Brazil

Silvia Maria Baeta Cavalcanti
Laboratory of Virological Diagnosis, Biomedical Institute, Universidade Federal Fluminense, Niterói, Brazil

Solange Artimos de Oliveira and Renata Artimos de Oliveira Vianna
Department of Maternal and Child, School of Medicine, Universidade Federal Fluminense, Niterói, Brazil

Claudete Aparecida Araújo Cardoso
Multiuser Laboratory for Research in Nephrology and Medical Science, School of Medicine, Universidade Federal Fluminense, Niterói, Brazil
Department of Maternal and Child, School of Medicine, Universidade Federal Fluminense, Niterói, Brazil

Alba Grifoni and Daniela Weiskopf
Center for Infectious Disease and Vaccine Research, La Jolla Institute for Immunology (LJI), San Diego, CA, United States

Alessandro Sette
Center for Infectious Disease and Vaccine Research, La Jolla Institute for Immunology (LJI), San Diego, CA, United States
Division of Infectious Diseases and Global Public Health, Department of Medicine, University of California, San Diego, San Diego, CA, United States

Eszter Toth, Diana Csala, Nikolett L. Szenasi and Kata Juhasz
Systems Biology of Reproduction Momentum Research Group, Institute of Enzymology, Research Centre for Natural Sciences, Hungarian Academy of Sciences, Budapest, Hungary

Andrea Balogh
Systems Biology of Reproduction Momentum Research Group, Institute of Enzymology, Research Centre for Natural Sciences, Hungarian Academy of Sciences, Budapest, Hungary
Department of Immunology, Eotvos Lorand University, Budapest, Hungary

Janos Matko
Department of Immunology, Eotvos Lorand University, Budapest, Hungary

Roberto Romero
Perinatology Research Branch, Eunice Kennedy Shriver National Institute of Child Health and Human Development, National Institutes of Health, U.S. Department of Health and Human Services, Bethesda, MD and Detroit, MI, United States
Department of Obstetrics and Gynecology, University of Michigan, Ann Arbor, MI, United States
Department of Epidemiology and Biostatistics, Michigan State University, East Lansing, MI, United States
Center for Molecular Medicine and Genetics, Wayne State University, Detroit, MI, United States

Katalin Parej
Systems Biology of Reproduction Momentum Research Group, Institute of Enzymology, Research Centre for Natural Sciences, Hungarian Academy of Sciences, Budapest, Hungary
Structural Biophysics Research Group, Institute of Enzymology, Research Centre for Natural Sciences, Hungarian Academy of Sciences, Budapest, Hungary

Istvan Hajdu and Peter Zavodszky
Structural Biophysics Research Group, Institute of Enzymology, Research Centre for Natural Sciences, Hungarian Academy of Sciences, Budapest, Hungary

Arpad F. Kovacs and Eva Pallinger
Department of Genetics, Cell and Immunobiology, Semmelweis University, Budapest, Hungary

Petronella Hupuczi
Maternity Private Clinic of Obstetrics and Gynecology, Budapest, Hungary

Adi L. Tarca
Perinatology Research Branch, Eunice Kennedy Shriver National Institute of Child Health and Human Development, National Institutes of Health, U.S. Department of Health and Human Services, Bethesda, MD and Detroit, MI, United States
Department of Obstetrics and Gynecology, Wayne State University School of Medicine, Detroit, MI, United States
Department of Computer Science, Wayne State University College of Engineering, Detroit, MI, United States

Sonia S. Hassan
Perinatology Research Branch, Eunice Kennedy Shriver National Institute of Child Health and Human Development, National Institutes of Health, U.S. Department of Health and Human Services, Bethesda, MD and Detroit, MI, United States
Department of Obstetrics and Gynecology, Wayne State University School of Medicine, Detroit, MI, United States
Department of Physiology, Wayne State University School of Medicine, Detroit, MI, United States

Hamutal Meiri
TeleMarpe Ltd, Tel Aviv, Israel

Offer Erez
Division of Obstetrics and Gynecology, Maternity Department "D", Faculty of Health Sciences, Soroka University Medical Center, School of Medicine, Ben Gurion University of the Negev, Beer-Sheva, Israel

Zoltan Papp
Maternity Private Clinic of Obstetrics and Gynecology, Budapest, Hungary
Department of Obstetrics and Gynecology, Semmelweis University, Budapest, Hungary

Simona W. Rossi and Sinuhe Hahn
Department of Biomedicine, University and University Hospital Basel, Basel, Switzerland

Nandor Gabor Than
Systems Biology of Reproduction Momentum Research Group, Institute of Enzymology, Research Centre for Natural Sciences, Hungarian Academy of Sciences, Budapest, Hungary
Maternity Private Clinic of Obstetrics and Gynecology, Budapest, Hungary
First Department of Pathology and Experimental Cancer Research, Semmelweis University, Budapest, Hungary

Elizabeth Q. Littauer and Ioanna Skountzou
Emory Vaccine Center, Emory University School of Medicine, Atlanta, GA, United States
Department of Microbiology and Immunology, Emory University School of Medicine, Atlanta, GA, United States

Jürgen Pollheimer, Sigrid Vondra and Martin Knöfler
Department of Obstetrics and Gynaecology, Medical University of Vienna, Vienna, Austria

Jennet Baltayeva and Alexander Guillermo Beristain
British Columbia's Children's Hospital Research Institute, Vancouver, BC, Canada
Department of Obstetrics and Gynecology, University of British Columbia, Vancouver, BC, Canada

Leticia Reyes
Department of Pathobiological Sciences, School of Veterinary Medicine, University of Wisconsin-Madison, Madison, WI, United States

Thaddeus G. Golos
Department of Comparative Biosciences, Wisconsin National Primate Research Center, School of Veterinary Medicine, University of Wisconsin-Madison, Madison, WI, United States

Petra C. Arck
Laboratory of Experimental Feto-Maternal Medicine, Department of Obstetrics and Fetal Medicine, University Medical Center Hamburg-Eppendorf, Hamburg, Germany

Steven Schepanski
Laboratory of Experimental Feto-Maternal Medicine, Department of Obstetrics and Fetal Medicine, University Medical Center Hamburg-Eppendorf, Hamburg, Germany
Developmental Neurophysiology, Institute of Neuroanatomy, University Medical Center Hamburg-Eppendorf, Hamburg, Germany

Ileana L. Hanganu-Opatz
Developmental Neurophysiology, Institute of Neuroanatomy, University Medical Center Hamburg-Eppendorf, Hamburg, Germany

Claudia Buss
Institute of Medical Psychology, Berlin Institute of Health, Charité-Universitätsmedizin Berlin, Corporate Member of Freie Universität Berlin, Humboldt-Universität zu Berlin, Berlin, Germany
Development, Health, and Disease Research Program, University of California, Irvine, Orange, CA, United States

A. Inkeri Lokki
Research Programs Unit, Immunobiology Research Program, University of Helsinki, Helsinki, Finland
Bacteriology and Immunology, University of Helsinki and Helsinki University Hospital, Helsinki, Finland

Jenni K. Heikkinen-Eloranta
Obstetrics and Gynecology, University of Helsinki and Helsinki University Hospital, Helsinki, Finland

Hannele Laivuori
Medical and Clinical genetics, University of Helsinki and Helsinki University Hospital, Helsinki, Finland
Institute for Molecular Medicine Finland, Helsinki Institute of Life Science, University of Helsinki, Helsinki, Finland
Faculty of Medicine and Life Sciences, University of Tampere, Tampere, Finland
Department of Obstetrics and Gynecology, Tampere University Hospital, Tampere, Finland

Sandra Šućurović and Biserka Mulac-Jeričević
Department of Physiology and Immunology, Faculty of Medicine, University of Rijeka, Rijeka, Croatia

Janri Geldenhuys
Department of Medical Microbiology, Faculty of Health Sciences, University of Pretoria, Pretoria, South Africa

Julia Szekeres-Bartho
Department of Medical Biology and Central Electron Microscope Laboratory, Medical School, Pécs University, Pécs, Hungary
János Szentágothai Research Centre, Pécs University, Pécs, Hungary
Endocrine Studies, Centre of Excellence, Pécs University, Pécs, Hungary
MTA-PTE Human Reproduction Research Group, Pécs, Hungary

Theresa Marie Rossouw
Department of Immunology, Institute for Cellular and Molecular Medicine, University of Pretoria, Pretoria, South Africa

Index

www.ingramcontent.com/pod-product-compliance
Lightning Source LLC
LaVergne TN
LVHW082131200926
848484LV00008B/2039